£37.00

WATER DAMAGE NOTED
4/09

Aging, Physical Activity, and Health

Roy J. Shephard, MD, PhD, DPE
University of Toronto

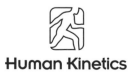

Human Kinetics

Library of Congress Cataloging-in-Publication Data

Shephard, Roy J.
    Aging, physical activity, and health / Roy J. Shephard.
        p.   cm.
    Includes bibliographical references and index.
    ISBN 0-87322-889-8
    1. Aging.   2. Physical fitness.   3. Age factors in disease.
    4. Exercise for the aged.   I. Title.
    QP86.S478   1997
    613.7'0446--dc20   96-43852
                                                                              CIP

ISBN: 0-87322-889-8

Acquisitions Editor: Becky Lane; **Developmental Editor:** Kristine Enderle; **Assistant Editors:** Sandra Merz Bott and Coree Schutter; **Editorial Assistant:** Laura Majersky; **Copyeditor:** Joyce Sexton; **Proofreader:** Debra Aglaia; **Graphic Artist:** Julie Overholt; **Graphic Designer:** Judy Henderson; **Cover Designer:** Jack Davis; **Illustrator:** Studio 2-D; **Printer:** Braun-Brumfield

Printed in the United States of America   10   9   8   7   6   5   4   3   2   1

Human Kinetics
Web site: http://www.humankinetics.com/

United States: Human Kinetics, P.O. Box 5076, Champaign, IL 61825-5076
1-800-747-4457
e-mail: humank@hkusa.com

Canada: Human Kinetics, Box 24040, Windsor, ON N8Y 4Y9
1-800-465-7301 (in Canada only)
e-mail: humank@hkcanada.com

Europe: Human Kinetics, P.O. Box IW14, Leeds LS16 6TR, United Kingdom
(44) 1132 781708
e-mail: humank@hkeurope.com

Australia: Human Kinetics, 57A Price Avenue, Lower Mitcham, South Australia 5062
(08) 277 1555
e-mail: humank@hkaustralia.com

New Zealand: Human Kinetics, P.O. Box 105-231, Auckland 1
(09) 523 3462
e-mail: humank@hknewz.com

Contents

Preface

When the monograph *Physical Activity and Aging* was published, in 1977, it represented the first systematic attempt to explore the implications of regular physical activity for population health in a rapidly aging society. It looked not simply at the prevalence of disease, but also at physical, social, and psychological well-being in older segments of the population. It detailed the progressive decrease in functional capacity and the loss of independence that commonly accompany aging. Further, it discussed the potential to stem and/or reverse these age-related changes through habitual physical activity, whether this was pursued at a low level (through household chores and community fitness programs), or on a more vigorous basis (for example, by participation in Masters athletic competition).

Public interest in the issues of physical activity and aging soon led to a rapid increase in the number of research studies involving geriatric populations. Thus, it became necessary to write a second, and greatly expanded, edition of *Physical Activity and Aging* in 1987. The years since 1987 have seen an exponential growth in our understanding of how regular physical activity can maintain functional abilities, well-being, and independence in the older person. A further consolidation of knowledge is thus urgently required.

Issues that in 1977 and even in 1987 seemed remote, theoretical possibilities have now become harsh realities. Governments need new and imaginative solutions to cope with the ever-growing numbers of seniors who are becoming dependent upon costly institutional care. The active labor force has itself aged, and these workers face increasing problems at the work site as their functional capacity declines. However, in some jurisdictions, human rights activists have successfully disputed the use of calendar age as a criterion governing the hiring, promotion, and retirement of workers. Moreover, a rapid expansion in the numbers of old and very old people has left both public and private pension funds undersubscribed. Thus, it has become necessary to consider raising the average age of retirement by several years.

Governments and society are confronted by the aging of physical capacity in a very broad context. It is necessary to view aging as a process that begins at birth, but accelerates progressively as we pass through working life. Many questions remain to be answered. What are the underlying causes of functional loss at various points in the life cycle? How far can such processes be controlled by the adoption of a prudent lifestyle, including regular physical activity? Why are there large interindividual differences in the biological age of older individuals? Can fair methods be established to determine such individual differences? And if so, can these techniques be applied to determine the continuing productive ability of a given employee?

These are some of the issues that have assumed importance since the two previous editions of *Physical Activity and Aging* were written. Rather than attempt an unhappy amalgam of new and old material, I have elected to write what is in essence a new monograph under the title *Aging, Physical Activity, and Health*. We begin with a chapter on demographics. This defines the elderly, looks at interindividual differences in biological age and life span, and considers the respective contributions of gender, inheritance, socioeconomic influences, and physical activity to these differences. It notes the health and socioeconomic consequences of an aging society and discusses the potential importance of maintaining an active lifestyle. We then move to current theories of aging, considering metaphors of the process together with its molecular, microstructural, and cellular manifestations. The third chapter details age-related changes in the major physiological systems, with a particular emphasis on those variables that influence the exercise response. The following chapter examines the ability of regular physical activity, continued athletic involvement, and training to limit these changes; it notes possible dangers of excessive physical activity and explores whether there is an age ceiling beyond which function can no longer be restored.

The second section of this book offers four chapters that explore the interactions between regular physical activity and health in older people. It covers in turn cardiorespiratory diseases, musculoskeletal diseases, metabolic health, and function and well-being, including the overall quality of life. Individual segments of each chapter look at the prevalence and incidence of various forms of ill health, commenting on the value of physical activity in primary, secondary, and tertiary prevention, together with potential applications in quaternary treatment.

The final two chapters turn to the economic and social consequences of an aging society. They deal with issues presented by aging of the labor force and a growing demand for medical services, noting the potential of regular physical activity to alleviate a number of these important problems of the late 20th century.

The book concludes with an extensive bibliography for those who wish to read further. In the interests of space, however, I have eliminated all except the most important of the references cited in earlier editions.

The material presented will serve primarily as a reference source for graduate students, upper-level undergraduates, and practicing professionals in exercise science, gerontology, and geriatric medicine. Nevertheless, many of the topics discussed will also appeal to other professionals with an interest in the interactions between age and human functional capacities: the physiologist, the physical educator, the ergonomist, and the physiotherapist. I have thus adopted a cross-disciplinary approach, avoiding obscure technicalities without sacrificing rigor in the analysis of important issues.

In preparing the new monograph, I have been fortunate to enjoy the generous support of Canadian Tire Acceptance Limited through an appointment as Resident Scholar in Health Studies at Brock University. I have also been privileged to draw upon the wisdom and experience that I have absorbed from many close colleagues, co-investigators, and former graduate students, including Drs. Kenneth Sidney, Veli Niinimaa, Gaston Godin, and Bill Montelpare. No magic solutions to the decline in biological function are offered. Even a physically active individual will continue to age. Nevertheless, either regular physical activity or moderate training can set the deterioration in physiological work capacity back by 10 to 20 years. Given that such activity has only a small impact upon the life expectancy of the elderly, it could greatly reduce that proportion of the population who must accept extended institutionalization. I hope the present volume will encourage senior citizens and their advisers to exploit this possibility!

Toronto and St. Catharines, Ontario
Roy Shephard

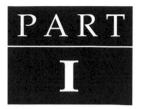

PART

I

Aging: Demographics and Biological Aspects

In the first part of this monograph, we start by taking a brief look at the demographics of aging, recognizing it as a continuous process that affects function progressively throughout the adult life span. We define the several categories of elderly people and discuss group and individual differences in the rate of aging. Next we consider changes in average life span and the age distribution of populations, noting the influences of inheritance, gender, socioeconomic status, and level of habitual activity on both survival and health. Finally, the first chapter examines briefly the health, economic, and social consequences of an aging society.

We then turn to current theories of aging, noting that metaphors are sometimes helpful in describing what remains a poorly understood process. Gross and cellular manifestations of aging and interindividual differences in biological age are discussed in relation to both the problems of physiological assessment and the ability to perform physical and mental tasks.

Having laid this groundwork, we turn to a more detailed examination of the impact of aging upon each of the major physiological systems.

We conclude part I by considering how far regular physical activity can moderate age-associated changes in each physiological system, noting that there are both risks and benefits from an active old age and that the response to a program of regular exercise depends on the stage of aging the individual has reached.

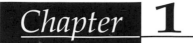

Demographics of Aging

In this chapter we define the elderly person, noting that the average age boundaries between the several categories of elderly individuals differ among nations and among socioeconomic classes. Classification at any given age is also affected by secular influences such as advances in medical treatment. The task of the gerontologist is further complicated by substantial interindividual differences in the rate of aging.

We thus examine the possibility of developing an index of biological age that can quantify such differences. Next we consider the overall life span of various populations, as well as the influence of life span on the age distribution of these populations. Communities that have claimed an unusual average longevity are discussed in the context of the maximal potential human life span, the typical human life span, and changes in these numbers over the present century. We then explore the influence of gender, inheritance, socioeconomic status, and habitual activity on an individual's life span and health prospects during the later years of life. Finally, brief consideration is given to the health, economic, and social consequences of an aging society. In particular, it is stressed that people can reverse many of the potentially unfavorable trends associated with aging by maintaining a physically active lifestyle.

Definition of the Elderly

Dividing points in any system of age classification show an almost direct relationship to the age of the writer. Some reports on the exercise tolerance of the elderly have discussed subjects in the age range from 40 to 60 years. Such a choice makes any research easier and somewhat safer to conduct, but from my vantage point, the individuals who have been studied no longer seem old! In many countries, demographers, insurers, and employers have set the threshold of old age at 65 years. In contrast, geriatricians often see their specialty as commencing at an age of around 75 years, depending upon the biological age of the individual, the environment in which he or she must live, and the resources available to potential care providers within the geriatric health service (Hazzard 1985).

Classification

Function provides one objective basis of age classification. We may thus place individuals into the following categories:

Middle age.   Middle age encompasses the second half of a person's working career; major biological systems show a 10% to 30% loss of function relative to peak values observed as a young adult. Typically, this phase extends from 40 to 65 years of age.

Old age.   Old age refers to the immediate postretirement period; there is usually some further loss of function, but no gross impairment of homeostasis. Typically, this phase extends from 65 to 75 years of age, and it is sometimes described as young old age.

Very old age.   In very old age, a person notices a substantial impairment of function when undertaking many daily activities; however, the individual can still live a relatively independent life. Typically, this phase extends from 75 to 85 years of age, and it is sometimes described as middle old age.

Oldest old age.   At this stage, institutional or nursing care, or both, are usually needed. Typically, the individuals concerned are over 85 years of age.

The average person spends some 15% of his or her total life span in an unhealthy state. Much of the impairment in health is due to disability, injury, or disease incurred in old age (U.S. National Center for Health Statistics 1993). In a typical scenario, an elderly person spends about 10 years in the very old age category (when there is a growing limitation of physical capabilities) and about a year in extreme old age (when there is at best a severe limitation of physical activity, and commonly total incapacitation) (Health and Welfare, Canada 1982). Because women survive for a longer total period than men, they usually experience a longer period of partial or total disability (see table 1.1).

National and Regional Differences

The boundaries that separate the several functional categories of old age vary substantially from one country to another.

This is perhaps most obvious in terms of the threshold of old age. A retirement age of 65 years has been traditional in most parts of North America, but retirement ages as low as 55 were adopted by some former Eastern bloc communist countries. There seem to have been no strong biological grounds for either choice. Rather, the retirement age was determined by considerations of economics, politics, and administrative convenience.

In the third world, in contrast, a lifetime of malnutrition, hard physical labor, frequent bouts of disease, and (for the women) repeated pregnancies have given strong biological reasons for early onset of the various categories of old age (Kalache 1991).

Table 1.1   Total survival (T) and disability-free (DF) survival (average in years, measured from birth).

Sample	Men		Women		Author
	T	DF	T	DF	
Canada	73.0	61.3	79.8	64.9	Health and Welfare, Canada (1982)
Québec	70.3	59	78.2	60	Dillard (1983)
United States *(not distinguished by gender)*					
Actual 1980	73.7	62			U.S. Public Health Service (1991)
Target 2000	75	65			

Socioeconomic Gradients

Within a given country, there have been substantial differences in the aging of older people from one socioeconomic group to another. In some situations (for example, ghettoes in the United States, or isolated circumpolar communities), limited access to modern medical treatment remains a factor, but such gradients also persist in countries that provide universal medical care.

For example, British people have benefited from a National Health Service for almost 50 years. However, in the wealthiest part of Britain (the region surrounding London), people still live about eight years longer than those in Scotland and northern England (Black 1980). Moreover, there exist corresponding regional gradients in health experience and thus the age of transition from one category of old age to the next.

Secular Trends

Secular trends in patterns of aging reflect changes in legislation, employment, medical practice, nutrition, and habitual physical activity.

Equal opportunity and human rights legislation has recently outlawed a fixed retirement age for many North American states and provinces, except in circumstances under which the continuing employment of older individuals endangers public safety (Shephard 1985b, 1991d). However, the practical impact of such legislation on the average length of the working career is less clear, given the opposing challenges of automation-related decreases in the availability of traditional forms of employment and pension funds that seem inadequate to support a growing population over a long period of retirement. Some professionals greatly enjoy their work and are reluctant to retire even when they have reached an advanced age, but for the average employee the main motivation to continued employment is economic. If legislation allows a free choice of retirement age, the worker's decision will thus be influenced heavily by the current cost of living and the security of financial provisions for retirement. Statistics Canada (1991) estimated that in Canada the labor force participation of men aged 55 to 64 years decreased by 25% between 1966 and 1991; moreover, almost half of the "baby-boomer" generation indicated that they planned to retire before reaching the age of 65 years. Despite recent legislation, negative stereotypes still discourage employers from hiring, retaining, or retraining older individuals (International Labor Organization [ILO] 1992). Only 4% of Canadian companies provide incentives that encourage employees to postpone retirement, but 33% of companies encourage early retirement. Some 57% of Canadian seniors who are living on farms continue in the labor force, but this is true of only 8% of other seniors (Statistics Canada 1984). Deteriorating health is the main factor that ultimately precipitates retirement for much of the population (Shephard 1995b). A combination of the economic pressures associated with an aging society and success in the prevention and treatment of chronic disease may thus lead to further secular changes in the average age of retirement.

In the past, institutional support of the elderly was more common in North America (8% of those over the age of 65) than in Britain (still only 4.7% of seniors, "Institutional Care" 1993). However, North American governments are now providing the very old with increased domestic help and residential nursing care in an attempt to increase the effective age of transition from the relative independence of the very old to the total dependence of the oldest old category.

Advances in medical practice are continually increasing the likelihood that a given individual will survive to very old and even to oldest old age (a phenomenon that Fries [1980a] has described as a squaring of the mortality curve). Fries (1980a, 1980b, 1992) has suggested that because preventive medicine has also delayed the average age of onset of disability, people may expect to live longer in good health (a compression of morbidity). Nevertheless, a realization of this hope depends on the compression of morbidity proceeding faster than any compression of mortality. It is not altogether clear that this is happening, or that current technology is augmenting the likely number of disability-free years (Colvez and Blanchet 1983; Wilkins and Adams 1983). Furthermore, new medical treatments have had little influence on the longevity of the longest-surviving members of society.

Interindividual Differences

At any given point in history, people age at differing rates even within a given country and a given socioeconomic class. Whereas some 70-year-old people are completely bedridden, some 90-year-olds remain extremely active. Statistics Canada (1985) noted that among those individuals aged 80 to 98 years who remained in good health, a lower proportion (40%) needed help with their grocery shopping than was the case among those who already reported poor health at an age of 55 to 59 years (55%). The magnitude of interindividual differences in functional status seems to increase with age. It would thus be very useful if we could develop some objective index of an individual's biological or functional age to correlate with that person's calendar age. Such an index would facilitate our understanding of the aging phenomenon, and would make it easier to determine whether the rate of functional deterioration can be manipulated by such measures as regular physical activity or adoption of a special diet (Heikkinen et al. 1994; Skinner 1988).

Concept of Biological Age

The ideal index of biological age would combine scores for items representative of function in each of the major biological systems of the body. Items included in the test battery would each show a regular, detectable, and age-related change when observations were repeated on the same person at 5- to 10-year intervals.

Unfortunately, functional status depends on a wide range of physiological, psychological, and sociological variables. The choice of appropriate items to include in such an index thus remains quite a subjective decision. Inevitably, different people ascribe differing relative values to the conservation of particular body functions. Moreover, there is still no agreement on how very disparate pieces of information should be weighted and combined to yield an overall measure of biological or functional age (Bourlière 1982; Comfort 1979; Heikkinen et al. 1994; Ries 1994).

Potential Measurements

The measurements that composed Comfort's (1979) classic suggested index of biological age included anthropometric data (standing, sitting, and trunk height; biacromial diameter; body mass; and hair graying score), physiological test scores (vital capacity, tidal volume, maximum voluntary ventilation, blood pressure, heart size, and grip strength), observations on the integrity of bone and connective tissue (osteoporotic index, skin elasticity, and nail calcium), sensory tests (visual acuity, dark adaptation, vibrometry, and audiometry), biochemical data (serum cholesterol, albumin, copper, elastase, and RNAase), cellular characteristics (lymphocyte RNA/DNA, serum growth promotion, clonal viability, and auto-antibody titers), intelligence tests (Wechsler test, digit span, digit symbol, and vocabulary), and psychomotor tests (reaction time and a light extinction test).

Borkan (cited by Costa and McCrae 1985) suggested evaluating individual measurements of body function against separate, age-related norms. A standardized score could then be derived for each item, and a composite score could be calculated by summing individual deviations from the respective norms.

Others have noted that the biological age is higher in individuals with chronic disease than in healthy members of the same general population (Furukawa 1994). Likewise, cardiovascular morbidity is greater among those who are functionally older (Borkan and Norris 1980). There have thus been proposals to rate age in terms of health risks (Hutchins 1994) or accumulated pathology. Applying this last approach to each of 13 body systems, Linn (1975) found that a cumulative "illness score" gave a good prediction of subsequent mortality.

Critique of Biological Age

Given the paucity of longitudinal data, calculations of biological age have generally been based on the loss of function as seen in cross-sectional measurements. Such information is vulnerable to cohort effects, such as changes in diet or habitual physical activity, from one generation to another.

If there were an unequivocal *a priori* index of biological age, it might be possible to develop an appropriate listing and weighting of test items by multiple regression analysis (Comfort 1979). Unfortunately, there is no such gold standard. In consequence, investigators have been forced to evaluate their indexes against calendar age. Thus, the equations generated have tended to become little more than a complicated and rather inaccurate method of predicting a person's calendar age. Fozard (1972) found a prediction error as large as 7.2 years. Although biological age may be a useful concept to apply to a population or a substantial group of subjects, any measurement with such a large error variance has little value when interpreting events in a given individual.

Moreover, it is difficult to comprehend the meaning of a composite biological age that is based on (for example) a combination of age-standardized scores for hair color and vital capacity. When functional scores have been submitted to factor analysis, the data have generally shown little tendency to group around a primary component of "general aging" as the concept of biological age assumes—rather, a host of lightly weighted, independent factors have emerged.

Many departures of individual test scores from anticipated values reflect an unusual value that was already present in the person as a young adult, the subsequent impact of illness, or even measurement error, rather than an unusually rapid aging of the test variable. There have been few attempts to determine whether people with a low biological age relative to their calendar age show either a slow rate of overall aging or an enhanced absolute or quality-adjusted life span (Shock et al. 1984). Discouragingly, the deterioration of a particular function may show a poorer correlation with the person's overall index of biological age than with calendar age *per se*. Paradoxically, Borkan (cited by Costa and McCrae 1985) found that the most rapid longitudinal changes occurred in the subjects he had initially classed as the most youthful on the basis of his index of biological age!

Medical analogues such as premature senility and Werner's syndrome provide some support for the idea that genetic influences can cause an unusually rapid rate of aging in specific individuals, but the link between such disorders and the normal aging process is tenuous. It also seems quite improbable that a diverse range of body processes would age at a common rate in any given person (Ludwig 1994). Thus, the whole concept of citing a single biological age for an individual has been vigorously questioned (Costa and McCrae 1985).

Life Span and Overall Age Distribution

In recent years, the proportion of very old and extremely old people has been increasing quite rapidly in most developed countries (ILO 1992). For instance, in the United States there are currently some 36 million elderly people, but this figure will almost double to 70 million by the year 2030 ("Geographic Profile" 1993). In 1900, only 40% of U.S. citizens survived to an age of 65 years, but by 1990, 80% reached this age and 50% lived to an age of 79 years (U.S. National Center for Health Statistics 1992). Likewise, in England and Wales the number of people aged 75 to 84 years increased by 16% between 1981 and 1989, and the number of those over the age of 85 increased by 39% during the same interval (Evans 1991). Reasons for the increasing fractions of old and very old people include (1) a decline in the birth rate, a decrease in childhood mortality, and the control of infectious disease over the first half of the 20th century; (2) a decrease in the proportion of premature adult deaths (as the prevention and treatment of ischemic heart disease and cancer have improved); and (3) a more general increase of average life span among the elderly (probably due to both enhanced living conditions and advances in medical practice). Other factors that influence the course of aging and the resultant demographic picture include gender, inheritance, socioeconomic status, and habitual physical activity.

The maximal human life span has changed little over the past 200 years, but the life span of the average person has generally increased. Demographers classify countries in terms of the proportions of the population who currently fall into the various age categories discussed in the preceding paragraphs.

Communities Claiming an Unusual Life Span

Much excitement was aroused some years ago by reports that several isolated communities had an unusually long life span; this was attributed to either a quirk of inheritance or the adoption of an unusual lifestyle (Leaf 1985). Subsequently, the claims of extreme age that had been made by Georgians in the Caucasus, Hunzas in the mountains of west Pakistan, and Ecuadorians living in the Andean village of Vilcabamba were painstakingly investigated. However, such studies showed that the true ages of the supposed centenarians had been either poorly documented or deliberately misrepresented.

Various sociocultural reasons (attempts to avoid military service, respect for the elders of the community, and even a wish to attract tourists and anthropologists) had encouraged villagers over the age of 70 to overstate their ages by 10 to 30 years. In Vilcabamba, the proportion of people over the age of 60 years had been augmented relative to the Ecuadorian average by the inward migration of a few elderly individuals, and the outward migration of many young people in search of paid employment. However, when individual ages were checked against church records, it was found that the overall longevity of the Vilcabamba residents was actually poorer than in many developed Western societies (Mazess and Mathiesen 1982).

Until recently, poor birth records have hampered the verification of many claims of extreme age. Even in the United States, the 1970 census was content to estimate the number of centenarians from either the assertions of those who were interviewed or the claims of relatives—an approach that may have overestimated the true prevalence as much as 20-fold (Leaf 1985). Most societies have now introduced unequivocal birth records. Where such data are still lacking, recourse may be made to biological dating, using such markers as the extent of racemization among L-amino acids in the stable proteins of the teeth and the lens of the eye (Helfman and Bada 1976).

Maximal Life Span

The maximal human life span has changed little over at least two centuries (Cutler 1985). The survival record was held for many years by Pierre Joubert, a French Canadian bootmaker. He was born in Charlesbourg, Québec, on 15 July 1701 and died in Québec City in 1814 at the age of 113 years, 124 days.

There have been several recent reports of longer survival. Nieman (1995) claims that a resident of Oakland was cycling on his 100th birthday and lived to 124 years; Nieman also cites a Japanese citizen who claimed to have reached an age of 121 years. Likewise, in February 1993, an international television station (TV-5) broadcast a program from an old people's home in Arles, France, where a woman was reputedly celebrating her 118th birthday. However, even where such unusual longevity has been well documented, the individuals concerned remain rare exceptions. The average life span is still considerably shorter than that of recent record holders.

Normal Human Life Span

In 1910, a male in the United States who survived birth lived for an average of 46.3 years, and a female child had a life expectancy of 48.3 years at birth. Corresponding figures were for 1930, 58.1 and 61.6 years; for 1950, 65.6 and 71.1 years; and for 1970, 67.1 and 74.6 years. In the United States, current life expectancies at birth are around 72.1 and 79 years for males and females, respectively (Kinsella 1992; Spirduso 1988; U.S. National Center for Health Statistics 1994). From 1900 to 1960, the life expectancy of a 65-year-old person increased by only 2.4 years, but a further 2.9 years was added between 1960 and 1990 (U.S. National Center for Health Statistics 1994).

Rather similar gains of average life span have been observed in other developed nations (see table 1.2). Thus, in 1930 the total life span of the Canadian male averaged 60.0 years and that of the Canadian female averaged 62.1 years, but by 1990 the respective figures had increased to 74.0 and 80.7 years (Kinsella 1992). In the first half of the 20th century, the largest factor contributing to a longer life span was a reduction of infant mortality. Gains in life expectancy were much smaller and less consistent for the elderly. In 1921, a 65-year-old Canadian man had the expectation of living to 78.0 years, but by 1986 his expectation had increased only to 79.9 years (Statistics Canada 1986, 1990).

Other factors that have improved prognosis include the control of major communicable diseases, the development of new medical and surgical techniques, the wider availability of comprehensive health care, improved programs of public health and sanitary engineering, the closer control of working conditions, better nutrition, a higher standard of living, and more general knowledge of the principles of hygiene.

Table 1.2 Average years of life expectancy at birth in selected countries.

	1900		1950		1990	
Country	Male	Female	Male	Female	Male	Female
United States	48.3	51.1	66.0	71.7	72.1	79.0
Canada			66.4	70.9	74.0	80.7
England/Wales	46.4	50.1	66.2	71.1	73.3	79.2
France	45.3	48.7	63.7	69.4	73.4	81.9
Sweden	52.8	55.3	69.9	72.6	74.7	80.7
Switzerland	45.7	48.5	66.4	70.8	75.2	82.6
Hungary	36.6	38.2	59.3	63.4	67.2	75.4
Spain	33.9	35.7	59.8	64.3	74.8	81.6
Australia	53.3	56.8	66.7	71.8	73.5	79.8
Japan	42.8	44.3	59.6	63.1	76.4	82.1

Based in part on data collected by Kinsella (1992).

Unfortunately, much of the potential for an increase in adult longevity promised by such advances has been dissipated through an increased prevalence of diseases such as arteriosclerosis, chronic obstructive lung disease, and lung cancer. The increased prevalence of these conditions seems attributable to problems of affluence: overnutrition, a lack of exercise because of ready access to automobiles, and indulgence in cigarettes. Probably because of these new causes of poor health, statistics for adult males in the United States, Australia, and a number of European countries showed very little improvement in life expectancy from the 1950s through to the early 1970s, when the popularity of fitness programs, smoking cessation clinics, low fat diets, and other preventive health measures began to yield further improvements in average life span.

A deterioration in economic conditions can still bring about a substantial increase in the prevalence of chronic disease, earlier movement into a given age category, and an overall shortening of life span. Thus, the deteriorating economic situation of Russia subsequent to the collapse of the state economy has been associated with a decline in life expectancy from a peak of 65 years in men (1986) and 73.8 years in women (1989) to recent values of 59 years in men and 73.2 years in women ("News Item" 1994; Ryan 1988).

Classification of Population Types

The United Nations (1981) distinguished among aged populations (in which 7% or more of people were older than 60 years), mature populations (in which 4% to 7% of people were over the age of 60), and young populations (in which less than 4% of people were over the age of 60). Demographers predict that irrespective of current categorization, most populations are likely to age further for the foreseeable future (see table 1.3).

If current trends are maintained, by the year 2025 some 20% of the population in North America and in many parts of Europe will be over the age of 55 years. Even in developing countries such as India, China, and those on the African continent, the proportion of late middle-aged and older individuals will be increasing rapidly (see table 1.3). Perhaps even more dramatic will be the increase in numbers of those who have reached extreme old age, most of whom will have become totally dependent. In 1940, the United States had slightly more than a million people who were over the age of 85 years. By 1980, this number had grown to 2.2 million, and it is estimated that by the year 2050 there will be 16 million people (5% of the national population) in this phase of aging (Spirduso 1988).

Nevertheless, demographic predictions can be upset by many unforeseen factors. The birth rate may fall (for example, there was a dramatic decrease of family size in Québec in the 1960s, when most women in that province rejected Roman Catholic doctrines opposing birth control). Immigration (legal or illegal) may lead to a selective increase in the proportion of young adults,

Table 1.3 Estimated percentages of the population over the age of 55 years in selected countries.

Country	1990 Male	1990 Female	2000 Male	2000 Female	2010 Male	2010 Female	2025 Male	2025 Female
Canada	9.6	13.0	10.4	14.0	11.5	15.4	16.2	21.3
United States	10.1	14.2	9.8	14.1	10.2	14.4	14.7	19.6
Poland	7.7	12.2	9.5	14.4	9.5	14.3	14.4	19.7
United Kingdom	12.6	18.4	12.6	18.0	13.0	18.2	15.8	21.5
Costa Rica	3.7	4.5	4.4	5.5	5.2	6.5	8.5	10.3
Brazil	4.4	4.9	5.1	5.8	5.8	6.8	8.4	10.2
China	5.3	6.6	6.6	7.8	7.6	8.9	11.7	14.0
India	4.5	4.8	5.3	5.9	6.2	7.1	9.1	10.3
Japan	9.4	13.3	13.1	17.0	15.9	20.1	17.8	22.8
Algeria	3.0	3.8	3.1	4.0	3.1	4.4	5.2	6.3
Nigeria	2.2	2.7	2.2	2.7	2.3	2.7	2.7	3.2

Based in part on data of ILO (1992).

particularly single males. Major wars may lead to selective loss of a substantial cohort of marriageable young men, as in Russia during World War II. Finally, large segments of a community may be killed by epidemics involving a microorganism for which the population concerned has neither immunity nor effective therapy (for instance, the outbreaks of measles and tuberculosis that decimated circumpolar communities during the early part of the 20th century, and currently, the widespread prevalence of AIDS in Central Africa).

Influences of Gender and Inheritance

The issues of gender and inheritance are closely intertwined, but there are also socially determined differences of lifestyle that contribute to differences in the rate of aging between men and women.

Gender Differences

Women survive longer than men in all countries (see tables 1.2 and 1.3). Recent years have widened the gender gap in life span to somewhere between five and nine years (Seely 1990; United Nations 1988). Thus, a large fraction of the elderly and an even larger fraction of the very old and extremely old are women. In 1975, the United States had only 64 men for every 100 women over the age of 65 years (Siegel 1981), and in 1992 the ratio was still under 68:100 (U.S. Department of Commerce 1994).

Genetic factors probably confer much of the survival advantage of women, since, as has been long recognized, animal species also show sex differences in average life span (Comfort 1979). Human females show a lower mortality than males from an early age, this being true for most of the common causes of death (Kinsella 1992). Gender discrepancies for cardiovascular disease and lung cancer are particularly marked (World Health Organization 1984). Until recently, many more men than women were killed in warfare. Again until recently, such adverse habits as cigarette smoking were the prerogative of men. Moreover, the gender-related secretion of estrogens (Shephard in press-b) apparently offers some protection against what among males is one of the most common causes of premature death (ischemic heart disease).

Despite longer survival, the deterioration of many aspects of function (particularly aerobic power and muscle strength) proceeds at least as rapidly in women as in men, so that women have a substantially longer average period of partial and total disability than men (Colvez and Blanchet 1983). Already, among those aged 55 to 64 years, 31% of Canadian women have noted a limitation of physical activity compared with 25% of Canadian men. In those 65 years and older, the corresponding values are 37% and 31% (National Health and Welfare 1989).

A progressive loss of the female advantage in life span may now be anticipated. Further medical advances are allowing the average person of either sex to approach a biologically determined "ceiling" of life span (Kinsella 1992). Moreover, women are increasingly adopting such adverse habits as cigarette smoking and fast driving. Nevertheless, the impact of these adverse changes in lifestyle upon female life expectancy may possibly be tempered by a decrease in the average number of pregnancies and their resulting complications.

Genetic Factors

Goodrick et al. (1983) estimated that half of the variance in the life span of inbred mice was attributable to genetic factors. However, inbreeding is an artificial situation, and when two different inbred strains are mated, the offspring live longer than either of the parents.

Human life insurance statistics have long shown a strong association between the life span of parents and that of their immediate male offspring (Dublin, Lotka, and Spiegelman 1949). Likewise, Vaillant (1991) noted that the longevity of parents and grandparents was a strong predictor of a person's risk of chronic illness at the age of 60 years, and of mortality by the age of 68 years. But such findings could reflect either the transmission of specific genetic information that determines survival, or the acquisition of behavior patterns such as cigarette smoking or obesity from parental contacts. There is the further possible complication that when a woman becomes pregnant at an advanced age, any acquired genetic abnormalities that curtail life span can be transmitted through several subsequent generations.

Comparisons between identical (monozygotic) and nonidentical (heterozygotic) twins (Carmelli 1982) provide more convincing evidence of a genetic influence on life span. The classic study of Kallman and Sander (1948) demonstrated that if identical twins died between the ages of 60 and 75 years, the average interpair difference in age at death was 47.6 months for male twins and 24.0 months for females. However, in the case of nonidentical twins, the corresponding interpair differences were 107.9 and 88.7 months. Puzzlingly, Jarvik et al. (1960) found that the difference in concordance of longevity between heterozygous and homozygous twins actually diminished as the twins grew older. Differences in concordance of life span between similar and dissimilar twins seem to offer quite strong proof that genetic factors influence survival prospects, perhaps by increasing susceptibility to sudden cardiac death (Wright 1988). But as with other twin studies, it could also be argued that identical twins experience unusually comparable environments over much of their life span, or that they suffer more grief than the heterozygotes on bereavement.

Finally, recent studies have shown substantial genetic contributions to the risk factors for such causes of aging and premature death as ischemic heart disease. For example, Bouchard and Després (1988) estimated that after standardizing their data for age, gender, and fatness, some 58% of the variance in a centripetal distribution of subcutaneous fat was transmissible from the parents, 32% of intersubject variation in scores being due to sociocultural inheritance and 25% to genetic inheritance.

Socioeconomic Influences

Socioeconomic factors make a major contribution to differences in the demographics of aging between rich and poor countries; poverty and sociocultural deprivation are also important determinants of ethnic and regional differences in longevity within a given country.

Developing Countries

In developing countries, there is often little governmental provision for social security in old age. The birth rate remains high, in part to ensure support in the final years of life, and a very high proportion of the total population are currently children (ILO 1992). Malnutrition, disease, and sheer hard work lead to rapid aging and an early average age at death (Kalache 1991), so the population pyramid is very steep.

Ethnic Differences

Among the developed nations, the demographics of aging differ from one ethnic group to another, although the observed differences probably have a sociocultural rather than a genetic basis. Thus, a population pyramid as steep as that of the developing nations can be observed among the Inuit of the northeastern Arctic (see fig. 1.1; Rode and Shephard 1996). This particular population still has a very high birth rate, and until recently many members of the community died before reaching the age of 60 years (a consequence of an extreme environment, with many natural hazards and limited access to medical care).

Likewise, in the United States, some 11% of the white population are 65 years of age or older, but this is true of only 3.6% of Hispanic Americans and 2.4% of African Americans.

Regional Differences

Because of patterns of urban growth, the elderly of North America are concentrated in the core of large cities, and in rural communities with a population of

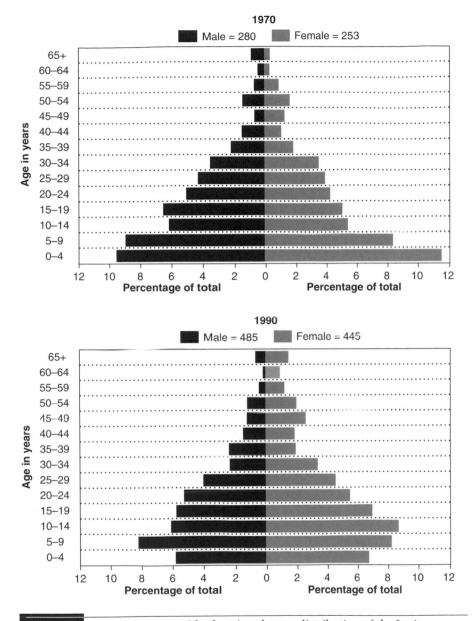

Figure 1.1   Population pyramids showing the age distribution of the Inuit population of Igloolik, Northwest Territories, Canada, in 1969/1970 and 1989/1990.
Reprinted from R.J. Shephard, and A. Rode, 1996, *Effects of modernization on the health of circumpolar populations*. (London: Cambridge University Press).

less than 2500. In Canada, senior citizens currently compose as much as 25% of the population in small towns and villages (Hodge 1987).

Other regional differences in health and average life span reflect corresponding socioeconomic gradients. This is well illustrated by data from the United Kingdom, where mortality statistics for the period 1970 to 1972 disclosed an eight-year difference between the affluent counties immediately around London and the northern half of the country (Black 1980). Chronic unemployment, poor nutrition, a lack of physical activity, and a high prevalence of smoking and alcoholism were thought to be factors that had contributed to the poor survival prospects of those living in Scotland and the north of England. Although it was first described some 16 years ago, the gap in prospects between the north and south of Great Britain has widened in subsequent years (Smith, Bartley, and Blane 1990).

Gradients of health status and life expectancy with socioeconomic status have been found by all countries that have collected relevant data (Smith, Bartley, and Blane 1990). Among Canadians over the age of 65 years, 40% of those in the lowest income group report limitations in physical activity, compared with only 11% of those in the upper and middle income groups (Health and Welfare, Canada 1989). A review of all known studies from the United States, Canada, and Europe (Robine and Ritchie 1991) noted that at age 65, the difference in life expectancy between the wealthiest and the poorest quintiles was 6.3 years for men and 2.8 years for women. Moreover, differences in disability-free life expectancy were 14.3 years for men and 7.6 years for women. Unemployment has particularly adverse effects on health and life expectancy. It is associated with downward social mobility, loss of owner-occupied housing, the breakdown of marriages, chronic poor health, and an adverse mortality experience (Moser et al. 1987). Analysis of various data sets shows higher rates of accidents, cardiovascular disease, cancer, respiratory disease, and cerebrovascular disease among the poorer members of society, all of these problems hastening the transition to older age categories.

Marital status is another important variable (Connidis 1989; McPherson 1990). Canadian men who are married live some 8 years longer than bachelors, and 12 years longer than widowers or men who are divorced. Likewise, married women live 3 years longer than women who never married, and 6 years longer than widows or divorcees. At least 75% of elderly men in Canada and the United States are married, but this is true of only about 40% of elderly women.

Physical Activity Patterns

It is unclear whether a decrease in habitual activity is a normal part of the aging process. Certainly, many animals become less active as they age. However, humans also offer cultural reinforcement to the idea that physical activity should diminish with aging. In developed societies, a senior citizen is expected to slow down and "take a well-earned rest." Equally, in "primitive" populations, young adults assume the responsibilities of hunting and gathering for older members of the community (Shephard and Rode 1996).

Prevalence of Physical Activity

Methods used to estimate the prevalence of physical activity generally have not distinguished the age of the subject, and questionnaires appropriate for young adults may not always have elicited details of the more vigorous activities undertaken by the middle-old and the oldest-old. Collection of population data on physical activity patterns began in the mid-1970s. There have been some subsequent changes in activity preferences, but only small changes in the proportion of active individuals (Powell et al. 1991). In recent years, the most prevalent forms of voluntary activity among adults over the age of 55 years in the United States (DiPietro et al. 1993) have been walking, gardening, cycling, golf (in men), and aerobics (in women). The respective figures for Canadian men and women over the age of 65 years (Stephens and Craig 1990) reflect participation *at least once* during a 12-month period: walking (77%, 81%), swimming (< 20%, 57%), cycling (< 20%, < 15%), and dancing (22%, 15%).

All of the available data are cross-sectional in type, so it is not possible to distinguish between the true effects of aging and possible cohort effects. Nevertheless, it appears that voluntary activity is most prevalent among the young, the better-educated, and the more affluent members of society. The age-related decline in participation rates is more marked for sport than for other active pursuits, and the proportion of walkers (in men) and gardeners (of both sexes) actually increases with age (Stephens and Craig 1990).

Estimates of the prevalence of physical activity depend on the rigor of the criteria applied. Many early reports suggested that a substantial proportion of senior citizens were active: 40% of those over the age of 60 years were "now doing" walking (U.S. President's Council on Physical Fitness and Sports 1973), and 47% of men and 39% of women over the age of 65 years were regularly participating in one or more of six listed activities (U.S. National Center for Health Statistics 1975). General Mills (1979) claimed that 39% of those over 65 years engaged in some planned physical exercise at least several times a week, and the National Health Interview Survey of 1984 estimated that the prevalence of regular physical activity declined from 30% of men and 28% of women aged 65 to 74 years to 23% of men and 15% of women over the age of 85 years (U.S. National Center for Health Statistics 1987).

Others who applied more exacting criteria of significant physical activity reported a much lower prevalence (Blair, Brill, and Kohl 1988); only 3% of subjects over 65 years were spending 6 MJ/week on sport and conditioning

(Perrier 1979), and only 7.5% of subjects over the age of 65 years were engaging in "appropriate" amounts of physical activity (U.S. National Health Interview Survey of 1985 [Caspersen, Christenson, and Pollard 1986]). The U.S. Centers for Disease Control (1986) estimated that no more than 10% of their sample exercised at 60% of maximal oxygen intake or more, 20 min/session, three or more times per week, and that only 15% of men and women over the age of 55 years reached a leisure energy expenditure of 12.5 kJ/kg per day. However, in Canada, 42% of men and 23% of women over the age of 65 years met this same standard (Stephens and Craig 1990).

Perhaps because the climate is better on the west coast than in other parts of the United States, a limited survey of 82 men and 111 women aged 65 to 74 years, randomly selected from five California cities (Sallis et al. 1985), found that moderate, vigorous, and very vigorous leisure activities added an average energy expenditure of as much as 8 MJ/week for men and 4 MJ/week for women; activities demanding > 5 METs occupied about 2 h/week in the men, but only 0.4 h/week in the women.

Parallel age-related decreases of habitual physical activity have been described in other developed countries. The Norwegian Confederation of Sport (1984) estimated that sport participation decreased from 69.2% of those aged 15 to 24 years to 32.9% of those aged 60 years and more. The proportion of joggers declined from 55.9% to 11.6% of the sample, that of weight lifters from 26.1% to 3.3%, and that of football players from 32.6% to 0%. In contrast, Nordic skiing (39.8% vs. 29.3%) and swimming (33.1% vs. 22.9%) showed smaller changes in participation rates with age, and the proportion of hikers (33.6% vs. 59.0%) actually increased in older members of the population.

The Canada Health Survey (Health and Welfare, Canada 1982) developed an arbitrary physical activity index based on the individual's reported frequency, duration, and intensity of habitual physical activity. Study participants were classified on a five-level scale ranging from sedentary to very active. When compared with adults aged 20 to 24 years, only about half as many of those over the age of 65 years were classed as moderately or very active (see table 1.4). Moreover, an increased proportion of the elderly (probably mainly those who were inactive) did not report their physical activity patterns. In the 1988 survey, age and gender differences were smaller; respective percentages of active and moderately active individuals (leisure energy expenditures > 6.3 kJ/kg per day) being 68% and 59% in men and 54% and 46% in women (Stephens and Craig 1990).

Daily Energy Expenditures

An increase of body mass and a decrease of mechanical efficiency tend to increase the energy expenditure of an older person during performance of physical activity at any given intensity. Added costs of movement are par-

Table 1.4   A comparison of physical activity levels between adults aged 20-24 years and those aged 65 years and older.

Activity level	Age 20-24 years		Age 65 years or older	
	Men	Women	Men	Women
Sedentary	16.0%	14.3%	29.1%	28.7%
Moderately inactive	13.9	24.2	14.1	21.5
Moderate	15.4	18.7	11.4	11.3
	45.3	57.2	54.6	61.5
Moderatively active	18.3	18.6	11.6	9.8
Very active	27.3	15.7	10.6	5.2
	45.6	34.3	22.2	15.0
Unknown	9.2	8.4	23.2	23.6

Based on the Canada Health Survey (Health and Welfare, Canada 1982).

ticularly likely if arthritis, hemiplegia, limb deformity, or an amputation distorts normal movement patterns (Lorentz 1985; Shephard et al. 1994, 1995). However, these same handicaps generally make people less active, so the overall trend in daily energy expenditure for a person who has developed some type of physical impairment is in a downward direction (McGandy et al. 1966).

The daily energy requirement of the average adult male decreases by some 0.8 MJ/day from age 45 to age 75, with a further decrease of 1.2 MJ/day in those who are even older. The U.S. National Research Council (1980) thus recommended dietary allowances of 12.6 MJ/day for men and 9.2 MJ/day for women aged 20 to 39 years, but decreased the respective allowances to 10.0 and 7.4 MJ/day for those aged 60 to 69 years. The most recent dietary recommendation (U.S. Food and Nutrition Board 1989) applies to all people over the age of 51 years, with an allowance of 9.6 MJ/day for men and 8.0 MJ/day for women. Energy needs may also vary with the local environment; thus, early estimates for elderly French women were 0.9 to 1.2 MJ/day higher for country than for urban environments (Debry, Bleyer, and Martin 1977).

In their classic study of the city of Tecumseh, Michigan, Cunningham et al. (1969) found that the ratio of working to basal metabolic rate declined slightly from 3.1 in subjects aged 16 to 29 years to 2.9 in those aged 50 to 59 and 60 to 69 years of age. However, it is likely that this trend has been reversed in recent years as young adults have accepted highly sedentary, automated jobs.

In the first few months after retirement begins, daily energy expenditures may rise, as a person who has been accustomed to working 8 h a day attempts to fill spare time. The Canada Fitness Survey estimated that the recreational energy expenditures of men dropped from 6.3 kJ/kg per day at 20 to 29 years to 2.5 kJ/kg per day at 50 to 59 years, but increased to 4.2 kJ/kg per day at age 60 to 69 years; corresponding figures for the women were 4.2, 2.9, and 2.9 kJ/kg per day (Stephens and Craig 1986).

Influence of Physical Impairments

Much of the decline in physical activity is self-determined, but a growing prevalence of physical impairment is also an important factor among the very old.

The U.S. National Center for Health Statistics (1993) estimated that 15% of the elderly who are living in the community suffer from some type of disability. Other data suggest that 40% to 50% are limited in either the amount or the kind of activity that they can perform; 18% have limited mobility, and 5% are confined to their homes (U.S. Department of Health and Human Services 1981).

The National Health Interview Survey found that 41% of men and 53% of women aged 65 to 74 years never walked as far as 1.6 km without taking a rest (Guralnik et al. 1989; U.S. National Center for Health Statistics 1987). Among those over the age of 85 years, the corresponding figures were 49% and 59%. Substantial fractions of those over the age of 55 years also had difficulty in walking a distance of 0.4 km or carrying 11 kg (Kovar and LaCroix 1987; see table 1.5). By the age of 80 to 84 years, 31% to 57% of men and 54% to 70% of women were unable to do heavy housework; 12% to 15% of men and 17% to 31% of women were unable to climb stairs; 8% to 12% of men and 9% to 23% of women were unable to walk across a room; and 1% to 8% of men and 8% to 14% of women were unable to rise from a chair or a bed (Coroni-Huntley et al. 1986; Manton, Corder, and Stallard 1993).

Such limitations of physical activity plainly reduce the quality of life for the affected individual, although the precise impact depends greatly upon the coping mechanisms that are adopted. A surprising 85% of Canadian seniors who report activity limitations also indicate that they are either very happy or pretty happy (Health and Welfare, Canada 1989).

Health, Economic, and Social Consequences of an Aging Society

Accepting that the proportion of elderly people will increase in most countries over the next 50 years, it is necessary to consider the consequences of such a trend in terms of health policy, economics, and social change.

Health Policy

Much of the decrease in habitual physical activity, as well as the development of disability and dependency noted in the previous section, is due to a pro-

Table 1.5   Percentages of people who have worked since the age of 45 years who have difficulty (D) walking or are unable (U) to walk 0.4 km or to carry 11 kg.

Age (years)	Men Walking 0.4 km D	U	Carrying 11 kg D	U	Women Walking 0.4 km D	U	Carrying 11 kg D	U
55-59	12.3	5.0	12.6	5.8	11.6	3.5	22.9	9.1
60-64	17.0	7.9	15.8	8.0	15.4	3.8	31.0	8.7
65-69	20.1	9.4	19.9	7.9	16.8	5.6	33.8	9.3
70-74	23.3	8.7	25.6	10.2	23.1	7.5	40.8	10.7

Source: U.S. National Center for Health Statistics (1987), *Aging in the eighties: Ability to perform work-related activities. Data from the supplement on aging to the National Health Interview Survey: United States, 1984,* Advance Data from Vital and Health Statistics, No. 136, DHS Publication PHS 87-1250 (Hyattsville, MD: U.S. Public Health Service).

gressive loss of biological function with age rather than to the development of any specific pathological condition. Nevertheless, additional restrictions on both habitual physical activity and the quality of life are imposed by pathological changes, disease, and illness; moreover, such problems become progressively more prevalent in older segments of the population.

It is often difficult to distinguish functional limitations from the restrictions imposed by disease (a pathological process), or by illness (the individual's reaction to the pathological process). For example, systemic blood pressures rise progressively with aging. This is largely a consequence of biological changes in the structure of the arterial wall. However, when the systolic or the diastolic pressure exceeds a certain threshold value, the clinical condition of hypertension is diagnosed, and this can predispose to a variety of subjective disturbances such as severe headaches. Equally, all adults show a progressive reduction in bone mineral content with aging, but when a certain cumulative loss has been incurred, the clinical condition of osteoporosis is diagnosed and treatment with estrogens may be initiated. Further, the weakening of bone structure may permit obvious clinical events such as a "spontaneous" bone fracture. On occasion, there may also be discrepancies between an objective assessment of the extent of disease and clinical symptomatology. For example, a person may have minimal radiographic evidence of osteoarthritic change and yet severe subjective disability (or vice versa).

The main perceived health problems of Canadian seniors (Statistics Canada 1990) are arthritis and rheumatism (46% of men, 63% of women), hypertension (33% of men, 43% of women), "heart trouble" (28% of men, 24% of women), respiratory problems (26% of men, 23% of women), and diabetes (9% in both sexes). The experience in the United States is somewhat similar, with 50% of the elderly reporting arthritis, 39% hypertension, 30% a hearing impairment, 20% a deformity or orthopedic impairment, 15% sinus problems, 10% visual problems, and 9% diabetes (U.S. National Center for Health Statistics 1993).

It is difficult to determine the pathological cause of disability in the elderly, since many conditions coexist; in the young-old and middle-old, chronic disease and limitations of mobility are dominant, but in the oldest-old a substantial proportion of people are limited by deterioration of the intellect and the special senses (Pope and Tarlov 1991). An early study by Hunt (1978) identified the causes as arthritis and rheumatism (36%), pulmonary conditions (17%), strokes and paralysis (15%), blindness and failing sight (14%), circulatory conditions (14%), cardiac conditions and abnormalities of blood pressure (13%), sequelae of accidents (10%), and neurological problems (5%). The resulting subjective problems include muscle weakness, joint stiffness, breathlessness, lack of control of movements due to tremor or spasticity, and disorders of balance.

The proportion of the population who are unsteady on their feet rises progressively with age (Lucy and Hayes 1985), from 22% of people between the ages of 65 and 74 years to 49% of those over the age of 75 years. The corresponding figures are, for poor eyesight, 32% and 42%; breathlessness after any effort, 29% and 35%; giddiness, 23% and 31%; tiredness, 25% and 29%; and arthritis or rheumatism, 50% and 58% (Abrams 1977).

The aging of the population will undoubtedly contribute to increases in the future costs of medical care (Fries 1980b). For example, in the Netherlands, men over the age of 75 years consume 6.5 times the medical resources used by those aged 15 to 44 years (ILO 1992). The type of treatment required will also change, with an increased need for preventive and rehabilitative services that can contain the burden of chronic disease. During the 20th century, effective treatments have been developed for many conditions that previously would have caused the death of an elderly person (for example, the use of antibiotics in pneumococcal pneumonia). This raises an important issue of health policy. Patterns of disease in the final years of life have changed. Whereas pneumonia once led to a relatively rapid death, modern treatments of terminal illness by repeated renal dialysis or blood transfusion allow quite lengthy periods of moribund survival. Difficult ethical questions then arise regarding the costs of advanced life support (Fries 1980b), the quality of the final life years (Evans 1991), and ceiling ages beyond which it is undesirable to prolong life by heroic measures (Spiegelhalter et al. 1992). It is useful to calculate the patient's quality-adjusted survival after application of various treatments; this is given by the product of years survived and a quality-of-life multiplier. Donaldson and Mooney (1991) point out that home chiropody can offer seniors an extra year of quality-adjusted life for a cost of $400. In contrast, a kidney transplant costs $12,000 per quality-adjusted life year, and home hemodialysis $26,000 per quality-adjusted life year.

Economic Consequences of an Aging Society

The productivity of the labor force and the ratio of dependents to active workers are two important determinants of the economic health of any given society.

We need to notice that dependents include not only those who have retired from the labor force but also children, full-time caregivers, and the unemployed. In most developed societies, the number of elderly dependents has been increasing rapidly, but this has been partially offset by a decline in the child population and a dramatic drop in the number of full-time caregivers as the birth rate has declined and as both "baby-boomers" and a higher proportion of women of older generations have entered the labor force.

Nevertheless, the ratio of dependents to active workers has increased progressively over the second half of the 20th century, because of a longer total period of education prior to employment, an earlier average age of retirement, a rising unemployment rate, and a growing number of individuals who survive to very old and extremely old age.

The average economic cost of supporting a child or a retiree is some 70% of that for an active member of the labor force. However, the calculation of dependency costs is complicated because figures are particularly high for (a) young dependents when they are attending a college or university, and (b) elderly dependents during the final months of their lives when full institutional care may be required (Fries 1980b). The costs associated with the very old are becoming particularly critical, because advanced life support systems now enable a large proportion of the population to survive to an advanced age, even if their functional abilities have become extremely restricted. One gloomy report from the United States predicted that by the year 2012, Medicaid nursing home payments could be expected to have increased 280%, to an annual burden of $6.3 billion (Ray et al. 1987).

The optimal economic solution might seem to counter a growing dependency ratio by increasing the productivity of the labor force. Possible options might include a greater investment in automation, more effective training programs for workers, a decrease in unemployment and underemployment, a full use of the potential of female employees, and immigration policies that favor the admission of skilled young workers. Many western nations have indeed made giant strides in productivity during the past two decades, giving a margin of wealth that in theory should satisfy both the growing consumer demands of the employed and the needs of an increasing number of dependents. However, it is less certain that the growth in productivity will continue, as work is displaced to parts of the world where labor is cheaper, and as production costs are increased by a depletion of nonrenewable resources.

What are the alternatives? Personal taxation now seems near the maximum that the employed public is willing to pay. A second option, currently being pursued by many governments, is a critical review of all expenditures. Geriatricians and gerontologists hope that such a review will allow the needs of a growing number of dependents to be met from cuts in defense or other "less worthy" programs, but many taxpayers would like a reduction in all social spending (including support of the elderly). A final possibility is the perpetuation of current budget deficits; this then reduces the effective value of pensions and savings through inflation. Such a "remedy" is becoming ever less practicable, since the elderly are the major holders of savings and they now form a powerful sector of the electorate, well-organized through groups such as the American Association of Retired Persons, and particularly prone to exercise their franchise (Shephard and LaBarre 1978).

Social Consequences of an Aging Society

The aging process entrains many social consequences, some of which have particular relevance to exercise and fitness programs.

Social Contacts

Many elderly people lead very lonely lives. Group exercise programs offer an important means of addressing the need for a greater number of social contacts.

An early survey from Britain (Shanas et al. 1968) reported that when there were children, 70% of elderly parents had seen at least one of their offspring in the previous 48 hours, and 86% had made contact over the previous week. When those living in the same home as their children were excluded, the corresponding figures were still 50% and 87%. However, social isolation was a problem for the 16% of seniors with no spouse or surviving children, and for a further 7% who were married but had no children. Among this 23% of the elderly population, almost a fifth had no close relatives. Shanas et al. (1968) estimated that 7% of old people were often lonely, and that a further 21% were sometimes lonely. The problem was particularly prevalent in widows, the recently bereaved, and those in poor health. Some 2% to 3% of seniors had received no visitors during the previous week and had made no human contacts on the previous day. More recently, the Health and Lifestyle Survey of 1987 found that 10% of men and 14% of women felt lonely (Sidell 1995). Blaxter (1990) developed an arbitrary scale of social contacts that was based on visits, letters, and phone calls. The respective percentages of men and women with a score of less than 6 out of a possible 30 points rose from 13% and 9% for respondents aged between 18 and 29 years to 33% and 33% in those over 70 years of age.

Differences in the extent of social isolation are influenced by the scale of a city and by traveling distances. Isolation is greater in London than in smaller British cities (Blaxter 1990). In California, contacts are apparently even less frequent than in Britain; Burch and Collot (1972) noted that 36% of seniors saw their relatives daily, 29% weekly, and 11% less than once a month. A further 4% of old people saw friends on a daily basis, and 48% did so once a week.

In suburban Paris, 43% to 55% of family who live in the same municipality pay daily visits to their aging parents, but figures drop to 19% to 35% if children live in a neighboring municipality, and to 10% to 19% when they live even further away. The full-time employment of most women, smaller numbers of offspring, aging of children who might offer support (Shanas 1980), the breakup of the nuclear family, and the shift to a global economy have progressively eroded family contacts. In North America, it is now quite common for the children of a senior citizen to live several thousand kilometers away, so that visits are paid no more than once a year. Nevertheless, four out of five of the 6 million North American seniors who require some care still live at home rather than in an institution (U.S. Senate Special Committee on Aging 1987).

Perceptions of loneliness are not directly related to the degree of social isolation. Burch and Collot (1972) noted that 75% to 81% of those living in Paris, and 83% of those living in California, felt a part of their respective communities. Where there are no surviving children, the elderly often develop substitute relationships with more remote kin or with neighbors. However, the efforts of such individuals do not usually match those of close family members, either in duration or in frequency of contact and support (Brody 1985).

Social Structures

On average, the elderly tend to be more conservative than younger people, and since seniors form a growing fraction of the active electorate, it seems likely that solutions to social needs will be sought through a right-wing rather than a left-wing agenda.

The physical structure of cities will be substantially modified as the elderly seek small, labor-saving apartments, and as large family homes with a substantial garden lose their popularity. Wealthy retirement communities will flourish in resort areas, and poorer old people will make up a growing fraction of the population in the core areas of large established cities. The growing numbers of the disabled and frail elderly will place heavy pressures on a variety of institutions and services: hospitals and extended care institutions, adapted forms of transportation, physicians, nurses, and ambulatory home-care services.

There will be an increasing need to retrofit public buildings to accommodate elderly people. The hockey arenas, gymnasiums, and swimming pools that were built to accommodate the "baby boom" will see diminishing utilization, but there will be a growing need for such recreational resources as lawn-bowling greens, aqua-fitness classes, libraries, and senior day-care facilities. Such changes in leisure behavior will have implications not only for municipal planners, but also for private sector resorts and for those who manufacture recreational equipment.

Potential Importance of Maintaining an Active Lifestyle

Among many arguments for encouraging the maintenance of an active lifestyle into old age, the regular exerciser may anticipate an increase of social contacts, enhanced physical and emotional health, a reduced risk of chronic disease, and a conservation of function. These gains not only enhance the health of the individual senior, but (by reducing the need for medical care and institutional support) also do much to contain the social costs of an aging society.

Increased Social Contacts

It is possible to pursue exercise in total social isolation, for instance by a personal program of cycle ergometry or chair exercises. Nevertheless, exercise participation is usually a group process that provides contact with others. As discussed in the preceding pages, such contact often is otherwise lacking in a senior's life.

Enhanced Physical and Mental Health

Exercise has an immediate arousing effect, so that the participant's perceived health is usually enhanced: the exerciser "feels better." This tends to counter the anxiety, sleeplessness, and mild depression that are the lot of many seniors (Morgan and Goldstone 1987). Appetite is enhanced, increasing the intake of key minerals and vitamins, and bowel function is increased (Shephard 1986d). Perhaps in part because of a new interest in life, many aspects of cognitive functioning are improved (Chodzo-Zajko and Moore 1994; Tomporowski and Ellis 1986).

The improved overall health is accompanied by enhanced immune function, possibly increasing resistance to acute infections (Brenner, Shek, and Shephard 1994) and the active person has a reserve of energy that improves prognosis if surgery is required (Young 1988).

Prevention of Chronic Disease

Regular physical activity counters many chronic disorders and helps to restore function after symptoms have appeared (Bouchard, Shephard, and Stephens 1994). This seems true of ischemic heart disease, peripheral vascular disease, hypertension, congestive heart failure, chronic obstructive lung disease, moderate obesity, maturity-onset diabetes mellitus, osteoporosis, and certain forms of cancer (colon, breast, and female reproductive tract).

Conservation of Function

Perhaps most importantly, regular physical activity ensures that function at any given age is some 20% higher than in a sedentary person. Thus, although the inherent rate of aging has changed very little, the active person has a level of function sufficient to reduce his or her biological age by 10 to 20 years relative to that of a sedentary individual (Shephard 1991c).

Residual function remains sufficient to allow an active person to walk up a moderate slope without extreme fatigue, to lift a bag of groceries, to open a jar, to lift the body mass from a chair or toilet seat, and to move the main joints through a sufficient range of motion to dress unaided—the many abilities that together enable the senior citizen to live a good quality, independent life (Shephard 1991c; in press-a).

Scientists have yet to discover the philosopher's stone that will confer immortality. However, the ability of regular exercise to reduce biological age by 10 to 20 years is no mean miracle. Indeed, I know of no other therapy that could achieve comparable results.

Conclusions

The population of seniors is far from homogenous. The likelihood of falling into one of three broad categories (young-old, middle-old, and oldest-old) depends not only on age but also on gender, lifestyle, health, socioeconomic factors, and constitutional influences. There is thus an urgent need for an effective measure of biological age. Medical advances are allowing a growing proportion of seniors to survive into the oldest old category, with major economic and social consequences for developed nations. It is important to ensure that enhanced survival is matched by an increase in the quality of life, and it appears that maintenance of regular, moderate physical activity through to an advanced age is a cost-effective method of attaining this objective.

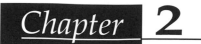# Chapter 2

Current Theories of Aging

In this chapter we consider some metaphors that enhance our understanding of the aging process and also examine molecular and cellular manifestations of aging.

Metaphors of Aging

A wide range of metaphors of aging has developed in both science and the humanities (Kenyon, Birren, and Schroots 1991). Study of these metaphors can facilitate research, clarify theoretical understanding of the aging process, and help in achieving such practical outcomes as an increase of quality-adjusted life expectancy (Schroots, Birren, and Kenyon 1991).

Humanist Perceptions

Humanists often see the life course as a journey or a circle (Cole and Meyer 1991; Kenyon 1991), personal in character, opaquely perceived, and of finite but unknown duration. Time is viewed as the "messenger of the gods" (Achenbaum 1991). The collective experience of the life cycle is more often a contest than a convoy (Dannefer 1991). Positive aspects of aging include a sense of completeness, fulfillment, self-meaning, wisdom, and connectedness (Manning 1991), but too often lack of employment after retirement leads to narcissism and life with little personal meaning (Mader 1991).

Perceptions of the Scientist

In contrast to the humanist, the physician and the exercise scientist see aging in terms of disease, decline, and degeneration (Davidson 1991). Taking a positivist approach, the scientists ask questions that often seem determined by available technology. In accordance with Black's (1979) interactive view of metaphor, aging becomes defined in terms of a decline in measurable numbers—maximal oxygen intake, muscle strength, flexibility, and balance—largely because such items are easy to quantify.

Specific medical metaphors of aging have included the "wear and tear" that is imposed upon a machine and the obsolescence that develops in a computer system (Shephard 1991b). The human body has also been seen as a target, prone to attack by various noxious agents. Others have visualized a programmed senescence, a failure of homeostasis, or an increased probability of death.

The Human as an Aging Piece of Machinery

Physicians and exercise scientists often view the human body as a very complex piece of machinery. A parallel can be drawn to a series of partially interlinked clocks (Schroots 1991). Like most clocks, the body tends to "run down," or become exhausted; also as with household clocks, not all of the timing mechanisms in the body run at the same speed! Some systems mature and age faster than others, and the speed of operation of individual timing mechanisms can be adjusted by specific types of treatment.

As with much machinery of human design, the body is designed for durability, but nevertheless is subject to "wear and tear," with ultimate irreversible breakdown (the *Abnutzungstheorie* of German gerontologists). Bellamy (1991) has likened the system to a machine-operated assembly line. In his analogy, "wear and tear" can lead to an error in one of the machine tools that controls the assembly of body proteins. The error is insufficient to prevent operation of the tool, but nevertheless the products that are assembled (enzymes and other proteins) do not reach an appropriate standard of quality for effective function.

Social critics of the machine metaphor and its derivatives have objected that it encourages both immediate robot-like exploitation of workers and rejection of them once their apparent usefulness as a part of the larger machine of society has passed (Shephard 1991b). From the biological perspective, the main weaknesses of the machine metaphor are the implied adverse effects of increased use (as seen in the exerciser), the anticipation of a sudden, catastrophic failure of the system, and the poor representation of both normal and abnormal repair processes.

Changes of Metabolic Rate

Pursued to its logical conclusion, the machine metaphor would indicate a prolongation of human survival if the body were subjected to less "wear and tear"—for example, if the number of metabolic cycles or the number of heart beats were reduced by studied inactivity.

In fruit flies, metabolic rate is not closely linked to longevity (Arking et al. 1988). However, experiments with small mammals have given some credence to such a hypothesis (Weindruch and Walford 1988; Yu, Masoro, and McMahan 1985). The life span of animals is reduced if the metabolic rate is increased by exposure to either high or low temperatures; conversely, survival is enhanced by hibernation or dietary restriction (Weindruch and Walford 1988). Nevertheless, such maneuvers do more than alter metabolic rate; they also reduce the energy available for cell proliferation (Weindruch and Walford 1988) and reproduction (Merry and Holehan 1981). Dietary restriction delays maturation, decreases adult size, and reduces the likelihood of obesity. Such changes (rather than a reduction of "wear and tear") probably account for most of the enhanced survival that has been reported in food-restricted animals. Much of the longer average life span may even reflect a smaller proportion of deaths before the animals reach maturity. If dietary restriction is begun during adult life, mortality seems to be increased rather than decreased (Holloszy 1993).

Regular exercise improves the average life span of both male and female rats without extending their maximal life span (Holloszy and Schectman 1991). Young male animals do not augment their food intake to compensate for running. Thus, it could be argued that (like food-restricted animals) exercisers mature more slowly, do not grow to as large a size as their sedentary peers, and avoid obesity. However, female rats increase their food intake to compensate for the added energy costs of regular exercise, yet they also improve their survival rate relative to sedentary controls (Holloszy 1993). This suggests that an increase in regular physical activity exerts some unique and beneficial influence upon survival prospects that is independent of increased energy usage.

Available human studies support the suggestion that the quantity and type of food that is consumed have a major influence upon population mortality. If food consumption is excessive relative to habitual activity, obesity develops. Obesity predisposes to both atherosclerosis and certain forms of cancer—common causes of premature death. Moreover, a diet rich in animal fat (as is common in the United States) predisposes to atherosclerosis, whereas a diet rich in polyunsaturated oils (fish oil or olive oil) has a protective effect (Kesteloot 1991). The *Abnutzungstheorie* would require that exercise shorten life span, but in fact for any given diet, regular, moderate bouts of endurance exercise increase the average life span. If 8 MJ/week of leisure activity is performed from early middle age (around 35 years), then survival relative to that of sedentary individuals is extended by as much as two years (Paffenbarger et al. 1994). Survival curves for active and sedentary individuals progressively converge over adult life (Pekkanen et al. 1987), and in the oldest age categories, any advantage of the active subjects is no more than 0.3 to 0.4 years (Paffenbarger et al. 1994).

Breakdown and Repair

The traditional *Abnutzungstheorie* anticipated a sudden, major breakdown in the body machinery. Humans do occasionally suffer a terminal catastrophe, such as the rupture of an aorta or a massive stroke, but more often death is preceded by a gradual deterioration of function in most of the body tissues.

The *Abnutzungstheorie* developed through observation of the mechanico-chemical deterioration of colloids *in vitro*. It is reasonable to expect some physical deterioration of bones, joints, and even blood vessels, if these are subject to rough usage. However, the concept that "wear" will result from moderate activity is at variance with our current understanding of the body tissues and normal repair processes. The individual elements of most tissues undergo continuous remodeling as the human machine operates. The turnover of liver proteins, for example, is such that the half-life of a given molecule is no more than 10 days. Moreover, although exercise leads to an immediate increase in the breakdown rate of body protein, the long-term effect of physical activity is to augment tissue synthesis and rebuilding (Blumberg and Meydani 1995).

Abnutzungstheorie nevertheless introduces the useful concept of "fair" wear and tear. The life span of most machinery is shortened by rough treatment. Likewise, although moderate exercise can enhance many aspects of body function, excessive physical activity can have negative consequences for both function and overall survival.

A Modified Machine Metaphor

Despite its weaknesses, the machine metaphor can perhaps be sustained if we think of a second-generation machine. In such a device, useful life is greatly prolonged by regularly scheduled maintenance and the replacement of key components.

As in second-generation machines of human design, certain body components are difficult or impossible to replace. For example, the proportion of actively functioning cells decreases progressively with age, and in the central nervous system there is no mechanism to replace damaged cells; nevertheless, neuroplasticity may allow some continuing compensation through changes in the functional connections of residual cells (Will, Schmitt, and Dalrymple-Alford 1985).

Tissue enzymes become exhausted after a finite number of reactions have been processed. In cells that remain capable of division, the enzymes can be replaced at mitosis, but post-mitotic cells such as nerve and muscle either have developed some non-mitotic mechanism to replace enzymes, or contain enzymes that are very resistant to spoilage.

The Human as an Aging Computer

A computer is in essence a late-20th-century machine. Many of the arguments that surround the machine metaphor thus apply to consideration of the human as an aging computer.

One immediate philosophical implication is that a person becomes a "black box," programmed to respond uniformly to certain input signals. All too often, a modern company expects its personnel to behave like computers, implementing policies and procedures according to a program predetermined by the organization. There is no potential for individuality of thought. The emphasis of the computer is on speed in the mindless processing of neat and conventionally ordered data. Such a metaphor is particularly damaging to the older person. It denies the tremendous innovative potential of senior citizens—people who have accumulated a wealth of personal experience, and finally can give full rein to this knowledge because they have escaped the conformist pressures of paid employment.

The computer ages by becoming obsolete, a process that occurs even faster than the "wear and tear" that destroys a traditional machine. And unfortunately, older workers also become obsolete—they have skills that are no longer relevant to the automated workplace.

The function of a computer is compromised by information loss. Aging, likewise, is marked by various manifestations of information loss—a departure from the intended mechanical properties in inert materials such as collagen, a structural deterioration of cell membranes that restricts the transfer of messenger substances, a confounding of the master template of protein synthesis (DNA), and a death of the cells responsible for neural impulses, hormone production, and cytokine secretion.

One further feature of the computer metaphor is that it assumes an absence of gross movement. Again, this is a disturbingly accurate metaphor of life in modern society. However, there are strong anthropological arguments favoring the hypothesis that the human body was "designed" by evolutionary pressures to engage in regular, moderate physical activity. Thus, we should regard as inappropriate any computer metaphor of aging that neglects this fundamental characteristic of human life.

The Aging Human Body as a Battered Target

This metaphor sees the human body as a target, battered from a number of sources: ultraviolet and other external forms of radiation, internally produced reactive chemicals, and invading viruses (Harman 1981). Individual cells receive fatal "hits" and are no longer able to transcribe proteins accurately. Whole organs and eventually the whole body die because of an accumulation of such "hits." One negative implication of the metaphor is that the process appears as random and stochastic, with little scope for preventive measures. In fact, many of the "hits" arise from human activities, such as creation of the air pollution that has depleted the ozone layer and augmented ultraviolet irradiation.

Early studies gave empirical support to the hypothesis implicit in the battered target metaphor, but recent research suggests that enzymes for the repair of DNA templates function equally well in young and old cells (Rothstein 1987).

Programmed Senescence

The concept of programmed senescence (Grigliatti 1987) sees aging and death as evolutionary adaptations that have prevented overpopulation of the world (Rose and Graves 1989). Prolonged survival after procreation of a sufficient number of offspring places an excessive burden on any given habitat. Starvation thus tends to eliminate variants of a species that show unusual longevity. Declining numbers of the variant in turn reduce the number of potential gene combinations, limiting the ability of the long-lived variant to adapt to any future change in the environment, and thereby hastening its demise. Each species develops an optimum life span, determined by the time to reach reproductive maturity, the number of offspring, and the likelihood that offspring will survive to reproductive maturity.

In order to ensure survival of the species, most mammals produce a number of litters over an extended time. Given the weight of adverse environmental pressures, there is no evolutionary advantage to the premature onset of senescence. Rather, a premium is set on variants that maintain health and vigor until the reproductive task has been completed (Sacher 1982). Indeed, if a gene enhances early reproductive or adaptive capacity, it may be selected even though it carries disadvantages for later life. In essence, natural selection favors a strategy whereby the body invests fewer resources in the maintenance of somatic tissues than would be needed to ensure their indefinite survival (Kirkwood 1992).

Empirical Evidence

Although there is a sense in which the germ plasma is immortal, aging and death are characteristic of living cells, unless they have been modified by exposure to chemical carcinogens or viruses (Hayflick 1985; Monti et al. 1992; Smith, Ning, and Pereira-Smith 1992). Even during embryonic development, tissue growth and remodeling are based upon an orderly death of some cell lines and an activation of others.

Under *in vitro* conditions, a culture of fibroblasts gradually reaches a phase of extended, irregular cell cycles and dies out after about 50 cell divisions have been completed. The critical factor in death of the culture seems to be an aging of the cell nucleus. Death can be accelerated by transplantion of an aging nucleus to young cytoplasm; conversely, the process can be slowed by transplantation of a young nucleus to aging cytoplasm. *In vivo*, much seems to depend on the environment, and if tissue is transplanted into an appropriate young host, it can outsurvive the donor animal.

Body cells differ in their capacity to multiply *in vivo*. Nerve and cardiac muscle cells have already ceased cell division by the time of birth; initially, there is considerable redundancy, and an adequate complement of cells usually survive over the life span. Regeneration is no longer possible, but neuroplasticity offers some potential to compensate for cell death (Strong and Garruto 1994; Strong, Wood, and Samorajski 1991). One major advantage that neurons gain from their post-mitotic state is that a sophisticated memory can be developed; this helps in coping with a multiplicity of environments. A second category of cells, for example hepatocytes, are also post-mitotic under normal conditions, but they can revert to a proliferative phase if the need arises. Other cells such as the erythrocyte and leucocyte stem lines are normally inter-mitotic: they retain a capacity to proliferate rapidly in response to appropriate growth signals such as an antigen challenge (Murasko et al. 1991).

Cells from older individuals are in general capable of fewer divisions than those from younger subjects (Cristofalo, Phillips, and Brooks 1985). A lesser capacity for cell multiplication also seems to be characteristic of individuals with an acceleration of aging due to such pathologies as childhood progeria (Brown, Zebrower, and Kieras 1985) and its adult form (Werner's syndrome; Salk, Fujiwara, and Martin 1985).

Genetic Control Mechanisms

The life span is marked by a relentless progression of the morphogenetic process of determination, differentiation, and pattern formation that built the individual from a single zygote (Yates 1991). This process is universal in nature, although it has specific features characteristic of a given species and a given individual (Birren and Lanum 1991; Kirkwood 1992).

The predetermined pattern of maturation and aging is presumably dictated by the genome (Gelman et al. 1988). There are a variety of "biological clocks" that could cause the loss of function in one or more key cell populations: the repression of growth-stimulating genes and the expression of growth-inhibiting genes, a loss of redundancy in the DNA molecule, a failure of repair processes with a resultant buildup of metabolic errors, and a depletion of key enzymes such as those dealing with reactive oxygen species (Goldstein 1990; Rothstein 1990; Turner and Weiss 1994). At least in fruit flies, certain mutations can accelerate aging (Grigliatti 1987), and artificial selection can increase life span by as much as 50% (Arking 1987).

The biological clocks in turn cause a loss of adaptability to environmental change, contributing to the exponential increase of mortality that we associate with the terminal phase of aging.

Failure of Homeostasis

The human body is "designed" to function in a closely regulated *milieu intérieur*. Thus, the capacity to regulate the internal environment (homeostasis) is closely interrelated with prospects for survival, and senescence can be viewed as a progressive loss of physiological adaptability to the external environment.

The elderly person responds more slowly and less effectively to environmental change through a deterioration in both control and effector mechanisms. On the effector side, functional reserves are progressively reduced; for example, resting metabolism accounts for an increasing fraction of peak oxygen intake, the gap between resting and peak heart rate diminishes progressively, and resting ventilation accounts for an ever-larger fraction of maximal ventilatory effort.

The person thus becomes increasingly vulnerable to such environmental threats as extremes of heat and cold, fluctuations of blood sugar, and the circulatory disturbances associated with exercise or blood loss.

Hypothermia

To take thermoregulation as a specific example (Kenney 1995), one early study found that 3.6% of old people who were admitted to English hospitals during the winter months showed unsuspected hypothermia. Likewise, United States death certificates indicate from 350 to 900 cold fatalities per year, with a particularly high incidence in those over the age of 75 years (Exton-Smith and Collins 1991; Macey and Schneider 1993). Sometimes the problem is a lack of funds to buy home heating fuel or immobilization by a fall, but other factors predisposing to hypothermia include the use of drugs that impair thermoregulation and diseases that decrease heat production, increase heat loss, or impair thermal regulation. Further, because of a deterioration of sensory receptors and impaired central processing of information, an old person may not realize that he or she is becoming cold. Whereas young people can detect an 0.8 °C difference in body temperature, the old person can only detect a change of 2.5 °C (Collins 1987).

Obesity offers partial protection to some seniors, but in general, adjustment to a cold environment is compounded by a low rate of resting metabolism, a limited ability to increase metabolism, and a deterioration in mechanisms that limit heat loss (Wagner and Horvath 1985). A decreased food intake limits the postprandial increase of resting metabolism, and the capacity to generate heat by physical exercise becomes progressively reduced with age. The shivering response is also decreased, peripheral blood flow is initially low, and the capacity for vasoconstriction is diminished.

Hyperthermia

In the summer months, old people are also vulnerable to hyperthermia. Heat waves in New York City, St. Louis, Pittsburgh, and most recently Chicago have led to a substantial increase in the death rate among the elderly population (Ramlow and Kuller 1990). The major immediate pathologies are ischemic heart disease and cerebrovascular disease. In Britain, ambient temperatures are less extreme. Nevertheless, the death rates of seniors reach their nadir when the mean daily temperature is 17 °C to 18 °C, and an increased mortality is observed at ambient temperatures above 20 °C (Office of Population Censuses and Surveys 1976).

Environmental Control

Although occasional incidents of both hypothermia and hyperthermia still demonstrate the declining ability to maintain homeostasis in an elderly person, air-conditioned vehicles, enclosed shopping malls, and centrally heated homes have now reduced the external challenge to thermoregulation for many elderly people.

The main threats to homeostasis now arise from within the body, in the form of responses to infections and vigorous physical activity. Vigorous exercise increases the demand on many body systems by a factor of at least 10, and a complicated system of feedback loops must be activated if constancy of the internal environment is to be preserved. Unfortunately, the functional speed and effectiveness of these cybernetic systems deteriorate with aging.

Increased Probability of Death

Several of the metaphors discussed above—"wear and tear," programmed senescence, and failure of homeostasis—point to the concept that aging is an increased probability of death. How far do survival curves support this view?

We could envisage life in a very hazardous environment, where death occurred from accident, starvation, disease, or other forms of stress before the aging process had opportunity to cause any important deterioration of homeostatic function. Under such conditions, a constant proportion of the residual population would die in each successive time interval (see fig. 2.1). This type of survival curve is thought to have been typical of neolithic communities. It is still observed in many animal populations (Cutler 1985), and was typical of isolated Inuit populations until quite recently.

The alternative possibility, characteristic of modern society, is to live in a well-protected environment. Premature deaths are then avoided, and almost all deaths are due to senescence. The survival curve becomes rectangular in form, with a precipitous drop in the percentage of survivors (and thus a rapidly increasing probability of death) once a critical age has been passed (Fries 1980a, 1992).

Gompertz Relationship

Beginning with Gompertz (1825), mathematicians have found much amusement in fitting equations to the curves that describe survival and/or death rates. Gompertz suggested that the death rate (Rm) at any given age (t) was an exponential function, determined by a hypothetical death rate at birth (Ro) and a slope coefficient (a):

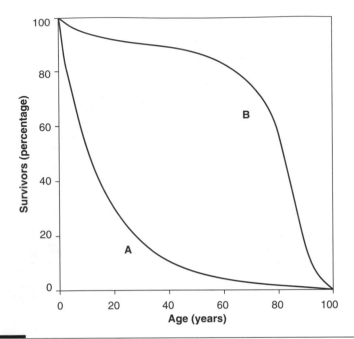

Figure 2.1 Survival curves showing two different scenarios. Population A shows a constant and random mortality due to natural causes. Population B experiences a sudden increase of mortality with the onset of senescence.

$$Rm = Ro \ e^{at}.$$

The implication of such an equation is that a linear function can be obtained on plotting the logarithm of the death rate against age (see fig. 2.2). In other words, aging is associated with a logarithmic increase in the probability of death, and the slope function (a) indicates the average rate of aging for a given cohort of the population.

Subsequent authors have attempted to improve on the basic Gompertz formula, either by adding a second component of mortality (Rb) that is independent of age,

$$Rm = Ro \ e^{at} + Rb,$$

or by allowing an interval of early adulthood (c) before senescence begins to take effect:

$$Rm = Ro \ e^{a(t - c)}.$$

However, it seems unlikely that any simple formula will do more than approximate the many age-related factors that can modify the form of the mortality curve: success in the control of infant mortality, immunization against the diseases of childhood, the adoption of traffic control measures

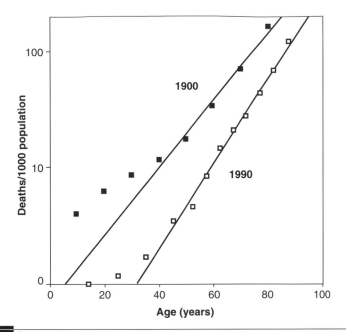

Figure 2.2   Gompertz plots relating deaths per 1000 of the population (logarithmic scale) to age of the population. Data for the United States, 1900 and 1990.

that increase the safety of automobile operation, and fitness and dietary programs that reduce the likelihood of developing chronic disease later in adult life. Gradual elimination of the causes of early death has displaced the Gompertz curve progressively toward the right, without much change in the final slope of the relationship (see fig. 2.2). Some authors have interpreted the rightward displacement of the line as evidence that biological age has decreased in relation to calendar age. However, there is little question that the main gains have resulted from a control of external threats to homeostasis, rather than a change in the intrinsic process of senescence.

One analytic and one semantic complication limit acceptance of aging as an increased probability of death. From the analytic viewpoint, the death rates applicable to any given cohort are derived from cross-sectional data, and external threats to survival have been decreasing as the survivors have aged. The slope of the Gompertz relationship thus reflects the combined influence of senescence and diminishing environmental hazards on any given cross-section of a population.

From the semantic standpoint, several biological systems age without obvious impact on the risk of dying. For example, many men lose their scalp hair at a fairly early age, and in women, reproductive function ceases around 50 years of age. Both phenomena are manifestations of aging, but they seemingly bear very little relationship to the likelihood of death. To overcome this problem of terminology, some authors distinguish between aging as a general phenomenon and senescence (a change that manifestly contributes to the probability of death). However, the distinction between aging and senescence is not clearcut. For example, osteoporosis can contribute to death, and in women the decline of reproductive function seems to accelerate the development of osteoporosis.

Critique of Concept

An increased probability of death has been a popular metaphor with biologists. They have noted that senescence brings a greater likelihood of death not only for the body as a whole, but also for organs and individual cells. However, this immediately tends to suggest that senescence is a disease, rather than a normal biological process. It also revives the inappropriate expectation of Paracelsus: discovery of a philosopher's stone that will confer immortality— either some anti-aging drug that will counter the destructive potential of reactive molecules, or a form of genetic engineering that can speed repair of any errors that develop in the DNA template.

In fact, recent medical advances have not extended the life span of the average person who remains in good health (Fries 1992). There remains a rapidly increasing probability of death around the age of 85 years. Moreover, the specter of impending death encourages a focus upon seeking survival at all costs, while ignoring the important issue of the quality of the individual's remaining years of life.

Molecular Changes

The several metaphors discussed in the preceding sections presage molecular expressions of aging. "Wear and tear" may cause molecular damage that is hard to repair, leading to an accumulation of undesirable waste products within a cell. "Targeting" by noxious agents may induce some irreversible chemical alteration in the DNA template, and programmed senescence may lead to either a progressive lack of key molecules or unwanted immune reactions to normal cell constituents.

Molecular "Wear and Tear"

Molecular aging is associated with progressive damage to key constituents of the cell and the accumulation of unwanted intracellular debris.

Repair Failure

According to this hypothesis, spontaneous hydrolysis and the action of free radicals lead to age-related errors in DNA structure and thus in the flow of genetically controlled information (Gensler and Bernstein 1981). However, it is uncertain whether the rate of mutation is sufficient to have serious consequences in the absence of exposure to ionizing radiation.

The DNA of a resting cell is contained within the nucleosome, in combination with several histones and other less well-identified proteins. Reactions such as acetylation uncoil the DNA sequence and activate it as a prelude to its replication. Effector molecules are then able to interact with sensor regions of the DNA sequence, and the sensor regions in turn activate adjacent integrator genes that begin to produce messenger RNAs. These carry the code for synthesis of a range of activator proteins that can react with receptors elsewhere on the DNA molecule.

Given the extended chain of command, there are a multiplicity of sites where functional deterioration and errors of replication could occur with aging. The type, amount, and structure of the histones or nonhistone proteins might become inappropriate. The normal unfolding of the DNA chain might be modified by changes in the rate of acetylation, methylation, or phosphorylation, allowing mutations, cross-linkages, breaks, and other errors to develop along the DNA chain. There might also be a decreased production of effector molecules. The DNA chain might show a loss of sensitivity in its sensor region, a poor transmission of information from the sensor to the integrator, or a faulty receptor sequence. Finally, the synthesis of messenger RNA might be deficient in amount or erroneous in its structure (Bellamy 1991).

Empirical studies have to date had little success in identifying the main site of the lesion when a DNA chain sustains a "hit." Possibly, the available methods of analysis are too crude, or the damaged cells are quickly eliminated. Pertinent age-related changes that have been identified to date include alterations in the association of DNA with nonhistone proteins such as collagen, procollagen, and fibronectin (Goldstein et al. 1990; Timiras 1988); a shortening of the chromosomes (Osiewacz 1995), with loss of some highly reiterated sequences in the DNA chain (Goldstein et al. 1985); and some loss of brain messenger RNA, exacerbated by Alzheimer's disease (Finch et al. 1987). However, there do not seem to be any substantial age-related changes in the fidelity of protein synthesis (Goldstein et al. 1985), and early suggestions of an inverse association between the life span of animals and the ability to detect, excise, and/or repair DNA faults have not been confirmed (Hanawalt, Gee, and Ho 1990).

Replication of gene sequences and redundancy in the DNA template reduce the likelihood of problems in protein transcription. Even if an error does develop in the DNA chain, it is speedily corrected. Conceivably the repair process could become slower or less effective with aging (Hanawalt, Gee, and Ho 1990). Eventually the redundancy of coding would then be exhausted, and an accumulation of metabolic errors along the length of the chain would make it impossible for the cell to survive.

Let us suppose that an accumulation of 30 errors in replication is sufficient to cause the death of a cell. The time needed to accumulate this ceiling depends on the repair rate; a doubling of the repair rate would extend life span by 40%, and a tripling in the speed of repair would be enough to guarantee immortality. Evolution has thus favored the development of a repair rate that allows a sufficiently prolonged survival to meet the needs of reproduction, without diverting an excessive amount of energy from the reproductive process itself (Kirkwood 1992). Corollaries of this hypothesis are that the longevity of a species is reflected in the repair rate for that species, and that fecundity is inversely related to longevity.

Accumulation of Debris

In theory, large molecules of metabolic debris could accumulate within a cell if they formed complexes with vital components of the cell, or if they were sufficiently altered to escape normal turnover processes. Some substances might even appear as precipitates.

In practice, age-related intracellular accumulations of calcium ions and pigments such as lipofuscin seem to be consequences rather than causes of aging. Calcium accumulates irreversibly in the cell membrane as it undergoes an age-related decrease in its phospholipid content. The rate of pumping of calcium ions in muscle and brain also decreases with age (Gwathmey et al. 1990; Landfield, Pitler, and Applegate 1986).

Accumulation of lipofuscin is particularly marked in the brain and heart (Timiras 1988). At various times, lipofuscin was thought to distort cell membranes, to chelate toxic products of metabolism, or to provide a matrix for immobilization of enzymes (Strong, Wood, and Samorajski 1991). In itself, it is probably no more than an extremely inert end product of the peroxidation of lipids (del Roso et al. 1990; Sohal and Wolfe 1986; Tsuchida, Miura, and Aibara 1987). A heart that is well impregnated with this pigment can still function very well, and indeed it can retain a normal capacity for hypertrophy (Timiras 1988). However, the underlying peroxidation of membrane lipids can have adverse consequences for brain function, as is seen in the pathological condition of ceroid lipofuscinosis (Armstrong 1991).

The accumulation of lipofuscin can be reduced by the administration of some antioxidants such as centrophenoxine (dimethylamino-p-chlorophenoxyacetate), but somewhat surprisingly, large doses of vitamin E have no effect on the storage of this pigment (Hayflick 1985).

"Targeting" and Molecular Damage

The complex molecular structure of the cell may be damaged by (1) a spontaneous hydrolysis of molecules, (2) exposure to external sources of ultraviolet or other irradiation, (3) the intracellular generation of reactive oxygen species during normal metabolism, (4) exposure to mutagenic chemicals, ozone, or metallic ions, or (5) the development of abnormal cross-linkages between key molecular components of the cell.

Targeting can cause a distortion of molecular information within the cell: as discussed above, errors in protein transcription may arise from a chemical alteration in the master template of protein synthesis (DNA) and changes elsewhere in the chain of command (alterations in other constituents of the chromosome, mRNA, or protein synthetases).

Role of Free Radicals

The harmful effects of both external radiation and a high metabolic rate seem to be attributable to the formation of free radicals (Mehlhorn and Cole 1985; Sohal and Allen 1985; Swartz and Mäder 1995). Both types of challenge cause an electron pair to separate temporarily into two independently moving electrons, with a large increase of free energy. This then allows adjacent molecules to be attacked.

The reactive species may cause a destruction of thiol groups, with adverse effects upon thiol-containing enzymes. A peroxidation of lipids occurs, with damage to mitochondrial enzymes, lysozomes, and the plasma membrane. Malonaldehyde is also produced, and this can cause the development of cross-linkages within a variety of substances, including collagen, elastin, and the DNA chain (see fig. 2.3).

An irradiation-induced "fault" was originally conceived as a cross-linkage that caused a mutation in one of the 3000 genes that are essential to normal cell function. A "hit" was a more major event, rendering inactive all of the genes on a single chromosome. An irradiation of 19 rad is usually sufficient to

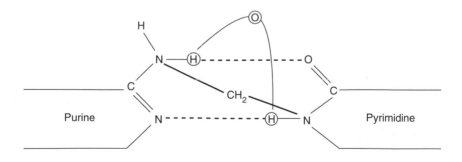

Figure 2.3 Example of cross-linkage. Two nucleosides are initially linked by weak hydrogen bonds (dotted lines) that connect the nitrogen atom of purine with the hydrogen molecule of pyrimidine, and the oxygen atom of pyrimidine with the hydrogen atom of purine. The aggressor molecule is here formaldehyde (but it could equally be a free radical). The bonding hydrogen atoms combine with the oxygen of formaldehyde to yield a molecule of water, and a strong methylene bridge is formed between the purine and pyrimidine radicals.

cause a chromosomal break, and 86 rad is the mean lethal dose for a human cell at the interphase stage in its life history.

Cross-linkage not only may unite two nucleoside chains of DNA, but may also bind the DNA more tightly to its associated protein, repressing its capacity to induce enzymes (Magnani et al. 1990). Cross-linkages that link other types of molecules yield amorphous deposits of hyaline and amyloid tissue that cannot be cleared by normal enzyme systems. Young collagen molecules consist of three helical chains, twisted around one another to form a super-helix and held together rather loosely by hydrogen bonds between carbonyl, imino, and amino acid groups (Shephard 1983a). However, the cross-linkage of aging (Eyre, Paz, and Gall 1984; Vlassara 1990) leads to a rigid bonding of two collagen chains (dimer formation) or all three chains (trimer formation), with a progressive loss of elasticity in the affected fibers.

Given the supposed role of peroxidation in the development of cross-linkages, it is surprising that antioxidant agents such as vitamin E have little preventive value.

Empirical Evidence of Molecular Damage

Any abnormalities of DNA that develop tend to be recessive. Errors of protein transcription are thus brought to light only if the homologous chromosome has already received a "hit" or is carrying a fault at a comparable point in its structure. Nevertheless, there is a progressive accumulation of abnormal DNA molecules as a person becomes older. The effects of such abnormalities are particularly serious at loci where there is no redundancy in the DNA coding sequence. A mis-specified enzyme could induce a cascade of faulty molecules, and the multiplication of a cell that has become abnormal could lead to an exponential accumulation of malfunction within an organ.

Despite the theoretical logic of this analysis, it is hard to demonstrate an accumulation of abnormal enzymes; some mutations do reduce levels of antioxidant enzymes such as catalase and peroxidase, but this does not seem to accelerate the aging process (Mehlhorn and Cole 1985). Moreover, on the basis of the considerations mentioned, one would expect homozygosity to mask many faults and allow the continued copying of important proteins (Hayflick 1985). But in practice, heterozygotes usually live longer than homozygotes. In partial explanation of this paradox, it has been argued that critical mutations are dominant rather than recessive and that they occur on control genes rather than on the genes that code for enzyme structure.

Prevention and Repair Processes

Free radical formation can be reduced by an increased intake of antioxidants such as vitamin E or vitamin C, or by an increase in the enzymes that break down peroxides. Some animal experiments have suggested that survival can be enhanced by the consumption of large doses of vitamin E, but it is unclear how far its antioxidant properties contribute to this effect. Vitamin E depresses appetite, with a slowing of growth and maturation (as in food restriction; Comfort 1979; Goodrick et al. 1983), and the administration of antioxidants also slows the development of tumors, which are a frequent cause of death. As noted previously, antioxidants do not have any obvious effect in reducing the extent of cross-linkage formation despite their ability to scavenge free radicals.

Regular exercise certainly increases the production of free radicals (Jenkins 1988; Ohno et al. 1988), but this disadvantage is compensated by an increase in the activity of oxidant-scavenging enzymes such as glutathione reductase (Ohno et al. 1988).

The body is able to correct many of the simpler faults of DNA structure, whether due to hydrolysis or to cross-linkage of the chains, by standard repair mechanisms (endonucleases, repair polymerases, and ligases; see fig. 2.4).

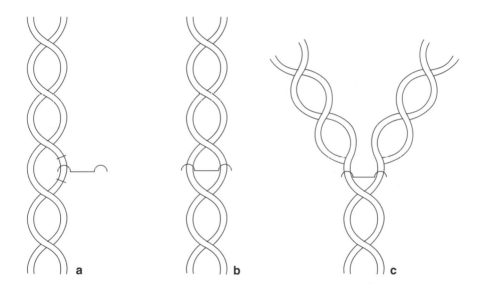

Figure 2.4 Illustration of three possible consequences of cross-linkage. (a) Cross-linkage attached to single DNA chain. Repair can be effected by excision of the affected segment, using its partner as a template for accurate resynthesis of the excised zone. (b) Cross-linkage attached to both filaments of DNA molecule. Excision is still possible, but the affected segment has been irreversibly damaged. (c) Failure to excise the cross-linkage, so that at the next cell division, separation of the nucleoside chains is incomplete, and a Y-shaped monstrosity is formed.
Adapted from J. Bjorksten, 1974, "Cross-linkage and the aging process," In M. Rockstein (Ed.), *Theoretical aspects of aging*. (New York: Academic Press).

The critical issue from the viewpoint of maintaining cell and organ function in an older person is any difference between the rates of damage and the rates of repair relative to the normal life span of the individual.

Implications for Survival

In terms of survival of the organism as a whole, several scenarios may be envisaged (Comfort 1979). Irradiation could be seen as an environmental hazard, decreasing a person's ability to survive over a given time interval, irrespective of the individual's initial age. This would increase the death rate of all adults, thus displacing the linear portion of the Gompertz plot (see fig. 2.2) to the left without changing its slope. Irradiation might also modify the rate of aging during adult life, so that those who were exposed would begin the linear portion of the Gompertz plot at a similar starting point, but their death rates would increase with a steeper slope than for those not exposed to this hazard. Finally, irradiation could cause all-or-none damage in a stochastic fashion, so that some members of the irradiated population would die prematurely, while others would enjoy an unchanged rate of aging.

The main empirical evidence regarding the effects of irradiation on aging and survival is drawn from the victims of the Hiroshima atomic explosion (Hollingsworth et al. 1969). This group seems to have experienced an increased incidence of leukemias and cancers, without any dramatic effect on other manifestations of aging.

Programmed Senescence

A number of authors have linked programmed senescence to a depletion of enzyme systems in post-mitotic cells, or to age-related changes in endocrine and paracrine function.

Enzyme Systems

A decrease of enzymic activity could reflect not only a depletion of active protein but also a failure of homeostasis, the local environment (pH, ionic concentration, concentration of activators and inhibitors, or temperature) becoming unfavorable to activity of the enzyme in question.

The overall rate of metabolism declines slightly with aging (Masoro 1985), but after one allows for an age-related increase in the proportion of adipose tissue, metabolic rates per unit of cell mass for the seventh and eighth decades of life are usually only about 10% lower than the values found in young adults. The main explanation for the decrement is probably an involution of the thyroid gland (Legros and Brunier 1982). However, differences of this magnitude are hard to interpret, and can in some instances arise from no more than a difference in diet between younger and older individuals (Rode and Shephard 1995).

Findings on age-related changes in enzyme activities in individual tissues have been inconsistent and inconclusive (Bellamy 1991). Fibroblast cultures show no decrease in the activity of key enzymes until toward the end of their life. In the liver, the activity of 50% of enzymes remains unchanged, while 25% of enzymes show an increase and 25% show a decrease (Timiras 1988). In muscle, a post-mitotic tissue, the oxidative power shows little change with age, but it is conceivable that a decrease in aerobic enzyme activity is masked by a selective loss of type II (glycolytic) fibers (Aoyagi and Shephard 1992). Likewise, inconsistent changes in lactate dehydrogenase seem to reflect an unchanged activity of the aerobic form of the enzyme (LDH-H), but a decrease in activity of the anaerobic form (LDH-M) that is found mainly in type II muscle fibers (Cress et al. 1984). The ATPase activity of skeletal muscle diminishes with age, but once again it is hard to separate this change from the selective loss of type II muscle fibers (Grimby et al. 1982). In cardiac muscle, ATPase activity decreases from neonatal to adult life, but there is surprisingly little change thereafter (Lakatta 1987). In the brain, there are age-related decreases in the activity of enzyme systems that synthesize catecholamines and regulate the formation and breakdown of acetylcholine (Poirier and Finch 1994), but again it is difficult to disentangle such observations from changes in the cellular composition of the material that is classified as brain.

In summary, there is as yet little evidence to support the idea of a progressive depletion of intracellular enzyme levels with aging.

Endocrine Changes

The substantial changes of endocrine balance at menopause suggest a possible relationship between aging and exhaustion of the endocrine system. Administration of androgens and estrogens can reverse some of the secondary cellular and molecular manifestations of aging, such as the loss of elasticity in the skin, osteoporosis, and atrophy of the vaginal epithelium. Such treatment may also increase the synthesis of protein, with a net cellular retention of nitrogen. However, aging seems to proceed at a normal rate in eunuchs, and there is no evidence that animals can be made senescent by the removal of any of their endocrine glands.

Some authors have maintained that food restriction slows the aging of animals because it induces a form of dietary hypophysectomy. Nevertheless, neuroendocrine theories cannot explain why aging occurs in simpler organisms that lack the relevant hypophyseal structures (Hayflick 1985).

Immune Disturbances

At one time, it was postulated that "hits" from irradiation modified body constituents until they became "other than self," provoking an immune response (Comfort 1979). However, the quantity of protein that is thus modified seems insufficient to provoke any substantial immunological reaction.

The concept that the antigenic characteristics of certain cells are modified by a viral infection is also now largely discounted.

Nevertheless, aging is associated with a deterioration in various aspects of immune function (Shephard and Shek 1995a), and the elderly become increasingly prone to autoimmune disorders such as rheumatoid arthritis (Calkins, Reinhard, and Vladutiu 1994). As Galen recognized, a progressive decrease in size of the thymus begins in late childhood. This seems to retard the development of T cells, and in particular to upset the normal balance between CD4 (helper) and CD8 (suppressor) T cells, decreasing the individual's resistance to infections and tumor cells and leading to formation of auto-antibodies by the B cells.

Russell (1978) and Walford (1980) have suggested that a specific site on chromosome 6 (the main histocompatibility complex) regulates both immune function and aging. But if the loss of immune function and the development of autoimmunity are truly age-linked phenomena, it is puzzling that autoimmune disorders are twice as common in women as in men. Another argument against a central role for immune disturbances is that aging occurs in animals that lack an immune system. The observed deterioration of human immune function is thus likely to be an effect rather than a cause of aging (Adler and Nagel 1994). Given the close reciprocal linkage of immune and endocrine systems, much of the immune change could merely be mirroring a deterioration of endocrine function.

Microstructural and Cellular Changes

Microstructural features of aging include alterations of intracellular water content, glycogen storage, fatty infiltration or degeneration, changes in the properties of connective tissue, and changes in cell structure and cell turn-over rate.

Water Content

Isotopic exchange studies suggest that as much as 30% of exchangeable body sodium is lost between 20 and 90 years of age, reflecting a progressive decline in body water content. There is a similar loss of exchangeable body potassium, mainly from within the cells. This begins as early as 30 years of age and continues at an unchanged rate through to 90 years of age. The timing suggests that a significant deletion of cells begins long before the body reaches the senescent phase, when there is a rapid increase in the probability of cell death (Cox and Shalaby 1981).

The aging cell becomes less efficient at retaining potassium and excluding sodium, although it is unclear whether this change reflects altered membrane permeability (secondary to lipid peroxidation), a decrease in cellular respiration with impaired functioning of the "sodium pump," or a deterioration in the sodium-regulating capacity of the kidneys (Rowe 1985).

The classic observations of Yoshikawa et al. (1978) described a progressive decrease of intracellular water, from 42% of body mass at age 25 years to 33% at age 75 years. A part of this change could reflect a replacement of lean tissue by fat. There is also a displacement of fluid from the intracellular to the extracellular compartment. In the brain, the atrophy index is calculated from the ratio of the volume of extracellular water to the volume of the bony cavity as seen by computed tomography (Takeda and Matsuzawa 1985). Further alterations in the distribution of water arise as active tissues are replaced by fibroblasts.

When observations are based on postmortem specimens, it is difficult to draw a line between the true effects of aging and the immediate concomitants of death such as heart failure, hypoproteinemia, renal disease, and endocrine malfunction. Some postmortem studies have linked aging to an intracellular accumulation of water, particularly in the mitochondria and the endoplasmic reticulum. Pathologists report this as a slight "cloudy swelling" of the tissues.

Glycogen Storage

Hepatic glycogen storage is often increased in the elderly, perhaps because of their tendency to diabetes and high blood glucose readings (Timiras 1988). Visible vacuoles of glycogen can be seen in both the hepatic and the renal cells. Likewise, aging cultures of fibroblasts accumulate glycogen (Kenney 1982). However, the glycogen content of both the mitochondria (Bourlière 1982) and the muscle fibers as a whole (Kenney 1982) is lower than in a young adult.

Fatty Infiltration

Observations on intracellular fat content have been limited mainly to pathological and postmortem specimens and *in vitro* cell cultures. Tissues such as the heart, liver, and kidney may show an unusual accumulation of fat (fatty degeneration or fatty metamorphosis), and aging fibroblast cultures also show an accumulation of fat (Kenney 1982; Timiras 1988). Although potentially reversible, the accumulation of fat is often followed by cell death.

Some suggested explanations would not account for the fat accumulation that is seen *in vitro*, for instance an increased transport of fat from the periphery, an increased capture of circulating chylomicrons, or an increased synthesis of fat by the liver. Other possibilities include a decreased utilization of fat associated with impending death, and an alteration in the form of stored fat, from the dispersed (micellar) form seen in the young adult to visible fat globules.

Connective Tissue

Connective tissue comprises collagen, elastin, reticular fibers (converted to collagen with maturation), a polysaccharide ground substance in the form of a hydrated gel, and (in the elderly) pseudoelastin and cellulose (Shephard 1983a). Maturation and aging lead to changes in the properties and relative proportions of these several constituents, owing to functional changes in the fibroblasts that secrete the tissue and alterations in molecules that have a slow turnover rate (Courtois 1982; Robert 1982).

Collagen

The collagen content of some tissues (such as ligaments and tendons) decreases with aging (Haut, Lancaster, and DeCamp 1992), but in other tissues the fibers increase in number and size (Kenney 1982). There is also an increase in the density and stability of collagen, due in part to an increased cross-linkage of fibrils but possibly also to a diminished activity of the collagenases (Bloomfield 1995). The result is a diminished excretion of hydroxyproline. The development of cross-linkage leads to changes in both the mechanical and the chemical properties of collagen. At first, aging is associated with an increased stiffness of the tendons (a loss of elasticity over the range where Hooke's law applies), an increase in the time required to regain the original dimensions after stretching (hysteresis), and a more limited range of lengths over which full recovery is possible (Viidik 1986). Cross-linked molecules also become resistant to collagenases and other lytic enzymes, although in the later stages of senescence (possibly as a consequence of inactivity), there may be an increase of collagenase activity and a resultant weakening of the tendons (Bloomfield 1995).

In some tissues, the collagen is linked to large structural glycoprotein molecules such as fibronectin (Pearlstein, Gold, and Garcia-Pardo 1980) or laminin (Timpl et al. 1979). Age-related changes in such anchorage may make an old person more vulnerable to certain types of tumor (Robert 1982).

Elastin

Elastin is some 15 times as extensible as collagen. It confers elasticity on a tissue, whereas the collagen protects against overextension. Electron microscopy and x-ray diffraction studies do not reveal any characteristic structure for elastic tissue; the fibers appear to have a random orientation.

Occasional reports of an increase in elastin content with age (Orentreich and Orentreich 1985) probably reflect confusion between elastin and pseudoelastin. As a person ages, the elastic fibers lose water, fray, undergo fragmentation, and gradually disappear (Maurel et al. 1980), leaving little except a dispersed granular material. Fluorescence increases, and the color becomes more yellow. Chemical analysis shows increased cross-linkage, sometimes with a deposition of calcium. Cross-linkages are formed through three amino acids: desmosine, isodesmosine, and lysinor-leucine. Some binding is important to the stability of elastic tissues, but excessive cross-linkage causes even greater changes in their mechanical properties than does the development of cross-linkages in collagen (Spina, Volpin, and Giro 1980). Elasticity decreases greatly in old age, although changes in the ground substance may contribute to this change.

Plasma levels of elastase fall throughout adult life, and the increasing breakdown of elastin in an old person seems attributable to a simultaneous decrease in the levels of plasma elastase inhibitor. Particularly after a stroke, high elastase levels indicate an adverse prognosis and early death (Hall et al. 1980).

Pseudoelastin

Elastin preparations from aged tissue contain a third protein that has been termed pseudoelastin. In amino acid composition, it is intermediate between collagen and elastin. Departures from the normal molecular appearance of collagen are largest in the dermis of the neck, where the normal 64 nm cross-striations are completely obliterated by an amorphous coating. It is unclear whether pseudoelastin is a degradation product of collagen, or whether it is an incorrectly synthesized form of collagen.

Cellulose

Old and pathological specimens of connective tissue contain anisotropic fibers that have a protein core similar to pseudoelastin, surrounded by a pair of opposed polysaccharide helices that are indistinguishable from cellulose. Such fibers resist attacks from both collagenase and elastase. Fibers of this type first appear around 20 years of age, and their number increases progressively as a person becomes older.

Polysaccharide

Complexes of protein and polysaccharide (proteoglycans) play an important role in cartilage, synovial fluid, and skin (Robert 1982). They have a strong negative charge, which excludes large molecules and imparts elasticity because of an extreme hydrophilia. Interstices in a network of linked chains of collagen are filled with polysaccharides, smaller fibers being "glued" to larger elements by a cement continuous with the ground substance.

The main constituents of the ground substance are hyaluronic acid and proteoglycans. Hyaluronic acid is a highly viscous lubricant, formed from disaccharides, n-acetylglucosamine, and glucuronic acid. It allows elastic tissue, collagen, and muscle fibers to slide over each other with minimal friction. The proteoglycans are peptide chains carrying chondroitin sulfate, which functions as the "cement." Aging leads to a loss of water from the ground substance, with an increase in density of the gel and a decrease in its volume (Kenney 1982).

Although aging increases the collagen content of tissues, the amount and the degree of polymerization of the proteoglycan ground substance diminish, reducing the stability of tissues such as cartilage (Robert 1982). The loss of polysaccharide may reflect a diminished formation by the connective tissue cells, an increased turnover of ground substance, or both. A progressive loss of the plasticizing function of the ground substance may also make the tissue stiffer and less permeable to nutrients.

Functional Sequelae

Connective tissues make a major contribution to the dynamic properties of many tissues. Alterations in the amount or mechanical properties of individual constituents lead to a loss of elasticity in the skin; altered pressure/volume relationships in the lungs, heart, and great vessels; tendon ruptures; and joint and back problems associated with shrinkage and greater rigidity of hyaline and fibrocartilage.

The aging sequence may be illustrated by changes in the blood vessel wall. Frayed elastic fibers and degenerated smooth muscle are progressively replaced by collagen. Initially, the collagen fibers are arranged in parallel with the elastin, but after repeated cycles of elongation and shortening, they do not resist distension until a substantial force is applied. Moreover, unlike elastin (which returns to its original length as soon as the distending force is released), collagen shows a substantial hysteresis, retaining as much as two-thirds of its elongation for a substantial period. The capacity of the peripheral blood vessels is thus increased, making it difficult for an elderly person to sustain a large central blood volume and a high cardiac output during vigorous exercise.

Cell Structure

Aging is associated with a progressive decrease in the number of functional cells, as shown by the decreased mass of most organs, and a decline in overall lean mass. The communication between individual cells also becomes less effective (Bellamy 1991), and organ function is progressively impaired.

Aging leads to changes in the appearance of many of the intracellular organelles, although the functional significance is less clear. The nucleus becomes larger and may show invagination of its membrane, with various inclusions. The nucleoli are increased both in size and in number. The chromatin material may show clumping, shrinking, fragmentation, or dissolution, and there is an increased likelihood of finding chromosome abnormalities. The cytoplasm shows an accumulation of pigments, and sometimes of fat. Other features include vacuole formation, the appearance of hyaline droplets, and alterations in the size, shape, cristal pattern, and matrix density of the mitochondria.

The exercise physiologist is perhaps most concerned with any deterioration in muscle cells. Analyses of muscle structure (Aoyagi and Shephard 1992) are complicated by an increase in the number of fibers per square millimeter (due to overall atrophy) and a selective loss of type IIa fibers, associated with a loss of terminal sprouting of the motor nerves (Aoyagi and Shephard 1992). Lexell, Henriksson-Larsson, and Sjöstrom (1983) found 1.1 $\times 10^5$ fewer fibers in the vastus lateralis of 70- to 73-year-old subjects relative to young adults, but most studies have reported only small changes in the number of capillaries per muscle fiber (Aoyagi and Shephard 1992). Likewise, the loss of motoneurons is less than the loss of muscle fibers, so that the number of fibers per motoneuron diminishes with aging. The area occupied by the motor endplate also decreases, and a decreased frequency of miniature endplate potentials suggests a diminished release of neurotransmitter chemicals. As in other tissues, there is an accumulation of lipofuscin and lipids. Other changes include a thickening of the sarcolemma and sarcoplasmic reticulum, streaming of the Z lines, disorganization of the myofibrils, proliferation of the T system, and a vacuolation of the mitochondria with a shortening of their cristae (Cress and Schultz 1985). One particularly important feature of aging muscle is a reduction in the number and growth potential of the satellite cells. In a young animal, these cells have the potential to regenerate an entire muscle three to four times, but in old age the regenerative capacity drops to 30% to 70% of normal muscle volume (Gibson and Schultze 1983).

Cell Turnover

Three distinct phases of cell turnover can be distinguished in tissue culture: an early rapid multiplication, a period of decreasing cell proliferation, and eventual death. As the culture ages, an ever-increasing proportion of the cells show nuclear abnormalities and chromosome aberrations. The life of the culture is sometimes prolonged by the presence of other varieties of cell, which possibly contribute nutrients that the main tissue is no longer able to synthesize. However, there is also a general relationship between the age of the donor and the age of the resultant culture, whether one is dealing with fibroblasts taken from the skin or with satellite cells from muscle (Schultz and Lipton 1982).

In vivo, muscle and nerve cells have already lost the capacity to proliferate at birth, and despite some neuroplasticity (Strong and Garruto 1994), the capacity for compensation through formation of new synapses diminishes with aging (Black, Polinsky, and Greenough 1989). Other cells continue to multiply until the person dies, but the time interval between successive cell divisions becomes progressively prolonged. For example, the bone marrow of an elderly person can still respond to blood loss by an increased production of red cells, although the rate of red cell replenishment diminishes with aging, in part because the marrow becomes infiltrated by fat (Oberling and Sengler 1982). Aging cells also have an increased 5-nucleotidase activity, which limits the availability of nucleotides for cell proliferation (Kenney 1982).

The brain shows a selective decrease in cell count with aging (Timiras 1991). Losses occur particularly in the superior temporal gyrus of the cortex, the substantia nigra, the corpus striatum, the locus coeruleus, the dorsal nucleus of the vagus, and the dentate nucleus. Often there is an associated and possibly a compensatory proliferation of glial cells (Diamond et al. 1985). Between the ages of 20 and 50 years, the predominant loss is of cells, but in older age groups there is also a neuroaxonal degeneration, marked by loss of myelin and swellings on the fibers. The rate of loss of fibers becomes greater than that of loss of cells, so the ratio of gray to white matter begins to increase again.

Depending on location, aging nerve cells show various signs of impaired metabolism: an accumulation of lipofuscin, protein fibrils, hyaline bodies, and vacuoles. However, it remains uncertain how far the loss of nerve cells is due to an accumulation of such metabolic errors, and how far it is caused by external factors such as atherosclerosis of the cerebral blood vessels or an action of glucocorticoids (Landfield 1987).

Damage to one specific region of the brain may lead to an imbalance of neurotransmitter substances. For example, a loss of midbrain dopamine production leads to a dominance of acetylcholine and the clinical pictures of Parkinson's disease (Moore, Demarest, and Lookingland 1987; Timiras 1991). Fortunately, there is an enormous redundancy of cells in the brain, and the functional consequences of cell death are usually difficult to perceive except in pathological conditions such as Alzheimer's disease, neurodegenerative disease, and cases in which a massive destructive lesion, due to a tumor or a stroke, has occurred.

Conclusions

Various hypotheses have been advanced to explain the aging process. One dominant feature is an increased probability of both cell death and death of the organism. Cell death is in part a genetically controlled, programmed event, "designed" to prevent overpopulation. Free radical damage, whether due to metabolism or external irradiation, also seems a part of the process. Other possible influences include endocrine and enzyme depletion and disturbances of immune function. Microstructural manifestations include alterations of intracellular water content, glycogen storage, and fatty infiltration. There are also changes in the properties of connective tissue, cell structure, and cell turnover rate.

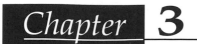

Chapter 3

Impact of Aging on Major Physiological Systems at Rest and During Submaximal and Maximal Exercise

Having examined current theories of aging and explored certain molecular and cellular manifestations of the aging process, we must now examine the impact of these changes on some of the major physiological systems of the body. Our particular focus will be on the continued ability of these systems to respond to the acute disturbances of homeostasis induced by a bout of vigorous physical activity.

General Considerations

Age-related changes in biological function may be examined using either cross-sectional or longitudinal data. With either approach, problems of interpretation may arise because of an incomplete sampling of the population, age-related changes in habitual physical activity and body build, secular changes in lifestyle, and an age-related increase in the prevalence of chronic disease.

Sampling Problems

The proportion of individuals who volunteer for cross-sectional surveys of physical fitness and physical activity generally decreases with age (Kannel and Brand 1985; Shephard 1993a). Thus, it is difficult to obtain data on either a random or a representative cross-section of a population. In the seemingly optimal conditions of the Canada Fitness Survey (in which the observers made their measurements during visits to the homes of selected families), some 50% of seniors either did not volunteer for testing or were excluded by survey personnel on grounds of safety (Shephard 1986c). If the required measurements involve vigorous exercise, it is likely that the older half of those composing a given population sample will include a disproportionate number of people with an above-average level of physical fitness. Those who volunteer for testing also tend to have adopted such healthy habits as a prudent diet and abstinence from cigarette smoking. Furthermore, survey participants are drawn predominantly from the upper end of the socioeconomic spectrum: people who have had less than average exposure to environmental pollutants, either at work or in their domestic environment. For all these reasons, cross-sectional data are likely to underestimate the average age-related loss of function within a population.

Migration into or out of a community may also create apparently age-related changes in the average size and fitness of local residents. For instance, an early study by Miall et al. (1967) described a selective emigration of taller young men from the Welsh mining valleys, thus exaggerating the normal decrease in height with age. If a region is rich in employment, there is an inward migration of healthy individuals, whereas if it is a favorite place for retirement it attracts those who are less fit than their peers and/or those who are suffering from manifestations of chronic disease.

A few longitudinal surveys, such as the Framingham study (Kannel and Brand 1985) and our study of the Igloolik Inuit (Shephard and Rode 1996), have followed the characteristics of a stable, circumscribed population for 20 years or longer. But in general, longitudinal studies have been sustained only for a relatively short time. Unfortunately, the standard error of the slope of gerontological data (the rate of aging) is inversely proportional to the duration of a study. It also varies inversely as the square root of the number of people examined. The choice of an appropriate study duration and size is further complicated by the likelihood of dropouts and a growing number of exclusions for disease as a study progresses. Nevertheless, it is generally better to have a small, protracted survey than a large-scale but short-lived study. Those who enroll in sustained longitudinal studies often have an above-average interest in health and fitness, and sometimes enrollment itself serves as a stimulus to adoption of an improved lifestyle. If the person who is recruited to such an investigation stops smoking, reduces body fat content, or increases habitual physical activity, then the functional consequences of aging are likely to be underestimated, particularly if the study duration is short (Shephard 1988). On the other hand, if those recruited are extremely active at the outset of the study, then they are likely to become more sedentary as they age, and the change in activity may exaggerate the inherent influence of age on biological function. In sustained longitudinal studies, the initial sample is further modified by defections due to both a loss of interest in repeated evaluation and the onset of disease; both of these factors bias the residual sample toward above-average levels of health and fitness.

Effects of Age-Related Changes in Habitual Physical Activity and Body Build

The habitual physical activity of the general population diminishes with aging, and even if an older individual continues to participate in some form of sport, it is likely that training sessions become shorter and less intense than when that person was younger. Thus, a part of any age-related decrease in muscle strength or aerobic power is usually attributable to a decrease of habitual physical activity rather than to some inherent manifestation of the aging process. Most people also accumulate 5 to 10 kg of body fat over the course of adult life, and this further reduces both aerobic power and muscle force when data are scaled per unit of body mass. Jackson et al. (1995) have estimated that a reduction of habitual physical activity and an increase of body mass can in themselves account for as much as one-half of the usually reported age-related decrease in aerobic power, expressed in ml/[kg · min].

Scores on a number of key variables, for example lung volumes, are usually interpreted relative to height-based norms. The standing height decreases by 30 to 50 mm during later adult life, due to an increasing curvature of the spine (kyphosis), a compression of the intervertebral disks, and (in extreme old age) an osteoporotic collapse of one or more vertebrae. A decrease of standing height is particularly important when one is interpreting volume measurements (since these are usually scaled in relation to the cube of stature).

Secular Changes

In developed societies, secular changes such as widespread car ownership, universal access to television, and the extensive automation of factories have substantially reduced daily energy expenditures among all age groups over the last 50 years. If the rate of aging is estimated from a cross-sectional survey, the older cohorts thus have had a physically active lifestyle for a greater proportion of their lives than those who are younger. This fact, in turn, may modify the rate of deterioration of biological function relative to values that would be found if a longitudinal study were to be initiated on the present generation of young adults.

In longitudinal studies, the lifestyle of many of the participants has changed over time. The losses of physical condition that are observed with the aging of such individuals thus tend to be greater than would be seen if a person were to maintain a consistently active lifestyle throughout the adult life span.

Onset of Disease

Perhaps the greatest problem in the interpretation of gerontological data is to distinguish true aging from the ravages of disease. For many variables, the dividing line between normal aging and pathology is very fine and indeed quite arbitrary.

For example, if a subject's diastolic blood pressure increases from a youthful level of 76 mmHg to a figure of 88 mmHg in old age, this is accepted as a normal expression of changes in the elastic properties of the arterial wall. But if the pressure exceeds a threshold value of 90 mmHg (or 95 mmHg, for some authors), the subject is regarded as having developed hypertension and is excluded from a normal sample. Likewise, most senior citizens show some subendothelial deposition of cholesterol in their major arteries, but in only a proportion of these individuals is the change large enough to cause a distinct pathology such as angina pectoris or myocardial infarction. Again, most people show some decrease of bone density with aging, but this change crosses the threshold for a clinical diagnosis of osteoporosis in only a minority of individuals. A final example concerns lung volumes. Anderson et al. (1968) noted that by the age of 65 years, the predicted vital capacity for a man with a height of 1.70 m was 4.23 L BTPS if respiratory health had remained good, but the prediction dropped to 2.96 L if there had been a pathological acceleration of aging due to previous respiratory disease.

Unfortunately, in large part the available cross-sectional data refer to aging as seen in the very sedentary and overfed population of North America. This exacerbates the problem of determining whether any observed loss of function is an inevitable expression of aging, or is instead the consequence of an adverse lifestyle and resulting chronic disease.

One early suggestion was that pathological changes be distinguished from the inherent aging process on the basis that the former had at least a potential for correction by appropriate therapy (Korenchevsky 1961). Exceptions to this generalization come to mind, but such a distinction may yet be upheld if the proviso is made that a treatment has yet to be discovered for some of the pathologies that affect the elderly. A second possible option is to make separate analyses of aging rates for a healthy elite (isolated by a preliminary rigorous health screening) and for the general population (Andres 1985). A third possibility is to define as "normal" all those who are well enough to engage in full-time work or (if they have passed the normal age of retirement) are able to carry out the activities of daily living without restriction.

As age advances, an ever-increasing proportion of the total population are affected by one or more chronic pathologies. This leaves only a small residual population who still have good clinical health. Is it realistic to base estimates of the rate of aging on findings for this minority, and if so, what relevance do the data have for the general population?

Aging, Body Build, and Body Composition

Aging is associated with a progressive decrease in standing height. Most people also show an increase of body fat content and a decrease in lean tissue mass. There is a progressive atrophy of the skeletal muscles, a loss of bone mineral, and often a restriction of joint mobility.

Body Stature

Several artifacts can distort estimates of both a person's current standing height and age-related changes in stature. The standing height can decrease by as much as 10 to 20 mm over the waking hours, particularly if a person has remained standing for a large part of the day. Thus, it is important that repeat measurements be obtained at a consistent hour, standardizing the period of standing prior to measurement. Over the past century, many populations have shown a secular trend to an increase in height, averaging as much as 1 mm/year (Shephard 1986c). Such a trend could in itself make 25-year-old adults 40 mm taller than 65-year-olds. Height is also related to socioeconomic status, to the choice of occupation (for instance, a professional basketball player is extremely tall, whereas the typical underground miner is a short individual), and to race; the shape of a cross-sectional aging curve can thus be changed by a selective migration into or out of the community (Miall et al. 1967).

Even when due allowance is made for such artifacts, most populations still show an age-related decrease in stature. In urban communities, this begins around 40 years of age, and it is at first more marked in women than in men. Cross-sectional data from the U.S. National Health and Nutrition Examination Survey (NHANES I) indicated that by the age of 65 to 74 years, men were on average 61 mm shorter, and women 50 mm shorter, than their counterparts in the age range 18 to 24 years (U.S. National Center for Health Statistics 1981); several cross-sectional Canadian surveys showed essentially similar findings (Shephard 1986c). However, such estimates include also an effect from the secular trend toward an increase of stature. In the past, this has amounted to about 1 cm/decade, although the trend is now diminishing in developed nations (Shephard 1986c). Thus, longitudinal estimates have suggested a much smaller loss than have cross-sectional data; the early observations of Rossman (1977) showed lifetime losses averaging 29 mm in men and 49 mm in women, and about half of this change was attributable to a decrease in sitting height. Some analyses have assumed a linear rate of decrease in height with age, but Svänborg, Eden, and Mellstrom (1991) found an acceleration of loss after the age of 70 years; over the age range of 70 to 82 years, the height of their subjects (both men and women) decreased by an average of 2 mm/year.

The main reason behind the true age-linked decrease in stature is a change in structure of the intervertebral disks. In a young adult, an outer shell of fibrous tissue and fibrocartilage encloses a soft yellow core of elastic tissue (the nucleus pulposus). With aging, the latter becomes desiccated and the disk is compressed or collapses. This shortens the spine and exaggerates any initial kyphosis. Other factors that increase kyphosis in the elderly include a weakening of the back muscles, physiological or pathological degeneration of the vertebrae ("senile osteoporosis"), and osteoarthritis of the vertebral joints. If the kyphosis becomes severe, even the effort of supporting the head can become very fatiguing. Marked kyphosis can also lead to low back pain and respiratory problems.

Other age-related changes in body dimensions normally include decreases in sitting height, shoulder width, and chest depth. However, in individuals who develop chronic chest disease, the trend is rather toward an increase in the postero-anterior diameter of the chest, the so-called "barrel-shaped" chest deformity. This deformity reflects the difficulty that the affected individual has in expelling air from the lungs.

In isolated northern communities such as those of the Laplanders and Inuit, the rate of decrease of stature with age currently seems to occur more rapidly than in urban white populations. Possible factors that have influenced cross-sectional data for the circumpolar regions include a rapid secular trend toward an increase of stature in recent generations of children (Rode and Shephard 1994b), a diet poor in calcium and vitamin D, limited exposure of the skin to sunlight and thus a slowing of endogenous vitamin D synthesis (Harper, Laughlin, and Mazess 1984; Jeppesen and Harvald 1985), and (particularly in the men) vertebral trauma from the prolonged operation of high-speed snowmobiles over rough ground (Hassi et al. 1985; Rode and Shephard 1994b; Shephard et al. 1984).

Body Mass and Body Fat

An individual's body mass commonly increases from age 25 to age 45 or 50 years, and thereafter shows a slow but progressive decline (Bray 1979; Metropolitan Life 1983; Shephard 1986c). The increase in body mass during middle age generally reflects an accumulation of fat, and in most people a simple question about weight gain during adulthood gives a crude estimate of how much fat they have accumulated. However, the true extent of the increase in body fat content is usually underestimated by the response, because fat accumulation has been masked by concomitant muscle wasting. More accurate estimates of body fat content can be obtained from determinations of skinfold thicknesses, underwater weighing, and other laboratory techniques.

In a classic longitudinal study of champion runners (Dill, Robinson, and Ross 1967), those whose body mass had increased by no more than 5 kg since their final competition carried only 15% body fat, but those who had gained 6 to 12 kg had 20% fat, and those who had gained 15 to 22 kg averaged 30% body fat.

The accumulation of fat generally has an adverse impact upon a person's health, although the optimal body mass for survival is somewhat greater in the elderly than in a young person (Andres 1994). Drenick et al. (1980) studied a sample of 200 men with morbid obesity. Body mass averaged 143 kg. The excess mortality in this population decreased from 1200% in those aged 25 to 34 years to 550% in those aged 35 to 44 years, 300% in those aged 45 to 54 years, and 200% in those over 55 years of age.

Interpretation of Body Mass

Total body mass is widely used to provide a simple index of obesity. The observed value may be assessed relative to a figure that is ideal from the actuarial standpoint. People with a heavy bone structure tend to weigh more, and data interpretation is thus facilitated by the use of elbow intercondylar breadth (Frisancho and Flegel 1983; Metropolitan Life 1983) or a radiographic estimate of bony chest breadth (Garn, Leonard, and Hawthorne 1986) to allow for interindividual differences in body frame size.

Alternatively, the BMI (kg per m^2 of standing height) may be calculated, or (as in analysis of the female NHANES data) weights can be presented as kg per $m^{1.5}$ (Kohrs and Czajka-Narins 1986). If body mass is expressed as a function of height, the average value for the population generally reflects the fatness of that population. On the other hand, the BMI is not very helpful in assessing the obesity of an individual, since the score may be distorted downward by muscle wasting or a general loss of bone mineral, and upward by a well-developed musculature or a decrease in stature as well as by an increase in body fat content.

Several specific pitfalls arise in interpretation of the body mass of elderly subjects:

1. Many of the published norms of body mass are based on data that were collected for insurance purposes. The samples are thus biased toward young adults from a favored socioeconomic class; those with initial ill health are excluded; and the mass may have been simply reported to a physician rather than measured. People commonly make errors when recollecting their body mass (Boutier and Payette 1994), and such errors tend to be larger in older people.
2. An age-related accumulation of body fat may be masked by a concomitant decrease in bone mass and atrophy of the skeletal musculature. Thus, in the example of table 3.1, the excess body mass relative to the actuarial ideal was smaller in subjects who had reached the sixth and seventh decades of life, although the skinfold thicknesses of these individuals were similar to or even greater than the values found in younger adults.

3. Obese individuals have a higher mortality than those of "ideal" body mass, in part because of an association between obesity and such chronic conditions as high blood pressure and diabetes mellitus (Andres 1994). Inevitably, the premature death of obese subjects increases the proportion of lighter individuals in the oldest segment of the population.

4. Volunteer bias recruits an excessive proportion of health-conscious individuals to a study. As they become older, such subjects accumulate less body fat than would have an unselected population.

5. The interpretation of body mass relative to stature is inappropriate if aging has led to a substantial decrease in standing height through kyphosis, or if the elderly person has difficulty in standing erect while his or her height is being measured. One potential alternative is to scale the body mass of an older person relative to the arm span, although such ratios may also be complicated by a chest deformity or problems in extending the arms. Other possible indexes of body size are provided by arm length (Mitchell and Lipschitz 1982) or knee height (Chumlea, Roche, and Mukherjee 1984).

6. The ideal mass reported in actuarial tables necessarily applies to the age when life insurance was purchased, commonly during young adulthood. There is no guarantee that maintenance of this "ideal" value will maximize survival later in life.

7. Even if any age-related increase of body mass is attributable entirely to fat, the mass/height ratio provides no information concerning the distribution of this fat. A "female" pattern of accumulation (over the hips and thighs) seemingly carries a much lower risk of cardiovascular and all-cause mortality than an abdominal or visceral accumulation of fat (Björntorp, Smith, and Lönnroth 1988; Schwartz et al. 1991).

Table 3.1 Influence of age on excess body mass (relative to the actuarial ideal) and the thickness of subcutaneous fat (an average of eight skinfold readings).

Age (years)	Men		Women	
	Excess mass (kg)	Skinfold (mm)	Excess mass (kg)	Skinfold (mm)
20-30	1.7 ± 8.7	11.2 ± 5.9	8.3 ± 5.3	15.2 ± 3.8
30-40	6.4 ± 8.5	16.1 ± 10.6	1.4 ± 5.3	13.5 ± 5.2
40-50	9.3 ± 9.5	14.0 ± 5.8	6.8 ± 8.4	17.3 ± 5.4
50-60	8.8 ± 7.7	15.2 ± 6.7	4.9 ± 7.2	18.2 ± 5.1
60-70	5.1 ± 7.3	15.4 ± 2.7	4.5 ± 9.5	22.5 ± 7.9

Reprinted, by permission, from R.J. Shephard, 1977, *Endurance fitness*, 2d ed. (Toronto, ON: University of Toronto Press).

Changes in "Ideal" Body Mass With Age

Actuarial data suggest that from the viewpoint of mortality, the "ideal" body mass increases substantially over the course of adult life. Andres (1994) found that the initial BMI associated with the lowest mortality experience increased from 21.4 kg/m^2 for the age range 20 to 29 years to 26.6 kg/m^2 for the age range 60 to 69 years.

In reaching their conclusion that the "ideal" value increases in older individuals, most investigators have covaried the BMI for current smoking habits (since smoking commonly reduces a person's body mass by several kilograms, but also shortens their anticipated life span by up to eight years). However, there remains the potential artifact that symptoms from a smoking-related disease may have caused both a low body mass and a recent cessation of smoking, so that the individual concerned has been counted as a nonsmoker (Roche 1994). Most studies of longevity screened participants for disease at entry, but nevertheless, undetected subclinical pathologies could also account for a part of the actuarial disadvantage that is associated with a low initial body mass. However, the main explanation for the data seems to be that some older adults have sustained a low body mass by the disadvantageous practice of combining a sedentary lifestyle with excessive dieting. Thus, one might anticipate better survival prospects in those who maintain their lean tissue, even if the cost is some increase in total body mass.

There may be more direct disadvantages of a low body mass, such as an adverse effect on the immune system (Roche 1994). However, an analysis of causes of death does not offer any great support to such a suggestion. Approximate values (kg/m^2) at the nadir of the BMI curve in older men are, for deaths from vascular lesions of the central nervous system, 25; for diabetes mellitus, 20; for malignant neoplasms, 27; for suicides, 31; for nephritis, 24; for pneumonia and influenza, 30; for the heart and circulatory diseases, 20; for coronary artery disease, 18; and for hypertensive heart disease, 23 (Andres 1994).

Measurement of Subcutaneous Fat

The measurement of chest and abdominal circumferences and/or skinfold thicknesses provides a more direct approach to the determination of body fat than do estimations of body mass. Some have argued that circumferences are easier to determine than skinfolds (Larsson et al. 1984). However, our data for an experienced observer (Murray and Shephard 1988) showed that the sum of four skinfolds had a substantially closer correlation ($r^2 = 0.626$) with the hydrostatic criterion of fatness than did waist circumference measurements on the same subjects ($r^2 = 0.478$).

The waist/hip ratio was for a time used to indicate an abdominal accumulation of fat. Values in excess of 1.0 for men and 0.9 for women were taken as indicators of increased cardiovascular risk, although recent evidence (Garn, Sullivan, and Hawthorne 1988) suggests that the simple measurement of waist circumference may constitute a more reliable measure of abdominal fat accumulation than a determination of the waist/hip ratio.

Skinfold thicknesses may be interpreted in their own right, although unfortunately there are as yet no norms for subjects over the age of 75 years (Kohrs and Czajka-Narins 1986). Alternatively, data may be converted to an estimate of the body density and thus the percentage of body fat, using widely accepted prediction formulas such as those of Durnin and Womersley (1974), although again equations suitable for the very old and oldest-old are lacking (Blumberg and Meydani 1995; Durenberg et al. 1988). There is some evidence that older people carry a greater proportion of their body fat internally (Shephard 1991a), and the density of the lean tissue compartment is also changed by osteoporosis and a loss of muscle mass. It is thus important to ensure that the skinfold formulas used in such predictions are indeed age-specific. Because of aging of the underlying connective tissue, the skin of an elderly person tends to move independently of subcutaneous fat. It is therefore vital to ensure that both skin and subcutaneous tissue are included between the jaws of the calipers as skinfold thicknesses are measured. There are also uncertainties about the distribution of subcutaneous fat (Eveleth 1994) and the thickness and compressibility of the skin in an elderly person (Eveleth 1994; Mernagh et al. 1986).

Age-Related Changes in the Distribution of Subcutaneous Fat

As women become older, they accumulate fat preferentially over the hips and thighs, whereas in men the abdomen is the preferred site of deposition (Bemben et al. 1995). Some authors have also suggested that men accumulate more fat than women as they age, thus narrowing the gender difference in body fat content. Heitmann (1991) noted that the average body fat content of men had increased substantially before they reached the age of 55 years, whereas in women fat accumulation usually occurred mainly after the age of 55 years. Men certainly have a greater age-related accumulation of fat if attention is focused on the trunk and abdominal skinfolds. However, if the changes that develop between 25 and 65 years of age are averaged across 7 to 10 skinfolds, then men show an overall increment of about 43%, whereas in women the increase is about 75% (see table 3.2).

At the cellular level, aging is associated with an overloading of existing fat cells rather than adipocyte hypertrophy (Shephard 1991a).

There is no strong reason to suppose that adults eat more as they become older. Potential reasons for the accumulation of fat in older individuals include a decrease in habitual physical activity, a decrease in resting energy expenditure, and a decrease in the thermic effect of food. Taken together, these three factors could lead to a substantial decrease in daily energy requirements. One study found that the adiposity of older adults was unrelated to reported habitual activity over the energy expenditure range 0 to 6 kJ/day (Reed et al. 1991), but this might merely reflect difficulties in measuring activity patterns

Table 3.2 Skinfold thicknesses at selected sites.

Skinfold	Male		Female	
	Ideal (mm)	Elderly (%)	Ideal (mm)	Elderly (%)
Chin	5.8	+39	7.1	+67
Subscapular	11.9	+31	11.3	+77
Triceps	7.8	+12	15.6	+26
Suprailiac	12.7	+8	14.6	+59
Waist	14.3	+62	15.3	+109
Suprapubic	11.0	+111	20.5	+68
Chest	12.0	+49	8.6	+106
Knee	8.6	+37	11.8	+90
Average (8 folds)		+43		+75

Reprinted, by permission, from R.J. Shephard, 1982, *Physiology and biochemistry of exercise*, (New York: Praeger). An imprint of Greenwood Publishing Group, Inc., Westport, CT.

with sufficient precision. The resting metabolic rate decreases with age, and the decrease persists if the data are covaried for both body fat content and fat-free mass (Poehlman, Melby, and Badylak 1991). The thermic effect of eating represents no more than 10% of total daily energy expenditure, but it is probably quite important to the overall energy balance of the body. Aging does not of itself alter this component of energy expenditure, but if the level of habitual physical activity is smaller in an older person, then the thermic effect of a meal is also likely to be decreased (Poehlman, Melby, and Badylak 1991).

There have been suggestions that fat accumulation usually ceases after a person has reached the age of 40 years (Silver et al. 1993) and that the amount of subcutaneous fat actually decreases after the age of 65 years. But it remains unclear whether such observations reflect sampling artifacts, a decrease of skin thickness, an altered distribution of fat between superficial and deep depots, or a true decrease in body fat content among elderly people. If the last explanation is correct, possible causes could include a loss of interest in cooking subsequent to bereavement, a lack of teeth or adequate dentures, and a poor gastrointestinal absorption of food.

Estimation of Body Fat Content by Underwater Weighing

Underwater weighing is often regarded as the gold standard against which other measures of body fat content should be judged. But because of uncertainties regarding the residual lung volume in an elderly person, it is necessary to determine the residual volume while the subject is submerged, rather than estimating it as a fixed fraction of the vital capacity. Measurement is often complicated by a slow equilibration between alveolar and marker gas, and in addition there is difficulty in maintaining a good seal at the spirometer mouthpiece because of age-related changes in jaw structure. Even if an accurate estimate of overall body density can be obtained, the calculation of body fat from this value is hampered because a decrease of bone density and an atrophy of the skeletal muscles cause substantial departures from the usually assumed average density of the lean tissue compartment (Mernagh et al. 1986; Shephard et al. 1985).

Alternative Methods of Estimating Body Fat

There are several alternative methods of estimating body fat content, but none is entirely satisfactory in an elderly person. Impedance measurements have been widely used to determine body fat content in recent years (Chumlea and Baumgartner 1990). The principle underlying the calculation is that the impedance offered to a high-frequency electrical signal depends upon the average cross-section of lean tissue that is interposed between the measuring electrodes. The values obtained by this methodology are vulnerable to unusual body proportions, muscle wasting, alterations of body hydration, and distortion of the electrical signal by fascial membranes. The accuracy of impedance estimates is thus questionable even in young adults, and many of the sources of error associated with this technique become exaggerated in an older person (Blumberg and Meydani 1995).

Other methods of body composition analysis that are available in specialized centers include ultrasound, magnetic resonance imaging, soft tissue radiography, computerized tomography, dual photon absorptiometry, and infrared interactance (Shephard 1991a). Most of these approaches are very costly, and as yet there is no convincing evidence that they are more effective than underwater weighing or the use of skinfold calipers.

The percentage of body fat can finally be estimated as the difference between lean and total body mass. Nevertheless, this approach cannot be recommended; since the body contains only 15% to 35% fat, a small error in the estimate of lean tissue mass leads to a large error in the prediction of body fat.

Lean Body Mass

The lean body mass may be estimated by subtracting fat mass from total body mass, although the value thus obtained is imprecise since one must accept all the errors of fat determination that arise in an old person. Calculations can also be based on the external dimensions of the limbs (Overend et al. 1993; Shephard et al. 1988), although an internal accumulation of fat and connective tissue often causes anthropometric methods to overestimate muscle mass in the elderly (Rice et al. 1989). Alternatively, the lean mass may be measured more directly with use of the techniques next described.

Direct Determination of Lean Body Mass

Most methods for the direct determination of lean tissue mass (Shephard 1991a) are problematic when applied to elderly subjects (Going et al. 1994).

About 98% of body creatine reserves are found in muscle, so a linear relationship is sometimes assumed between the resting excretion of creatinine and lean body mass (Shephard 1991a). However, old people have difficulty in resynthesizing creatine, and thus they may show a substantial increase of creatinine excretion if they have engaged even in mild exercise prior to data collection (Manfredi et al. 1991). The relationship between lean tissue mass and creatinine excretion is also distorted if aging has led to a deterioration of renal function. Similar criticisms apply to estimates of lean tissue mass that are based on the excretion of 3-methyl-L-histidine (Mendez, Lukaski, and Buskirk 1984), 90% of which is found in muscle.

The naturally occurring isotope ^{40}K is a third potential marker of muscle mass. In a young adult, some 60% of body potassium is found in muscle. Unfortunately, other tissues account for an increasing fraction of the total body content of ^{40}K in older individuals. Moreover, the potassium content varies from one tissue to another (Morgan and Burkinshaw 1983): muscle (87 mE/kg), other lean tissue (49 mE/kg), and adipose tissue (15 mE/kg). The average relationship that is assumed between radioactive emissions and the available mass of potassium (22 counts/g of potassium) can be influenced by alterations in body dimensions and by overlying adipose tissue, which tends to screen out radiation. Finally, as noted in chapter 2, the potassium content of most cells decreases with age. Thus, although the ^{40}K method is often regarded as providing a well-equipped body composition laboratory with one of the better estimates of lean tissue mass, it is by no means an infallible method in the elderly.

Neutron activation of nitrogen is another option for determining lean tissue in a well-equipped laboratory (Ellis et al. 1982; Shephard et al. 1985). Once again, the difficulty is that the ratio of total nitrogen to lean mass varies with such factors as muscularity, body hydration, and the protein content of the skeleton.

The technique of dual photon absorptiometry has gained popularity in recent years (Gotfredsen et al. 1986). Its main limitation is that information on body composition is obtained from only one region of the body. The same criticism applies to computed tomography (Overend et al. 1993), although this last method can give a useful indication of cross-sectional changes in lean tissue mass at any one location (Fiatarone et al. 1990; Häkkinen and Häkkinen 1991).

Nuclear magnetic resonance (Lewis et al. 1986) can identify such tissue constituents as creatine, but when this approach is applied in an elderly person, estimates of muscle mass are probably subject to errors similar to those seen with estimates based upon creatinine excretion.

Finally, estimates of lean tissue mass can be derived from body water determinations (using, for example, deuterium or tritium dilution methods). However, it is then necessary to assume that the lean tissue contains a fixed fraction of body water, and it is difficult to guarantee that this figure remains constant in an elderly person.

Age and Lean Body Mass

One would expect the lean mass to be less in older people, partly because the elderly are on average smaller than younger individuals, and partly because aging is associated with muscle wasting. Despite the methodological problems just discussed, there is fair agreement between the estimates of age-related changes in lean body mass that are based on determinations of ^{40}K (Noppa et al. 1979; Shephard et al. 1985), creatinine excretion (Rowe et al. 1976), limb circumferences (Kallman, Plato, and Tobin 1990), ultrasound (Vandervoort and McComas 1986), and computerized tomography (Fiatarone et al. 1990).

The main sites of lean tissue loss are muscle, liver, kidneys, and adrenal glands, but in the very old there is also a significant decrease of brain mass. Masters athletes may show little or no loss of lean tissue until the seventh or eighth decade of life (Pollock et al. 1987; Shephard 1991c). The general population tend to sustain a plateau of lean tissue mass through to about 40 years of age, with an accelerating rate of loss thereafter. Aniansson et al. (1983) saw an earlier decline in women than in men, and Bemben et al. (1995) did not find any significant changes in male subjects before 70 years of age; in contrast, Flynn et al. (1989) observed a large loss in men between 40 and 60 years, whereas the loss in women occurred mainly after 60 years of age. The cumulative loss by 80 years amounts to more than 40% of the young adult mass in men, and to some 20% of the young adult value in women (Rogers and Evans 1993).

Local ultrasound estimates of lean tissue loss, made in muscular regions of the body, are generally of an order similar to those for the whole-body measurements. For example, the quadriceps muscle of older subjects commonly loses about 0.5% to 0.7% of tissue per year (Young, Hughes, et al. 1980), a figure that seems compatible both with the rate of loss of muscle strength (Aniansson and Gustafsson 1981) and with cadaver estimates of overall muscle wasting (Haggmark, Jansson, and Svane 1978).

Changes in Enzymes and Hormonal Activity

The loss of lean tissue is accompanied by a decrease in myofibrillar protein synthesis and mitochondrial protein concentrations (Welle et al. 1993). The muscles show a resulting decrease in activity of aerobic enzymes (Aoyagi and Shephard 1992; Farrar, Martin, and Ardies 1981; Keh-Evans et al. 1992) as well as phosphofructokinase, a key enzyme in glycolysis (Keh-Evans et al. 1992).

There is an association between the decline in lean tissue mass and decreasing plasma levels of IGF-1, the peptide that mediates the anabolic effects of growth hormone (Copeland et al. 1990; Kelly et al. 1990). It is less certain whether the decline in plasma IGF-1 is an inevitable consequence of aging or whether it also is due to changes in lifestyle such as a decrease in habitual physical activity. Fasting plasma levels of IGF-1 can be increased by training (Poehlman et al. 1994). Older adults usually show a loss in sensitivity to a given concentration of IGF-1, although the young adult response can be restored by an appropriate training program (Dardevet et al. 1994; Willis and Parkhouse 1994). Despite these observations, the administration of recombinant human growth hormone does not increase muscle strength over what can be realized by a regular exercise program alone (Taaffe et al. 1994). Moreover, at least one study has found no relationship between one indicator of plasma growth hormone secretion (the plasma concentration of somatomedin C) and muscle performance (Capuano-Pucci, Rheault, and Rudman 1987). In contrast to these negative findings, the loss of grip strength in elderly men can be retarded by the administration of testosterone (Morley et al. 1993).

Muscle Strength, Endurance, and Coordination

The muscle atrophy that accounts for so much of the decrease in lean mass with aging reflects both a decrease in average fiber size and a decrease in the number of muscle fibers (Aoyagi and Shephard 1992). However, it remains unclear how large a fraction of the total loss of muscle tissue is due to aging *per se* and how much reflects a decrease of habitual physical activity with aging (Lexell 1993). In support of the latter explanation, individual examples have been cited of very active individuals in whom little loss of lean mass has occurred over an extended period of observation (Bemben et al. 1995; Forbes 1987).

Muscle endurance is generally better preserved than peak muscle strength as people age (LaForest et al. 1990), although some authors have also described age-related decreases in endurance (for example, Clarke, Hunt, and Dotson 1992). The strength of most muscle groups shows a pattern of decline similar to that described earlier for lean tissue mass, although in part because of measurement problems and in part because of alterations in composition of the lean compartment, the correlation may not be very close (Shephard et al. 1991). Much of the muscle atrophy and associated loss of strength seems to reflect a selective denervation of muscle fibers, with reinnervation by axonal sprouting from an adjacent unit that has retained its nerve supply (Brooks and Faulkner 1994; Aoyagi and Shephard 1992). The greatest functional losses occur among the largest and fastest motor units (Doherty, Vandervoort, and Brown 1993; see table 3.3). Accordingly, some authors have found that the decrease in strength is most obvious at high speeds of muscle contraction (LaForest et

Table 3.3 Age-related changes in muscle contractile properties.

Reference	Muscle	Sex	Age (y)	MVC (N)	P_t (N)	CT (msec)	1/2RT (msec)	CV (m/sec)	M wave (mV)	PAP (/control)
Campbell et al. (1973)	EDB	M+F	3-58		?	64	53	48.1	5.7	
			60-96		?	93	109	44.2	2.7	
Davies and White (1983)	TS	M	21	1759	102	113	78			
			67-71	1152	89	148	99			
Davies et al. (1983)	TS	M	22	2109	137	121	76			
			69	1210	92	151	98			
Davies et al. (1986)	TS	M	22	1932	120	118	82			
			70	1199	96	147	100			
		F	22	1441	152	132	98			
			69	1043	118	143	126			
Klein et al. (1988)[a]	TS	M	19-32	1579	87	105	91			
			64-69	1085	64	128	92			
McDonagh et al. (1984)	TS	M	26	1895	133	119				
			71	1141	86	146				
	EF	M	26	330	39.1	71				
			71	263	27.2	76				
Vandervoort and McComas (1986)[b]	ADF	M	20-32	43.5	4.2	101	84		9.4	1.71
			40-52	37.2	4.5	111	100		9.7	1.45
			60-69	36.2	3.3	104	102		7.0	1.42
			70-79	31.6	3.3	115	122		7.8	1.31
			80-100	24.2	2.6	125	125		5.4	1.31

		Age						
	F	20-32	26.6	2.7	96	84	9.1	1.75
		40-52	25.8	3.7	113	110	10.5	1.46
		60-69	23.8	2.8	115	120	7.9	1.35
		70-79	21.5	1.8	110	119	6.3	1.35
		80-100	16.7	1.7	128	131	5.2	1.28
APF	M	20-32	171	15.5	144	109	20.7	1.52
		40-52	171	16.3	169	122	18.6	1.56
		60-69	136	13.4	170	117	13.3	1.29
		70-79	121	13.4	178	133	12.2	1.22
		80-100	94	11.9	186	144	9.5	1.15
	F	20-32	113	13.6	146	123	18.9	1.35
		40-52	127	14.5	179	139	15.0	1.20
		60-69	96	11.9	182	133	10.5	1.12
		70-79	94	13.0	183	143	8.8	1.12
		80-100	54	8.6	195	169	6.4	1.17

[a]Subjects were physically active.

[b]Data on MVC and P_t are expressed as N · m.

ADF = ankle dorsiflexor; APF = ankle plantarflexor; CT = contraction time; CV = maximal impulse conduction velocity; EDB = extensor digitorum brevis; EF = elbow flexor; MVC = maximal voluntary contraction; PAP = postactivation potentiation; P_t = maximal twitch tension; 1/2RT = half-relaxation time; TS = triceps surae.

Reprinted, by permission, from Y. Aoyagi and R.J. Shephard, 1992, "Aging and muscle function," *Sports Medicine* 14: 376-396. (Note: See original article for details of references.)

al. 1990). However, Harries and Bassey (1990) reported a similar age-related loss of isokinetic strength at all speeds over the range 0 to 5.24 rad/sec.

Effects of Gender and Occupation

The loss of isokinetic force with age proceeds more rapidly in women than in men (Freedson et al. 1993), with the largest losses of strength occurring in the perimenopausal period (Sandler et al. 1991). Gender differences in the rate of loss of peak isometric and isokinetic muscle force may reflect, in part, differences in the influence of age upon habitual physical activity patterns between men and women.

Perhaps in part because manual workers were strong as young adults, Era et al. (1992) found a greater age-related loss of strength in this group than in men in white collar occupations; however, the strength of older women was unrelated to a history of heavy physical employment (Rautanen, Sipilä, and Suominen 1993).

Strength Per Unit of Muscle Cross-Section

The strength per unit of muscle mass or muscle cross-section decreases with age (Frontera et al. 1991; Kallman, Plato, and Tobin 1990; Reed et al. 1991), although changes in dimensions do not account for all of the decrease of peak muscle power in older individuals (Ferretti et al. 1994). Factors contributing to the change in force per unit of cross-section include the following:

1. An infiltration of the muscle by fat and connective tissue (Davies, Thomas, and White 1986; Rice et al. 1989)
2. Greater stiffness of the resting muscle (Kovanen 1989), perhaps due to residual fatigue (Davies, Thomas, and White 1986)
3. A slower pumping of calcium ions by the sarcoplasmic reticulum (Gafni and Yu 1989; Klitgaard, Ausoni, and Damiani 1989; McCarter 1990), with a less rapid relaxation of antagonists opposing a given movement
4. Suboptimal patterns of motor unit recruitment and a poorer synchronization of neuronal firing (Fiatarone et al. 1990)
5. A selective decrease in the number or size of fast-twitch motor fibers (Aoyagi and Shephard 1992; Lexell, Taylor, and Sjöstrom 1988), with a greater prevalence of slow myosin isoforms and a decrease of myosin ATPase activity (Klitgaard et al. 1990)
6. An increase of internal resistance to contraction, associated with a loss of elastic tissue and alterations of collagen structure in both intracellular and extracellular compartments (Alnaqeeb, Zaid, and Goldspink 1984; Purslow 1989; Wang et al. 1991)

Most people accept that there is a selective loss of fast-twitch fibers with aging (see fig. 3.1), although it remains just as conceivable that there are changes in the size and contraction characteristics of both fast- and slow-twitch fibers, causing strength and twitch speed to decrease without any alteration in the relative proportion of the two fiber types. Fast fibers may be lost simply because old people rarely exert forceful muscle contractions against resistance. The important contribution of the loss of fast fibers to the overall functional change is suggested by a lengthening of the time to peak tension, a decrease of peak tension, a lengthening of the half-relaxation time, and an increase in the fatigue resistance of muscle (Doherty, Vandervoort, and Brown 1993; Keh-Evans et al. 1992). An age-related decrease of energy reserves was also once postulated, but nuclear magnetic resonance studies suggest similar intramuscular stores of ATP and creatine phosphate in adults aged 20 to 45 years and 70 to 80 years (Taylor et al. 1984).

Empirical Data

The deterioration in muscle function with aging can be seen in athletic performance, simple field tests, and more sophisticated laboratory measurements.

Athletic performance and simple field tests. Both cross-sectional and longitudinal studies of weight lifters have shown a decrease in the weight lifted of about 1.5% per year between 30 and 60 years of age, with a steepening of the

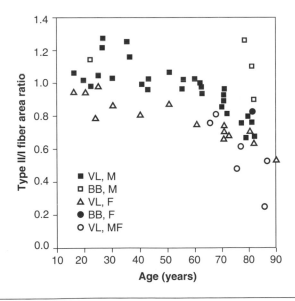

Figure 3.1   Fiber area ratio (type II/type I fibers) in relation to age. *Note*: Results of selected authors for vastus lateralis (VL) and biceps brachialis (BB) in male (M) and female (F) subjects. For sources, see original paper.
Reprinted, by permission, from Y. Aoyagi and R.J. Shephard, 1992, "Aging and muscle function," *Sports Medicine* 14: 376-396.

deterioration in performance in those over the age of 70 years (Meltzer 1993). However, it is unclear how far these changes in performance are due to a lessening of training with advancing age.

There are also age-related decreases in the scores for field tests such as push-ups and timed leg lifts (Israel 1992). The power of a vertical jump is 65% lower in 50-year-olds than in young adults (Ferretti et al. 1994). Cycle ergometer power output decreases 6% per decade, and anaerobic power (as assessed by a staircase sprint; Dummer et al. 1985; Makrides et al. 1985) shows a total loss of 45% to age 65 years, although a part of this loss reflects poorer coordination.

Laboratory tests. The great majority of empirical laboratory studies on the aging of muscle function are based upon cross-sectional changes in the peak isometric force that can be developed by selected muscle groups at various ages. Kallman, Plato, and Tobin (1990) maintained that losses are similar in cross-sectional and longitudinal data, but an early study by Clement (1974) found a more rapid decrease of strength in the longitudinal data.

Reproducible maximal isometric testing of the major muscle groups seems possible to at least 80 years of age (Bemben et al. 1992). However, at least two trials may be needed if a subject is to reach maximal force on either a handgrip dynamometer or the isokinetic apparatus (Frontera et al. 1993). The age-related decrease in peak force does not seem due simply to a decrease in motivation, since losses of a similar order are observed if the contraction is evoked by electrical stimulation (Davies, Thomas, and White 1986; Doherty, Vandervoort, and Brown 1993; Klein et al. 1988).

In young adults, hand dynamometer scores can be enhanced by a local development of the forearm muscles, but in subjects over the age of 60 years, hand dynamometer scores are highly correlated (r = .72 to .85) with scores for more sophisticated isokinetic measurements of strength in other parts of the body (Reed et al. 1993). There are also age-related decreases in the maximal *rate* of force production and the total force impulse that can be generated by a given muscle group (Bemben et al. 1991).

In general, isometric force peaks at around 30 years of age, remains fairly constant to about 50 years, and shows an accelerating decline thereafter (Aniansson et al. 1983; Danneskold-Samsoe et al. 1984; Kallman, Plato, and Tobin 1990). The classic observations of Quetelet (1835) found a 40% loss of both handgrip and back strength in men by the age of 65 years (1.6% per year). A number of recent authors have suggested that the loss of function is somewhat slower than Quetelet postulated, with an 18% to 23% deterioration of strength by 65 years (0.7% to 0.9% per year) and an average loss of 37% (0.8% per year) by 80 to 90 years of age (Aniansson et al. 1988). In support of these figures, Shephard et al. (1991) noted a loss of 6% to 8% per decade in cross-sectional comparisons over the age range 45 to 75 years. Others, such as Vandervoort (1992), have found no significant change prior to the age of 60 years (see fig. 3.2). Bassey and Harries (1993) repeated tests over a four-year

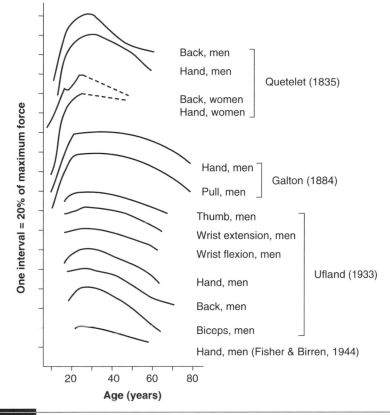

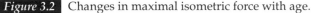

Figure 3.2 Changes in maximal isometric force with age.

interval; perhaps because their subjects were initially quite old (either 65 to 74 or over 75 years of age), losses of grip strength averaged as much as 2% per year in both men and women.

Despite the age-related decrease in peak grip strength, the grip force exerted during the lifting of a given object may be much higher in the elderly than in someone younger (Cole 1991; Cole and Beck 1994). This reflects a diminished tactile sensitivity, impaired dexterity, and difficulties in maintaining a stable grip.

Differential Losses of Muscle Function

Strength may be better preserved in the upper than in the lower extremities, this difference reflecting differential changes in activity patterns with aging (Aniansson et al. 1986). Thus, Grimby et al. (1982) found larger losses for the back and knee (40%, 1% per year, assuming a plateau to age 40 years) than for handgrip (23%, 0.6% per year) over the age span 30 to 80 years of age.

However, some authors have observed similar age-related losses of isometric strength in muscle groups other than those of the hand. Vandervoort and McComas (1986) found that by 80 to 100 years of age, maximal plantar extension torque had declined by 44% and 37% in men and women, respectively (0.9%, 0.7% per year, assuming a plateau to age 40 years), and maximal plantar flexor torque showed similar losses of 45% and 52% in men and women. Young, Stokes, and Crowe (1985) reported that at an age of 70 to 79 years, quadriceps force was 39% less than in subjects aged 21 to 28 years (1.1% per year). Viitsala et al. (1985) reported the strength of several muscle groups from 33 to 73 years of age; respective losses over this age range were 47% for knee extension (1.4% per year), 42% (1.3% per year) for handgrip and trunk extension, and 35% (1.1% per year) for trunk and elbow flexion.

Discrepancies between the various studies reflect the influence of technical considerations such as initial joint angle (and thus muscle length), habitual physical activity, and even socioeconomic status. The loss of isometric force seems to be greater if the muscle is initially extended (Fisher, Pendergast, and Calkins 1990).

Differences Between Isometric and Isokinetic Tests

The early studies of Shock and Norris (1970) indicated greater losses in dynamic than in static tests. In their 80-year-old subjects, the maximum power output on a cranking test was 45% smaller than in a young adult (a loss of 1.1% per year), but isometric strength showed a difference of only 28% (0.7% per year) relative to its peak at middle age. Likewise, Young and Skelton (1994) suggested that over the age range 65 to 84 years, strength was lost at a rate of 1.5% per year, whereas power was lost at a rate of 3.5% per year.

Stanley and Taylor (1993) further found that in postmenopausal women the loss of isokinetic function was greater for the flexors than for the extensor muscles. In contrast, Shephard et al. (1991) found similar losses of isokinetic strength (knee extension and knee flexion) and of handgrip force (all 6% to 8% per decade) over the age range 45 to 75 years.

Concentric Versus Eccentric Contraction

Poulin et al. (1992) found losses of peak torque of 31% (elbow) and 32% (knee extension) when 60- to 75-year-old subjects were compared with those aged 23 to 32 years. In their sample, eccentric strength seemed to be better maintained than concentric force.

Clarke, Hunt, and Dotson (1992) applied a 6 min bout of rhythmic arm contractions to subjects aged 20, 35, and 50 years. By the age of 50, subjects showed lower values not only for initial strength, but also for endurance, even if an active lifestyle had been maintained.

Functional Consequences

Bassey et al. (1992) demonstrated the practical value of conserving strength in terms of continued ability to undertake the activities of daily living independently. Among nursing home residents in the ninth decade of life, the maximal power output of leg extension over a 1 sec interval was correlated with the speed of rising from a chair, with stair-climbing speed, and with the rate of walking. Strength also has important implications for bone mass, gait, balance, and the risk of falls (discussed in chapter 8).

Booth, Weeden, and Tseng (1994) further suggested that as much as half of the age-related decline in aerobic power was attributable to a loss of muscle mass.

Bone

There is general agreement that senescence is associated with a progressive loss of both minerals and matrix from the bones, although as with so many other issues of aging, it is less clear to what extent this is an inevitable process and to what extent it reflects a decrease of habitual physical activity or some pathological change.

Osteoporosis implies a low bone mass and associated microarchitectural deterioration in the bone tissue (Kiebzak 1991). During the perimenopausal period, the process affects mainly trabecular (spongy) bone, predisposing to compression fractures of the vertebrae and fractures of the wrist on falling. However, in older individuals there is a progressive loss of both trabecular and compact bone, predisposing to hip fractures.

Some authors distinguish osteomalacia (a pathological deficiency of calcification, but a normal bone matrix) from osteoporosis (in which the amount of bone is reduced, but its characteristics are unchanged). Common causes of osteomalacia are a lack of magnesium, boron, and vitamins C and D (a dietary deficiency, a lack of exposure to sunlight and thus reduced endogenous synthesis of vitamin D, or a poor intestinal absorption of calcium and phosphorus); hepatic disease (leading to impaired 25-hydroxylation of vitamin D); and renal problems or a high intake of protein or sodium (all of which lead to an increased excretion of calcium, vitamin D, or both).

Other investigators distinguish osteopenia (a loss of bone mass—for example 2.5 SD below the reference standard for a young adult) from osteoporosis (a combination of osteopenia with a mechanical failure of the skeleton). A third basis of classification distinguishes primary osteoporosis (due to aging) and secondary osteoporosis (where there is some additional cause such as immobilization of a body part, a nutritional deficiency, an endocrine disorder, a malignancy, a genetic abnormality, or the prolonged use of drugs such as corticosteroids).

Genetic factors have a major influence on peak bone mass, possibly accounting for as much as 60% to 80% of interindividual variability (Slemenda and Johnson 1994; Slemenda, Miller, Hui, et al. 1991; Slemenda, Miller, Reister, et al. 1991). On the other hand, interindividual differences in the subsequent rate of bone loss seem to be determined more by environmental factors. A number of authors in the United States have stated that African Americans have a higher peak bone density than white or Asian subjects, although it is difficult to establish how far racial differences in socioeconomic status and lifestyle contribute to these observed differences.

Bone loss is a well-recognized complication of bed rest (Krølner and Toft 1983) and immobilization of a limb (Chi et al. 1983). Many cross-sectional comparisons have found better conservation of bone mass in active than in sedentary subjects (Drinkwater 1994). Muscle development (a marker of habitual activity) is also inversely related to bone loss (Cottreau et al. 1995; Sandler 1989).

Measurement Techniques

The overall age-related loss of bone calcium can be followed by neutron activation measurements of total body calcium, computerized tomography, or ultrasound (Shephard 1991a). Biopsy specimens taken from the iliac crest allow laboratory determinations of calcification rates. Local measurements of bone density at a specific site can also be made by soft tissue radiographs and single or dual photon spectrophotometry. Biochemical estimates of bone resorption can be made from a nonspecific measure of collagen breakdown (urinary hydroxyproline excretion), or more specifically from urinary pyrinoline and deoxypyrinoline concentrations (Uebelhart et al. 1991). Serum osteocalcin concentrations in turn provide an index of the rate of bone formation (Brown et al. 1984).

Effects of Aging

The process of bone mineral depletion occurs more rapidly in women (36 g/decade) than in men (30 g/decade), and women are also more vulnerable because they commence the aging process with a smaller peak calcium content. Moreover, women show an accelerated loss of calcium for about five years around menopause (Riggs and Melton 1992). Losses are more marked in the spine than in the limbs (Genant, Cann, and Faul 1982), and in early old age the losses are also more marked in trabecular than in cortical bone (Riggs and Melton 1992). However, there is no evidence of a selective loss of bone from low-stress regions such as the trabeculae or Ward's triangle (Kawashima and Uhthoff 1991).

Smith, Sempos, and Purvis (1981) reported that in women the loss was typically 0.75% to 1.0% per year, starting at an age of 30 to 35 years. Seto and Brewster (1991) suggested that in men, losses did not begin until 50 to 55 years of age, and the initial rate of loss was no more than 0.4% per year. In contrast, Jahng et al. (1991) found an average loss of 0.9% per year in men and 1.1% in women. One reason for these discrepancies is that the rate of bone loss accelerates in the perimenopausal period and again in older age groups. The reported values thus depend on both the measurement site and the age span of the sample. By the age of 80 years, the bone mineral content has dropped to some 55% of the young adult level in men and to 40% of the young adult level in women.

Osteoporosis is less marked in those individuals who maximized their bone mineral by an adequate intake of milk (Murphy et al. 1994) and vigorous exercise as young adults (Välimäki et al. 1994) and who have persisted with heavy weight- or load-bearing exercise into later life (Slemenda, Miller, Hui, et al. 1991; Suominen and Rahkila 1991). However, programs of aerobic activity seem to confer less protection than resisted exercise (Chilibeck, Sale, and Webber 1995), and neither running nor swimming can prevent bone loss from the vertebrae after menopause (Drinkwater 1994). Losses are less marked in obese individuals (mainly because they support a larger total body mass when performing the activities of daily living, but also because body fat is an important site of estrogen formation; Cottreau et al. 1995; Dequeker et al. 1991; Stini, Chen, and Stein 1994). Other variables with a favorable impact on bone density include, in women, the administration of exogenous estrogen (Riggs and Melton 1992; U.S. Department of Health and Human Services 1991b), progestogen (Lee 1991; Nordin et al. 1985), and anabolic steroids (Need et al. 1989). Osteoporosis is exacerbated by a sedentary lifestyle; androgen deficiency (Slemenda et al. 1987); a low intake of calcium both currently and as a young adult (Nordin and Heaney 1990; Slemenda, Miller, Reister, et al. 1991); an increased excretion of calcium (possibly a consequence rather than a cause of osteoporosis; Horowitz et al. 1993); an overall dietary deficiency; and possibly the use of alcohol, caffeine, and cigarettes (Chappard et al. 1991; Hasling et al. 1992; Hernandez-Avila et al. 1992; Hollenbach et al. 1993; U.S. Department of Health and Human Services 1991b).

Cellular Basis

One possible explanation of osteoporosis is that with aging, the normal process of bone turnover (resorption by osteoclasts, followed by the synthesis of new bone by osteoblasts) becomes uncoupled (Kiebzak 1991). According to this hypothesis, the rate of bone formation is unchanged, but the ability of the osteoblasts to modulate osteoclast activity is reduced (Armbrecht, Perry, and Martin 1993). Bone resorption is thus increased (Seto and Brewster 1991). Extreme protein deprivation, dietary calcium lack, a poor intestinal absorption of calcium (Horowitz et al. 1993), and an adverse calcium/phosphorus ratio could all contribute to such a phenomenon.

Mechanical stress seems to stimulate osteoclast activity (Carter 1984), but as long as this remains well coordinated with osteoblastic activity, the bone becomes strengthened along the lines where stress has been applied (Lanyon

1984). An age-related decrease in renal mass and a deterioration in renal function reduce blood levels of vitamin D but increase serum levels of parathyroid hormone (Armbrecht, Perry, and Martin 1993). Moreover, aging reduces the ability of parathyroid hormone to stimulate the formation of 1:25-dihydroxy vitamin D (Armbrecht, Perry, and Martin 1993). In women, a loss of estrogens is a further factor accelerating bone mineral loss following menopause (Drinkwater 1994; Notelovitz et al. 1991). Together, a lack of estrogens and low blood levels of vitamin D may reduce calcium absorption, thus stimulating the secretion of parathyroid hormone and osteoclast activity. Conversely, the risk of osteoporosis is decreased by an adequate calcium intake. Estrogens reduce the response of osteoclasts to parathyroid hormone (Chestnut 1994).

Other suggested factors contributing to osteoporosis include low circulating levels of calcitonin (MacIntyre et al. 1988) and prolactin (Chestnut 1994), and (in men) testosterone (Baylink and Jennings 1994; Kasperk et al. 1989; Slemenda et al. 1987).

Risk of Fractures

As bone loses calcium, it becomes increasingly vulnerable to fracture (Chestnut 1994; Cummings et al. 1989; Erickson, Isberg, and Lindgren 1989; Gardsell, Johnell, and Nilsson 1991; Heaney 1989; Hui, Slemenda, and Johnston 1989; Martin, Silverthorn, et al. 1991; Perloff et al. 1991). The classic studies of Garn (1975) showed that the cumulative probability of fractures at the wrist increased in parallel with the reduction in cortical thickness of the metacarpal bones, although there was a lag period of some 10 years between the onset of bone loss and an increase in the risk of fractures. In the femur, Hoiseth et al. (1991) found that the amount of calcified bone rather than the radiographic bone density was the important determinant of resistance to fracture.

Reductions in bone mass and bone quality narrow the safety margin between applied stresses and the point of failure (Biewener 1993; Bloomfield 1995). Thus, in advanced osteoporosis, minimal trauma such as a cough, a brisk muscular contraction, or a fall becomes enough to cause a fracture. Common sites of injury are the dorsal and upper lumbar vertebrae, the wrist (Colles fracture), the hips, and the proximal humerus (Biggemann et al. 1991; U.S. National Institutes of Health 1984).

Fractures of the hip have a particularly grave prognosis, with a fatality rate of at least 15% to 20% in one year (Keene, Parker, and Prtor 1993; Star and Hockberg 1993). Among those Americans who have survived to an age of 90 years, one-third of the women and one-half of the men have already sustained a hip fracture (Star and Hockberg 1993). Such an event shortens the survival of the affected individual by at least 15%, and as many as a half of those affected subsequently need help in performing the activities of daily living.

The potential contributions of osteoporosis to senile kyphosis and vertebral collapse have been noted already. Quantitated computed tomography can be used to predict the risk of such fractures. Spinal loads of 3 to 4 kN are common in daily life. Thus, if the compressive strength of the vertebrae is less than 3 kN, there is a high risk of vertebral fracture, but if the strength is greater than 5 kN, the risk is almost zero (Biggemann et al. 1991). Others have defined a threshold bone density (110 mg/cm^3) that the spine must have in order for a person to avoid fractures (Richardson et al. 1985). As many as a third of elderly women in North America have one or more vertebral fractures. Often the affected individuals remain unaware of this development.

Joints and Tendons

Problems in one or more of the joints are perhaps the most common complaints of the elderly person (Calkins and Challa 1985).

Incidence of Arthritis

As many as 80% of seniors have some form of rheumatic complaint (Pullar and Wright 1991), and in about one-fourth of old people this leads to a moderate or severe limitation of daily activities. Moss and Parsons (1986) found that 47% of those over the age of 65 years complained of arthritis and that more than 17% had deformities or orthopedic impairments.

Existing osteoarthritis gradually progresses as a person becomes older (Kallman et al. 1989), but in the oldest age categories the increase in prevalence seems to slow down. Thus, Bagge et al. (1991) observed no difference in the prevalence of osteoarthritis between 79- and 85-year-old subjects. In a surprising number of individuals, symptoms disappear at reexamination (Bagge, Bjelle, and Svänborg 1992). It is unclear whether this reflects a compensatory decrease in physical activity, problems of memory, a masking of arthritic complaints by other more serious conditions, or a real regression of the osteoarthritic lesion.

Causes of Osteoarthritis

Heredity, previous acute joint disease, and metabolic disorders are all thought to speed the rate of joint degeneration. Lesions can be produced by repeated heavy loading of a joint (Radin and Rose 1986), and overuse and trauma have often been suggested as important contributory causes of osteoarthritis. For example, problems are concentrated in the elbows and shoulders of those operating pneumatic drills, in the hands of boxers, and in the ankles and feet of professional dancers (Panush 1994).

Two other possible causes of osteoarthritis may be noted. Obesity increases the risk of an osteoarthritic knee, but this may reflect an alteration in joint alignment rather than the added body mass that must be carried (Leach, Baumgard, and Broom 1985). In some instances, the lesion may be an autoimmune response or a reaction to the release of lysosomal enzymes as damaged cartilage is being phagocytosed (Abbas, Lichtman, and Pober 1995).

Pathological Changes

Problems of joint function reflect changes in the structure of collagen (as seen in chapter 2), including a loss of its regular fiber orientation (Seto and Brewster 1991) and the formation of stiffer and less resilient bone. There is also an increased liability to degeneration of joint cartilage, exacerbated if body mass increases. At first there is a compensatory increase in the synthesis of proteoglycans, but later synthesis is checked by a failure of the chondrocytes. The color of the articular cartilage changes from white to yellow, its elasticity decreases, it becomes thinner, and frank defects appear over weight-bearing areas.

Degenerative joint changes can first be detected from the second decade of life. Aging can be distinguished from a pathological osteoarthrosis only in terms of the severity of the lesion.

Changes in the synovial lining of the joints include an increase in the number of villi and a decrease in vascularity of the underlying stroma, occasionally with the development of cartilaginous areas in the synovial membrane.

Functional Consequences

The most common functional problems of the arthritic joint are a stiffening ("gelling") after a period of immobility and (at the knee) a loss of stability because the joint cannot be locked in full extension. By the age of 55 to 64 years, some 85% of people have radiographic changes that could be interpreted as osteoarthrosis, but only about a quarter of these individuals complain of symptoms.

The proportion of people with functionally significant limitation in the range of motion at major joints is much smaller than might be inferred from the stated prevalence of arthritis. Bergstrom et al. (1986) found that in 79-year-old subjects, hip motion was limited in 11% of men and 5% of women. Moreover, 8% lacked full extension of the right knee.

Nevertheless, the range of motion at many of the large joints does diminish progressively, beginning in early adult life. This has been documented most fully for the simple sit-and-reach test. The Canada Fitness Survey (Fitness Canada 1983) found that the forward reach at age 20 to 29 years was 0.33 m in women and 0.30 m in men, but that by the age of 60 to 69 years it had decreased to 0.28 m in women and 0.22 m in men. Shephard, Berridge, and Montelpare (1990) documented decreases in the range of motion at other joints over the age range 45 to 75 years (see table 3.4). Unfortunately, although the sit-and-reach test is easy to perform, the data thus obtained in an older population bear only a limited relationship to the deterioration of function in other joints (Shephard, Berridge, and Montelpare 1990).

Lesions of Tendons and Ligaments

Loss of resilience in both collagen and bone makes strains, sprains, and tendon rupture frequent complications of overvigorous or unfamiliar activity in

Table 3.4 Influence of age (A, yr) and gender (G, male = 1, female = 2) on the range of motion at selected joints.

Joint movement	Regression equation
Head rotation	
Right	$75.2° - 0.18(A)°$
Left	$87.5° - 0.31(A)°$
Shoulder	
Extension	$27.6° - 0.29(A)°$
Internal rotation	Not significant
External rotation	$252.2° - 5.54(A)° + 0.045(A^2)°$
Ankle	
Plantar flexion	$14.1° - 0.20(A)°$
Dorsiflexion	Not significant
Hip	
Flexion	Not signifcant
Sit and reach test	$32.4° - 0.31(A)° + 0.12 (A \times G)°$

Linear regression equations fitted to cross-sectional data for subjects aged 45 to 75 years of age.

Reprinted with permission from *Research Quarterly for Exercise and Sport*, 61, 326-330, Copyright 1990 by the American Alliance for Health, Physical Education, Recreation and Dance, 1900 Association Drive, Reston, Virginia 20191.

the elderly. However, such problems can be checked by an extended warm-up, the gradual progression of an exercise program, and an emphasis on activities such as walking on a smooth surface, where tendon strain is minimized.

The capillary supply to the tendons decreases with age, and some authors have suggested that localized ischemia may be a factor contributing to tendon rupture. A further consequence is that any injuries incurred are slow to heal. Aging modifies the insertion of tendon into the bones. The cortex of the bone becomes thinner, and the marrow extends into the tendon through small fissures, allowing bone formation to occur in the proximal part of the tendon. As with changes in the tendon proper, it is often difficult to decide whether such lesions are an inevitable consequence of aging, or whether they may be blamed on reduced activity and intercurrent disease.

Aging of the Cardiovascular System

As in other tissues, it is very difficult to draw dividing lines between normal cardiovascular aging, the effects of age-related decreases in habitual physical activity, and the pathology that develops with advancing years. Autopsy studies show that as many as 60% to 70% of older subjects have some evidence of coronary vascular disease (Elveback and Lie 1984). Moreover, the exercise responses of this majority of the older population differ substantially from the reactions seen in the disease-free minority of elders (Fleg et al. 1993; Rozanski et al. 1984).

Anatomical Changes

In part because of increased systolic pressures and in part because of an increase in end-diastolic volume, the left ventricular wall thickness (see fig. 3.3) and ventricular mass are greater in a senior than in a younger person (Di Bello et al. 1993). The total number of cardiac myocytes decreases, but there is a reactive hypertrophy of the remaining tissue (Olivetti et al. 1991). Moreover, the fibrous component of the heart wall (as evaluated by hydroxyproline concentration) doubles over the span of adult life (Lakatta 1987).

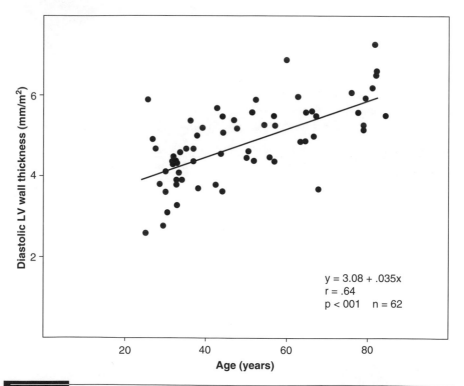

$$y = 3.08 + .035x$$
$$r = .64$$
$$p < 001 \quad n = 62$$

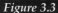 *Figure 3.3*   Increase in thickness of left ventricular (LV) posterior wall with age. Cross-sectional echocardiographic data for men enrolled in the Baltimore Longitudinal Study of Aging (Gerstenblith et al. 1977). Reproduced with permission. *Circulation* 56: 273-278. Copyright 1977 American Heart Association.

A progressive loss of elasticity in the large arteries leads to an increase of systemic blood pressure, an alteration in form of the arterial pulse wave, and an increase of the pressure against which the ventricle must empty (the cardiac afterload). The capacity of the venous system is also increased by a progressive reduction in venous tone and the development of numerous varicosities.

Functional Changes

We will examine in turn heart rate, stroke volume, cardiac output, arteriovenous oxygen difference, and blood pressure, for each of these variables looking at resting data and responses to submaximal and maximal exercise. Many of the changes in cardiovascular function seem linked to a down-regulation of beta-adrenoceptors, with a decrease in the chronotropic and inotropic responses to exercise that are seen in a younger person. A decrease of the maximal arteriovenous oxygen difference may further reduce peak oxygen delivery for a given cardiac output.

Heart Rate

Aging leads to some changes of resting heart rate, but there are more marked age differences in the response to submaximal and maximal exercise.

Resting Data

The average resting heart rate changes surprisingly little with aging (Fagard, Thijs, and Amery 1993; Gerstenblith, Weisfeldt, and Lakatta 1985; Lakatta 1993a). On the other hand, there are diminutions in the power spectrum of cardiac frequency variations (Fouillot et al. 1992), particularly a decrease in the vagally mediated sinus rate variations over the respiratory cycle, in spontaneous variations of heart rate over a 24 h period (Kostis et al. 1986), and in the intrinsic sinus rate that is observed after blockade of sympathetic and parasympathetic nerves.

Submaximal Exercise

During submaximal exercise, the relationship between heart rate and oxygen consumption is often much as in younger adults (Dempsey and Seals 1995; Lakatta 1993a). Because the peak oxygen intake is reduced, one might anticipate that the heart rate would be increased at any given fraction of aerobic power. Nevertheless, some authors have found a slower, rather than a faster, heart rate in old people during submaximal effort, both dynamic (Kohrt et al. 1993; Sachs, Hamberger, and Kaijser 1985) and isometric activity (Sachs, Hamberger, and Kaijser 1985; Taylor et al. 1991). This could reflect a lesser resting vagal activity (with a correspondingly higher resting heart rate and less scope for a reduction in vagal tone and increase of heart rate during exercise). One pointer in this direction is a lessening of the vagally-linked high-frequency component of heart rate variability in older subjects (Lakatta 1993a; Shannon, Carley, and Benson 1987). Older individuals may also show a smaller chronotropic response to catecholamines, due to a down-regulation of the beta-adrenoreceptors. Finally, any apparent decrease in the heart rate response at a given fraction of the individual's peak oxygen intake could be an artifact, a poor peak effort by an older person leading to the testing of responses at a smaller fraction of the subject's true maximal oxygen intake.

The increase of heart rate and of oxygen intake at the beginning of exercise occurs more slowly as people age (Babcock et al. 1994; Paterson, Cunningham, and Babcock 1989). Young adults show a progressive upward drift of heart rate if the activity continues for several minutes or longer, but any drift is much smaller in an elderly person (Chick et al. 1991). This may reflect a lesser chronotropic action of circulating catecholamines on the cardiac pacemaker (Stratton et al. 1992), together with a decrease in catecholamine-mediated glycogenolysis, and a selective decrease in the availability of glycogen-rich type II skeletal muscle fibers that modify peripheral feedback to the cardioregulatory centers of the medulla.

Maximal Effort

The maximal heart rate decreases substantially with aging. One easily remembered formula suggests that the maximal heart rate is 220 minus the person's age in years. A steady maximal value of 195 to 200 beats/min is certainly typical of a healthy young adult, but by the age of 65 years, some authors (myself included) have found average readings up to 20 beats/min higher than the 155 beats/min suggested by the simple formula (Dempsey and Seals 1995), provided that the individuals concerned made a good maximal effort. It remains unclear how far the low peak heart rates reported in some early studies were due to an incomplete stressing of the cardiorespiratory system, and how far they reflected a high level of fitness in the subjects examined. Certainly there is some tendency to an inverse gradient between aerobic fitness and peak heart rate in subjects at all ages.

Reasons for the age-related decline in maximal heart rate have yet to be fully resolved, but possibly include alterations in catecholamine release and response, and an increased stiffness of the heart wall.

Sympathetic activity and catecholamine release.   Sympathetic nerve activity may increase with age, in a bid to maintain arterial blood pressure and the perfusion of vital organs during exercise (Hajduczok, Chapleau, and Abboud 1991). Various investigators have reported that the associated spillover of norepinephrine into the blood is decreased (Hagberg et al. 1988; Jensen et al. 1992; Taylor et al. 1992), unchanged (Kastello, Sothman, and Murthy 1993), or even increased (Fleg, Tzankoff, and Lakatta 1985; Lehman and Keul 1986; Meredith et al. 1991) at any given relative intensity of dynamic or isometric exercise.

Factors contributing to the variations in response include prejunctional inhibition of norepinephrine release, a decrease in neuronal re-uptake of norepinephrine, a variable rate of clearance of norepinephrine from the plasma (Seals, Taylor, et al. 1994), possible errors in the calculation of relative work rate due to a poor maximal effort, and a potential dependence of the sympathetic response on absolute rather than relative work rate. Those authors who find an increased norepinephrine spillover have debated whether this should be viewed as an attempt to compensate for diminished receptor responsiveness, or whether the primary event is an increased norepinephrine spillover, with a secondary down-regulation of beta-adrenergic receptors (Bristow et al. 1990).

Chronotropic response to catecholamines. The older subject undoubtedly shows a decline in the chronotropic response to catecholamines. Most authors find that the beta-adrenergic receptor density remains unchanged in older adults (Lakatta 1993a, 1993b; Scarpace 1986), although Böhm and Erdmann (1989) described a decrease. In contrast, there is good evidence of a postsynaptic down-regulation of the beta-adrenergic-sensitive adenylate cyclase system (Böhm et al. 1993; Lakatta 1993a, 1993b; Seals, Taylor, et al. 1994; Stratton et al. 1992).

Ventricular compliance. Greater stiffness (a reduced compliance) of the heart wall (due to both myocardial hypertrophy and increasing cross-linkage of collagen fibers) likely contributes to the reduction in peak heart rate. A resultant slowing in the early phase of diastolic relaxation lengthens the time required for ventricular filling (Schulman et al. 1992) and modifies the feedback of information about cardiac preloading to the cardioregulatory system.

Other factors. Other possible factors influencing heart rate include a slowing of the intrinsic cardiac rhythm (Jose and Collison 1970), a lesser potential for the withdrawal of vagal tone (Seals, Taylor, et al. 1994), in some instances a decrease in drive to the sympathetic pacemaker (Lakatta 1993a), and (in pathological cases) a decrease in oxygen supply to the cardiac pacemaker (Wei 1994).

Stroke Volume

Except in extreme old age, the heart volume is well maintained. Echocardiography shows some increase in the thickness of the left ventricular wall (see fig. 3.3; Lakatta 1993a). This reflects the joint influences of an increased resting systolic pressure, a decrease in distensibility of the aorta, and (in some situations) an increase of stroke volume that attempts to compensate for the decrease in maximal heart rate.

Resting Data

Many early studies described a small decrease of resting stroke volume with age (Fagard, Thijs, and Amery 1993), but it was not always clear whether older members of the test sample were in normal cardiac health. In contrast, Weisfeldt, Gerstenblith, and Lakatta (1985) reported a small age-related increase of resting stroke volume in subjects who were free of both electrocardiographic and scintigraphic evidence of myocardial ischemia.

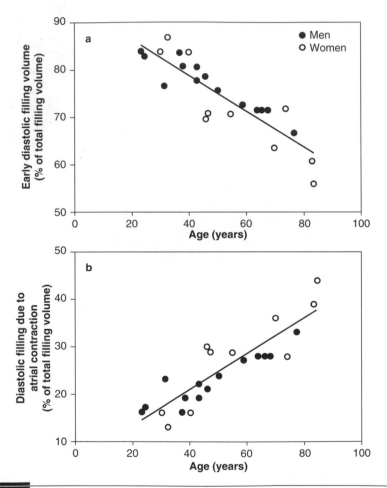

Figure 3.4   Influence of age on mechanism of ventricular filling. Upper panel: early diastolic filling volume as percentage of total filling volume. Lower panel: diastolic filling due to atrial contraction as percentage of total filling volume. Based on data of Swinne et al. (1992).

Reprinted, by permission, from J.L. Fleg, 1994, "Normative aging on the cardiovascular system," *American Journal of Geriatric Cardiology* 3: 27.

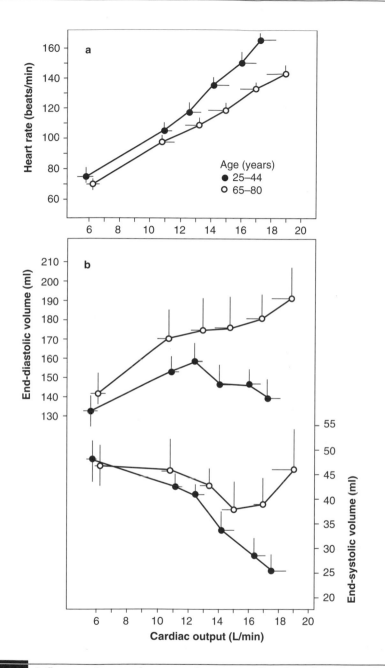

Figure 3.5 Influence of age on heart rate (upper panel) and stroke volume (lower panel) at various cardiac outputs. Cross-sectional data from Baltimore Longitudinal Study of Aging (Rodeheffer et al. 1984).
Reproduced with permission. *Circulation* 69: 203-213. Copyright 1984 American Heart Association.

Submaximal Exercise

During normal upright exercise, the stroke volume of a young adult increases progressively with work rate. During moderate activity, elderly subjects usually increase their stroke volume to 110 to 120 ml/beat, much as in younger individuals. However, the ejection fraction is less well maintained as peak effort is approached, particularly if there has been a loss of physical condition with aging (Ogawa et al. 1992). Whereas fit individuals tend to increase their stroke volume by an increase of end-diastolic volume (see figs. 3.4 and 3.5), subjects who are unfit or obese seek to maintain or increase their stroke volume by the less effective mechanism of decreasing end-systolic volume (O'Connor et al. 1994). Port et al. (1980) noted that when subjects were exercising at 85% of maximal heart rate, the ejection fraction was less than 0.60 in 45% of individuals over the age of 60 years, compared with only 2% of young adults; in those with severe cardiac disease and congestive failure, the ejection fraction may drop to 0.20 or lower. Abnormalities of ventricular wall motion are also increasingly prevalent in those over the age of 50 years.

Maximal Effort

As maximal effort is approached, the stroke volume of an elderly person often actually declines (Ogawa et al. 1992; Tate, Hyek, and Taffet 1994). Fleg et al. (1993) examined a group of 74-year-old subjects; the ejection fraction during peak effort on a cycle ergometer was 0.76 in those who were free of myocardial ischemia, and 0.66 in those with silent ischemia, as compared to 0.85 in young controls. Moreover, the ejection fraction of the elderly subjects did not increase relative to the values observed at 50% of peak power output, even in those who were free of myocardial ischemia. In others who also were clinically healthy but showed ECG evidence of silent ischemia, the left ventricular ejection fraction actually declined as work rate increased.

Difficulty in sustaining ventricular ejection at high power outputs may reflect, among other factors, a poorer perfusion of the myocardium in an older heart, a lesser inotropic response of the myocardium to catecholamines (Schulman et al. 1992), a lesser compliance of the ventricular wall and thus impaired diastolic filling, a change in the contractile characteristics of the cardiac muscle, a progressive replacement of ventricular muscle by fibrous tissue, and increased afterloading (due to a high vascular impedance).

Impaired myocardial perfusion.   Weisfeldt, Gerstenblith, and Lakatta (1985) argued strongly that any decrease of stroke volume at high work rates was due to impaired coronary flow and resultant myocardial ischemia. In their heavily selected population (all with a normal coronary circulation as established by exercise ECGs and scintigrams), the stroke volume was actually larger in older than in younger age groups. However, their heart rate data suggest that subjects were tested at substantially less than maximal aerobic effort, and it is conceivable that if the older individuals had been encouraged to make a greater effort, a decrease of stroke volume would have been observed as in most studies of true maximal performance. Any increase of stroke volume that these authors observed was obtained at the expense of a decrease in cardiac reserve. Moreover, as Fleg et al. (1993) demonstrated, the myocardium was functioning less effectively in the older subjects, since the gain of stroke volume for a given increase of end-diastolic volume was poorer in such individuals, even if they showed no evidence of exercise-induced myocardial ischemia.

Myocardial ischemia and fibrosis are frequently observed in older individuals. These changes undoubtedly reduce peak stroke volume, but are pathological rather than normal manifestations of aging.

Altered myocardial properties.   Aging is associated with a decrease in the mRNA for alpha-myosin, with no change in the beta-myosin mRNA. There is thus a progressive conversion of the contractile protein in the heart wall from the fast (alpha-myosin) to the slow (beta-myosin) isoform. There is an associated decrease in actomyosin ATPase activity. These changes have some adaptive value for the aging coronary circulation, since the slower isoform of myosin produces a given ventricular wall tension at a lower energy cost (Holubarsch et al. 1985). Aging is also associated with an increase in the duration of calcium activation of the myofibrils, and with a prolongation of the myocardial action potential (Lakatta 1987).

Animal experiments with isolated cardiac muscle show a 15% to 20% age-related increase in the time to development of peak force, and a parallel slowing in subsequent relaxation. The slowing of myocardial relaxation reflects a delay of Ca^{2+} sequestration following contraction (Lakatta 1987; Tate, Hyek, and Taffet 1994). Tate, Hyek, and Taffet (1994) attributed this delay to a decrease of calcium-dependent ATPase activity, but Narayanan (1981) suggested that the problem arose mainly because the energy released by the ATPase had become uncoupled from the Ca^{2+} pumping process.

Despite these alterations in the fundamental contractile properties of the ventricular muscle, echocardiographic observations on healthy human subjects have shown surprisingly little influence of age on the velocity of circumferential fiber shortening, either at rest or after systolic pressure is increased by the administration of phenylephrine (Lakatta 1987).

Altered catecholamine response.   In a young adult, exercise leads to a substantial, catecholamine-mediated increase of myocardial contractility, the inotropic response. In an elderly person, the change of function induced by propranolol administration is less than in the young adult (Fleg et al. 1994), showing an impairment of the response of the ventricle to catecholamines; the response may be further limited by changes in the inherent contractile properties of the myocardium (Lakatta 1993a; Port et al. 1980), as discussed above.

Animal data suggest that the density of beta-adrenergic receptors does not change with aging; indeed, because of ventricular hypertrophy there may even be an increase in the total number of beta-receptors (Scarpace, Lowenthal, and Tümer 1992). Nevertheless, the inotropic response is attenuated by a down-regulation of receptors in the cardiac muscle, and this is not entirely offset even if there is an increase of beta-adrenergic nerve activity (Port et al. 1980; Seals, Taylor et al. 1994).

A lesser increase in the speed of ventricular contraction during exercise not only tends to limit peak stroke volume, but also lengthens the systolic phase of the cardiac cycle, when coronary perfusion is restricted by the tension in the heart wall.

Venous filling.   Several factors tend to reduce preloading of the ventricles in an elderly person: a general loss of physical condition with a poor resultant venous tone and a reduction of blood volume, a pooling of blood in varicosities, and a slow diastolic relaxation of the ventricles. One important practical manifestation of reduced venous filling is that many older people show a significant drop in systemic blood pressure on moving rapidly from the supine to a vertical position (Fagard, Thijs, and Amery 1993).

Under resting conditions, relaxation of the ventricular wall may be slowed not only by the delays in calcium ion sequestration already discussed, but also because of hypertrophy or collagen cross-linkage (Guenard and Emeriau 1992; Tate, Hyek, and Taffet 1994; Thomas et al. 1992). The catecholamine-mediated increase of ventricular filling rate during exercise seems to be of a similar absolute magnitude in the young and the elderly, but because older individuals begin from poorer resting values, they show slower filling during both rhythmic (Stratton, Levy et al. 1994) and isometric (Swinne et al. 1992) exercise.

Delays in venous filling suggest a latent problem for the cardiac performance of an older person, but under most circumstances there is adequate compensation by an enhanced atrial contribution to filling late in diastole (see fig. 3.4; Downes et al. 1989; Green and Crouse 1993; Kitzman, Higginbotham, and Sullivan 1993; Miller et al. 1986; Miyatake et al. 1984; Takemoto et al. 1992). Echocardiography has not demonstrated any decrease of end-diastolic volumes in older individuals, either at rest or during near-maximal exercise (Lakatta 1993b).

Afterload.   Under resting conditions, elderly individuals may show an overall peripheral resistance similar to that of younger people, but during vigorous exercise there is a larger increase of systemic blood pressure at any given power output (Martin, Ogawa, et al. 1991; White and Carrington 1993), so the impedance to ejection of the ventricular contents is substantially greater than in a younger person. Several factors contribute to this change. The aorta and major arteries are less compliant in the elderly person. Aging is also associated with a greater vasoconstriction in the blood vessels supplying inactive muscle (Seals,

Taylor, et al. 1994; Taylor et al. 1992). Finally, perfusion of the active limbs is specifically impeded because the weakened skeletal muscles develop a given effort at a larger fraction of their maximal force (Sun, Eiken, and Mekjavic 1993).

Cardiac Output

Age has little influence on cardiac output at rest or during submaximal exercise, but it leads to a progressive reduction of peak cardiac output.

Resting Data

Early reports suggested that there was some reduction of resting cardiac output with aging, associated with a decrease of resting metabolism. However, Weisfeldt, Gerstenblith, and Lakatta (1985) found that after all subjects with latent ischemic heart disease had been eliminated from their sample, resting cardiac output was unrelated to age. It may thus be the case that in the earlier studies results were biased by the choice of unfit, convalescent hospital patients as subjects.

Submaximal Exercise

During light submaximal exercise, age continues to have only a minor influence on heart rate and stroke volume, and most authors thus find little change in cardiac output at a given oxygen intake, although McElvaney et al. (1989) claimed that the cardiac output of 65-year-old subjects was somewhat lower than in a younger individual at any given absolute level of power output.

Maximal Exercise

The peak cardiac output is reached at a lower work rate and a lower peak heart rate than in a younger person. Thus, the maximal cardiac output at an age of 65 years is typically 17 to 20 L/min (100-120 ml × 170 beats/min), some 20% to 30% less than in a young adult (Fagard, Thijs, and Amery 1993; Fuchi et al. 1989; Higginbotham et al. 1986; Kitzman, Higginbotham, and Sullivan 1993; Ogawa et al. 1992; Seals, Taylor, et al. 1994). As Paterson (1992) has pointed out, the decrease in maximal cardiac output commonly runs in parallel with a loss of lean tissue, so that the peak blood flow per unit of active muscle tends to remain adequate in an older person.

Weisfeldt, Gerstenblith, and Lakatta (1985) aroused considerable interest by their suggestion that subjects who had reached an average age of 71 years, but who were free of electrocardiographic and scintigraphic abnormalities, could compensate for a low peak heart rate by exploiting the Frank-Starling mechanism. In their series, the resulting increase of stroke volume was said to be sufficient to maintain the maximal cardiac output at the level observed in young adults (see fig. 3.5), albeit at the cost of an increase in end-diastolic volume and thus a decrease in cardiac reserve. However, it is important to emphasize that the response the authors observed (a peak cardiac output of 17.3 L/min, based on a stroke volume of 125 ml and a heart rate of 143 beats/min) is not in disagreement with traditional views on the maximal cardiac output of the elderly. It seems likely that if they had pushed their subjects to a truly maximal heart rate (160-170 beats/min), they would have seen a decrease in stroke volume similar to what others have reported. Even their data show a substantial drop of ejection fraction with age, from an average of 0.835 at an age of 35 years to 0.761 at an age of 71 years.

Arteriovenous Oxygen Difference

The volume of oxygen that a given cardiac output transports to the tissues depends upon the magnitude of the mean arteriovenous oxygen difference.

Rest and Submaximal Exercise

At rest and at any given submaximal rate of working, the arteriovenous difference seems unchanged in active men, but tends to be 20 to 50 ml/L greater in older women (Dempsey and Seals 1995; Spina et al. 1993). This reflects some reduction in the mechanical efficiency of exercise and thus an increase in the oxygen cost of any given task, together with a stroke volume and cardiac output that are slightly smaller than those seen when a young person exercises at the same intensity of effort.

Maximal Exercise

Many healthy 65-year-olds can still develop the maximal arteriovenous oxygen difference of 140 to 150 ml/L expected in a young adult, but values tend to be lower in the elderly (Weisfeldt, Gerstenblith, and Lakatta 1985). Potential factors contributing to a reduction of maximal arteriovenous oxygen difference include a reduction of arterial oxygen content, a poorer peripheral distribution of the available cardiac output, and a loss of activity in tissue enzyme systems.

Reduced arterial oxygen content.   In some seniors, chronic chest disease leads to a decrease in pulmonary diffusing capacity and thus a reduction of arterial oxygen saturation. In others, anemia is responsible. Although a small volume of oxygen is carried in physical solution, the oxygen-carrying capacity of oxygenated blood is almost directly proportional to its hemoglobin content.

An early study by Elwood (1971) found relatively normal hemoglobin levels (male, 14.5-14.9 g/dl; female, 12.9-13.3 g/dl) in a community survey of healthy subjects over the age of 65 years. Likewise, Garry (1994) found normal values in a wealthy community in New Mexico. Nevertheless, several epidemiologic studies have shown an increased prevalence of anemia in the elderly (Lipschitz 1994).

Elderly individuals are particularly vulnerable to a number of the causes of anemia: (1) a poor diet or gastrointestinal atrophy may limit the absorption of iron or vitamin B12; (2) internal bleeding from an undetected ulcer or neoplasm may reduce hemoglobin levels; and (3) red, hemopoietic bone marrow is progressively replaced by fatty tissue (Lipschitz 1994). The prevalence of anemia thus increases with age (Lipschitz 1994), although most elderly people retain an ability to respond to hemorrhage by a brisk erythropoiesis.

Blood flow distribution. A large arteriovenous oxygen difference depends on a large fraction of the cardiac output passing to the active skeletal muscles (where oxygen extraction is high), and a small fraction passing to the viscera and the skin (where oxygen extraction is much smaller). A combination of aging and a low level of fitness alters the ratio of muscle to visceral and skin blood flow, thus tending to reduce the arteriovenous oxygen difference.

If maximum oxygen intake is developed by exercising a relatively small muscle mass (as in cycle ergometry and, more obviously, in short crank arm ergometry), the heart encounters some difficulty in pumping blood through the strongly contracting muscles. The older person is at particular risk of this type of peripheral flow limitation. Because the skeletal muscles have become weaker, the remaining tissue must contract at a high percentage of maximal voluntary force in order to achieve a given power output. Thus, despite a lower heart rate (143 vs. 174 beats/min), Weisfeldt, Gerstenblith, and Lakatta (1985) noted that the systemic vascular resistance in 71-year-old subjects was 30% greater than in those with an average age of 35 years. In an attempt to compensate for difficulties in muscle perfusion, both systolic and diastolic pressures were some 10 mmHg higher in the elderly group. Such compensation is often enough to sustain arteriovenous oxygen difference during submaximal exercise, but muscle blood flow and thus oxygen extraction may drop as maximal effort is approached.

Part of the greater increase in systemic blood pressure of the older person is developed by a progressive restriction of blood flow to parts of the body that are not involved in exercise—particularly inactive muscle. Thus, when leg exercise is being performed, the peripheral resistance in the arm vessels at any given fraction of peak oxygen intake is greater in the elderly than in a young adult (Taylor et al. 1992).

Another factor that tends to reduce oxygen extraction in the older person is a greater demand for skin blood flow than in a younger exerciser. This reflects (1) a thick layer of subcutaneous fat that impedes the direct conduction of heat to the skin surface, and (2) a lesser sweat rate and thus a smaller evaporative heat loss in older people (Cable and Green 1990). Nevertheless, the additional skin blood flow is not readily available (Havenith et al. 1995). Indeed, if young and older subjects are matched for habitual activity patterns, the older individuals show less extensive cutaneous vasodilatation and a poorer heat tolerance when exercising (Tankersley et al. 1991).

The resting renal blood flow is lower in the elderly than in younger individuals (Kenney and Zappe 1994). However, during exercise in the heat, the reduction of renal blood flow is much smaller in fit elderly subjects (13% to 15%) than in young adults who have a similar maximal oxygen intake (37% to 50%), so this factor also predisposes to a narrowing of the maximal arteriovenous oxygen difference.

Tissue oxygen extraction.   A proportion of elderly subjects develop frank oxygen want in their muscles during vigorous physical activity. This is exemplified by the acute calf pain (intermittent claudication) that develops during walking in a person who has a poor blood supply to the lower limbs. However, such acute muscle ischemia is due mainly to obliterative disease in a major artery rather than to difficulty in oxygen extraction within the tissues (Thiele and Strandness 1994).

There may be a reduction in the number of tissue capillaries with aging (Aoyagi and Shephard 1992; Celli 1986; see table 3.5a and b), but because there is also some wasting of the muscle fibers, the diffusion pathway from the capillaries to metabolic sites within the mitochondria remains relatively constant (Aoyagi and Shephard 1992; Celli 1986). Many muscle enzymes also show a reduction of activity in older subjects (see table 3.6), although it is unclear how far this is attributable to aging and how far it reflects an age-related decrease in physical condition.

As in a younger person, the main argument against a significant peripheral limitation of oxygen extraction is the very low oxygen content of blood leaving the active skeletal muscles (Shephard 1993a). Since the overall arteriovenous oxygen difference for healthy seniors is 140 to 150 ml/L, the local arteriovenous difference across the working muscles must be at least 160 to 170 ml/L. The corresponding oxygen pressure in venous blood draining from the active muscles would then be no more than 10 to 12 mmHg (1.3-1.6 kPa). Evidently, the main pressure gradient and thus the main impedance to oxygen transport remains in the cardiorespiratory system rather than within the contracting muscles (Shephard 1993a).

Blood Pressure

Old age is associated with both an increased prevalence of episodes of low blood pressure (orthostatic hypotension), and a progressive increase in systolic pressures (hypertension) at rest as well as during exercise.

Hypotension

The circulatory system of an elderly person shows a reduced tolerance to change. On moving suddenly from a supine to an upright position, on rising from a sitting position in a hot environment, or after emerging from a swim-

Table 3.5a   Influence of age upon muscle capillarity.

Group		Capillaries (mm^{-2})	Capillaries (fiber^{-1})	CC		
				type I	type IIA	type IIB
Men	Young[a]	270-369	0.81-1.80	3.90-4.76	4.20-4.84	2.94-3.00
	Old[b]	247-347	0.59-1.61	3.70-4.56	3.08-3.92	2.64-3.20
Women	Young[c]	301-348	1.11-1.39	4.00-4.11	3.40-3.70	2.33-2.90
	Old[b]	296-358	1.10-1.40	3.40-4.38	2.60-3.80	2.75-2.90

Table 3.5b   Influence of age upon muscle capillarity relative to fiber area.

Group		Capillaries (mm^{-2})	Capillaries (fiber^{-1})	CC relative to fiber area (μ.m$^{-2} \times 10^{-3}$)		
				type I	type IIA	type IIB
Men	Young[a]	270-369	0.81-1.80	1.03-1.25	0.86-0.95	0.78-0.84
	Old[b]	247-347	0.59-1.61	0.90-1.54	1.03-1.72	1.07-1.38
Women	Young[c]	301-348	1.11-1.39	1.07	0.99	0.84
	Old[b]	296-358	1.10-1.40	1.11-1.31	1.05-1.30	0.80-1.26

[a]18 to 34 years.
[b]67 to 81 years.
[c]18 to 40 years.
CC = capillaries in contact with each fiber.
Reprinted, by permission, from Y. Aoyagi and R.J. Shephard, 1992, "Aging and muscle function," *Sports Medicine* 14: 376-396.

ming pool, there is a marked drop in systemic blood pressure (postural hypotension). This causes complaints of dizziness, confusion, weakness, and fainting (Fagard, Thijs, and Amery 1993; Halter 1985). Between 10% and 30% of community-dwelling seniors show a drop in pressure of 20 mmHg (2.7 kPa) or more with a change of posture (Lipsitz 1989; Mader 1989). Postural hypotension is one factor contributing to the prevalence of falls in the elderly. A sudden drop in blood pressure immediately after a bout of exercise may also precipitate myocardial infarction or cardiac arrest.

Hypotension reflects an increase of venous pooling due to varicosities and a poor venous tone, together with an impaired baroreceptor reflex, and sometimes a less than normal increase in the secretion of norepinephrine as posture is changed (Polinsky et al. 1981). Tonkin et al. (1991) have suggested that one important problem is a dysfunction in the afferent limb of the baroreceptor reflex. Possibly, receptors that would otherwise sense a fall in blood pres-

Table 3.6 Changes in enzyme activity in the vastus lateralis muscle with age.

Reference	Age	n	Oxidative				Glycolytic							Mg++ ATP
			SDH	HAD	CYTOX	CS	PFK	PHOSP	LDH	MK	HK	TPDH	CPK	
Aniansson et al. (1980b)	16-78	113	↕				↕	↕						
Aniansson et al. (1981)[a]	66-76	47							↕	↕				↕
Aniansson et al. (1986)	73-83	22							↕	⇉				
Borges and Essen-Gustavsson (1989)	20-70	14		↕		↕			(↕)				↕	
Essen-Gustavsson and Borges (1986)	20-70	34		(↕)	(↕)	→ (↓)			(↕)		↕ (↕)	→	(↓)	
Grimby et al. (1982)[a]	78-81	34		↕		↕			↕		↕			
Larsson (1978)[a]	22-65	55	⇈ ↑	⇈ ↑	↑	↑ ↕	↕ ↕		→ →	↕				↕
Örlander and Aniansson (1980)[a]	70-75	5							→ →					

Data mainly for men, with findings for women indicated in parentheses.

[a]Based on cross-sectional comparisons with data published by other investigators.

CPK - creatine phosphokinase; CS = citrate synthase; CYTOX = cytochrome oxidase; HAD = 3-hydroxyacyl-CoA-dehydrogenase; HK - hexokinase; LDH = lactate dehydrogenase; MG++ ATP = Mg++-stimulated adenosine triphosphatase; MK = myokinase; PFK = phosphofructokinase; PHOSP = phosphorylase; SDH - succinate dehydrogenase TPDH = triose phosphate dehydrogenase; ↑, ↓ = tendency to increased or decreased activity; ⇈, ⇊ = significantly (p < 0.05) increased or decreased activity; ←→ = unchanged activity.

Reprinted, by permission, from Y. Aoyagi and R.J. Shephard, 1992, "Aging and muscle function," *Sports Medicine* 14: 376-96.

sure are "splinted" by noncompliant arterial walls. Often the problem also seems to occur in subjects with a high resting blood pressure (Lipsitz 1989), although the prescription of antihypertensive medication may be a factor in this association.

Barrett-Connor and Palinkas (1994) have noted an association between a low diastolic pressure and the depression that is such a common feature of old age.

Hypertension

Aging is associated with both increases in average systolic blood pressures and an increased prevalence of clinical hypertension.

Resting data. In developed societies, the resting systolic blood pressure may rise on average by as much as 35 mmHg over the adult life span (Kannel 1980). Early studies of indigenous communities such as the Navajo (DeStephano, Coulehan, and Wiant 1979) and the Pacific Islanders (Page, Damon, and Moelleriag 1974; see fig. 3.6) showed little increase in systolic blood pressure with age, and this still seems true in isolated Inuit populations (Rode and Shephard 1995b). Differences of personal lifestyle that apparently have protected the indigenous populations include a high level of habitual physical activity, a low body mass, a low salt intake, and (in some cases) a high intake of omega-3 fatty acids from dietary sources such as fish and marine mammals (Rode et al. 1995).

The rise in blood pressure that is seen in urban populations reflects a progressive decrease in the elasticity of the major blood vessels. There is an atrophy of the elastic lamellae, with both diffuse and focal increases in collagen content. The aorta also becomes progressively larger, and radiographs may show patchy calcification. The more rigid arteries expand less readily to accept the cardiac stroke volume.

The interpretation of blood pressures in older population samples is complicated by selective mortality, an underrepresentation of hypertensive individuals, and an increase in the intraindividual variability of pressures that leads to an age-linked overdiagnosis of hypertension (Forette, Henry, and Hervy 1982). Both the resting pulse pressure and the systolic pressure tend to be higher than in younger subjects. Weisfeldt, Gerstenblith, and Lakatta (1985) noted respective differences of 11 and 18 mmHg between 35- and 71-year-old subjects. In some cross-sectional studies, systolic pressure has continued to increase over the life span (Applegate 1994), but in others the increase has ceased at around 65 years (Miall and Brennan 1981; Whelton 1985).

In addition to the overall increase in resting systolic pressure, there is a change in the shape of the pulse wave with aging. Thus, recordings from the carotid artery show a late augmentation of systolic pressure in older subjects. This is thought to be due to an increase in the magnitude of reflected pressure waves as the arteries become more rigid (Vaitkevicius et al. 1993).

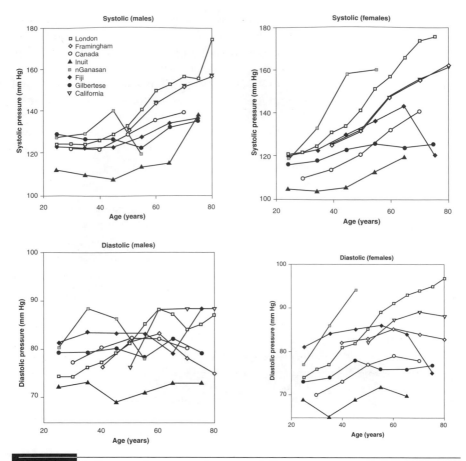

Figure 3.6   Influence of age on various populations.

Submaximal and maximal exercise.   Vigorous rhythmic, isometric, and isokinetic exercise lead to increases of blood pressure in all age groups, but the increase tends to be larger in those with high resting values (Zerzawy 1987). Thus, although old people have a smaller peak stroke volume and peak cardiac output, many reach a higher peak blood pressure than their younger peers during exercise. Whereas a maximum systolic reading of some 180 mmHg (24 kPa) would be anticipated in a young adult performing aerobic exercise, Sidney and Shephard (unpublished data) found average aerobic maxima of 217 ± 38 mmHg (28.9 ± 5.1 kPa) in elderly men and 206 ± 32 mmHg (27.5 ± 4.3 kPa) in elderly women. Incidentally, these figures are substantially higher than the peak systolic pressure of 195 mmHg observed by Weisfeldt, Gerstenblith, and Lakatta (1985) in what they claimed was a near-maximal work rate.

The cardiovascular strain is greater for concentric than for eccentric muscle contractions (Horstmann et al. 1994), concentric activity being associated with larger increases of heart rate, blood pressure, and noradrenaline output. The elderly person who has developed substantial hypertension usually shows a correspondingly greater ventricular hypertrophy than a normotensive senior. In the hypertensive individual, a more rapid fractional shortening usually indicates an increase of systolic function under resting conditions, but the ventricular relaxation time is increased. Moreover, when exercise is undertaken, systolic function deteriorates relative to that of normotensive individuals (Suzuki et al. 1991).

Aging of the Respiratory System

Despite occasional reports that respiratory function can limit the maximal oxygen intake of top athletes (Dempsey, Powers, and Gledhill 1990), the respiratory system, in general, does not appear to limit the performance of aerobic exercise in a young adult (Shephard 1993b). Does respiratory function meet the demands of exercise less adequately in older subjects? We examine this question in terms of anatomical changes in the chest wall, the bronchial tree, the microstructure of the lungs, and the pulmonary vessels, along with related changes in compliance, static lung volumes, pulmonary dynamics, gas exchange, and the oxygen cost of breathing. In general, the respiratory function appears to remain adequate for the needs of exercise in the elderly, despite some increase in ventilatory demand. However, dyspnea becomes more common, and reasons for this are discussed.

Anatomical Changes

The skeletal muscles as a whole undergo extensive wasting as aging develops, but constant recruitment by the breathing process tends to spare the muscles that perform the mechanical work of quiet breathing (Gosselin, Bohlmann, and Thomas 1988). Nevertheless, it has yet to be demonstrated that the accessory muscles recruited for respiration during vigorous exercise also escape age-related wasting. Moreover, aging also brings anatomical changes in the chest wall, bronchi, and pulmonary vessels that have adverse consequences for respiratory function.

Chest Wall

A "barrel-shaped" deformity of the chest wall often develops with aging. There is an increase in the depth of the chest which reflects a loss of or an alteration in the properties of elastic fibers in the lungs (D'Errico et al. 1989). The work required to modify the volume of the thorax is augmented by kyphosis (the "dowager's hump" of osteoporotic older women), a loss of elasticity in the ribs, and a stiffening or even an ankylosis of the joints about which the ribs rotate (Crapo 1993). Age-related alterations in thoracic shape (and in women, a weakness of the abdominal wall with a resulting descent of the diaphragm) adversely affect length-tension relationships for many of the respiratory muscles (Road et al. 1986; Zadai 1985). Breathing thus depends increasingly on diaphragmatic activity (Teramoto et al. 1995).

Bronchial Tree

Aging may lead to some increase in the number and/or size of mucous glands in the bronchial mucosa, although it is hard to draw a line between "normal" changes and effects that should be attributed to chronic bronchitis. There is also a progressive decrease in ciliary function (even in nonsmokers), together with an increased risk of aspiration of food (due to altered swallowing reflexes and impaired coughing; Tockman 1994), and sometimes a deterioration of immune responses (Abbas, Lichtman, and Pober 1995). Taken together, these changes leave the older person increasingly vulnerable to both bacterial and viral infections (Goodwin, Searles, and Tung 1982; Roghmann 1987). Aging does not necessarily increase the intrinsic dimensions of the larger airways at any given alveolar volume, although there is generally some increase of anatomical dead space. A progressive loss of cartilaginous support also leaves the large air passages more vulnerable to collapse during a forceful expiration.

Lung Tissues

Postmortem specimens show a progressive rise in the volume/weight ratio of the lungs at any given inflation pressure (Andreotti et al. 1983). Gross analyses of the lungs may reveal little change in collagen, elastic tissue, or fibrous protein content (Andreotti et al. 1983), but changes of lung elasticity imply a dramatic change in either the location or the properties of the supporting tissues (Davies 1991). In particular, there is a decrease in the number and thickness of the radial alveolar elastic fibers that maintain the patency of both the smaller air passages and the dimensions of the alveoli (D'Errico et al. 1989). The smaller airways thus become progressively narrowed, although the diameter of the terminal alveolar ducts is increased.

The fine structure of the aging lung suggests a rapid disintegration of supporting structures. There is some thickening of the basal membrane, due to an accumulation of type IV collagen and laminin (D'Errico et al. 1989). On the other hand, the overall thickness of the alveolar membrane is decreased. At the same time, alveolar size is increased, and there is a progressive increase in the number and the size of window-like openings (Kohn's pores) that connect adjacent alveoli (Reiser, Hennesy, and Last 1987). Destruction of alveoli and pulmonary capillaries causes the effective functional area of the lungs to decrease from a peak of about 70 m^2 at 20 years of age to 50 to 60 m^2 at 80 years (Thurlbeck 1991).

Elastic forces are reduced with aging (Reiser, Hennesy, and Last 1987; Thurlbeck 1991). Type II alveolar cells show some decrease in the number of lamellar bodies (Shimura, Boatman, and Martin 1986), but the rate of incorporation of ^{3}[H]-palmitic acid into lecithin is unchanged, suggesting little alteration in the production of alveolar surfactant (Dempsey and Seals 1995). The total elastin and collagen content of the lungs is also unchanged, as are the number and size of the elastic fibers (Thurlbeck 1991). By exclusion, the decreased elasticity seems attributable to molecular changes such as an increased cross-linkage of collagen molecules (Reiser, Hennesy, and Last 1987).

Pulmonary Vessels

Aging of the pulmonary arteries is marked by alterations in the structure of the vessel walls, much as in the systemic circulation. Nevertheless, pulmonary pressures are low in young adults, so the magnitude of age-related increases of pressure is generally smaller than in the systemic circulation (Davidson and Fee 1990).

Compliance

The aging process is marked by an increasing stiffness of the chest wall and an opposing loss of elasticity in pulmonary tissue.

Chest Wall Compliance

By the age of 60 years, the elastic resistance of the chest is double that of a young adult. It is probable that the viscous resistance of the chest wall also increases with age, although here precise statistics are needed. In consequence, older people make increasing use of the diaphragm, particularly when emptying the lungs to less than functional residual capacity (Teramoto et al. 1995). By the eighth decade of life, changes of chest circumference account for only about a quarter of the resting tidal volume, and for an even smaller fraction of exercise ventilation.

Lung Compliance

Elastic tissue is lost progressively from the tissues of the aging lung. In consequence, pulmonary compliance increases (Cotes 1993; Murray 1981). The greater compliance of the lungs leads in turn to an increase of residual volume, with a corresponding decrease in the expiratory reserve volume (the difference between the functional residual capacity and the residual volume).

Because of the subtle shading from normality into chronic chest disease, it remains unclear whether the loss of pulmonary elastic tissue should be regarded as an intrinsic effect of aging. A substantial fraction of the functional loss is commonly due to cigarette smoking (Adair 1994), prior respiratory disease (Rode and Shephard 1994a, 1996), and exposure to air pollutants (observed by Shephard and Lavalleé [in press] and Rokaw et al. [1980], but not by Buist et al. [1979]). In some populations, there are also cohort effects (for example, when making observations on an isolated Inuit community, Rode and Shephard [1994a] noted the distortion of cross-sectional data by the aging of a cohort with extensive respiratory disease).

There may thus be substantial differences in the apparent rate of aging between cross-sectional and longitudinal studies (McClaran et al. 1995; Vollmer et al. 1988; Ware et al. 1990), even when observations are compared over the same age range. Nevertheless, there is good evidence that healthy, physically active nonsmokers who have been exposed to only low concentrations of air pollutants (including environmental cigarette smoke) either in their occupation or in their leisure time show a much smaller cumulative loss of lung function than other members of the same population with a less favorable life history.

Static Lung Volumes

As a person ages, there is a decrease in vital capacity that is roughly matched by an increase in residual lung volume, so that there is little change in total lung capacity (Burrows et al. 1986; Cotes 1993). The functional residual capacity also shows little change (Cotes 1993; Culver and Butler 1985; Murray 1981).

Vital Capacity

Many of the commonly used equations for the prediction of lung volumes have assumed a linear loss of function over the span of adult life, continuing steadily from 20 to 60, 65, or even 70 years of age (Cotes 1993). However, the early studies of Anderson et al. (1968) demonstrated that vital capacity and related volumes continued to increase until the subject reached an age of about 24 years. There is then a relatively linear loss of function through middle age, with an accelerating decrease of lung volumes in the final years of life (McClaran et al. 1995). Thus, data are not well represented by a regression equation that assumes a linear loss throughout adult life.

Anderson et al. (1968) found that although smoking influenced the age-related rate of loss of vital capacity significantly, the effect of this variable disappeared if subjects with a history of chronic respiratory disease were excluded from the analysis. Their data are compatible with the view that although smoking has a cumulative adverse effect upon the elastic tissue of the lungs, much of its impact is concentrated in a genetically vulnerable segment of the population who lack alpha-1-antitrypsins and are thus particularly vulnerable to chronic chest disease. When subjects with chest disease were excluded from their analysis, Anderson et al. (1968) found that the annual loss of vital capacity was only 17.4 ml/year in men and 10.5 ml/year in women.

At least one-half of the gender difference in aging rate could be explained by the shorter stature of the female subjects. The residual difference may have arisen from an effect of smoking in those who were free of chest disease, since until fairly recently smoking has been more common among men than among women.

Most studies on the aging of vital capacity have been cross-sectional in type, with resulting complications from cohort effects and other artifacts (McClaran et al. 1995; Rode and Shephard 1994a; Vollmer et al. 1988; Ware et al. 1990). The older portion of a typical cross-sectional sample differs from the younger subjects in smoking history (the proportion of smokers, the age at which smoking began and/or ceased, and the type of cigarettes consumed). Those who were born 60 to 80 years ago also lived a substantial part of their lives before the introduction of modern antibiotics. They thus had a much greater chance of developing lung damage from acute episodes of respiratory disease. Finally, vital capacity tends to be a cubic function of stature (Shephard 1982c), so the fitting of linear regressions based on age and height may not be appropriate to the analysis of cross-sectional data that cover a period when adult height has been increasing by 10 mm/decade.

Keeping in mind the limitations of cross-sectional results, one may note that the aging of vital capacity in six studies of urban men, mostly aged 20 to 65 years, averaged 24.4 ml/year. In 13 assorted ethnic populations who were living in remote regions with little exposure to air pollutants, the loss was surprisingly similar (an average of 25.4 ml/year, Shephard 1978a). The consequences of this loss for ventilatory function and the sensation of dyspnea are discussed later in this section.

Residual Volume

Most of the age-related increase of residual volume reflects an expansion of the alveolar space. One disadvantage of a large resting alveolar gas volume is that its gas composition changes only slowly in response to an increase of ventilation. The alveolar oxygen pressure of an old person thus climbs more slowly at the beginning of exercise, with a potentially negative influence on the time course of the oxygen intake on-transient (Babcock et al. 1994). Greater practical importance attaches to indirect functional consequences of the enlarged chest volume: a decrease in mechanical efficiency of the chest muscles, a reduction of vital capacity, and a resulting tendency to dyspnea during exercise.

An increase of residual volume has only a small direct impact upon the steady state gas exchange of a young old person (age range 65 to 75 years), even during vigorous exercise. To the extent that the expansion of residual volume occurs in the terminal alveolar ducts rather than in the alveoli proper, there is an increase in series dead space; this slows diffusional mixing between inspired air and alveolar gas.

Pulmonary Dynamics

The ability to develop large air flows during exercise depends on such factors as the strength of the chest muscles, any voluntary inhibition of their contraction, and the impedance presented by compliance, airway resistance, and collapse of the airways.

Respiratory Muscle Performance

Wasting of the accessory muscles may reduce peak respiratory forces, thereby limiting the peak, effort-dependent portion of ventilation. Further, the weakened muscles may develop earlier fatigue if ventilatory demand is sustained over a prolonged bout of exercise.

Empirical data generally show that the peak ventilatory pressures that a person can develop diminish with age, but there is much interindividual variation. In the report of McElvaney et al. (1989), the average difference between young adults and 70-year-olds was not statistically significant. In another study of very fit 69-year-old patients (maximal oxygen intake 204% of age-predicted norms!), there was no decrease of peak inspiratory pressures when such individuals carried out 3 min of all-out exercise (Johnson, Reddan, Pegelow, et al. 1991; Johnson, Reddan, Scow, et al. 1991).

There remains a need to test the ability of more typical older people to develop peak pressures over substantial time periods.

Voluntary Inhibition of Contraction

The sensations reported by the respiratory muscles as they contract depend on an appropriate balance between the change in muscle length and the resulting change in muscle tension. An age-related decrease in the strength of the respiratory muscles and an increase in the impedance to ventilation are likely to augment tension, thereby increasing the sensation of effort for a given ventilation.

Airway Impedance and Collapse

The thickening of the mucosal lining in the smaller air passages and the decrease of thoracic compliance tend to narrow the small air passages of an older person. This increases the resistance to both inspiratory and expiratory airflow (Johnson, Reddan, Scow et al. 1991). It also augments the pressure gradient from the lungs to the extrathoracic portion of the airway for any given flow rate. Collapse of the airway occurs if the pressure gradient from the alveoli to the larger bronchi substantially exceeds the opposing force offered by the elastic recoil of the lung tissues.

Aging progressively increases the likelihood that a person who exercises vigorously will reach the effort-independent portion of the expiratory flow/volume curve, where more forceful expiratory efforts cause a collapse of the airways without augmenting airflow (Johnson and Dempsey 1991). The increase of end-expiratory lung volume expands the airways, partially offsetting the trend to airway collapse, but this advantage is won at the cost of a considerable decrease in the mechanical efficiency of the inspiratory muscles. The overall dynamic compliance also decreases, since the older subject tends to use the less compliant part of the pressure/volume curve (near maximal inspiration) during tidal breathing.

Dynamic Lung Volumes

The narrowed airways and expiratory collapse of the air passages lead to an age-related decrease in various indexes of dynamic function such as the maximal voluntary ventilation, the peak expiratory flow rate, and the 1 sec forced expiratory volume (Anderson et al. 1968; Cotes 1993; Dempsey and Seals 1995). Aging is commonly linked to a larger loss of 1 sec forced expiratory volume than of vital capacity (Burr, Phillips, and Hurst 1985; Coe et al. 1989). Thus, the proportion of the vital capacity that can be expelled in 1 sec drops from 82% to 86% in a young adult to 75% to 79% by the age of 65 years (Shephard 1978a). As with forced vital capacity, the aging of the 1 sec forced expiratory volume is exacerbated by exposure to tobacco smoke and other air pollutants. But even nonsmokers living in an area where air pollution is light show a steady loss of the 1 sec volume over the span of working life (about 32 ml/ year in men and 25 ml/year in women; Burrows et al. 1986; Knudson et al. 1983; Tager et al. 1988).

When the dynamic lung volumes observed at an age of 65 years are expressed as a percentage of young adult values, losses are seen to be similar to the age-related decrease in maximal oxygen intake. Pulmonary dynamics thus seem no more likely to limit oxygen transport in the healthy young old person than in a young adult. Nevertheless, the margin of ventilatory reserve is small. Johnson and Dempsey (1991) noted that fit 70-year-old subjects reached their limiting expiratory flow rate over 40% to 90% of the vital capacity range, and many of their subjects were unable to increase ventilation further if the inspired carbon dioxide concentration was deliberately increased while they were exercising maximally.

Gas Exchange

Aging hampers gas exchange through an impaired distribution of inspired gas, with a worsening of alveolar ventilation and pulmonary diffusion, and an increase in alveolar-arterial pressure gradients.

Gas Distribution

By the age of 65 years, airway closure occurs over at least a quarter of the vital capacity range (Cotes 1993; Tockman 1994). For hydrostatic reasons, closure restricts ventilation mainly in the dependent parts of the lungs. Unfortunately, a large fraction of the total pulmonary blood flow is distributed to the lower third of the lungs, also for hydrostatic reasons. Thus, airway collapse leads to a progressive worsening of the matching between ventilation and perfusion of the lungs, with an increase in the alveolar component of pulmonary dead space (Dempsey and Seals 1995).

In part because of airway closure, and in part because of patchy changes in lung compliance and airflow resistance, the distribution of an inspired breath of oxygen, xenon, or krypton becomes progressively less uniform as age increases. However, observations concerning gas distribution have generally been made under resting conditions, and the findings do not necessarily apply to vigorous exercise.

As tidal volume is increased by exercise, a greater volume of air becomes directed to the lower part of the lungs, and there is a corresponding decrease in the vertical nonuniformity of ventilation (Shephard 1982c). Nevertheless, exercise also increases the respiratory rate, and it may become so rapid that there is no longer adequate time for gas to diffuse from the terminal alveolar ducts into the alveolar space proper. Such a problem is particularly likely to occur in an elderly person, since gas mixing is hampered by an age-related expansion of the terminal alveolar ducts and an inhomogeneity of time constants for the ventilation of individual alveolar spaces. Thus, although vigorous exercise usually reduces the vertical nonuniformity of ventilation due to airway closure, it may increase the extent of nonuniformity in the horizontal axis (Shephard 1982c).

Alveolar Ventilation

Aging usually leads to some increase in the anatomical dead space of the conducting airways. Cotes (1993) has estimated the increase in bronchial volume at 10 ml/decade. However, this change is small relative to the increase of physiological dead space that arises from airway closure, expansion of the terminal alveolar ducts, a slow equilibration of gas between the airways and the alveolar spaces, and a poor matching of ventilation with perfusion.

The age-related loss of pulmonary capillaries leaves a large number of alveolar spaces ventilated but poorly perfused, and this inevitably increases the physiological dead space. A small increase of pulmonary arterial pressure may improve perfusion of the apical regions of the lungs, but marked pulmonary hypertension (as seen in some emphysematous patients) restricts peak pulmonary blood flow, further worsening the match between alveolar ventilation and perfusion.

In view of these various problems, a substantial worsening of the normal matching of ventilation and perfusion might be anticipated in elderly subjects (Davies 1991). In practice, the resting ventilation/perfusion ratios for healthy old people are surprisingly normal. Johnson and Dempsey (1991) suggested that under resting conditions, the overall dead space/tidal volume ratio was 15% to 20% larger in elderly subjects, but that even this handicap diminished progressively during exercise. Derks (1980) reported that in vigorous exercise, alveolar ventilation was some 70% of external ventilation, as compared with 75% to 80% in a young adult.

Pulmonary Diffusion

Pulmonary diffusion $(\dot{D}_L)$ depends on both the diffusing capacity of the pulmonary membrane $(\dot{D}_m)$ and the product of the pulmonary capillary blood volume (V_c) and a hemoglobin reaction constant (Θ):

$$1/\dot{D}_L = 1/\dot{D}_m + 1/(\Theta)V_c.$$

Resting values for $\dot{D}_m$ decrease after 40 years of age, and there is also a decrease of V_c because pulmonary capillaries have been destroyed. Expressing $\dot{D}_L$ in traditional units, the annual loss of diffusing capacity is about 0.15 ml/min per mmHg (Horvath and Borgia 1984). As with many other body functions, there is thus a cumulative loss of about 25% over the span of working life.

The change corresponds roughly with the decrease in functional area of the gas exchanging surface (Thurlbeck 1991), although a part of the deterioration of gas exchange is probably due to a poor distribution of inspired gas rather than to a loss of alveolar surface. Because exercise increases the uniformity of both ventilation and perfusion, healthy and relatively fit 65-year-old subjects show little loss of maximal diffusing capacity, and as will be noted in the next section, arterial oxygen saturation is generally well maintained during maximal exercise.

Alveolar-Arterial Pressure Gradients

In most young adults, there is almost no gradient of oxygen partial pressure between the alveolar spaces and arterial blood. Paradoxically, equilibration is poorer in top-level endurance athletes. Such individuals sometimes develop a significant alveolar-arterial pressure gradient during vigorous exercise because blood passes so rapidly through some of their capillaries that it does not have time to equilibrate with alveolar gas (Dempsey, Powers, and Gledhill 1990).

It might be thought that the age-related decrease in the pulmonary capillary bed would exacerbate the problem of incomplete equilibration, but in practice this is generally offset by a smaller peak cardiac output in older individuals. Thus, the time available for equilibration does not decrease very much with age. Johnson and Dempsey (1991) found that the resting alveolar-arterial oxygen partial pressure gradient of fit 70-year-old subjects was only 2 to 5 mmHg greater than their values for young adults. Even during maximal exercise, only 4 of the 19 elderly subjects had an arterial oxygen pressure of less than 75 mmHg, or an arterial oxygen saturation of less than 92%.

As in younger subjects, the continuing athletes are the elderly group who are at some risk of a reduction in oxygen saturation during vigorous exercise (Préfaut et al. 1994).

Work of Breathing

The magnitude of the work of breathing depends upon ventilatory demand and the mechanical efficiency of the chest bellows.

Ventilatory Demand

The sensitivity of the respiratory centers to stimuli such as carbon dioxide and lack of oxygen may diminish by as much as 50% relative to that of a young adult (Dill, Hillyard, and Miller 1980), but nevertheless the resting respiratory minute volume changes little with age.

During submaximal exercise, in contrast, the ventilation per unit of external work seems to increase by 3% to 5% per year (McConnell and Davies 1992). Many factors augment the ventilatory demand of an old person. The oxygen cost of a given activity is increased, as we will note in the next section. There is a greater accumulation of lactate during submaximal work, due to the slower increase of oxygen consumption at the beginning of exercise (Babcock et al. 1994). There is also a poorer myocardial contractility, weaker skeletal muscles, and an impaired peripheral circulation. Finally, there is a reduction in the mechanical efficiency of the chest bellows.

In contrast, the respiratory minute volumes observed during maximal aerobic effort are less than in a younger person, perhaps because limiting expiratory flow rates have been reached (Dempsey and Seals 1995).

Oxygen Cost of External Work

The oxygen cost of skeletal muscle contraction during most forms of external work is increased by joint stiffness, poor motor coordination, increased body sway, and/or a lack of recent familiarity with the activity in question. This decreases mechanical efficiency. For example, we have noted that the net mechanical efficiency of cycle ergometry drops from 23% in a young adult to 21.5% in a 65-year-old. The total oxygen cost of physical activity is increased further in an old person because of the augmentation in respiratory work, as will be seen in the section that follows. The age-related rise of systemic blood pressure also causes some increase in the oxygen consumption of the heart relative to findings in a younger individual.

Mechanical Efficiency of Chest Bellows

Factors reducing the efficiency of ventilation in an older person include distortion of the rib cage by kyphosis and a barrel-shaped deformity, adoption of a smaller tidal volume with a more rapid respiratory rate, an increase in both airflow resistance and tissue resistance, a shift of ventilation to the mechanically unfavorable high-volume portion of the pressure/volume diagram, and an expiratory collapse of the airway (Johnson and Dempsey 1991). Ventilation is also increased to compensate (in a more or less direct fashion) for the increase of anatomical and physiological dead space.

Oxygen Cost of Respiratory Work

The age-related increase in rigidity of the thoracic cage is largely offset by a greater compliance in the lung tissues, so that there is little change in the elastic work performed during the breathing cycle. However, the work of ventilation is increased in an older person owing to a narrowing and/or collapse of the larger airways. Johnson and Dempsey (1991) estimated that whereas the chest muscles consumed only 6% of maximal oxygen intake in a young adult, the oxygen cost of breathing accounted for 13% of maximal oxygen intake in a fit 70-year-old man. Most old people are far from fit, and many have developed some emphysema. This quickly increases the oxygen cost of breathing 10- to 20-fold relative to that for a healthy person of similar age.

Prevalence of Dyspnea

Complaints of dyspnea are frequent when an older adult undertakes vigorous exercise, and respiratory sensations often become a significant determinant of the peak oxygen transport that is attained. However, it is less clear how far the increase in reported breathlessness has an anatomical or physiological basis, and how far it reflects simply a lack of recent familiarity with vigorous exercise. We will examine this question in terms of the dyspnea threshold and the resulting ventilatory comfort of an elderly person during vigorous exercise.

Dyspnea Threshold

Depending upon the subject's motivation and experience, unpleasant dyspnea develops at a tidal volume somewhere between 33% and 75% of vital capacity (Killian 1987; Killian and Jones 1988; Shephard 1987b).

The dyspnea threshold seems just as variable in fit 70-year-old men as in younger individuals (43% to 86% of vital capacity; Johnson, Reddan, Pegelow, et al. 1991; Johnson, Reddan, Scow, et al. 1991). Muscle weakness and a large functional residual capacity are likely to induce dyspnea at a reduced fraction of vital capacity in many seniors (Jones 1984). But even if the average elderly person remained able to use 50% of a vital capacity of 4.4 L, the peak tidal volume would still be limited to 2.2 L. Moreover, if the peak respiratory rate remained at 40 breaths/min, as in a younger person, then dyspnea might be expected at a respiratory minute volume of 88 L/min.

Implications for Oxygen Transport

If we assume a ventilatory equivalent of 30 L/L during maximal effort, then a respiratory minute volume of 88 L/min would permit an oxygen intake of 2.93 L/min, about 38 ml/[kg · min] in a man weighing 77 kg. Such a figure is slightly above the peak oxygen intake that is commonly observed at 65 years of age (see fig. 3.7). Thus, the vital capacity and the associated dyspnea threshold should not impose a major limitation on oxygen transport in a person of this age.

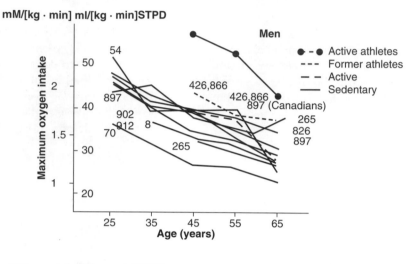

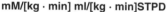

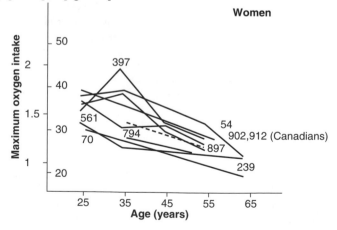

Figure 3.7   Changes in maximal oxygen intake with age.

Reprinted, by permission, from R.J. Shephard, 1987, *Physical activity and aging*, 2d ed. (London: Croom Helm). See original publication for sources of individual data sets.

In some situations, the ventilatory equivalent may exceed 30 L/L, bringing the elderly person closer to the dyspnea threshold. The increase of ventilatory equivalent reflects such factors as weakness of the skeletal muscles, an early accumulation of hydrogen ions, a poor distribution of inspired gas, and an enlargement of both the anatomical and the physiological dead space. During treadmill exercise, researchers in our laboratory found values of only 25.2 L/L in men and 27.4 L/L in women aged 65 years. However, when the same subjects exercised on a cycle ergometer, values rose to 34.0 L/L in men and 33.9 L/L in women. Johnson and Dempsey (1991) also found values as large as 38 L/L.

Let us now consider the case of a person who has reached the age of 85 years. The peak ventilatory equivalent has risen to perhaps 35 L/L. The vital capacity has also diminished by perhaps 70 ml/year between 65 and 85 years of age. Thus, the average vital capacity, even in a healthy 85-year-old, is no more than 3.0 L. If such a person were able and prepared to utilize 50% of his or her vital capacity for breathing, the peak respiratory minute volume would still not exceed 60 L/min, and the sensation of dyspnea would restrict oxygen transport to a peak of perhaps 1.71 L/min, or 22 ml/[kg · min]. At this stage in life, dyspnea thus becomes an important factor limiting exercise tolerance, even in a relatively healthy individual.

Factors Exacerbating Dyspnea

In practice, shortness of breath may limit exercise performance before a person reaches the age of 85 years, particularly if the individual uses a large fraction of his or her maximal inspiratory pressure in order to perform the test exercise (Johnson and Dempsey 1991).

Factors exacerbating the tendency to dyspnea include not only an increase of the ventilatory equivalent of oxygen, but also alterations in respiratory perceptions. Feelings of breathlessness are linked to a lack of recent experience of vigorous ventilation, weakness of the thoracic musculature, a poor mechanical advantage associated with the barrel-shaped chest, a collapse of the airways during vigorous expiratory efforts, and an alteration of sensory input or central neuronal processing linked to stiffening of the rib cage and an overall increase in the impedance to breathing.

Overall Metabolic Response to Exercise

To this point, we have considered mainly steady state cardiac and respiratory responses to aerobic exercise. However, with advancing age, a longer time is required for heart rate, blood pressure, and ventilation to attain equilibrium at any given power output (Babcock et al. 1994; Paterson, Cunningham, and Babcock 1989). In part, this reflects a deterioration in control mechanisms. Beta-receptors become less responsive to both agonist and antagonist drugs, and there are decreased responses to a Valsalva maneuver, facial immersion, and tilting (Lakatta 1993a).

The maximum power output decreases with age, so that at any given work rate an older person operates closer to his or her anaerobic threshold than someone who is younger. Finally, because fitness levels are low, the recovery period following exercise is prolonged. An increased proportion of the energy requirements of a given task are met by anaerobic metabolism, and metabolic heat is also eliminated more slowly than in a young person.

The great majority of published data (see fig. 3.7) show the maximal oxygen intake declining progressively with age, whether the data be expressed in absolute units (L/min) or relative to body mass (ml/[kg · min]). However, because aging is often associated with an increase of body fat content, the change becomes larger if it is expressed in relative units. It is also arguable that a part of the apparent decline in aerobic power reflects either unwillingness of the elderly person to reach a high intensity of effort, or an age-related decline in habitual physical activity and thus a loss of physical condition. Jackson et al. (1995) have estimated by multiple regression techniques that as much as half of the age-related loss of aerobic power is attributable to an accumulation of fat and a decrease of habitual physical activity.

The ideal criterion of maximal effort in a young adult is the attainment of an oxygen consumption plateau (an increase in oxygen consumption of less than 0.15 L/min with a further increase in power output). As maximal oxygen intake declines, this criterion necessarily reflects a growing fraction of an individual's maximal performance. Moreover, it becomes difficult to attain such a plateau in senior citizens. Particularly during cycle ergometry, a test may be halted by muscular exhaustion before the subject has reached a plateau of oxygen transport. Nevertheless, in our experience, three-fourths of healthy 65-year-old subjects reach an oxygen consumption plateau during their first treadmill test, and half of the remaining subjects are able to do so if they are allowed a second attempt. We found that in men who made a good maximal effort, final heart rates averaged 172 beats/min and blood lactate concentration early during the recovery period averaged 11.1 mmol/L. However, a low peak heart rate, a low respiratory gas exchange ratio, and (when measured) a low peak blood lactate point to a less satisfactory realization of maximal effort in the data sets obtained by some investigators.

Despite these problems, and substantial intersample differences in the mean level of maximal oxygen transport, cross-sectional data are consistent in showing that by the age of 65 years, aerobic power is 30% to 40% less than the young adult value in both sexes (see fig. 3.7). Expressed in relative units, the rate of loss in men averages 420 to 520 µl/[kg · min] per year, beginning around the age of 20 years. In women, the loss is 500 to 700 µl/[kg · min] per year, but the loss of function does not begin until as late as 35 years of age. Possibly the physical activity involved in caring for young children keeps young adult women from a deterioration of physical condition.

Estimates of loss based on longitudinal data are more variable; some greatly exceed the cross-sectional change, but others show almost no loss. Problems in the longitudinal data sets commonly include a small sample size, a relatively brief period of observation, and a correspondingly greater vulnerability to a change in habitual physical activity patterns subsequent to initial testing.

Further information on maximal oxygen intake and the changes induced by training is presented in chapter 4.

Visceral Functions

Age-related changes in the function of the gastrointestinal tract, the liver, and the kidneys all have important implications for energy reserves, synthesis of lean tissue, and the maintenance of fluid and nutritional balance during exercise.

Gastrointestinal Tract

Loss of the sensation of taste (Chauhan et al. 1987), lack of teeth (Carlos and Wolfe 1989), weakness of the orofacial muscles, physical problems limiting the ability to cook, and poverty and solitude (Chernoff and Silver 1993) are all possible factors that restrict the preparation and ingestion of food in the very old, although there is little good evidence that a decreased intake of food impairs physical performance.

The motor activity of the esophagus is poorly coordinated in the elderly, and sudden body movements may cause a reflux of the gastric contents (Minaker and Rowe 1982; Young and Urban 1986). The gastric emptying time is also prolonged in an older person (Horowitz et al. 1984; Moore et al. 1983), reducing the volume of fluids that can usefully be ingested when one is exercising under hot conditions. Colonic movements tend to become sluggish, particularly in those seniors who have limited mobility (Young and Urban 1986), but conversely, colonic function can be enhanced by a moderate exercise program. Poor function of the anal sphincters causes incontinence in an increasing proportion of the very old, and vigorous exercise can sometimes exacerbate this trend.

Aging is associated with a decreased production of a number of the enzymes that aid in the digestion of food: salivary ptyalin, gastric fluid and histamine, and pancreatic amylase and trypsin. Most nutrients continue to be well absorbed from the gut. Nevertheless, carbohydrate absorption is slowed (Feibusch and Holt 1982; Mayersohn 1982), and in the very old there may be an impaired absorption of iron (Young and Urban 1986), calcium (Gunby and Morley 1995), vitamin B1 (Kohrs and Czajka-Narins 1986), and vitamin B12 (Bidlack and Wang 1995), with implications for hemoglobin level and bone health.

Liver

The liver undergoes a substantial reduction in mass from age 60 to age 90 years, but in the absence of heart failure or alcoholism, hepatic function seems only marginally affected (Morris et al. 1991); any changes do not seem to influence exercise performance.

Kidneys

The kidneys reach their maximal size in early adulthood and show an accelerating decrease of mass after the age of 50 years. By the age of 80 years, the total renal mass averages only 70% of the young adult peak value (McLachlan 1987). Nevertheless, when assessing whether such a loss has occurred in an elderly exerciser, it is difficult to dissociate the effects of local ischemia and renal infections from the normal aging process (Cox, Macias-Nunez, and Dowd 1991). Moreover, when assessing function, one must take account of the overall decline in lean body mass and peak aerobic power. Thus, residual renal function usually remains adequate to meet the demands of a smaller peak rate of muscle metabolism until the senior reaches an advanced age.

The loss of renal tissue is accompanied by an obliteration of glomeruli, a reduction in the number of glomerular capillary loops, and a progressive deletion of entire nephron units. By the age of 80 years, renal blood flow is only 50% of the young adult peak. The glomerular filtration rate shows at least a parallel decline. The elderly person thus has increasing difficulty in correcting the disturbances of mineral (Macias, Bondia, and Rodriguez-Commes 1987; Suderam and Manikar 1983) and water balance (Bengele et al. 1981) that may arise when exercising in a hot environment. Correction of an acidosis also takes longer than it would in a younger person (Macias et al. 1983).

Aging of the Nervous System

The vast literature on aging of the central nervous system has been well reviewed in the context of physical activity (Ostrow 1989; Spirduso 1995). This section provides brief highlights of issues important to the performance of physical activity. Age-related changes in overall cerebral function, vision, hearing, and other senses are first discussed. A slowing of reactions is noted, and such possible causes as cell death, impaired cerebral perfusion, and an altered secretion of and sensitivity to neurotransmitters are explored. Further sections provide an overview of impaired gait, tremor, impaired balance, and falls. Finally, the overall perception of effort is examined.

Cerebral Function

Disturbances of overall cerebral function in the elderly person are shown by alterations of electrical activity, by decreases in memory, cognition, and learning capability, and by disturbed sleep patterns.

Electrical Activity

The alpha rhythm of the electroencephalogram slows from a speed of perhaps 10 Hz in a young adult to 8 to 9 Hz in the elderly, with a parallel increase in slow delta- and theta-wave activity. Loss of alpha waves and foci of rapid waves seem to be associated with loss of memory and impaired learning.

Visual and auditory evoked potentials recorded from the scalp show increases in both latency and amplitude, and a greater homogeneity across recording sites. Possibly there is more synchrony of discharge in an older person because there are fewer competing channels of information, or it may be that there is less inhibition of the cerebral response.

Memory, Cognition, and Learning Capacity

Many aspects of memory, cognition, and information processing deteriorate with age (Birren, Woods, and Williams 1980; Charness 1991). The recognition component of long-term memory is relatively well preserved, but there are difficulties in retrieving information from this store (Benham and Heston 1989). The short-term memory and short-term sensory store develop progressively larger deficits as age increases (Abourezk 1989; Salthouse 1982).

The pace of learning becomes slower in an old person, and a more single-minded approach leads to a reduction in learning of the peripheral elements of a task. The extent of functional loss can be illustrated by such measures as the chess performance of grand masters, which commonly peaks around 35 years of age.

Factors contributing to poor cerebral performance include not only conditions such as Alzheimer's disease but also a limited educational level, a lack of recent practice of specialized sensory and motor skills, a slowing in perceptual speed that is probably related to a deterioration of the special senses (Schaie 1989), a depression of mood state, a slowing in the synthesis of memory-specific peptides (McGeer and McGeer 1980), cardiovascular disease, the administration of sedative drugs, and changing levels of habitual physical activity (Poitrenaud et al. 1994). Cross-sectional studies suggest a strong association between cognitive neuropsychological performance and the level of habitual physical activity (Clarkson-Smith and Hartley 1989, 1990; Dustman, Emmerson, and Shearer 1994).

Sleep

Aging leads to both subjective and objective changes in sleep patterns (Buysse et al. 1991). Old people commonly take a long time to fall asleep. They also spend less total time asleep and are usually light sleepers, rousing more easily than a younger individual (Morgan 1987; Zepelin, McDonald, and Zammit 1984); deep, slow-wave sleep is increasingly replaced by shallow, stage 2 sleep. Because of problems such as nocturia, they may have to get out of bed more frequently than would a younger person, and they often waken very early in the morning (Mulder and Härmä 1992; Shaver, Giblin, and Paulsen 1991). Other pathological causes of sleep disturbance include anxiety and depression, various sources of pain, respiratory and cardiovascular disease, sleep apnea, and nocturnal muscle spasms (Spiegel, Azcona, and Morgan 1991). However, the quality of a senior's sleep can probably be enhanced by an increase in physical and mental effort during the day (Horne 1988).

Possibly as a corollary of the sleep disturbance, the amplitude of circadian rhythms decreases with age (van Gool and Mirmiran 1986). Beginning around the age of 40 years, the older worker experiences increasing difficulty in adapting to the demands of shift work (Härmä and Hakola 1992) and finds a reduced capacity to compensate for any accumulated sleep loss (Webb 1981).

Vision

Aging is associated with a progressive deterioration in various aspects of vision, many of which tend to limit the range and extent of physical activities and the performance attained (Makris et al. 1993). There is a reduction in the visual field, difficulty in focusing upon near objects (a lack of accommodation), and a steady diminution of visual acuity (Graham 1991; Stelmach and Worringham 1985). A substantial minority of the elderly population reach the legal definition of blindness, and most of the remainder need to wear some type of glasses. Weakness of vision in one eye, impaired proprioceptor function in the eye muscles, and poor retinal focusing lead to a deterioration of spectroscopic vision in many seniors. These various impairments lead to difficulty in distinguishing colors (particularly at night), an impaired performance of tasks that depend on visual skills, and a greater risk of collision with external objects.

Shrinkage of the visual field is caused in part by mechanical factors. Drooping of the upper eyelid (senile ptosis) restricts vision in an upward direction, while loss of fat from the rear of the eye socket causes a sunken eyeball, limiting vision in all directions. These external changes may be exacerbated by a pathological distortion of the retina itself, associated with an increase of intraocular pressure (glaucoma).

The near point at which small objects can be brought into focus increases from around 0.1 m for a young adult to 0.5 m for a person aged 50 years and 1 m for a person 70 years of age. The rate of accommodation of the eye to a change of focal length is also slower in an old person. Difficulties of refraction are compounded by an increase in the anteroposterior diameter of the lens, a yellowing of the lens substance, corneal astigmatism, an uneven refraction of light associated with the loss of retro-orbital fat, and an increased scattering of light both in the lens and in the vitreous fluid (Michaels 1994).

The cross-sectional area of the pupil is greatly reduced in an old person because of rigidity and atrophy of the iris. The ability of light to penetrate the eye is further diminished by changes in the optical properties of the lens, and the development of opacities in the vitreous fluid. The chemical constituents of the lens appear to be vulnerable to oxidation by superoxides, and changes can thus be minimized by a large intake of ascorbic acid, vitamin E, and other antioxidants (Graham 1991). Floaters in the vitreous fluid are commonly produced by sudden jarring movements that tear the posterior surface of the vitreous from the optic disk (Graham 1991). By the age of 60 years, the retina receives only about one-third as much white light and one-ninth as much blue light as in a young adult.

Hearing

Auditory acuity decreases with aging (Mills 1991). Often an old person has a poorer ability to understand speech than might be inferred from pure tone audiometry (Mills 1991). This leads to withdrawal of the senior from all types of social events, including those that generate physical activity.

Some investigators have ascribed a major part of hearing loss to environmental noise. This can be an important factor in certain industries, particularly if adequate ear protection is not worn; but in general, intrinsic age-related changes seem to be more important (Davis 1987). Effects from a thickening and loss of elasticity in the eardrum and from impaired articulation of the ossicles of the middle ear are small, but larger adverse effects stem from a progressive loss of receptor nerve cells in Corti's organ, a decrease of elasticity in the vibrating partition in the cochlea, damage to the auditory nerve, and a deterioration of function in the brainstem nuclei or the auditory cortex. Only about 1.6% of young adults have a significant hearing impairment, but by the age of retirement 12% to 30% of the population are affected, and by the age of 80 years more than 50% of people have a substantial hearing impairment. A hypersensitivity to sound (loudness recruitment) may also develop, so that noisy conversation or loud music for gymnastics class may cause annoyance and even pain.

The old person has particular difficulty in detecting high-frequency sounds (Moller 1981) and in distinguishing a true signal from random "noise." A part of the latter is generated internally in the auditory pathway (the sensation of tinnitus, a ringing or buzzing in the ears; Coles 1981). As a consequence of these various changes, the auditory reaction time increases, and the affected individual has difficulty in detecting the direction from which a sound originates.

Other Sense Organs

Age leads to a loss of function in many other sense organs, and these changes contribute to the progressive deterioration in skilled motor performance.

There is a decrease in the number of touch receptors, the Pacinian corpuscles, and Krause end-organs of the skin, as well as a degeneration of the associated nerve fibers. In consequence, there is a progressive deterioration in sensitivity to light touch. The loss of peripheral sensation is exacerbated by atherosclerosis and by alcoholic or diabetic neuropathies. Clinical evidence of greater vulnerability to hypo- and hyperthermia suggests that the sensitivity of receptors responding to heat and cold also decreases with advancing years. On the other hand, the pain threshold is unchanged, at least in the healthy older adult.

The proprioceptive organs in and around the joints have a diminished ability to detect small displacements of the limbs. Tests in which the subject is required to duplicate a forced movement are also performed less accurately, because function of the muscle proprioceptors is impaired.

Reaction Speed and Central Processing

The speed of response to signals (a combination of reaction speed and movement time) decreases progressively with aging (see fig. 3.8). The slowing of response is particularly marked if the subject must make generalizations, undertake a complex task (Lupinacci et al. 1993), or must distinguish between several competing signals (Charness 1991; Era, Jokela, and Heikkinen 1986; Stelmach 1994). Tasks that require effortful processing seem particularly sensitive to personal fitness (Chodzo-Zajko 1991).

Often the inherent loss of function with aging is exacerbated by an excessive use of depressant medications (Jarvik and Neshkes 1985), hormonal disturbances (Lavis 1981), or nutritional deficiencies (particularly a lack of B vitamins). In contrast, the slowing of reaction speed is sometimes less obvious in active individuals who have maintained or developed a large aerobic power (Era, Jokela, and Heikkinen 1986; Whitehurst 1991). Tasks with a heavy visuospatial demand seem particularly well preserved in the fit individual (Shay and Roth 1992).

Site of Slowed Responses

A slowing of nerve conduction accounts for no more than 4% of the deterioration in response times as a person ages. There is also some slowing of movement time (Wright and Shephard 1978) due to such factors as joint stiffness and a loss of muscle power. However, the main site of the slow response of an older person is within the brain, where there is a progressive decrease in the ability to process information and complete such operations as coding, retrieval, comparison, and selection (Spirduso 1995).

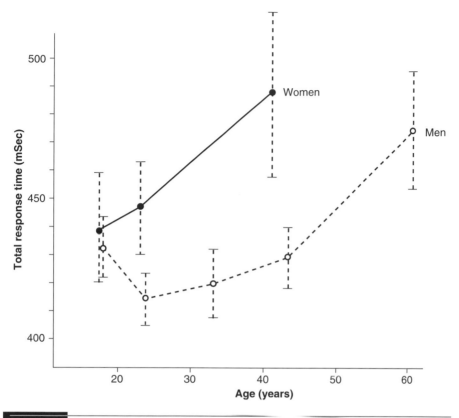

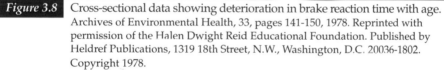 Cross-sectional data showing deterioration in brake reaction time with age. Archives of Environmental Health, 33, pages 141-150, 1978. Reprinted with permission of the Halen Dwight Reid Educational Foundation. Published by Heldref Publications, 1319 18th Street, N.W., Washington, D.C. 20036-1802. Copyright 1978.

It remains unclear to what extent such local changes should be attributed to vascular disease, the after-effects of viral infections, intoxication with heavy metals, or a lack of antioxidants rather than to aging *per se*. Possible contributing factors include a progressive death of neurons, a loss of interconnecting dendrites (Feldman 1976), a decrease of cerebral blood flow (Toole and Abourezk 1989), and various changes in enzyme activity, receptor structures, and neurohormonal function.

Changes in Cerebral Perfusion

The vertebral arteries become progressively more tortuous with age, and in consequence the cerebral blood flow decreases from its young adult peak of 50 to 60 ml/min per 100 g of tissue to around 40 ml/min per 100 g in a senior. The latter figure seems to be around the minimum level needed to maintain full neuronal function, and any additional disturbance of the cerebral circulation is enough to cause cell death. Some authors thus have argued that one of the important benefits of an acute bout of vigorous physical activity is an associated rise of central arterial pressure, with a resultant increase of cerebral blood flow (Pantano et al. 1983; Toole and Abourezk 1989). However, any exercise-induced increases in blood pressure are short-lived, and it is difficult to believe that they have a substantial influence on the rate of loss of brain function.

Cellular and Enzymatic Changes

The cerebral cells accumulate the pigment lipofuscin, and they also show various enzymatic changes as they become older. There is a significant loss of both Nissl granules and DNA and abnormal neurofibrils develop. A progressive death of cerebral cells leads to a 10% to 20% decrease in the total mass of cerebral tissue between the ages of 20 and 90 years.

Some parts of the brain show decreased levels of the enzymes that synthesize neurotransmitter substances (Strong, Wood, and Samorajski 1991), including dopamines, catecholamines, serotonin, acetylcholine, and (to a lesser extent) GABA (Allen et al. 1983; Gottfries 1986; Poirier and Finch 1994). At the same time, there are alterations in synaptic calcium ion transport (Sun and Seaman 1977), increases in activity of the monoamine oxidase that breaks down catecholamines, and alterations in the sensitivity and/or density of receptors for such neurotransmitters as dopamine (D2 type only; Morgan et al. 1987; Rinne 1987), noradrenaline (Maggi et al. 1979), serotonin (both S1 and S2 receptors; Morgan, May, and Finch 1988) and acetylcholine (Araujo et al. 1990).

The concentration of norepinephrine in the hindbrain of an elderly person may be as much as 40% below its young adult value. For this reason, there has been interest in the possibility that monoamine oxidase inhibitors such as procaine hydrochloride could delay the aging of brain function; however, to date such research has been inconclusive.

Losses of choline acetyltransferase, the enzyme responsible for the synthesis of acetylcholine, are most marked in the cerebral cortex and the caudate nucleus (Allen et al. 1983). A lack of acetylcholine in these regions of the brain is associated with certain forms of tremor and with Alzheimer's disease (Domino 1988; Morgan, May, and Finch 1988).

A reduction in activity of glutamic acid decarboxylase, the enzyme responsible for the synthesis of GABA, is most marked in the thalamus (Poirier and Finch 1994) and the temporal lobe of the brain (Allen et al. 1983). A lack of GABA may contribute to the age-related slowing in the processing of sensory information.

Low levels of dopamine in the substantia nigra are a marked feature of Parkinson's disease (Poirier and Finch 1994).

Reaction Speed and Memory

Whether reacting or remembering, the functional problem of the elderly brain is a deterioration in the signal/noise ratio. A deterioration in the various sensory receptors gives a weaker signal, and a reduction in the number of corti-cal cells gives less potential for a "smoothing" of occasional aberrant signals by an averaging process. The elderly person must thus delay any response until sufficient information has been accumulated to distinguish a signal from background noise (Welford 1984).

As noted earlier, short-term memory decreases with age (Poitrenaud et al. 1994; Schmidt 1987; Spirduso 1995). This limits the ability to develop new skills and concepts (Robertson-Tschabo and Arenberg 1985). The channel ca-pacity of the brain is also reduced, so the older person needs less arousal to assure optimum cerebral performance (expressed another way, an older per-son is more easily overaroused by a demanding task; Bäckman and Molander 1989).

Difficulty in task learning is likely if the number of items to be remembered exceeds the capacity of the short-term store, if information must be manipu-lated, or if attention must be divided (Ostrow 1989). Tactics for enhancing performance include the provision of written instructions, an extended an-ticipation interval, and a prolonged inspection period. Age has less influence on the performance of highly learned or automatic actions (Hoyer and Plude 1980).

In an apparent attempt to optimize residual performance, the emphasis of the elderly person usually shifts from speed to accuracy of performance. There is increased reliance upon experience (Charness 1991) and established pat-terns of problem solving, so that particular difficulty is encountered if the information does not conform to an existing "set."

Local lesions of the brain can also cause emotional problems, loss of coordi-nation (ataxia), and various forms of tremor (associated with overactivity of the extrapyramidal pathways).

Gait, Tremor, Balance, and Falls

As age advances, ambulation is progressively impeded by a deterioration of gait, the appearance of a variety of tremors, a loss of balance, and an increased vulnerability to falls.

Gait

The gait of an elderly person is usually mechanically less efficient than that of a younger individual. Assessment commonly uses a sophisticated force plat-form laboratory, with measurements of heel strike, midstance, push-off, swing, and double-support phases of the walking cycle (Buchner et al. 1993). How-ever, Dobbs et al. (1993) have recently developed speed- and height-specific criteria to assess the normality of free walking, using only a stopwatch.

The movement of a frail elderly person is typically slow; the base of sup-port is widened, and the limb movements become shuffling and hesitant rather than deliberate (Koller, Glatt, and Fox 1985; Sudarsky and Rosenthal 1983). Individual characteristics of the old person that contribute to the poor mechanical efficiency include a loss of confidence, deteriorations in vision and balance, weakened muscles, an impaired coordination of motor unit activation, and a stiffening of the joints.

Training programs can enhance the efficiency of movement. They reduce the oxygen cost of a given task such as walking, thus increasing the potential range of performance even in conditions such as chronic obstructive lung disease, where the underlying cardiorespiratory pathology is irreversible.

Tremor

As age increases, a growing proportion of the population shows some form of tremor (Griffiths and Pathy 1991). The tremor may be perceived at rest, as in Parkinson's disease, a condition in which there is an inadequate level of the neurotransmitter dopamine in the inhibitory nuclei of the midbrain. In other people, the abnormality takes the form of an "intention tremor," which first appears when an action is attempted. Such tremors reflect a deterioration of muscle proprioceptor activity, damage to the comparator function of the cerebellum, or both (Shephard 1982c).

Balance

A progressive loss of cells in the brainstem and cerebellum, a diminution of proprioceptor function in the joints and eye muscles, degenerative changes in the saccule and the utricle, and muscle weakness all limit the ability of an older person to control body movements, including the corrective movements that are needed when the center of gravity is displaced by some external force (Woollacott 1993). Balance thus shows a progressive deterioration with aging (Buchner et al. 1993; MacRae, Feltner, and Reinsch 1994; Pyykkö et al. 1988). Older people have particular difficulty in balancing under conditions of sensory conflict (for example, when walking near a stream of fast-moving vehicles).

Corrective responses to a loss of balance are initiated more slowly than in a younger individual and are sometimes disorganized, with a response of both agonist and antagonist muscles (a general stiffening of the limbs). Body sway reaches a minimum in the teen years and increases progressively thereafter. At any given age, women show more sway than men, because of a poorer muscle mass/body mass ratio and (possibly) because their shoes provide less ankle support. Poor balance and increased body sway not only increase the risk of falls, but also lead to a deterioration in the mechanical efficiency of movement, as discussed earlier.

Falls

One-third of community-dwelling seniors fall each year (Perry 1982), and the prevalence of falls becomes much higher following institutionalization

(Rubenstein et al. 1988). In the very old person in whom bone structure has been weakened by osteoporosis, a fall commonly leads to hip fracture, confinement to bed, and early death (Poor, Jacobsen, and Melton 1994).

The most common cause of falls (Overstall 1991) is tripping over some obstacle (see table 3.7). The likelihood of such an incident is increased by slippery or uneven floor surfaces, lighting that is inadequate for an older person, poor eyesight (Tinetti, Speechley, and Ginter 1988), a shuffling gait with reduced leg lift (Woollacott 1993), loss of proprioceptive sensation (Skinner, Barrack, and Cook 1984), a slow reaction speed (Stelmach 1994), and muscle weakness that makes it difficult to restore balance after stumbling. Subjects who have sustained multiple falls show significantly greater body sway than their age-matched peers (Crilly et al. 1987; Era and Heikkinen 1985), although this may be in part a consequence rather than a cause of their injuries.

Etiologies of falls other than tripping assume increasing importance in people over the age of 75 years (Pollock 1992). In addition to being affected by general cognitive impairment, specific neurological lesions, and joint pathologies such as rheumatoid arthritis or osteoarthritis (Nevitt et al. 1989), balance may be impaired by a variety of prescribed medications (including sedatives, antihypertensives, diuretics, phenothiazines, and benzodiazepines; Ray, Griffin, and Downey 1989).

Postural hypotension is seen in as many as 15% to 24% of elderly subjects (Overstall 1991). A proportion of the elderly are liable to "drop attacks," precipitated by a turning of the neck. The pathology underlying such episodes is often, but not always, a transient restriction of cerebral blood flow secondary to degeneration of the intervertebral disks and/or a kinking and tortuosity of the vertebral artery (Rubenstein and Josephson 1993). In the "subclavian steal" syndrome, there is a transient reversal of flow in the vertebral artery to compensate for a temporary narrowing or occlusion of the subclavian artery; such an attack may be initiated by exercise of the affected arm.

Table 3.7   Cause of falls in 146 elderly subjects.

Cause of fall	Percentage of incidents
Tripping	47.1
Drop attacks	12.2
Giddiness	8.7
Loss of balance	8.2
After rising	6.4
Turning head	5.2
Other	12.2

Reprinted, by permission, from P.W. Overstall et al., 1977, "Falls in the elderly related to postural imbalance," *British Medical Journal* 1: 261-264. (BMJ Publishing Group)

Other causes of a brief loss of consciousness include cardiac syncope induced by a prolonged bout of coughing, urinary straining, various cardiac disorders (heart block, dysrhythmias, paroxysms of tachycardia, and narrowing of the aortic orifice), epilepsy, anemia, and hypotension associated with Parkinson's disease.

Perception of Effort

Perception of exertion can be assessed from open-ended questioning, from observation of the self-selected walking pace, and from formal ratings of standard exercise tasks (Shephard 1989b).

Self-Assessment

Self-assessments of the ability to undertake the activities of daily living are generally related to objective measurements of an individual's physical abilities (Myers and Huddy 1985).

Occasionally, the stated or perceived abilities of an old person may exceed objective predictions because unanticipated tricks are used to accomplish a task (for instance, people may pull themselves upstairs by their arms if their legs are not strong enough to accomplish this task). More often, people state that they can accomplish less than would be predicted from objective assessment of their condition. Here, the discrepancy arises because perceptions of self-efficacy are strongly influenced by a lack of recent experience of the task, a deterioration in the sense of overall well-being, or a loss of self-esteem (Reker and Wong 1984).

Too often, common tasks have been avoided in recent years, not only because of the natural fears of the elderly, but also because of needless restrictions imposed by physicians and nursing staff.

Self-Paced Activities

The correlation between the self-selected pace of walking and maximal oxygen intake is quite low in the elderly (r = 0.25-0.30; Cunningham, Rechnitzer, and Donner 1986). This suggests that the speed of walking adopted by a person is strongly influenced by factors other than aerobic power. Determinants may include personal perceptions of the corresponding level of metabolic effort, and the individual's more general feelings of self-efficacy.

Ratings of Perceived Exertion

There has been much interest in the use of formal Borg scale ratings of effort as a means both of gauging an individual's fitness and of regulating the intensity of an exercise prescription. Such an approach has particular attraction in situations in which the heart rate does not show the anticipated increase with exercise (for instance, following cardiac transplantation, or in a person who is being treated with beta-blocking drugs).

We might anticipate that an older person would perceive a given intensity of effort as more difficult than a younger individual. The various factors contributing to the overall Gestalt of effort all increase with age. For instance, respiratory sensations are augmented because the breathing frequency is greater, and ventilation accounts for a larger fraction of the individual's maximal voluntary ventilation at any given power output. Likewise, as the muscles become weaker, they must exert a greater force per unit of cross-section, and a decline in cardiac function reduces muscle perfusion, allowing a greater buildup of tissue metabolites as exercise proceeds.

However, almost all these changes develop roughly in parallel with the decline in maximal oxygen intake and maximal heart rate. The classic study of Borg and Linderholm (1967) thus found that although the absolute heart rate associated with a given perception of cycle ergometer effort declined with aging, the rating of effort maintained a consistent relationship to the relative stress, expressed as a percentage of the individual's maximal oxygen intake or his or her heart rate reserve. Our laboratory has duplicated these findings when comparing the responses of young and elderly subjects to vigorous treadmill exercise.

The practical value of formal effort ratings as a means of regulating the intensity of prescribed exercise is nevertheless limited. If people are advised to reach an intensity of effort that they perceive as "moderately hard," they will adopt a relative loading that is 70% ± 10% of their maximal oxygen intake. Because of the large variance in perceptions, 1 person in 40 will exercise at an excessively low intensity (no more than 50% of his or her maximal oxygen intake), and another 1 in 40 will exercise at a dangerously high intensity (90% of his or her maximal effort; Shephard et al. 1992). The main value of an effort rating is not to set an exercise prescription; this is better achieved by recommending that a person walk a specific distance within a specified time. Rather, the rating serves to fine-tune a basic prescription in the face of factors that augment loading—for instance, adverse weather conditions.

Regulation of Homeostasis and Aging of the Endocrine System

Although aging is marked by a deterioration in the function of individual cells and organs, a more serious problem arises from a failure of the mechanisms that coordinate function between the various parts of the body. A weakening of both neural and hormonal control systems limits the ability to respond to both external and internal stresses. We have commented already on problems in maintaining blood pressure during sudden changes of body position (postural hypotension) and the excessive body cooling that occurs in cold environments. Regulatory problems are equally likely in a hot environment or during exercise.

Impaired Heat Tolerance

Causes of impaired regulatory responses to heat (Kenney 1995) include a smaller peak cardiac output, the administration of antihypertensive drugs such as beta-blocking agents, impairment of the sensation of thirst (Phillips et al. 1984), use of diuretic medications (Collins, Exton-Smith, and Doré 1981), a decreased output of vasopressin but an increased sensitivity to this hormone (Phillips et al. 1984), an impairment of renal concentrating ability, a slow onset of sweating plus a reduced secretion of sweat by atrophied eccrine glands, and an obesity-related decrease in the efficiency of peripheral heat loss despite (in some cases) a greater heat-induced vasodilatation (Kenney 1995; O'Reilly 1989).

Physical condition seems to be the most critical determinant of heat tolerance. If elderly subjects are matched with younger people in terms of their habitual physical activity, then an impairment of both sweating and vasodilatation is very evident; on the other hand, if matching is based upon maximal oxygen intake (that is, young men in average physical condition are compared with very fit old people), then no deterioration of thermoregulation is seen in the elderly (Tankersley et al. 1991).

Hormonal Adjustments to Exercise

Aging is associated with impairment in a number of hormonal regulatory systems that are important to maintenance of homeostasis during exercise.

A hormonal deficiency could arise at any stage in the process from nuclear synthesis of the hormone through its activation, bloodstream transport by carrier proteins, interaction with cell membrane receptors, and ultimate clearance from the bloodstream. Vascular or degenerative disease in the neuroendocrine pathways of the supraoptic nuclei and hypothalamus seem particularly likely to limit the production of many key hormones in the very old (Green 1991).

In the context of vigorous physical activity, hormones make particularly important contributions to (1) the regulation of circulating fluid volumes and cardiovascular performance in warm environments, (2) the mobilization of fuels for exercise (maintenance of blood glucose, liberation of fat, and breakdown of protein), and (3) the repair of body structures with the synthesis of new protein (anabolism) in response to an appropriate pattern of training.

Sympathoadrenal Activity

An age-related deterioration in function of the autonomic nervous system is shown by a decreased sensitivity to preganglionic stimulation. As noted earlier, the synthesis of acetylcholine is diminished in cholinergic parts of the system, but there are also offsetting decreases in choline esterase activity. In postsynaptic elements, an increased sensitivity to directly applied neurotransmitters might be anticipated (much as in a denervated organ). However, the myocardium of an elderly person, as discussed earlier, shows a decreased sensitivity to both excitatory and blocking agents.

Vigorous physical activity is associated with an increased output of epinephrine from the adrenal medulla and also of norepinephrine (derived largely from the sympathetic nerves regulating the circulatory system). Relative to younger individuals, the elderly show a two- to threefold increase in blood norepinephrine levels in response to such stresses as adoption of the upright posture (Young et al. 1980), a fixed rate of exercising (Kohrt et al. 1993), the ingestion of glucose, and mental activity (Barnes et al. 1982). However, at any given fraction of aerobic power, the effect of strenuous exercise is either the same in an older person as in someone younger (Jensen et al. 1994), or is less marked in the older person (Kohrt et al. 1993; Mazzeo, Colburn, and Horvath 1985).

One important factor limiting the sympathoadrenal response in an older adult is the decreased beta-adrenergic responsiveness at the end-organ (Kelly and O'Malley 1984; Lakatta 1993a). There does not seem to be any decrease in either the density or the affinity of adrenergic receptors. Possibly there is an impaired activation of adenylate cyclase (Feldman 1986; Halter 1985), or an increased prejunctional uptake of active catecholamines (Goldberg et al. 1986).

Adrenal Cortex

A slight loss of adrenal cortical tissue can be detected around 50 years of age. Connective tissue replaces parenchymal cells, the capsule of the adrenal gland becomes thickened, and pigment accumulates throughout the cortex.

In a young adult, the pituitary secretion of ACTH stimulates an increase of plasma cortisol levels during exhausting or emotionally stressful activity. The ACTH response remains intact in an older person, and a lower cortisol secretion rate is compensated by a lower plasma clearance rate of this hormone (Green 1991). The nighttime peaks of cortisol may actually be larger in elderly individuals, particularly if their sleep patterns are disturbed (Murray et al. 1981). At a given percentage of maximal oxygen intake, we have found rather similar exercise responses in young and elderly subjects, but the reaction at a fixed power output is greater in an older person.

Aldosterone secretion is controlled by the renin-angiotensin system, by plasma potassium levels, and (to a limited extent) by ACTH levels. Aldosterone secretion is diminished in the elderly, but this is partly counteracted by a decrease in metabolic clearance of the hormone. Thus, an elderly person can acclimatize to a combination of exercise and heat under desert conditions (Yousef et al. 1984), but homeostasis is impaired if there is a hemorrhage or other major disturbance of fluid or mineral balance (Reddan 1985).

Androgenic and Ovarian Hormones

In addition to their effects on the secondary sex organs, the androgens have important general metabolic effects, increasing protein synthesis in muscle and bone, promoting the storage of glycogen and retention of water, and reducing serum cholesterol.

The production of testosterone diminishes in older men, as the Leydig cells of the testes atrophy and increasing quantities of circulating androgens are converted to estrogens in body fat (Pirke, Sinterman, and Vogt 1980). Some physicians have thus prescribed androgens (Baron et al. 1978; Jackson et al. 1987; Morley, Kaiser, and Perry 1993) and recombinant growth hormone (Rudman et al. 1993) to the frail elderly in an attempt to counter muscle wasting, hypercholesterolemia, and senile osteoporosis. However, the benefits of such treatment remain debatable.

In women, the conversion of adrenal androgens to estrone in the liver and peripheral fat depots is particularly important after menopause. It has been suggested that those who develop early manifestations of osteoporosis have either a limited secretion of adrenal androgens or an impaired conversion of androgens to estrones. Some physicians advocate hormone replacement therapy for postmenopausal women as a means of countering osteoporosis and correcting the increasing risk of cardiovascular disease and Alzheimer's disease (Stampfer et al. 1991). The risk of breast cancer arising from such treatment remains, although problems are probably less than was once feared, particularly with modern patterns of replacement therapy (Baber and Studd 1989; Horowitz et al. 1993). Nevertheless, a combination of exercise, an adequate calcium intake, and calcitonin administration (where required) at least match the effect of estrogens in preventing osteoporosis. Moreover, such a physiological regimen is practicable for many patients (Kanis et al. 1992), and it carries other important dividends such as the prevention of cardiovascular disease.

Insulin and Glucagon

The incidence of clinical diabetes rises sharply with age (Horowitz 1986; Wilson, Anderson, and Kannel 1986). Prevalence of the disorder is particularly marked among indigenous populations that formerly were physically very active but now have become acculturated to a sedentary "western" lifestyle (Shephard and Rode 1996).

By the age of 70 years, some 20% of men and 30% of women show "abnormal" glucose tolerance curves. Nevertheless, the pathological significance of borderline cases is still debated (Goldberg, Andres, and Bierman 1985), and it may be necessary to increase "normal" ceilings of both resting blood sugar and responses to a standard glucose loading by as much as 0.5 mmol/L for each decade beyond the age of 50 years (Jackson and Finucane 1991).

A decline in habitual physical activity, a smaller lean mass for storing glycogen, an increase of adiposity, and a diet poor in chromium could all be important factors contributing to the increased prevalence of impaired insulin tolerance in older individuals (Horowitz 1986; Kirwan et al. 1993; Nordstrom 1982). However, responses to oral and intravenous test doses of glucose remain similar to each other, as in younger individuals, so that age-related changes in glucose absorption are not a factor (Jackson and Finucane 1991).

Plasma samples from some older subjects show a decreased production of insulin or an increased fraction of hormone remaining in the proinsulin form, but in many instances the resting levels of insulin secretion are apparently unchanged or even increased (Cononie et al. 1994). There is usually a decreased peripheral sensitivity to insulin, but in some subjects at least, insulin receptor binding remains normal (Jackson and Finucane 1991). In such individuals, the tissues (especially muscle) seem to become resistant to the metabolic effects of insulin at the post-receptor level (Wallberg-Henriksson 1992). Other factors adversely affecting the system of glucose homeostasis include an increase of sympathetic nerve activity in response to oral glucose (Rowe and Troen 1980), a slowing of insulin clearance from the bloodstream (Minaker et al. 1982), and a lesser response of the pancreatic beta cells to stimulating and inhibiting hormones under conditions in which the blood glucose is "clamped" at a fixed level (Elahi et al. 1982).

In subjects over 60 years of age, the blood glucose tends to fall rather than rise during performance of a bout of maximal exercise (Goldfarb, Vaccaro, and Ostrove 1989). This is unrelated to any loss of fitness, decrease of lean tissue mass, or accumulation of body fat. The reasons as yet remain obscure.

There is little information concerning possible changes in glucagon secretion with age. Fasting levels of glucagon show little alteration in an older person, and the response to a dose of arginine also seems to be unaltered. Glucagon may play an important role in tissue repair, and thus in countering the effects of aging (Timiras 1991).

Thyroid Hormone

The thyroid hormone weakens the metabolic coupling between catabolism and the resynthesis of ATP, thus increasing basal metabolism and contributing to thermoregulation during prolonged periods of cold exposure.

Aging is associated with a number of changes in the thyroid gland, including reductions in the follicular diameter, epithelial cell height, and colloid content of the gland. However, function seems to be affected but little by these changes. Some impairment of thyroid function might be inferred from the poor response of the elderly person to cold exposure, but at least when measured under standard conditions, the basal metabolic rate changes relatively little over adult life, provided that all data are expressed per unit of lean body mass.

A small proportion of elderly individuals show a significant impairment of thyroid function, but this is usually a consequence of autoimmune disease or earlier treatment of thyrotoxicosis (Green 1991). Occasionally, hypopituitarism may be to blame (Belchetz 1985).

Pituitary Secretions

The pituitary gland plays an important role in metabolic regulation, both through the secretion of its own active products such as growth hormone and also by stimulating the secretion of other glands, including the thyroid and the adrenal cortex.

The pituitary gland of an elderly person shows many morphological changes, including a decrease in vascularity, a diffuse fibrosis, a progressive loss of basophilic and eosinophilic cells, a proliferation of chromophobe cells, and an increased likelihood of adenoma formation. Overall function seems quite well preserved, although some authors have maintained that a progressive dysregulation of the hypothalamus, with corresponding changes in the secretion of pituitary hormones, plays a major role in the aging phenomenon (Timiras 1991).

Growth Hormone

Basal levels of growth hormone may change relatively little in old age, but (perhaps because of the decrease in slow-wave sleep) the elderly show less evidence of nocturnal bursts of secretion. Rudman et al. (1990) noted that in men aged 61 to 81 years there were low plasma levels of both growth hormone and IGF-1. Relative to age-matched controls, elderly subjects who received recombinant growth hormone for six months showed increased lean body mass (+8.8%) and decreased body fat (–14.4%), with a 1.6% increase of lumbar vertebral bone density.

Sidney and Shephard (1978b) tested the response of 65-year-old subjects to a 20 min bout of vigorous exercise. They observed an exercise-induced increase of secretion that was somewhat less than in their sample of young adults. Other investigators also have described a diminished response to both exercise and test doses of arginine in elderly people. Further information on growth hormone responses in the elderly is included in chapter 4.

Prolactin

Age does not affect plasma prolactin levels in men, but in women there is a decrease after menopause; this is probably secondary to decreases in blood levels of estrogen and dopamine (Timiras 1991).

The secretion of prolactin in response to thyrotropic hormone occurs more slowly in an old person, but it is also more prolonged (Blackman et al. 1986). This in turn could modify the secretion of endorphins, and thus the mood changes induced by exercise.

Antidiuretic Hormone

Opinions regarding the effects of aging on the secretion of antidiuretic hormone are conflicting. One study reported that there was a decreased output of the hormone (Legros and Brunier 1982), with a reduced sensitivity of the neural hypophysis to increases of plasma osmotic pressure (Hugonot, Dubos, and Mathes 1978). Another article suggested that there was an increased output of the hormone in an attempt to compensate for declining renal function (Helderman et al. 1978).

Parathyroid Hormone and Calcitonin

Concentrations of parathyroid (a hormone that favors the transfer of calcium from bone to plasma) rise with age, whereas concentrations of the opposing hormone (calcitonin) decrease (Kanis et al. 1992).

In men, plasma levels of parathyroid hormone reach a plateau of three times the young adult value by the age of 50 years, although they seem to decline thereafter. In women, levels of parathyroid hormone reach a minimum in the 40s and subsequently increase, particularly in those individuals affected by osteoporosis.

It is unclear how far the increase in parathyroid levels among older individuals represents an attempt to compensate for dietary deficiencies of calcium and vitamin D or for an inadequate endogenous synthesis of vitamin D (Pansu and Bellaton 1976).

Aging of the Immune System

Detailed reviews of aging and immune function have been provided by Mazzeo and Nasrullah (1992) and Shephard and Shek (1995b).

Anatomical Changes

The thymus is one of the first of the body organs to atrophy. The mass of this tissue decreases from late puberty onward (Makinodan et al. 1991, 1987). However, there is sufficient redundancy in the system that immune function is well preserved through to the retirement years. Only in the final phases of aging is there evidence of a gross failure in cellular immune reactions, with an increased risk of tumors and the development of autoimmunity (discussed in chapter 2).

Immunity and the Aging Process

Some authors have ascribed an important place to immune changes in the overall aging process. Russell (1978) and Walford (1980) both argued that a specific genome on chromosome 6 (the major histocompatibility complex) regulates both immune function and aging. However, several important pieces of evidence argue against the immune system's playing any fundamental role in aging. Aging can occur in organisms that seemingly lack an immune system, and in humans the deterioration of T-cell function seems to follow rather than to precede aging (Abbas, Lichtman, and Pober 1995).

An alternative hypothesis is that immune function is adversely affected by some other facet of aging, such as a decrease of habitual physical activity, poor nutrition (particularly a lack of protein, ascorbate, and vitamin E), the long-term effects of cigarette smoking, the progressive breakdown of mucocutaneous barriers in the skin and genitourinary tract, and an increase of chronic disease or depression. All these factors have an adverse influence upon immune responses. Other disturbances of immune function could arise from polypharmacy, including the prolonged administration of aspirin, cortisone, estrogens, and mood-altering drugs.

Cellular Changes

Information on changes in the cellular component of the immune defenses is limited to a small number of cross-sectional comparisons, and given the important influence of physical activity on the immune system, it is unfortunate that most studies have not controlled for associated age-related differences in habitual physical activity.

A number of reports suggest that natural killer cell activity remains unchanged in older subjects who remain normally active (Fiatarone et al. 1989; Murasko et al. 1991). Others have noted age-related decreases in the numbers and cytolytic activity of natural killer cells (Penschow and Mackay 1980; Sato, Fuse, and Kuwata 1979) and lymphokine-activated killer cells, with a diminished affinity for target cells (Effros and Walford 1983; Mariani et al. 1990; Nasrullah and Mazzeo 1992; Zharhary and Gershon 1981).

Some authors have noted a decrease in the proportion of helper T cells in older subjects, whereas others have found a decreased proportion of suppressor T cells (Shephard and Shek 1995b). Ben-Yehuda and Weksler (1992) suggested that the number of helper T (CD4+) cells was increased in elderly subjects, but that their activity was decreased. In contrast, the suppressor T (CD8+) count was depressed by aging, but the activity of the individual CD8+ cells was unchanged. Both the spontaneous proliferative activity of the T cells and their response to mitogens diminish in older subjects (Froelich et al. 1988; Hefton et al. 1980; Murasko et al. 1991). From the peak values that are reached around puberty, activity ultimately decreases by 5% to 30% (Erschler 1988; Froelich et al. 1988; Makinodan et al. 1991; Miller 1991), although peripheral blood specimens may not show a clear change until a person reaches 70 or 75 years of age (Adler and Nagel 1994).

Other indexes of immune function ultimately show a more drastic drop, to as little as 5% to 10% of their young adult value (Walford 1982).

Responses to Exercise

Exercise-induced changes in the output of a number of immunomodulatory hormones (catecholamines, cortisol, beta-endorphins, and prostaglandins) are modified by aging. Nevertheless, the natural killer cell response to an acute bout of moderate exercise seems remarkably normal (Fiatarone et al. 1989; Solomon 1991).

Animal experiments have suggested a larger exercise-induced stimulation of proliferative responses to phytohemagglutinin in young than in elderly mice (Delafuente et al. 1992). Older individuals also have a greater vulnerability to both microinjuries of the active muscles and the resulting acute-phase response, so it seems likely that when undertaking vigorous exercise they would more easily reach the point where an acute bout of exercise had a depressant rather than a stimulatory action upon the immune system (Cannon et al. 1991).

Conclusions

There are substantial technical difficulties in defining and sampling a healthy population of elderly individuals, and it is even more difficult to follow them longitudinally. Most body systems show an accelerating, age-related decline of function, but the extent to which this is due to a parallel decline in habitual physical activity remains unclear.

Standing height decreases with age, due mainly to kyphosis and compression of intervertebral disks. Body mass increases during middle age, but remains more constant in older age, as lean tissue is replaced by fat. The loss of muscle mass leads to a progressive decrease of strength and endurance. The bones show a progressive loss of both minerals and matrix with aging, and they become progressively more vulnerable to fracture. A deterioration in the joint surfaces leads to a high prevalence of arthritis; this often restricts daily activities. Loss of resilience in tendons and ligaments predisposes to strains and sprains. There is a progressive decrease in peak heart rate with age; an increase of stroke volume offers some compensation in submaximal effort, but the peak cardiac output decreases in parallel with the decline in maximal oxygen intake. There is a progressive rise in systolic blood pressure with age, but poor regulation of blood pressure leads to increasing prevalence of postural hypotension. The respiratory system shows a stiffening of the thoracic cage, but a loss of elasticity in the pulmonary tissue. Vital capacity decreases and residual volume increases, but there is little change of total lung capacity.

Airway collapse becomes increasingly probable during vigorous expiratory effort. Gas distribution also becomes nonuniform, but healthy elderly people are able to maintain their arterial oxygen saturation during vigorous exercise. Age-related gastrointestinal and renal changes have implications for fluid replenishment during exercise in the heat. Aging of the brain leads to difficulties with short-term memory, cognition, and the learning of new tasks. Deteriorations in vision and hearing also handicap some activities. Task performance may be compromised by poor gait, tremor, lack of balance, and a propensity for falls. Aging of the endocrine system hampers maintenance of the *milieu intérieur* during prolonged activity, and a deterioration in various components of the immune system may limit repair processes following very heavy bouts of exercise.

Chapter 4

Impact of Regular Physical Activity on Age-Associated Changes in Physiological Systems

Now that we have considered the changes in various physiological systems that are commonly associated with aging, the question arises how far these losses of function can be slowed or reversed by an increase of physical activity, whether through a deliberate exercise program, sport, or an active daily lifestyle. In principle, each physiological system merits extended discussion. However, constraints of space require that we focus on a few of the more important topics affecting functional health in the older adult.

The effects of regular physical activity can be tested both by comparisons between continuing athletes and sedentary individuals and by longitudinal training experiments of varying duration. Nevertheless, there remain a number of problems of data interpretation. Both cross-sectional and longitudinal studies tend to recruit fit, healthy, and wealthy subjects with an above-average interest in the adoption of a healthy lifestyle (Shephard 1993a). Both athletes and sedentary subjects show a varying but age-related decrease in habitual physical activity, and the interpretation of longitudinal fitness data may be further clouded by vigorous training either at recruitment or in anticipation of subsequent fitness evaluation.

Body fat increases with age; thus the question arises, should such items as aerobic power and muscle strength be evaluated in absolute units, or per kg of body mass? Likewise, if muscle strength or aerobic power (whether expressed in absolute or relative units) declines by 25% over the course of adult life, what constitutes a consistent and age-independent intensity of training? Should the level of conditioning also be reduced by 25% as a person ages, so that training proceeds at the same fraction of the individual's maximal voluntary force or peak aerobic power, or should a consistent absolute level of training be imposed? Finally, how can we allow for the fact that in old age a deterioration of physical condition and frank disease cause the weaker members of a population to defect from training programs?

Body Composition

An appropriate program of regular physical activity should be sufficient to control the accumulation of body fat, to maintain or increase the mass of lean tissue, and to maintain or increase bone density.

Body Fat

One major reason for the accumulation of body fat in older adults is an age-related decrease of habitual physical activity. We might thus anticipate that a moderate increase in physical activity would reverse this trend, without a need for any special dietary restrictions. We will first consider factors potentially complicating this simple reasoning, and we will then examine the empirical evidence in terms of correlational, epidemiological, cross-sectional, and longitudinal studies, concluding with some comments on the advantages of physical activity relative to dieting in the control of obesity.

Potential Limitations of Response to Increased Physical Activity

The anticipated decrease in body fat content with an increase of physical activity may be modified by exercise-induced changes of appetite, a decrease in both resting and exercise metabolism due to any reduction in body mass that is achieved (Weigle 1988), and exercise- and diet-induced changes in the resting metabolic rate. Furthermore, older people who have become obese may have more difficulty in losing body fat than younger adults, because they have a limited exercise tolerance. Finally, the decision to begin a deliberate conditioning program may lead to a voluntary or subconscious reduction of voluntary energy expenditure during other segments of the day (Goran and Poehlman 1992a).

In men, vigorous physical activity usually leads to a transient decrease in food intake, probably because of the secretion of catecholamines, with a resulting rise in blood sugar and a mobilization of depot fat. In contrast, exercise appears to enhance appetite in premenopausal women (Ballor and Keesey 1991), perhaps because fat depots are more stable in female subjects. It remains unclear whether this gender difference persists into old age.

Despite these various theoretical complications, a meta-analysis completed by Ballor and Keesey (1991) offers good evidence that fat loss is proportional to the frequency and duration of exercise sessions, the initial body fat content, and the total weekly energy expenditure.

Correlational Studies

Correlational studies have related resting metabolic rate or total daily energy expenditure to body composition and aerobic fitness. If a person exercises on a regular basis, some increase of total daily energy expenditure would be expected. However, the low intensity of most activities undertaken by the elderly limits the magnitude of such increases relative to the reductions in basal metabolism associated with a negative energy balance (which can amount to 10% to 15% of daily food intake).

Goran and Poehlman (1992a, 1992b) found an inverse correlation (r = 0.64) between the total daily energy expenditure of elderly subjects (as assessed by the accurate but expensive doubly labeled water technique) and densitometric estimates of body fat content. Others, who assessed energy intake from self-reports, failed to observe such an association, although the reason may have been an inaccurate estimation of habitual physical activity or a significant underreporting of food consumption by elderly people (Johnson, Goran, and Poehlman 1994).

Several studies (Poehlman 1989; Poehlman, Melby, and Badylak 1991; Webb, Poehlman, and Tonino 1993) have noted a positive association between aerobic fitness and resting metabolic rate. Possible reasons exercise might cause an immediate increase in resting metabolism include (1) the energy costs of repairing local muscle damage, (2) an increase of protein turnover and synthesis of lean tissue, (3) a need for glycogen resynthesis, (4) greater lipolysis, (5) an enhanced thermic effect of food consumption, and (6) increased sympathetic nerve activity (possibly inducing thermogenesis in brown adipose tissue, Keesey 1992).

Any stimulation of resting metabolism is probably quite short-lived. Tremblay et al. (1987) found that at 16 to 84 h post-exercise, the resting metabolic rate was reduced relative to control observations. The reported effect of an exercise program thus depends on the timing of the metabolic measurements relative to the last bout of physical activity.

Cross-Sectional Studies

Kavanagh et al. (1989) made a cross-sectional analysis of body composition in a large sample of Masters athletes who had sustained a moderate volume of training from the third to the eighth decades of life (see table 4.1). The types of activities that were represented covered a broad range of athletic endeavors, with distance running, cycling, and swimming being particularly popular. The group is interesting because the frequency, intensity, and duration of physical activity were of the order that the general public might be persuaded to accept (on average, four sessions per week; in the men, each session comprised 49 min of jogging over a distance of 8.6 km, and in the women, a session involved 40 min of jogging over 6.1 km). Moreover, training speeds and the duration of training sessions had remained relatively consistent until the

Table 4.1   Cross-sectional study of Masters athletes, showing changes in body composition across six decades of life.

Variable	20-29 yr	30-39 yr	40-49 yr
Female subjects			
Body mass (kg)	58.0 ± 7.0	61.2 ± 9.1	62.0 ± 8.6
Body fat (%)	27.2 ± 6.1	27.7 ± 6.1	27.2 ± 5.5
Lean body mass (kg)	42.0 ± 3.4	44.0 ± 5.9	45.4 ± 6.7
Male subjects			
Body mass (kg)	80.2 ± 6.7	75.9 ± 9.2	77.3 ± 10.8
Body fat (%)	19.0 ± 5.9	18.3 ± 4.9	19.8 ± 4.8
Lean body mass (kg)	64.9 ± 6.7	61.3 ± 6.6	62.1 ± 8.2

Variable	50-59 yr	60-69 yr	70-79 yr
Female subjects			
Body mass (kg)	62.0 ± 8.1	61.4 ± 11.0	56.5 ± 3.0
Body fat (%)	30.2 ± 5.4	27.3 ± 5.3	28.0 ± 4.7
Lean body mass (kg)	43.1 ± 4.8	45.2 ± 8.6	40.7 ± 2.8
Male subjects			
Body mass (kg)	77.3 ± 11.2	77.6 ± 9.9	72.0 ± 11.7
Body fat (%)	20.0 ± 5.5	20.4 ± 5.1	20.8 ± 4.5
Lean body mass (kg)	62.0 ± 8.7	62.2 ± 8.2	57.9 ± 7.2

The subjects in the various age categories maintained a relatively consistent level of daily training. Mean ± SD. Based on data of Kavanagh et al. (1989).

Reprinted, by permission, from Kavanagh et al., 1989, "Health and aging of Masters athletes," *Clinical Sports Medicine* 1: 72-88 (Chapman & Hall).

eighth decade of life, when speeds became slower and sessions shorter in duration.

The younger competitors of both sexes had a body fat content similar to that of the average young adult in urban North America. However, in contrast to their sedentary counterparts, the Masters athletes showed little increase of body fat content across six age decades. The lean mass likewise remained relatively constant until the eighth decade of life. At this stage, when the volume of training had become smaller, average values for lean mass were substantially less than in the younger competitors.

Kohrt et al. (1992) compared young adults and seniors, noting that elderly people who exercised not only had a lesser accumulation of body fat than their sedentary peers, but also showed less tendency to the centripetal fat deposition that is associated with the development of cardiovascular and metabolic disease. Other investigations have also shown lower total body fat (Hagberg et al. 1988; Poehlman et al. 1990; Voorips, van Staeveren, and Hautvast 1991) and truncal fat (Larsson et al. 1984) in active than in sedentary individuals.

Although such cross-sectional studies strongly suggest that benefit can be obtained from a modest program of regular physical activity, obesity has a substantial genetic component (Bouchard 1992), and it remains possible to argue that the type of body build that favored an active lifestyle or participation in Masters competition also limited an age-related accumulation of body fat.

Epidemiological Studies

The investigation by Lee and Paffenbarger (1992) provides a good example of epidemiological studies examining the role of habitual physical activity in the control of obesity. Self-reports of body mass were obtained from a large sample of initially middle-aged Harvard alumni over an 11- to 15-year follow-up. Energy expenditures were averaged for those who reported a decrease in body mass. Those who indicated losing > 5 kg had increased their habitual physical activity by an average of 1.2 MJ/week. Those who had a more modest weight loss (1 to 5 kg) had also increased their physical activity, by an average of 0.7 MJ/week.

Owens et al. (1992) likewise found that the weight gain of women over a three-year period was inversely associated both with physical activity as reported at baseline, and with increases in physical activity over the course of the study.

However, it remains difficult to be certain from such reports that the weight loss did not encourage an increase of habitual physical activity, rather than the converse. Moreover, because large samples were studied, most epidemiologists examined the reported or measured changes in total body mass rather than making a more direct examination of changes in body composition. Unfortunately, a decrease in body mass is a somewhat fallible criterion of fat loss. Indeed, with a well-designed physical activity prescription, fat may be replaced by an approximately equal mass of lean tissue, so that body weight remains unchanged.

Experimental Studies

There have been many experimental studies demonstrating the favorable effects of regular exercise on body composition in middle-aged subjects (Ballor and Keesey 1991), but observations on seniors have been fewer and less consistent (Butterworth et al. 1993; Kohrt, Obert, and Holloszy 1992; Morey et al. 1989; Pratley et al. 1994; Schwartz et al. 1991; Webb, Poehlman, and Tonino 1993). Occasional reports have shown either no change in body fat (Poehlman et al. 1994) or even an increase of adiposity despite training (Pollock et al.

1987). Unfortunately, some of the experimental studies have continued only for short periods (less than three months). This is an important criticism, since an obese person takes some time to begin exercising effectively, and little benefit may be seen over the first eight weeks of observation (Webb, Poehlman, and Tonino 1993). Moreover, even if an attempt is made to assign people to experimental and control groups, defections from the assigned treatment quickly lead to what is essentially a self-selection of experimental or control regimen. Finally, any early gains from exercising are soon dissipated if a person later stops the activity program.

Sidney, Shephard, and Harrison (1977) enrolled 65-year-old subjects in a regular lunchtime exercise program that stressed alternate fast and slow walking. There was no specific control of diet, but the energy expended in the training sessions amounted to a substantial 0.6 to 0.8 MJ/visit. The participants sorted themselves into four categories in terms of their attendance at exercise classes (high frequency, an average of 3.3 sessions per week; low frequency, 1.0 to 1.5 times per week) and the vigor of their participation (high intensity, progressing from 60% to 80% of aerobic power; low intensity, effort not exceeding 60% of aerobic power). Although the extent of program participation was self-selected, all categories of subjects showed a progressive decrease of average skinfold thicknesses and of predicted body fat over the course of the study. The largest effect (a loss of 3.1 mm, 2.7% body fat over the first 14 weeks of observation) was seen in the high-frequency, high-intensity exercisers (see table 4.2). The fat loss was sustained over 52 weeks of observation. Further (and in contrast to the effects of dieting), lean body mass increased by 1.2 to 1.7 kg, depending on the pattern of exercise that had been adopted during the year. The gains of lean tissue, as estimated from body mass and skinfold data, were confirmed by ^{40}K determinations of lean tissue mass; the latter technique showed a 1.2% gain of lean tissue at 14 weeks and a 4% gain after 52 weeks of training.

Mertens, Kavanagh, and Shephard (1995) recently demonstrated similar beneficial changes in body composition when middle-aged postcoronary patients (initial age 52 ± 7 years) were enrolled in a training program. Again, there was no specific restriction of diet. Nevertheless, over a year of observation, body mass decreased by 4.5 kg, and body fat decreased from 35.4% to 33.2%. The intensity of activity adopted in the postcoronary program was quite modest, and perhaps for this reason the subjects showed no change in lean body mass (57.7 vs. 57.8 kg). Mertens, Kavanagh, and Shephard (1995) obtained serial measurements of resting metabolic rate over the year of study. In keeping with the cross-sectional data already cited, they found that one feature contributing to development of a negative energy balance and thus a loss of body fat was a program-induced increase in resting metabolic rate, from 3.1 to 3.4 ml/[kg · min].

Kohrt, Obert, and Holloszy (1992) reported that over a 9- to 12-month program of walking, jogging, rowing, and cycling, 60- to 70-year-old men and

Table 4.2 Changes in skinfolds, percentage body fat, and lean body mass over 7 and 14 weeks of endurance training.

Variable	Group	7-week change	14-week change
Average skinfold (mm)	LF, LI	–0.8	–1.4
	LF, HI	–1.4	–1.9
	HF, LI	–1.5	–2.9
	HF, HI	–2.4	–3.1
Predicted body fat (%)	LF, LI	–0.8	–1.9
	LF, HI	–1.1	–2.4
	HF, LI	–0.9	–2.0
	HF, HI	–1.6	–2.7
Lean body mass (kg)	LF, LI	0.5	1.2
	LF, HI	0.7	1.6
	HF, LI	0.4	1.3
	HF, HI	1.0	1.7

Note: LF = low frequency (1.0-1.5 times/week); HF = high frequency (average, 3.3 times/week); LI = low intensity (no more than 60% of aerobic power); HI = high intensity (60%, progressing to 80% of aerobic power).

Adapted, by permission, from R.J. Shephard et al., 1977, *American Journal of Clinical Nutrition* 30: 326-333. © American Journal of Clinical Nutrition, American Society for Clinical Nutrition.

women showed a decrease of subcutaneous fat. In the men there was a selective loss of fat from central and upper body sites; this was not seen in the women, perhaps because they entered the study with less central fat deposition.

In summary, regular physical activity seems most likely to enhance body composition if it is viewed as a long-term project, to be pursued over a year or longer. There must be a clear increase in daily energy expenditure (500 kJ/ day), and it is helpful if this is accompanied by a small decrease of energy intake (500 kJ/day).

Advantages of Physical Activity Over Dieting Alone

If weight is lost by dieting alone, a substantial fraction of the total decrease in body mass is due to a loss of lean tissue. However, exercise tends to conserve lean tissue, except when the added energy expenditure is sufficient to create a large energy deficit (Donnelly 1992).

Dieting also induces a 10% to 15% reduction of resting metabolism, which can be enough to negate the benefits of all except very stringent energy restriction programs. In contrast, as noted above, exercise often stimulates an increase in metabolism after exercise, and this in itself makes a useful contribution to the reduction of body fat.

Furthermore, dietary restriction is often associated with a depression of mood state. In contrast, exercise often leads to an improvement of mood state, encouraging compliance with the prescribed regimen. However, more studies are needed to show that the elderly exerciser can experience the elevation of mood seen in the young exerciser (Foreyt 1992).

Lean Tissue Mass

The response of lean tissue to a training program depends not only on the type of activity performed, but also on hormonal factors and the quantity and quality of the food ingested.

Type of Activity

Aerobic exercise leads to an immediate increase of protein catabolism, although this is usually followed by a phase of enhanced protein synthesis (Zackin and Meredith 1989). Resistance training also augments the excretion of 3-methyl-L-histidine, suggesting an increased turnover of myofibrillar protein (Frontera et al. 1988). Moreover, the empirical evidence to be discussed shows that such training can induce substantial gains in muscle cross-section and muscle force in the elderly person, given appropriate hormonal and nutritional conditions.

Hormonal Factors

A decreased secretion of testosterone, growth hormone, and the insulin-like growth factor (somatomedin C) that mediates the effects of growth hormone (Florini and Roberts 1980; Sara and Hall 1990) may all contribute to muscle wasting with age. Conversely, for an optimal response of lean mass to a training program, it may be necessary to supplement blood levels of these hormones in elderly subjects.

Morley et al. (1993) tested men over the age of 70 years who initially had a low serum testosterone (< 70 ng/dl). Over a three-month period, those receiving 200 mg of testosterone intramuscularly every two weeks developed an advantage of grip strength relative to controls who did not receive the injections.

In the sedentary rat, aging is associated with a loss of tissue sensitivity to the insulin-like growth factor, but a normal response can be restored by a program of aerobic exercise; there is a corresponding increase in receptor mRNA (Willis and Parkhouse 1994). In elderly human subjects, the data are less consistent, but it appears that aerobic training may enhance the output of growth hormone and augment concentrations of serum IGF-1 (Borst, Millard, and Lowenthal 1994).

Dietary Influences

As in a younger individual, the older person needs an adequate protein intake to cover both the increased protein breakdown induced by exercise and the needs of tissue hypertrophy. Meredith et al. (1992) enrolled subjects aged 61 to 72 years in a program of resistance exercises. Many nutritionists would have regarded the initial protein intake (1.25 g/kg per day) as more than adequate. However, the experimental subjects received dietary supplements, bringing their protein intake to a final value of 1.55 g/kg per day. The lean mass of these subjects did not increase relative to that of controls who continued to receive only 1.25 g/kg of protein each day, but computed tomography of the mid-thigh suggested that the experimental subjects had developed a substantially greater increase in muscle cross-section than the controls who had performed the same exercises but had received only a standard diet.

Training Response

Cross-sectional studies of Masters athletes (see table 4.1) suggest that regular physical activity can conserve lean tissue mass. Several authors have also demonstrated that people as old as 90 years can follow programs of heavy resistance training (Charette et al. 1991; Cress et al. 1991; Fiatarone et al. 1990; Hagberg, Graves, et al. 1989). Substantial gains of muscle strength have been observed. At one time, such responses were attributed simply to an improved motor unit recruitment (Moritani and de Vries 1980); but observations based on limb circumferences, muscle fiber size (Charette et al. 1991), creatinine excretion (Yarasheski 1993), ^{40}K content (Sidney, Shephard, and Harrison 1977), and computed tomography and magnetic resonance imaging (Fiatarone et al. 1990) have now demonstrated that at least a part of the observed increase in muscle strength is attributable to muscle hypertrophy.

Nichols et al. (1993) found a 1.5 kg increase of lean tissue when 36 women over the age of 60 years completed 24 weeks of heavy resistance training. The percentage of body fat also decreased from 38.8% to 37.9%. Likewise, Brown, McCartney, and Sale (1990) saw a 30% increase of muscle cross-section over 12 weeks of weight lifting in a study of 60- to 70-year-old men. In the experiments by Fiatarone et al. (1990), frail nursing home residents aged 86 to 96 years showed a 180% increase of muscle strength and a 9% increase of thigh cross-section over as little as eight weeks of vigorous training (contractions at 80% of the one-repetition maximum, three times per week). Muscle biopsies showed a 34% increase in the area of individual type I fibers and a 28% increase in the area of type II fibers. The aerobic power also increased when measured during leg exercise, but it showed no change when measured during arm exercise; this finding suggests that local muscle strength is an important determinant of oxygen transport in the frail elderly. Other investigators, in apparent disagreement with Fiatarone et al. (1990), have noted that hypertrophy was concentrated in type II fibers (Cartee 1994; Pyka et al. 1994; Rogers and Evans 1993).

Some muscle biopsy studies have shown little change in aerobic enzyme activity after training, but this is probably because the intensity of training was light. After 12 weeks of vigorous cycling, 45 min/day, three days per week, Meredith et al. (1989) found a larger increase of oxidative capacity in the elderly (128%) than in young subjects (27%). Likewise, after 10 months of endurance training, Coggan et al. (1992) found increased activity in several markers of aerobic metabolism: succinate dehydrogenase, citrate synthase, and beta-hydroxyacyl-CoA dehydrogenase.

Thus, we may conclude that it is now well established that an appropriate program of resisted exercise can restore both muscle strength and lean tissue in even the oldest-old.

Bone

Studies in turkeys have suggested that repeated stressing of the ulna increases bone formation at the periosteal surface, augmenting its strength; however, this response is greatly reduced in old turkeys (Rubin, Bain, and McLeod 1992). In humans, also, an increase of bone density is seen in body parts that have been stressed by gravity or muscle contraction. It has been postulated that the application of force stimulates bone formation by a piezoelectric effect. The rate of bone formation (B) is related to both the number of loading cycles (N) and the applied force (F), expressed as a fraction of the critical force (F_c) needed to cause a fracture according to the equation (Carter, Fyhrie, and Whalen 1987):

$$B = N \, (F/F_c)^n$$

where n is an exponent between 2 and 6. The implication of this formula is that bone strength is influenced much more by an intense strain than by the repeated application of low-intensity forces, an important point when one considers exercise responses in the frail elderly.

Critique of Empirical Data

For reasons of convenience, many early measurements of human bone density—both in cross-sectional comparisons and in longitudinal interventions—were made on the wrist. Except among participants in a few sports such as tennis (Simkin, Ayalon, and Leichter 1987), such measurements are unlikely to reveal the full beneficial effects of exercise, and the conclusions from upper limb measurements have been correspondingly equivocal. Other variables that also were poorly controlled in many early studies included diet (both calcium and vitamin D intake), exercise-induced changes in energy balance and body mass, the use of hormone supplements (particularly by perimenopausal women), and involvement in physical activities unrelated to the experimental variable (for example, substantial amounts of walking or jogging undertaken by some of those classed as swimmers).

Cross-Sectional Studies

A large number of cross-sectional studies have indicated a higher bone density in athletic than in sedentary individuals (Ballard et al. 1990; Granhed, Johnson, and Hansson 1987; Heinonen et al. 1993; Stillman et al. 1986). Weight lifters, for example, have 10% to 13% more bone mineral than age-matched controls (Karlsson, Johnell, and Obrant 1993). Moreover, this effect apparently persists into senior age groups.

Barrett-Connor (1995) found a significant correlation between the density of the hip and reported physical activity as an adolescent and at ages 30 and 50 years. Likewise, Aloia et al. (1988) found that 16% to 25% of the variance in total body calcium and lumbar bone density could be explained by motion sensor measurements of habitual physical activity. Several authors (Cheng et al. 1991; Chow et al. 1986; Nguyen et al. 1994; Pocock et al. 1986; Vico et al. 1995) have all reported significant associations between the amount of calcium in the trunk and upper thighs and the individual's aerobic power. In principle, aerobic power provides a convenient objective index of a person's habitual physical activity. But if maximal oxygen intake is expressed in L/min, as in the study of Pocock et al. (1986), it (like bone density) is necessarily correlated with body size, and a spurious association results.

Krall and Dawson-Hughes (1994) found that women aged 43 to 72 years who walked 1.6 km/day had higher lumbar and whole-body bone densities than their peers who walked a lesser distance. Other investigators (Hatori et al. 1993; Nelson et al. 1991; Zylstra et al. 1989) have made similar observations on the benefits of walking. Zylstra et al. (1989) concluded that the femoral neck of a walker was effectively equivalent to that of a sedentary woman who was some four years younger.

Longitudinal Studies

Bloomfield et al. (1993) claimed that eight months of training increased the lumbar spine density of postmenopausal women by 2.5%, compared with a deterioration of 0.7% in controls over the same time interval; the advantage seen in the experimental group is interesting, since the subjects performed weight-supported aerobic training on a cycle ergometer. Chow, Harrison, and Notarius (1987) adopted the more sophisticated approach of measuring total body calcium by neutron activation; the readings in exercisers showed a moderate increase rather than the expected decrease. The response was almost twice as large in those who undertook a combination of aerobic and muscle-strengthening exercises as in those who undertook aerobic exercise alone.

Other programs with an aerobic emphasis have had only a limited influence on bone density. In an early study (Sidney, Shephard, and Harrison 1977), my colleagues and I measured whole-body calcium by neutron activation. After one year of progressive aerobic training (mainly fast walking), values averaged 99.7% ± 7.0% of initial levels. However, in the subjects who had exercised least, whole-body calcium had diminished by 9%, whereas there were substantial gains of density in those who had elected to exercise vigorously and frequently. Likewise, Martin and Notelovitz (1993) reported that 12 months of aerobic training did no more than attenuate the local loss of mineral density in the lumbar spine. Again, Cavanaugh and Cann (1988) found that brisk walking (30 min, three times per week) did not prevent a 6% decrease in lumbar bone density over a year of observation. Many of the participants in these studies were walking rather than jogging, and possibly the intensity of activity was insufficient to prevent osteoporosis; ground reaction forces are two to three times greater in jogging than in walking. In some instances, the subjects may also have needed calcium and/or hormonal supplements in order to realize the benefits of gravitational stimulation (Nelson et al. 1991).

Need for Weight-Bearing Activity

In terms of preventing osteoporosis, exercise that requires weight bearing (aerobic dance, calisthenics, walking, jogging, or stair climbing) has generally proven more effective than seated activity. Weight-bearing pursuits have increased the mineral density of the lumbar spine by 4% to 6% over eight to nine months in postmenopausal women (Chow, Harrison, and Notarius 1987; Dalsky et al. 1988; Krølner et al. 1983). In contrast, sedentary control subjects have lost 1% to 3% of bone mineral density over the same period.

Swim training has generally had little influence on the development of osteoporosis; this emphasizes the importance of applying mechanical force to the bones by gravity. In one cross-sectional study of swimmers, Orwoll et al. (1989) found benefit in men but not in women. Conceivably the men had engaged in a more vigorous swimming program and thus had applied substantial muscle forces to the skeleton, or possibly they had engaged in other forms of exercise as well as swimming.

Strength Training

Strength training provides an alternative method of applying mechanical force to the bones, thus stimulating mineral deposition. In some longitudinal studies, bone mineral content has remained unchanged when elderly subjects have enrolled in weight-lifting programs. Such a lack of response (for example, Smidt et al. 1992) may be attributed to the fact that the observation period was too short for subjects to progress to a substantial volume of physical activity. Over 16 weeks of training, strength training that increased muscle strength by 45% also increased femoral density by 3.8% and lumbar density by 2% in 59-year-old, previously sedentary men; there was an associated 26% increase in alkaline phosphatase and a 19% increase of osteocalcin (Menkes et al. 1993).

Estrogen Supplements

In women, gains have been largest in programs in which estrogens were also administered (Prince et al. 1991); Notelovitz et al. (1991) noted an 8.4% increase of bone density in a longitudinal study of such individuals. There has thus been a growing use of hormone replacement therapy for postmenopausal women, particularly in the United States. Nevertheless, there remains a need to evaluate the resulting benefits of increased bone remineralization and decreased cardiovascular risk (McDonald et al. 1995; Stampfer et al. 1991) relative to the long-term risks of breast cancer that are incurred when exercise is supplemented by estrogen administration, with or without progesterone.

Comparison of Cross-Sectional and Longitudinal Data

The magnitude of the active subject's advantage in bone density has usually been larger in cross-sectional comparisons (Granhed, Johnson, and Hansson 1987; Heinonen et al. 1993) than in longitudinal training studies (Bloomfield 1995; Chilibeck, Sale, and Webber 1995; Drinkwater 1994; Forwood and Burr 1993; Gutin and Kasper 1992; Suominen 1994). Even among participants in longitudinal studies that combined aerobics and weight lifting, increases in whole-body or lumbar calcium content relative to control subjects have usually been no more than 6% to 8% (Bloomfield 1995; Drinkwater 1994). In contrast, cross-sectional comparisons have shown a 40% advantage of bone mineral content in the lumbar vertebrae of distance runners (Lane et al. 1986) and an 18% advantage in an active population of frail elderly (Chow et al. 1986).

Cross-sectional studies cannot entirely rule out the possibility of selection bias, particularly when sedentary subjects are compared with participants in sports that favor heavily-built individuals. Nevertheless, changes in bone density have a relatively slow time course, so the full benefit of an active lifestyle is likely to be seen more clearly in comparisons between athletes and sedentary subjects than in short-term training studies (Kohrt and Snead 1993).

Clinical Implications

The risk of hip fracture approximately doubles for each 10% decrease in bone density (Drinkwater 1994). Thus, even a 6% to 8% increase in bone density would be important in preventing pathological fractures, and the 18% to 40% increase suggested by cross-sectional comparisons would have great practical significance for health.

The benefit obtained from a training program is reversible. Thus, Michel et al. (1992) noted that in runners aged 55 to 77 years of age, the loss of bone mineral over a five-year interval was greatest in those who had reduced their training by the largest amount. The implication is that physical activity must be sustained in order to preserve bone mineral content.

Finally, as with most aspects of exercise therapy, it is important to note that an excess of physical activity can have negative effects. Michel et al. (1992) noted that in older subjects who reported exercising more than 200 to 300 min/week, the bone density of the lumbar spine was extremely low relative to that of either sedentary controls or moderate exercisers.

Tendons and Ligaments

In general, tendons and ligaments are strengthened by a program of moderate physical activity. However, because of age-related deteriorations in the structure of collagen as discussed in chapter 2, a decrease in the diameter of the tendon fibrils (Amiel et al. 1991; Jones 1991; Naresh and Brodsky 1992), and a decrease in junctional strength at the point of insertion into the bone, there is a danger that overrigorous training will cause injuries to tendons and ligaments, including in some cases a frank tendon rupture (Kannus and Józsa 1991).

Whereas the ground matrix proteoglycans are readily increased by training in young rats, little benefit is seen in older animals; however, this may be because the older animals run a much shorter distance (Vailas et al. 1985). Kasperczyk et al. (1991) claimed that when subjects were matched for habitual physical activity, there were no differences in the elastic properties of the knee ligaments between 30- and 65-year-old individuals.

Cardiorespiratory System

Respiratory function is changed relatively little by either general aerobic training or specific breathing exercises. However, there is now little dispute that seniors can augment both their peak cardiovascular performance and their overall oxygen transport in response to an appropriate training regimen. Items that still arouse vigorous discussion are (1) the optimal pattern of training to enhance cardiorespiratory performance, (2) the extent of benefit relative to gains in younger individuals who exercise in similar fashion, (3) the influence of a physically active lifestyle on the rate of aging of cardiorespiratory function, (4) the influence of atherosclerotic disease on the ability to exercise and the resulting training response, (5) the ability of aerobic training to enhance the coronary circulation, and (6) whether there is a ceiling age beyond which training becomes dangerous and inadvisable.

Respiratory System

Training programs have little influence on either static or dynamic lung volumes. Nevertheless, beneficial ventilatory changes can result from a well-designed aerobic training program.

Lung Volumes

Cross-sectional studies comparing sedentary individuals with those who had a maximal oxygen intake 1.5 to 2 times greater have consistently shown that very fit older adults have a smaller functional residual capacity (a difference of about 10%), a greater 1 sec forced expiratory volume (an advantage of about

9%), and a greater maximal expiratory flow rate (an advantage of about 25%) (Dempsey and Seals 1995; Hagberg, Yerg, and Seals 1988; Johnson, Reddan, Pegelow, et al. 1991). Even habitual walking is associated with larger lung volumes (Frändin et al. 1991).

Some early longitudinal studies showed very little change of vital capacity in physical education teachers as they became older (Åstrand 1986). Since sedentary adults show a 20 to 30 ml loss of vital capacity per year of working life, such figures might seem to suggest that a sustained interest in physical activity could limit the age-related decrease of lung volumes. However, athletes are likely to be nonsmokers and thus they avoid the effects of chronic bronchitis and emphysema. Moreover, spirometer designs have improved substantially over the past 20 to 30 years; subjects may thus have been able to expel a larger fraction of their total lung capacity when measurements were repeated on a newer instrument.

In an early study of 60- to 76-year-old subjects with lung volumes that were normal or larger than normal, Niinimaa and Shephard (1978a) saw no gains in static or dynamic lung volumes, closing volumes, or pulmonary diffusing capacity over an 11-week aerobic training program that augmented maximal oxygen intakes by an average of 10%. More recently, McClaran et al. (1995) noted substantial declines in vital capacity and midexpiratory flow rate despite the continued daily training of very fit subjects.

Nevertheless, Dempsey and Seals (1995) have argued that the respiratory system is unlikely to limit aerobic performance in the elderly, except in the unusual situation where maximal oxygen intake is particularly well preserved and there has at the same time been a substantial decline in ventilatory performance.

Other Mechanisms of Benefit

Despite the lack of influence upon static and dynamic lung volumes, a training program can have several beneficial effects on the ventilation of an elderly person.

An improvement in the mechanical efficiency of movement may reduce what are initially a high oxygen cost and ventilatory cost for the performance of a given physical activity (McConnell and Davies 1992; Poulin et al. 1994). A strengthening of the skeletal muscles may also diminish acidosis and thus the ventilation demanded by a given bout of heavy physical work (the ratio $\dot{V}_E/\dot{V}_{O2}$; Ades et al. 1993; Massé-Biron et al. 1992; Yerg et al. 1985), although this latter type of adaptation is likely to be observed only if the oxygen cost of the task initially exceeds the individual's ventilatory threshold.

A combination of instruction in breathing techniques and specific development of the chest muscles may enable an elderly person to take a faster inspiration and thus a slower expiration during vigorous exercise. This in turn diminishes the tendency to expiratory collapse of the airways (Johnson, Reddan, Scow, et al. 1991), thereby increasing the uniformity of ventilation and reducing dead space ventilation.

Finally, the aerobic exercise of an elderly person is often halted by dyspnea, and a training program may habituate an individual to the sensation of breathlessness, allowing a greater ventilation to be developed.

Cardiovascular System

Given that the respiratory system is rarely the limiting link in the oxygen transport chain, even in the elderly, and that training has very little effect on respiratory function in this age group, any training-related increase in oxygen transport must arise from an augmentation of maximal heart rate and/or maximal stroke volume—with a resulting increase of peak cardiac output, a more effective distribution of the available cardiac output, an increased peripheral extraction of oxygen in the working muscles, or an enhanced coronary arterial flow. We will now examine each of these possibilities.

Heart Rate

In contrast with younger individuals, older adults in some studies have shown little change in resting heart rate in response to a moderate training program (Blumenthal, Emery, Madden, Coleman, et al. 1991). Nevertheless, more rigorous conditioning continues to have some effect. Thus, Pollock et al. (1987) found average resting heart rates of 42 beats/min in 60-year-old Masters athletes who were still competing, as contrasted with 52 beats/min in those who had ceased competing. Any decrease of resting heart rate is mediated largely by an increase of vagal tonus, although there may also be some reduction of intrinsic heart rate (De Meersman 1993; Denahan et al. 1993). There is an associated increase of resting stroke volume, so that the resting cardiac output shows little change.

Many of the frail elderly have difficulty in reaching an oxygen consumption plateau when they first attempt maximal effort. As their physical condition improves, they are able to exercise harder, so that a higher peak heart rate and respiratory gas exchange ratio may be attained (Pollock et al. 1987). However, with the exception of a few instances in which there is initially a pathological deficit of blood flow to the sinus pacemaker (the sick sinus syndrome), there is no physiological basis for a true increase of maximal heart rate with training, nor is such a change usually observed (Spina et al. 1994). Relative to that of sedentary individuals of similar age, the maximal heart rate of continuing athletes is either similar (Fleg et al. 1988; Fuchi et al. 1989; Hagberg et al. 1985; Ogawa et al. 1992; Saltin 1986) or slightly lower (Blumenthal, Emery, Madden, Coleman, et al. 1991; Spina et al. 1993).

Active and sedentary individuals thus show a roughly parallel decrease in peak heart rates as they become older (Saltin 1986). Kavanagh et al. (1989) found that the heart rate of Masters competitors decreased from 170 to 175 beats/min at age 35 years to 152 to 154 beats/min at age 65 years (a decrease of some 25 beats/min over 30 years). In a more general sample of the population, Sidney and Shephard (1978a) found maximal values of around 195 and 170 beats/min in 25- and 65-year-old men (a decrease of 25 beats/min over 40 years).

Stroke Volume

A training-induced increase of stroke volume may reflect increased preloading of the ventricles, ventricular hypertrophy, enhanced myocardial contractility, or a decreased afterloading. We will examine changes in these determinants before looking at empirical data on oxygen pulse, ejection fraction, and stroke volume.

Preloading. According to Lakatta (1993a), the elderly person has already exploited the Frank-Starling relationship before beginning training; this limits the possibility of augmenting stroke volume by a further increase of end-diastolic volume, whether this is caused by a training-induced increase of total blood volume or an enhanced peripheral venous tone.

Nevertheless, an early report by Benestad (1965) noted significant increases of both total blood volume and total hemoglobin when elderly subjects underwent five weeks of intensive training. At least one study also reported an increase of end-diastolic volume in 60- to 70-year-old subjects who trained sufficiently to augment their aerobic power by 18% (Ehsani et al. 1991). There is still disagreement about whether an increase in the rate of early diastolic filling is (Forman et al. 1992; Levy et al. 1993; Takemoto et al. 1992) or is not (Schulman et al. 1992) responsible for this increase.

The effect of increased preloading probably depends upon the oxygenation of the myocardium. If there is already some myocardial ischemia, the left ventricle reacts poorly to a further increase of end-diastolic volume, and it is quite easy for a few weeks of excessively heavy exertion to push a frail elderly individual into a state of either congestive heart failure or pulmonary edema. It is thus common for geriatric physicians to curtail salt and fluid intake and to prescribe diuretics for their elderly patients. Such measures tend to reduce ventricular preloading and stroke volume. Even if the coronary vessels have suffered little narrowing and the hazard of cardiac failure is avoided, an increase of blood volume might seem of limited value to an elderly person, because of a slow relaxation of the ventricular wall and thus a reduced rate of ventricular filling (Lakatta 1993a).

Cardiac hypertrophy and myocardial contractility. It is unlikely that a sedentary senior citizen will be persuaded to exercise with sufficient vigor to induce cardiac hypertrophy. In contrast, there is some evidence from cardiac radiographs that the large heart of the endurance athlete persists in those individuals who maintain their training schedules.

Early radiographic estimates of total cardiac volume showed that values in Masters athletes increased from 12 ml/kg in those under 40 years of age to

13.9 ml/kg at ages 60 to 70, and to 13.2 ml/kg at 70 to 90 years (Kavanagh and Shephard 1977). Likewise, Grimby and Saltin (1966) found that whereas the total heart volume of inactive orienteers had already dropped to 11.1 ml/kg by 45 years of age, those who persisted with their sport had maintained values as high as 15 ml/kg. More recently, Di Bello et al. (1993) noted a left ventricular volume of 319 ml/m^2 (8.8 ml/kg) in 65-year-old endurance athletes compared with 225 ml/m^2 (6.3 ml/kg) in sedentary controls of similar age.

Echocardiographic studies have shown matching increases in left ventricular end-diastolic diameter and posterior wall thickness over 12 months of vigorous training (Ehsani et al. 1991; Seals, Hagberg, et al. 1994).

Despite this evidence of ventricular hypertrophy, the age-related impairment in the beta-adrenergic (inotropic) response to exercise does not seem to be reversed by endurance training (Stratton et al. 1992).

Afterloading.   As in younger adults, cross-sectional comparisons between sedentary individuals and either actively training subjects (Kasch et al. 1993) or Masters athletes (Pollock et al. 1987) suggest that the normal age-related increment of resting systemic blood pressures is either abolished or reduced by training (see table 4.3). Moreover, Reaven, Barrett-Connor, and Edelstein (1991) maintain that in older women the association between physically active leisure and a low resting blood pressure is independent of any changes in obesity or plasma insulin level.

Longitudinal studies also suggest that a regular program of endurance exercise can induce a therapeutically useful decrease of resting systemic blood pressure (5-10 mmHg) in subjects as old as 70 to 79 years (Cononie et al. 1991), although it is puzzling that this change is not seen in nocturnal blood pressure readings (Gilders and Dudley 1992). In Masters athletes who continue their training regimen, blood pressures remain relatively constant over many years; however, in those who cease training as they become older, systolic pressures rise by as much as 10 mmHg over 10 years (Pollock et al. 1987). Other longitudinal observations have shown that small (5-10 mmHg) reductions in resting blood pressure can be induced by aerobic training, particularly when initial readings are high (Tipton 1991).

During exercise, the blood pressure at a given relative work rate is either unchanged (Ehsani et al. 1991; Ogawa et al. 1992; Spina et al. 1993) or lower (Martin, Ogawa, et al. 1991; Saltin 1986) in a well-trained person compared to a sedentary individual of similar age. The main explanation seems to be that if the muscles are strengthened, they are more easily perfused at any given rate of working and the rise of blood pressure is correspondingly smaller. Martin et al. (1990) used plethysmography to demonstrate that 31 weeks of training at 70% to 90% of maximal oxygen intake increased the maximal limb flow in 64-year-old men and women. Likewise, Makrides, Heigenhauser, and Jones (1990) found increases of vascular conductance in 60- to 70-year-old men after 12 weeks of high-intensity endurance training. However, because

Table 4.3   Resting systemic blood pressures for elderly athletes, compared with the values of Master et al. (1964) for the general population.

Age Years	Master et al. (1964)	Kavanagh and Shephard (1977)	Pollock (1974)	Asano, Ogawa, and Furuta (1976)	Kavanagh et al. (1989) Men	Kavanagh et al. (1989) Women
<40	127/80	124/79	—	—	125/78	117/73
40-50	130/82	120/77	117/76	117/70	128/82	118/77
50-60	137/84	127/77	129/81	132/79	132/82	129/80
60-70	143/84	128/77	122/78	135/82	142/86	133/82
70-80	146/82	140/86	141/83	157/78	143/82	135/81

All male data except for those of Kavanagh et al. (1989).

well-trained individuals can exercise to a higher peak work rate, trained subjects usually reach peak blood pressures that are as high as or higher than the values seen in their sedentary peers (Saltin 1986).

Oxygen pulse.   It is technically quite difficult to measure either stroke volume or cardiac output when subjects are exercising hard, and intergroup differences in stroke volume have often been inferred from a much-maligned statistic, the oxygen pulse (the ratio of oxygen consumption to heart rate).

In a cross-sectional comparison between younger and older individuals, Hagberg et al. (1985) revised their earlier view that oxygen pulse did not change with age, describing a small decline of this index in older individuals. Saltin (1986) also found a 23.8% decrease of oxygen pulse from age 26 to 66 years. Kavanagh et al. (1989) tested subjects who were maintaining a substantial volume of training; nevertheless, values for oxygen pulse declined from 21.2 to 17.8 ml/beat in the men and from 15.4 to 12.4 ml/beat in the women over the age range 35 to 65 years.

All studies have found larger oxygen pulse values in Masters athletes than in sedentary subjects of similar age. For example, Saltin (1986) observed no difference in oxygen pulse between elderly orienteers who were still increasing their training schedule and those who had allowed training to slip. Nevertheless, at an age of 65 years the mean value for the group (0.32 ml/kg per beat, about 23 ml/beat) was substantially larger than the average figure for 65-year-old men. Between 50 and 60 years of age, Pollock et al. (1987) saw no change of oxygen pulse in Masters athletes who were still competing at a high level; in others who continued to cover a similar mileage but who had ceased competition, the oxygen pulse decreased from 22.4 to 20.0 ml/beat.

Ejection fraction and stroke volume.   We have already noted the view of Lakatta (1993a) that the fit, well-trained older individual compensates for the age-related decrease in maximal heart rate by an increase of end-diastolic volume and thus of cardiac ejection fraction. In contrast, the person who remains inactive with some silent myocardial ischemia is unable to increase his or her ejection fraction by this mechanism, so that the stroke volume diminishes with aging. Fleg et al. (1993) found a left ventricular ejection fraction of 85% in young adults, 76% in fit 76-year-old men, and 66% in age-matched individuals with silent ischemia.

Endurance training may augment stroke volume by virtue of an increase in myocardial contractility, a decrease in collagen cross-linkage, or both. These changes are important to making good use of the increase in end-diastolic volume (Ehsani et al. 1991; Thomas et al. 1992).

Cross-sectional comparisons have shown a substantial 40 to 50 ml difference in the measured peak stroke volume between continuing athletes and sedentary subjects (Fuchi et al. 1989; Ogawa et al. 1992; Rivera et al. 1989; Saltin 1986). Early carbon dioxide rebreathing measurements (Niinimaa and Shephard 1978a) showed no increase of peak stroke volume in a group of elderly subjects over an 11-week period of aerobic training, despite a 10% increase of maximal oxygen intake. Other investigators (Makrides, Heigenhauser, and Jones 1990; Spina et al. 1993) have observed small gains over longer training programs. Seals et al. (1984b) noted a 6% increase in stroke volume over six months of vigorous aerobic training. Spina et al. (1993) had their 64-year-old subjects train five days per week for 9 to 12 months at an intensity rising to 75% to 85% of maximal heart rate. They used the acetylene rebreathing method to demonstrate a 15% increase of maximal stroke volume in male but not in female subjects. The gender difference may reflect hormonal factors—particularly a lack of estrogen in older women (Giraud et al. 1993; Pines et al. 1991). The echocardiographic data of Ehsani et al. (1991) suggested that stroke volume increased from 110 to 132 ml (a 20% gain) during 12 months of vigorous training; 17 ml of the increase was due to an augmentation of end-diastolic volume, with the exercise ejection fraction increasing from 67% to 78%.

Such studies support the inference from the oxygen pulse readings that continuing athletes have a large stroke volume. The advantage is partly genetic, but benefit has also been won by a long period of hard training. Nevertheless, it is difficult to increase stroke volume by a short-term training program.

Cardiac Output

Relative to a sedentary person, the elderly individual who has trained for many years shows a slightly lower maximal heart rate, but a substantially larger peak stroke volume. The active person thus has an advantage of maximal cardiac output (Saltin 1986; Seals et al. 1984b; Spina et al. 1993). However, this advantage can be realized only by long-term training that is effective in augmenting the peak stroke volume.

Training may also help to correct the slow on-transient of heart rate and oxygen consumption that is such a marked characteristic of the early exercise response in a sedentary older person (Babcock et al. 1994).

Arteriovenous Oxygen Difference

A training-induced increase of maximal arteriovenous oxygen difference could reflect a more efficient extraction of oxygen in the working muscles (because of greater capillarization or an increase of muscle enzyme activity, for instance), or it could be due to a more effective redirection of blood flow from the skin, viscera, and inactive muscles (where oxygen extraction is limited) to the working muscles.

There have been reports that training increases capillary blood supply and augments the activity of aerobic enzymes in skeletal muscle, as outlined in chapter 3. However, oxygen extraction is relatively complete in the working muscles even before such changes take effect. Saltin (1986) noted that the maximal arteriovenous oxygen difference of elderly orienteers (134 ml/L) remained quite low, and similar to that of sedentary individuals rather than to that of young athletes. Nevertheless, blood sampled from the femoral vein of these subjects had a very low oxygen content (18 ml/L). It thus appears that (1) the subjects had little potential to increase oxygen extraction in the working muscles and (2) they had little more success than sedentary subjects in redirecting blood flow from the inactive to the active tissues.

Studies from our laboratory (Niinimaa and Shephard 1978b) showed little increase of arteriovenous oxygen difference in 65-year-old subjects over 11 weeks of training. However, others have noted greater arteriovenous oxygen differences in cross-sectional comparisons between athletes and sedentary individuals (Ogawa et al. 1992; Rivera et al. 1989) and after prolonged training (Makrides, Heigenhauser, and Jones 1990; Spina et al. 1993). Indeed, Spina et al. (1993) attributed all of the training-induced increase of maximal oxygen intake in elderly women to an increase of arteriovenous oxygen difference (although they also found some increase of cardiac output in their male subjects).

The majority of authors have attributed the widening of the arteriovenous oxygen difference to an increase in capillary density and an augmentation of aerobic enzyme activity in the muscles (Coggan et al. 1992; Martin, Kohrt, et al. 1990; Martin, Ogawa, et al. 1991; Rogers and Evans 1993). However, other contributing factors include (1) a decrease in obesity and an increase in sweating, with a corresponding reduction in the need for a large skin blood flow (Buono, McKenzie, and Kasch 1991; Tankersley et al. 1991), and (2) a larger cardiac output, so that the fraction of the total blood flow directed to the skin and viscera has a smaller impact upon the overall arteriovenous oxygen difference.

Coronary Arterial Blood Flow

Because the coronary vascular supply is marginal for the peak metabolic needs of the heart in an older person, a narrowing of the coronary arteries can diminish aerobic power, increase dilatation of the left ventricle, and reduce the possibility of an effective training response (Fleg et al. 1993).

The Masters athlete may show many of the electrocardiographic features observed in a younger endurance competitor, such as a partial atrioventricular block and ST-segmental elevation (Thompson and Dorsey 1986). A substantial minority of competitors also show exercise-induced ST-segmental depression that would be regarded as clinically significant in a younger individual (Kavanagh et al. 1989).

As age increases, a growing proportion of the population, both active and sedentary, show changes in the exercise ECG (particularly depression of the ST segment) that have been linked statistically with an increased risk of coronary vascular narrowing and premature cardiac death. The sensitivity of treadmill testing in older individuals is 84% (Hlatky et al. 1984) or 85% (Newman and Phillips 1988), but the specificity is poor (70%, Hlatky et al. 1984; 56%, Newman and Phillips 1988); in other words, most diseased subjects will be identified, but there will also be many false-positive diagnoses. A physical training program reduces both the extent and the prevalence of ECG abnormalities at a given intensity of external work. A slower heart rate, possibly coupled with some reduction of systolic blood pressure, reduces the cardiac work rate and thus the oxygen demand of the heart at any specified submaximal oxygen consumption. A variety of factors facilitate coronary perfusion in the trained individual. The slower heart rate permits a longer diastolic phase (when most of the coronary blood flow occurs). If cardiac hypertrophy has resulted from prolonged training, a given blood pressure can be developed for a lesser tension per unit cross-section of the ventricular wall, further facilitating myocardial blood flow during systole. A well-trained individual may also release fewer potassium ions at a given intensity of muscular effort; this further reduces the tendency to ST depression and ventricular fibrillation. Finally, there are controversial reports that training broadens coronary vascular dimensions and encourages the development of coronary collateral vessels that bypass points of arterial narrowing (Kavanagh 1989).

In practice, it is uncertain how far training alters the prevalence of abnormal ECGs at a constant relative work rate or a constant heart rate. During maximal testing, the prevalence of ECG abnormalities in Masters athletes is similar to, or perhaps slightly less than, that in the general population of similar age (Kavanagh and Shephard 1978, Kavanagh et al. 1989). In longitudinal studies, a decrease in ST abnormalities often arises from a reduction of the exercise heart rate and thus the myocardial oxygen consumption at a given work rate. Some years ago, a colleague and I made a detailed study of changes in the ECGs of 42 elderly subjects over a program of aerobic training (Sidney and Shephard 1977b). One feature that complicated the interpretation of ECGs in the study was a progressive elevation of the resting ST segment as training continued. The increase in resting ST voltages averaged .03 mV at 7 weeks of training and .04 mV at 14 weeks; the largest changes were seen in those who were frequent participants in the program. The ST voltages at a fixed heart rate of 120 beats/min shifted in a favorable direction, from an average of −.03 to +.03 mV, over the 14 weeks of training. Initially, 11 of the 42 subjects showed a clinically significant exercise-induced ST depression (>.10 mV), but over the 14 weeks of observation, 5 of the 11 progressed to the point at which the depression was less than .10 mV. A further 2 of the 11 subjects resolved their ST depression after a full year of training.

One practical consequence of exercise-induced ischemia is an increased risk of cardiac arrest and/or myocardial infarction during vigorous exercise (Shephard 1981; Siscovick et al. 1984; Vuori 1995). The risk that exercise will provoke a cardiac incident rises with age, in part because coronary atherosclerosis is a progressive condition, and in part because a decline in peak performance increases the relative demand imposed by any given intensity of physical activity. Thus, the improvement in life span achieved by beginning a vigorous training program diminishes progressively with age (Paffenbarger et al. 1994; Pekkanen et al. 1987). As discussed later in this chapter, beyond the age of about 80 years, heavy training may actually shorten a person's life span (although possibly enhancing its quality).

Overall Oxygen Transport

Cross-sectional comparisons show that elderly athletes have a substantially higher maximal oxygen intake than sedentary individuals, and subjects who begin an appropriate training program develop substantial gains of aerobic power through to the ninth decade of life (Denis and Chatard 1992; Hagberg, Graves, et al. 1989). However, it is less certain how far maintenance of a consistent, physically active lifestyle can attenuate the age-related decrease in oxygen transport.

Cross-Sectional Comparisons

Many studies have simply compared the maximal oxygen intake of older athletes with that of their sedentary age-matched peers. Such investigations show that substantial training-related differences persist into old age, both in men (Kavanagh et al. 1989; Ogawa et al. 1992; Pollock et al. 1987) and in women (Kavanagh et al. 1989; Stevenson et al. 1995; Wells, Boorman, and Riggs 1992).

It is less certain how far the advantage of the athletes is due to the selection of sporting activities by individuals who are genetically well endowed and how far the high scores are a consequence of continued training. Pollock et al. (1987) observed an average aerobic power of 53.3 ml/[kg · min] in 60-year-old Masters athletes who were still competing; this value dropped to 45.9 ml/[kg · min] in other members of the same group who were still undertaking some training but had ceased competing.

Longitudinal Data

The gains seen with participation in an endurance training program depend heavily upon the initial fitness of the individual (Denis and Chatard 1992; fig. 4.1). As in younger individuals, the extent of gains also varies with both the frequency and the intensity of training, but because many seniors are extremely inactive, a training response is sometimes seen at an intensity of effort that would have little effect on younger individuals. One of the first systematic studies of training in the elderly was conducted by Sidney and Shephard (1978a). They noted that over the first 14 weeks of training, the response of 65-year-old subjects was largest in those who elected to undertake relatively high-intensity activity (a heart rate of 130-140 beats/min) on a frequent basis

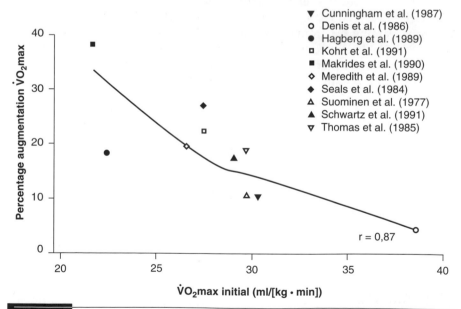

 Influence of initial level of maximal oxygen intake upon response to a program of endurance training.

Reprinted, by permission, from C. Denis and J.-C. Chatard, 1992, "Entrainabilité du sujet agé. La Revue de Gériatrie," *Proceedings of Euromedicine*, (Le Corum, Montpellier) 92: 203.

(two or more sessions per week). In such individuals, the percentage gain in maximal oxygen intake (around 35%) seemed at least as large as would be anticipated when younger persons participate in vigorous training (see fig. 4.2; Hagberg, Graves, et al. 1989; Kohrt et al. 1991; Makrides, Heigenhauser, and Jones 1990). However, many elderly people are either unwilling or unable to begin training at this intensity of effort. It is thus important that both Sidney and Shephard (1978a) and Cunningham et al. (1987) observed slow gains of oxygen transport in those who trained frequently at a heart rate of no more than 120 beats/min. It seems likely that if these subjects had persisted with such a regimen, substantial benefit might have resulted.

From the viewpoints of both safety and motivation, it is important to begin training the old person at a low intensity. Moreover, there is growing

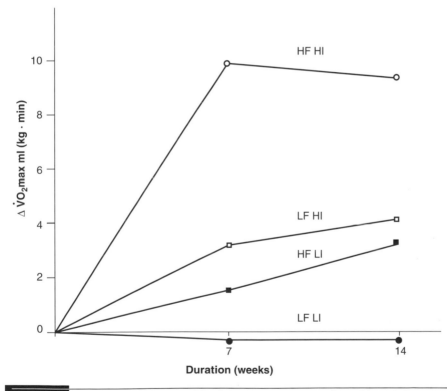

 Figure 4.2 Response of 65-year-old subjects to a program of aerobic training. Sample subdivided on basis of self-selected program: high (HI) or low (LI) intensity and high (HF) or low (LF) frequency of participation.
Reprinted, by permission, from K.H. Sidney and R.J. Shephard, 1978b, "Frequency and intensity of training for elderly subjects," *Medicine and Science in Sports and Exercise* 10: 125-131.

evidence (Badenhop et al. 1983; Belman and Gaesser 1991; Foster et al. 1989; Probart et al. 1991) that a large fraction of potential health gains can be realized from prolonged periods of moderate-intensity effort (for example, 1 h exercise sessions at 50% of maximal oxygen intake; American College of Sports Medicine 1995a). Seals et al. (1984b), working with a fairly sedentary elderly sample, claimed a 14% gain of maximal oxygen intake in response to six months of training at only 40% of maximal heart rate. After 12 months, the average response was a 30% increase in maximal oxygen intake, with a range from 2% to 49%.

Blumenthal, Emery, Madden, Coleman, et al. (1991) had subjects over the age of 60 years perform 1 h of cycle ergometry three times per week, beginning at 50% of the heart rate reserve and progressing to 70% of reserve as condition improved. Over the first 4 months, they saw a 10% to 15% improvement in aerobic power, with further gains of 1% to 6% when training was continued to 14 months. Likewise, Kohrt et al. (1991) reported an average 18% gain of maximal oxygen intake over 6 months of exercise at 75% to 80% of maximal heart rate, although there was a wide interindividual range in the training response. Others, who began their studies with subjects who had a higher fitness level (Cunningham et al. 1987; Denis and Chatard 1992), obtained correspondingly smaller responses. Govindasamy et al. (1992) further claimed that the half-time of response to training at 70% of aerobic power was only eight training sessions (14 days) in 66-year-old men.

There is thus good longitudinal evidence that endurance training can augment the aerobic power of elderly individuals. Nevertheless, the data of Posner et al. (1992) strike one note of caution. These investigators had 68-year-old men exercise at 70% of their peak heart rate (an average of 115 beats/min) for 40 min, three times per week. Over 16 weeks, maximal oxygen intake increased by 8.5%, but the oxygen intake at the ventilatory threshold increased by only 3.5%. The determination of ventilatory threshold requires less cooperation from an elderly person, and it may be that when subjects are tested to subjective exhaustion they move closer to their true maximal oxygen intake during a second test, thereby exaggerating the extent of the gain in aerobic power relative to estimates based upon the ventilatory threshold.

Continued Training and the Aging of Aerobic Power

Empirical studies have compared the rates of aging of aerobic power in both cross-sectional and longitudinal comparisons of aging rates between active and sedentary groups. Unfortunately, it has not always been clear to what extent the active group may have increased their training as a reaction to either initial testing or the prospect of reevaluation. Likewise, the extent of aging in sedentary individuals may have been exaggerated by an accumulation of body fat or a progressive decline in habitual physical activity as subjects became older (Jackson et al. 1995).

Cross-sectional data.   One tactic for evaluating interactions between regular exercise and the aging of aerobic power has been to compare the rate of decrease in aerobic power between sedentary individuals and Masters athletes who have maintained a consistent level of aerobic training. Kavanagh and Shephard (1977) found that between the ages of 35 and 65 years, the oxygen transport of Masters athletes decreased by an average of 0.28 ml/[kg · min] per year. A similar annual loss was found by Heath et al. (1981; 0.32 ml/[kg · min]). Slightly larger annual decreases were seen in other cross-sectional studies of athletes: Kavanagh et al. (1989; males 0.43 ml/[kg · min], females 0.41 ml/[kg · min]), Pollock et al. (1974; 0.42 ml/[kg · min]), and Saltin and Grimby (1968; 0.42 ml/[kg · min]). Saltin (1986) described a loss of 0.73 ml/[kg · min] per year in "still active" orienteers. In their investigation, the initial age of the subjects was higher (55 years); participants entered the trial with a very high level of aerobic power, and the authors could not rule out the possibility that the intensity of training had decreased during the 20 years of observation.

In general, the age-related losses of aerobic power in Masters athletes and regular exercisers seem somewhat smaller than the 0.50 to 0.60 ml/[kg · min] per year that has been described in cross-sectional analyses of average adults (Shephard 1986c). This is not an unexpected finding, since it has been estimated that when data are expressed in ml/[kg · min], half of the age-related decrease in aerobic power of the general population reflects the combined influence of a decrease of habitual activity and an increase in obesity (Bovens et al. 1993; Jackson et al. 1995; Marti and Howald 1990). When these factors are taken into account, the cross-sectional data do not suggest that continued aerobic training had any very large effect upon the age-related decline in maximal oxygen transport.

Longitudinal training studies.   Most longitudinal studies of the aging of maximal oxygen intake have been hampered by a short time frame, and thus have been particularly vulnerable to changes in the habitual physical activity of the participants as the study proceeded. Such data are also susceptible to errors resulting from day-to-day variation, to technical test-retest errors in determinations of maximal oxygen intake (possibly as large as 4% to 5% in older subjects), and to an increased willingness of the subjects to undertake maximal effort as physical condition improves.

Some early reports claimed that the annual loss of oxygen transport in athletes (0.5-0.7 ml/[kg · min]) was less than in the general population, but such claims rested upon exaggerated (and indeed unsustainable) estimates of loss in the nonathletic samples. In contrast, Kasch et al. (1993) claimed that their small sample of middle-aged men showed no loss of aerobic power with age. During the first 10 years of observation, the effects of aging were apparently obscured by a substantial training and/or test-confidence response, but the overall pattern (an average annual loss of 0.27 ml/[kg · min]) was not greatly disparate from the cross-sectional estimates already reviewed. Pollock et al. (1987) followed Masters athletes longitudinally between the ages of 50 and 60 years. They divided their sample into two arbitrary groups: those who continued vigorous competition (for whom the annual loss was only 0.09 ml/[kg · min]) and a group who maintained their training distance but no longer participated in competition (for whom the annual loss was 0.66 ml/[kg · min]). However, the post hoc classification of subjects was somewhat arbitrary, and as in many of the other studies, the average change in aerobic power was 0.28 ml/ [kg · min] per year.

Marti and Howald (1990) also divided their sample on the basis of current training, finding that while the aerobic power showed little age-related change in athletes who maintained their training program, there was a steep decline in those who halted or reduced training.

On present evidence, we may thus conclude that subjects who continue training lose aerobic power a little less readily than sedentary individuals (Dempsey and Seals 1995; Hagberg 1987; Rogers, Hagberg, et al. 1990). A part of their advantage arises because they avoid the trend toward an age-related gain in body mass that is commonly observed in sedentary people (Jackson et al. 1995; Toth et al. 1994). Nevertheless, the difference in aerobic power between an active and a sedentary senior at any given calendar age is substantial; there is a 10- to 20-year difference in biological age between the two groups, and some active 65-year-old individuals have as large a maximal oxygen intake as a sedentary 25-year-old.

Muscular Strength and Flexibility

Until recently, the prime emphasis of training programs for the elderly has been upon the development of aerobic function. Nevertheless, the maintenance and (where possible) the increase of strength and flexibility have at least equal importance for function and quality of life, particularly in the frail elderly. Recent observations have shown that muscle strength can be augmented by appropriately graded resistance exercises, without inducing an excessive and dangerous rise of systemic blood pressure. A part of the observed gain in muscular performance reflects such factors as improved coordination and greater neural activation (Moritani and de Vries 1980), but a suitable training program can also reverse muscle atrophy and induce gains of lean tissue mass (Brown and Rose 1985; Fiatarone et al. 1990).

Muscular Strength

Two large-scale studies from Norway (Avlund et al. 1994; Era et al. 1994) have demonstrated associations between the habitual activity of the elderly and their muscle strength.

Large gains of muscle strength would not be anticipated with typical aerobic training programs. Early studies of 65-year-old subjects (Sidney, Shephard, and Harrison 1977) noted gains of leg strength averaging 11% after seven weeks of aerobic conditioning and 13% after one year. Other longitudinal studies of aerobic programs involving treadmill running (Brown 1985; Stebbins et al. 1985) have shown similar benefits.

Coggan et al. (1992) had 64-year-old subjects exercise at 80% of maximal heart rate for 45 min, four days per week, for 9 to 12 months. This relatively strenuous aerobic program yielded a small increase in the percentage of type IIA fibers at the expense of type IIB; the cross-sectional area of types I and IIA fibers each increased by about 11%, capillary density increased 20%, and the activity of mitochondrial enzymes by 24% to 55%.

During the last few years, there have also been several well-controlled longitudinal studies of resistance training for seniors of various ages. Almost all investigators have demonstrated substantial gains of strength, but increments of muscle cross-section have been smaller and less consistent (Rogers and Evans 1993). Heislein, Harris, and Jette (1994) applied progressive weight-bearing exercise to a group of women aged 50 to 64 years. An eight-week program that involved one supervised and two unsupervised sessions of physical activity per week yielded significant gains in strength of the quadriceps (21%), the hamstrings (9%), and handgrip (14%). Dupler and Cortes (1993) adopted a relatively high-intensity weight training program; their participants exercised at loads that increased from 45% to 75% of the individual's one-repetition maximum force. Muscle strength increased by an average of 66%; this apparently reflected mainly improved coordination, since no significant increase of lean body mass was seen.

Cress et al. (1991) adopted weighted stair climbing as a technique to develop both strength and aerobic power in elderly subjects. Significant gains of thigh strength were seen over 50 weeks of training, and in this study the type IIB fiber area increased by 29%, as compared with a 22% decrease in controls. Frontera et al. (1988) gave men aged 60 to 72 years 12-week training of the knee extensors; this increased the one-repetition maximum force by 110%, but the cross-section of the quadriceps was augmented by only 9%. The area of individual muscle fibers in the vastus lateralis increased by 34% for type I and by 28% for type II fibers. Pyka et al. (1994) had men and women aged 61 to 78 years perform a circuit of 12 resistance exercises three times per week for 50 weeks. Significant increases in strength developed after 8 weeks of participation. The investigators also found that type I fiber area had increased after 15 weeks of training and that gains in type II fiber area were evident by 30 weeks of training.

McMurdo and Rennie (1993) recruited subjects of average age 83 years to a twice-weekly program of isometric exercise. The quadriceps strength of participants was increased relative to that of controls who undertook reminiscence therapy. Fiatarone et al. (1994) recruited an even older group of patients, aged 72 to 98 years. All were residents in a nursing home. Nevertheless, Fiatarone and her associates were able to obtain 94% adherence to a 10-week program of progressive resistance training. Nutritional supplements were also provided. Local muscle strength increased by 113% in the exercised group; moreover, there were associated gains in less specific measures such as gait velocity (11.8%) and stair-climbing power (28.4%). However, the cross-sectional area of the thigh muscles showed only a very small increment (2.7%).

Thus, there is good evidence that even the frail elderly can undertake programs of resisted exercise. Moreover, such programs can yield substantial gains of strength, with corresponding improvements in gait, balance, and overall functional ability; further, if programs are pursued consistently over long periods, at least small increments of lean tissue mass can be induced.

Flexibility

Two cross-sectional studies have examined associations between regular physical activity and the maintenance of adequate flexibility in older subjects. Several longitudinal studies have also examined the changes induced by programs of physiotherapy, general exercises, and specific range of motion exercises.

Cross-Sectional Studies

Duncan et al. (1993) demonstrated that walking ability was positively associated with goniometer measures of left knee flexion and right ankle dorsiflexion in a convenience sample of 39 men of average age 75 years. Likewise, Voorips et al. (1993) found an association between questionnaire reports of habitual physical activity and flexibility of the hip and spine in Dutch subjects whose average age was 71.5 years. However, it is unclear from these studies whether physical activity increased flexibility or whether flexibility permitted continued involvement in physical activity.

Longitudinal Studies

Mulrow et al. (1994) examined the impact of a standard physiotherapy program on 163 frail nursing home residents. Perhaps because of multiple comorbid conditions, those receiving physiotherapy showed no gains of flexibility relative to those who received merely a social visit.

Other studies of the young-old have had greater success. Morey et al. (1991) found that over a two-year program of aerobic, strength, and flexibility exercises, 65- to 74-year-old veterans showed an 11% increase in flexibility (as assessed by hamstring length). Brown and Holloszy (1991) had 65-year-old subjects perform general unsupervised exercise for three months. Relative to values in self-selected controls, significant gains were seen in forward bend, straight leg raise, hip extension, and hip internal rotation, but not in ankle range of motion. Rider and Daly (1991) carried out a program of specific flexibility exercises, assessing the sum of spinal flexion and extension; after 10 weeks of treatment, the experimental subjects showed a significant advantage over the controls who received more general forms of exercise. McMurdo and Rennie (1993) had 87-year-old subjects perform exercises to music; relative to reminiscence controls, the exercisers developed significant gains of spinal flexibility, but knee mobility did not change significantly. Blumenthal et al. (1989) compared the movements at various major joints between experimental and control subjects in a 16-week study of men and women aged 60 to 83 years. They found a substantial (80% to 90%) increase of flexibility in response to a program of either aerobic exercise or yoga plus flexibility exercises.

Other authors have tested the benefits of more specific range of motion exercises. Hopkins et al. (1990) found a small (9%) improvement of sit-and-reach scores relative to those of control subjects when 57- to 77-year-old women performed a program of stretching, walking, and dance movements for 12 weeks. Rider and Daly (1991) had 72-year-old women perform four specific spinal mobility exercises for a period of 10 weeks; their sit-and-reach scores improved by 14.8% compared with a 2.3% decrease in controls. The exercisers also showed small increments of spine extension. Misner et al. (1992) had a group of 12 women participate in comprehensive range of motion exercises plus water exercises for five years; at the end of this period, Leighton flexometer measurements showed significant increases in the range of motion at all joints except the shoulder, although unfortunately this study did not include controls.

We may conclude that there is fairly good evidence that both general programs of physical activity and specific range of motion exercises can enhance flexibility in old and very old subjects. Moreover, such programs seem to be more effective than conventional physiotherapy as a means of improving the range of joint movement.

Central Nervous System

Occasional reports have suggested that regular exercise can enhance cerebral function, particularly in the very old. There is more convincing evidence that such programs improve balance and protect the participant against falls.

Cerebral Function

The possible influence of exercise programs on the cerebral function of elderly individuals has been discussed in more detail by Howe, Stones, and Brainerd (1990), MacRae (1989), and Spirduso (1995). Cross-sectional comparisons have shown faster simple and complex reaction times in those who have remained vigorously active than in their sedentary peers (Dustman,

Emmerson, and Shearer 1994), but it is uncertain from such observations whether exercise is the cause or merely a consequence of enhanced cerebral function. Several months of aerobic exercise sufficient to increase the maximal oxygen intake of seniors by 20% to 30% has been associated with appreciable gains in a number of mental performance test scores, including critical flicker fusion frequency, the digit symbol test from the Wechsler intelligence scale, estimation of briefly presented dot numbers, and simple and complex reaction times. In contrast, no gains of cerebral performance have been seen in controls (Lord and Castell 1994; Rikli and Edwards 1991) or in those who performed strength and flexibility exercises (Dustman et al. 1994) or yoga programs (Blumenthal, Emery, Madden, Schniebolk, et al. 1991). Other authors have found little or no difference in cerebral function between exercisers and controls (Hill, Storandt, and Malley 1993; McMurdo and Rennie 1993; Panton et al. 1990; Roberts 1990; Stevenson and Topp 1990; Whitehurst 1991). Various explanations have been offered for the divergent response to training, including a task specificity of benefit (the gains in cerebral function seem greater for more complex tasks; Hawkins, Kramer, and Capaldi 1992), the transient nature of changes, the need for a minimum age-related deterioration of cerebral function before benefit can be demonstrated, ineffective exercise programs (for example, Hassmen, Ceci, and Backman 1992; Puggaard et al. 1994), or a ceiling of cerebral response when some as yet unspecified level of aerobic fitness has been attained (Chodzo-Zajko and Moore 1994; Stones and Dawe 1993).

The explanation of any gains in cerebral function is problematic (Shephard and Leith 1990). There is some evidence that dynamic (but not static) exercise increases overall or regional cerebral perfusion (Jorgensen, Perko, and Secher 1992; MacRae 1989; Rogers, Schroeder, et al. 1990). Since the rise of systemic blood pressure is at least equally great during resisted as during dynamic exercise, it is puzzling that cerebral flow is increased only by dynamic activity. In any event, a blood pressure effect would be quite short-lived, and would likely depend also on the relative intensity of any physical activity that was undertaken (Moraine et al. 1993). Exercise may also modify the secretion or the passage across the blood-brain barrier of chemicals important to mood state, neural transmission, and overall cerebral performance—endorphins, dopamine, and catecholamines, for instance (Emery and Blumenthal 1991; Etnier and Landers 1995; MacRae 1989). It is further likely that regular physical activity lessens anxiety and depression, increases self-esteem, optimizes cerebral arousal (Poon 1985), and focuses attention (Stelmach 1994). Finally, participation in an exercise program may simply sustain brain function by increasing the individual's overall interest in daily life.

Balance

Iverson et al. (1990) reported that both balance and strength were positively correlated with self-reported physical activity. Judge et al. (1993) and Hu and

Woollacott (1994) also observed improved balance and less postural sway after participation in a specific program of balance training.

Others have claimed benefit from quite short periods of more general training. Binder et al. (1994) reported that frail elderly people showed improved balance after attending group exercises three times a week for only eight weeks. Roberts (1989) found a significant improvement of balance when 72-year-old subjects participated in a six-week walking program; Hopkins et al. (1990) noted a 12% increase in balance time after completion of a 12-week program of walking, stretching, and movement to music; and Johansson and Jarnio (1991) found significant gains on six of nine balance tests over a five-week program of supervised walking to music.

Nevertheless, enhanced postural control is by no means a uniform finding. Brown and Holloszy (1991) found no significant improvement of either balance or gait in their study of 60- to 71-year-old subjects. Crilly et al. (1989) reported no difference in postural sway between controls and 85-year olds participating in a three-month strength, flexibility, and balancing program. Likewise, Mulrow et al. (1994) found no gains of balance from participation in a program of physiotherapy, and Jirovec (1991) noted no significant gains of balance when 15 elderly and cognitively impaired nursing home residents were given a month of assisted walking. Finally, although Topp et al. (1993) observed a trend to enhanced balance after 12 weeks of strength training, again this finding was not statistically significant.

Available data support the view of Buchner et al. (1993) that a regular exercise program can improve balance and thus gait in the elderly. However, such a program does not always accomplish this, perhaps because the intensity of activity undertaken is insufficient to increase muscle strength substantially.

Falls

Training is unlikely to correct all causes of falls. Indeed, some observers have argued that an increase in the movement of the frail elderly is likely to place them in a greater number of situations in which they can fall. Nevertheless, empirical data show that the various consequences of a regular exercise program—a faster walking speed, a longer stride, greater muscle strength, and enhanced aerobic fitness—are negatively associated with the risk of falling (Wolfson et al. 1990). Moreover, regular physical activity can reduce the likelihood of postural hypotension by increasing peripheral venous tone, reducing the need for hypotensive medication (Scarpace, Mader, and Tümer 1993), and increasing vasopressor reactions (discussed later in this chapter).

Regular physical activity also increases reaction speed, and because of greater muscle strength, a fit individual is likely to make any necessary corrective movements more rapidly than someone who is frail and weak (Rubenstein and Josephson 1993). Training programs commonly enhance proprioceptor sensitivity (Lord, Caplan, and Ward 1993; Meeuwsen, Sawicki, and

Stelmach 1993), gains at the ankle joint being particularly critical for balance (Anacker and Di Fabio 1992). Finally, because the bones are stronger and the greater bulk of lean tissue enhances physical protection against external forces, the active person is less likely to incur a fracture if a fall does occur.

Jaglal, Kreger, and Darlington (1993) compared 381 women aged 55 to 84 years with a first diagnosis of hip fracture against 1138 matched controls. After multiple regression analysis for confounding variables, the odds ratio of fracture was 0.66 for those with a history of past activity and 0.54 for those who had been very active. MacRae, Feltner, and Reinsch (1994) reported that over a year of observation, 36% of exercised seniors but 45% of controls sustained falls. Likewise, Hornbrook et al. (1994) commented that in subjects who had undertaken an unsupervised walking program, the risk ratio for falls decreased to 0.85 over the next 23 months. Province et al. (1995) also found a decreased incidence of falls among those enrolling in exercise programs. In contrast, Reinsch et al. (1992) found that 1 h/week of supervised exercise at a senior center was not sufficient to change the number of falls incurred over the following year.

Wolf et al. (1993) have argued that tai chi may offer an ideal form of physical activity for the elderly because it combines the development of muscle balance with muscle strengthening and cardiovascular demand. Some cerebral benefits have also been claimed from estrogen administration, particularly an enhanced central processing of proprioceptive information (Birge 1993).

We may conclude that there is growing evidence that participation in a program of regular physical activity, far from increasing the risk of falls, is an effective form of prophylaxis for the frail elderly.

Endocrine System and Metabolism

Training programs have a favorable effect on many parts of the endocrine system in the elderly person. Those hormones that have received particular attention include the insulin-glucagon system, growth hormone, cortisol, and catecholamines.

Insulin

One of the most immediate benefits of regular physical activity is an increased demand for carbohydrate; this in itself helps to maintain blood glucose at a more uniform level (Durak 1989). The cellular binding of insulin is increased by regular physical activity, further enhancing glucose disposal in the active individual (Hughes and Meredith 1989). The potential for muscle glycogen storage is also increased by training, and this provides a reserve of carbohydrate for periods when blood sugar might otherwise fall.

Cross-sectional comparisons show that whereas Masters athletes have a glucose tolerance similar to that of young adults, older people who are sedentary have much poorer glucose tolerance curves (Seals et al. 1984b). Long-term training appears to normalize glucose tolerance (Rogers 1989), and it decreases the insulin secretory response to a given dose of glucose independently of any changes in body composition (Cononie et al. 1994; Hughes and Meredith 1989). At the same time, training increases insulin sensitivity, so glucose tolerance is not compromised by a reduced secretion of insulin (Kirwan et al. 1993; Wallberg-Henriksson 1989).

We may conclude that most studies suggest that regular physical activity is beneficial to the regulation of blood sugar in older individuals (Reaven 1995). Unfortunately, the physical condition of some older diabetic patients may have deteriorated to the point where they find it difficult to sustain effective involvement in such programs (Schneider et al. 1992; Skarfors et al. 1987).

Growth Hormone

Growth hormone functions as a "biochemical amplifier," enhancing the exercise- and androgen-modulated synthesis of muscle protein. It also conserves existing reserves of protein by enhancing the mobilization of depot fat during periods of negative energy balance.

Protein conservation may require greater quantities of growth hormone in the elderly than in a younger person who is exposed to the same physical stress, since aging greatly reduces the secretion of androgens. Moreover, limited glycogen reserves and a poor peripheral circulation encourage the older person to use protein as a metabolic fuel during periods of sustained exercise. Rudman (1985) has estimated that as many as one-half of seniors suffer from a deficient secretion of growth hormone. Recombinant growth hormone or growth hormone-releasing hormone has thus been used increasingly in an attempt to reverse age-related changes in body composition.

There are unwanted side effects from the administration of synthetic growth hormone (including diabetes, carpal tunnel syndrome, and gynecomastia). If the subject has not become too frail, it may thus be better to exploit the ability of endurance training to stimulate the endogenous production of growth hormone (see fig. 4.3; Rogol et al. 1992; Weltman et al. 1992) rather than to administer exogenous growth hormone. In young adults, the response to growth hormone-releasing hormone is increased fivefold by concomitant exercise (de Vries et al. 1991). Little attention has yet been directed to possible interactions between training and growth hormone secretion in elderly subjects, although Willis and Parkhouse (1994) have demonstrated that in aged mice, regular training can restore the sensitivity of skeletal muscle to IGF-1.

Most of the endogenous secretion of growth hormone occurs at night. It may therefore be advantageous to arrange exercise sessions in the evening

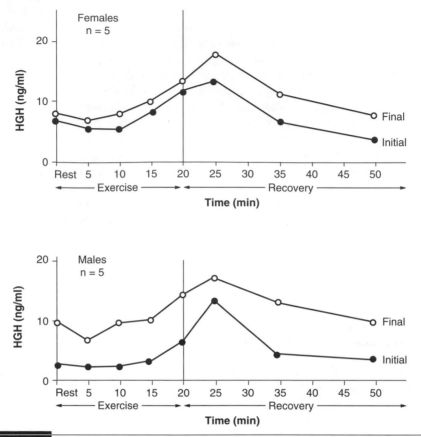

Figure 4.3   Influence of endurance training on the growth hormone response (HGH) of 65-year-old subjects to a bout of exercise (peak intensity 85% of maximal oxygen intake) before and after 10 weeks of aerobic conditioning.

Reprinted, by permission, from K.H. Sidney and R.J. Shephard, 1978b, "Growth hormone and cortisol: Age differences, effects of exercise and training," *Canadian Journal of Applied Sport Sciences* 2: 189-193.

hours, in order to maximize any stimulation of growth hormone release. Some investigators have combined endurance training with administration of growth hormone (Borst, Millard, and Lowenthal 1994), or have given doses of arginine or L-tryptophan in an attempt to boost the natural output of growth hormone (Ghigo et al. 1990). Such tactics are effective in young adults deficient in growth hormone, but they have yet to be exploited in seniors.

Cortisol

Heuser et al. (1991) found that cortisol responses to hCRH were significantly increased in endurance athletes; ACTH responses also tended to be increased in well-trained individuals. Heuser et al. (1991) suggested that a negative feedback signal initially decreased the sensitivity of the adrenal cortex to hCRH, but that later there was a switch to positive glucocorticoid feedback, an enhanced secretion of ACTH secretagogues such as vasopressin, or a combination of the two factors.

Nevertheless, basal cortisol and ACTH levels do not differ between elderly endurance athletes and sedentary controls (Heuser et al. 1991). Moreover, cortisol levels are not increased by an acute bout of exercise unless the activity is very prolonged and stressful. Finally, early longitudinal experiments have shown no change in the cortisol secretion of elderly subjects in response to training (Sidney and Shephard 1978b).

Catecholamines

It has been claimed that aging increases sympathetic nervous system activity during exercise, as evidenced by increased levels of circulating catecholamines. However, many cross-sectional comparisons have ignored possible differences in cigarette consumption between young and older samples (Jensen et al. 1994), and unfortunately, smoking increases catecholamine release. The response to a given dose of exercise also depends upon the individual's fitness. Age differences are largely abolished if young and elderly subjects are first matched for maximal oxygen intake per unit of body mass, and are then exercised at the same relative stress (Kastello, Sothman, and Murthy 1993).

Poehlman and Danforth (1991) examined the effects of an eight-week training program on the secretion of a number of metabolic hormones. The most striking change following training was a faster rate of norepinephrine appearance. This led to a 24% increase in circulating concentrations of norepinephrine at rest and to an associated 10% increase of resting metabolic rate, without change of body mass (Poehlman, Gardner, and Goran 1992). However, circulating levels of thyroxine and triiodothyronine remained unchanged. After training, increased resting levels of circulating catecholamines may also increase insulin sensitivity (Newsholme 1990) by enhancing beta-adrenergic-mediated lipolysis.

The main determinant of the catecholamine response to a given bout of exercise is the fraction of the maximal oxygen intake that is utilized. Thus, training at any age decreases the catecholamine that is released at a given absolute intensity of effort (Kohrt et al. 1993). However, it also permits exercise to a higher peak work rate, and it may thus increase the catecholamine concentration reached during a prolonged bout of all-out exercise (Jensen et al. 1994).

As in younger persons, endurance training reduces the baroreflex sensitivity of the elderly, increasing their vulnerability to postural hypotension, but this change is offset by an increase in alpha-adrenergic-mediated pressor responses (Spina et al. 1994). Training also helps to reverse the age-related slowing of diastolic filling, but apparently it achieves this through some mechanism other than an increase in the sensitivity of the beta-adrenergic receptors (Stratton et al. 1992).

Immune System

In theory, a moderate training program has a number of effects that could help to reverse the impact of aging on the immune system (Shephard and Shek 1995b; Uhlenbruck 1993). Benefits include a direct modulation of sympathetic activity in the neurohypophysis, a reduction of stress, a facilitation of sleep, and a diminution of free radical formation. However, empirical data are very limited.

Barnes et al. (1991) tested the ability of elderly rats to mount an antibody response to keyhole limpet hemocyanin; this was unchanged by 10 weeks of endurance training. Pahlavani et al. (1988) compared the responses of young, middle-aged, and elderly rats to six months of training. In the young animals, training had a depressant effect, reducing concanavalin-stimulated cell proliferation and the *in vitro* production of interleukin-2, but in elderly animals the immune responses were unchanged by what appeared to be a comparable volume of training. Nasrullah and Mazzeo (1992) found an even more favorable response in older animals: whereas training again depressed resting interleukin-2 production and cell proliferation in young rats, in elderly animals 15 weeks of moderate training enhanced both interleukin-2 production and mitogen-induced cell proliferation, bringing both up to the level observed in younger untrained animals. In contrast, Barnes et al. (1991) found that 10 weeks of training did not restore the age-related decline in production of IgG.

There have been only four human studies to date. Xusheng, Yugi, and Ronggang (1990) found that the resting percentage of rosette-forming (T) cells was lower in devotees of tai chi chuan than in controls. Crist et al. (1989) found that after a 16-week exercise program, moderately trained elderly women had a 33% greater natural killer cell activity than their untrained peers. Nieman, Henson et al. (1993) found that at baseline, highly trained women aged 67 to 85 years had circulating lymphocyte counts similar to those of their sedentary peers, although their peripheral mononuclear cells showed a 55% advantage of lytic activity, as well as a 56% greater proliferative response after stimulation with the mitogen phytohemagglutinin. Twelve weeks of exercise sessions at 60% of maximal oxygen intake proved insufficient to modify either their natural killer cell activity or T-cell function.

Shinkai et al. (1995) compared 17 elderly distance runners with 19 controls of similar age. They noted that relative to their control subjects, the runners had lower circulating counts of almost all immunocompetent cells. They also had a slightly lower CD4+/CD8+ (helper T/suppressor-cytotoxic T cell) ratio, but a significantly greater proliferative response to the mitogen phytohemagglutinin and higher rates of production of interleukin-2, interferon-gamma, and interleukin-4.

Further research is needed to test whether the immune function of an elderly person can be modified favorably by a moderate training program. However, current indications are that the response to regular physical activity remains much as in a younger individual. If this proves to be the case, then we are probably dealing with an inverted U-shaped response curve. Moderate training is likely to enhance immune function, potentially increasing resistance to both infection and tumor cells, but excessive physical activity could well have a negative impact on immune responses. This is one more reason for the necessity to regulate the dose of exercise undertaken by an elderly person.

Risks of Increased Physical Activity in Older People

One major fear of most physicians is that if they prescribe a significant amount of physical activity for an older person, it will provoke some form of heart attack, either myocardial infarction or cardiac arrest, and that the doctor will then be blamed for the incident. The risk that exercise will cause musculoskeletal injury is also greater than in a younger person, particularly if the bones have undergone extensive demineralization. Finally, exposure to various adverse environments—hot and cold weather, high altitudes, and deepwater diving—is less well tolerated than in a younger person. However, other hazards that are associated with exercise and sport participation in a young adult—overtraining, with suppression of the immune system, exercise addiction, and doping—seem much less likely to be incurred through the modest amounts of exercise that are undertaken by the average senior citizen.

Cardiac Risks

There are a variety of causes of exercise-related cardiac incidents and deaths in a young person (Chillag et al. 1990; Goodman 1995b; Torg 1995). But in the senior who dies during or immediately after a bout of physical activity, the underlying cause is almost always coronary vascular disease (Thompson and Fahrenbach 1994; Vuori 1995). We look here at the relative and absolute risk of such incidents, the impact on overall longevity, identification of vulnerable individuals, and immediate warning signs of a cardiac catastrophe.

Relative Risk of Exercise

In a young adult, the risk of sudden death is increased from 5- to 50-fold while the person is actually exercising (Shephard 1981; Siscovick et al. 1984; Vuori 1995), but this is offset by a 50% to 70% reduction of risk during the remainder of the day, so that the prognosis is generally improved by engaging in a regular exercise program (Powell et al. 1987). Although such concepts are now well established, the incidents are sufficiently rare that details of risks for the various types of exercise and sport have limited precision, even in young adults. Because few old people engage in vigorous exercise, the estimates of risk become even less precise when extended to the retirement years.

There does not appear to be any great increase in the relative risk of exercise as a person becomes older (Siscovick et al. 1984; Thompson et al. 1982; Vuori 1995). The careful analyses of Vuori (1995, see table 4.4) showed that both the risk relative to inactivity and the absolute number of deaths per million hours of participation in many types of physical activity were actually lower in those aged 50 to 69 years than in middle-aged people. Reasons for the reduced relative risk of exercise in older people include the prior death of some of the most vulnerable individuals, a large increase in the number of heart attacks while seniors are inactive, and the fact that elderly people are

Table 4.4   Influence of age on the risk of sudden cardiovascular death during exercise.

| Type of exercise | Age (years) | | | | | |
| | 20-39 | | 40-49 | | 50-69 | |
	D	R	D	R	D	R
Walking	0	0	37.9	0.2	11.7	0.5
Jogging	16.2	9.3	4.1	4.7	4.7	0.7
Nordic skiing	8.8	9.3	1.1	9.0	0.7	6.1
Ball games	17.8		3.3		10.3	
Nonstrenuous	26.0	3.4	5.2	3.7	3.4	3.0
Strenuous	6.1	11.8	1.2	12.8	1.2	6.2

Note: D = death rate per estimated 10^6 exercise sessions; R = relative risk (observed deaths/anticipated deaths for the same time interval).

Reprinted, by permission, from I. Vuori, T. Suurnäkki, and L. Suurnäkki, 1983, "Liikuntaan littyvän äkkikuoleman riski ja syyt" [Causes and risks of sudden death in exercise and sports], *Duodecim* 99: 516-526.

unlikely to embark upon a bout of very intensive physical activity for which they are ill prepared.

Mittelman et al. (1993) concluded that people over the age of 70 years were still at increased relative risk when undertaking strenuous activity, but they suggested that the main reason for this finding was that in North America people over 70 years of age rarely engaged in even mild physical activity. In their research, irregular exercise participation was a strong predictor of such incidents, irrespective of the individual's age.

Absolute Risk of Exercise

Whittington and Banerjee (1994) estimated that only 52 deaths occurred within 6 h of sport participation when a population of 1,130,000 were followed over a four-year period. Although the ages of the victims ranged widely from 8 to 84 years, the majority of incidents occurred in older male subjects. Bowling and golf were common antecedents of death, probably because these are common pastimes of the elderly. There were usually no warning symptoms that exercise was likely to precipitate death.

The absolute risk of a cardiac incident during unsupervised exercise is no greater for the elderly person than for younger patients who have previously sustained a myocardial infarction: perhaps one episode in 60,000 or 100,000 hours of exercise (Haskell 1994; Shephard et al. 1983). This would remain a somewhat more frequent occurrence than the one episode in 750,000 hours of supervised exercise reported for younger adults who were attending cardiac rehabilitation programs (Van Camp and Peterson 1986), but it would still be a very rare event.

Overall Risk of an Active Lifestyle

One method of comparing overall risks between sedentary and active individuals is to look at longevity data. Such statistics show that those who choose to engage in moderate physical activity live longer than their sedentary peers through to about 90 years of age (see table 4.5). Thereafter, the prognosis of the sedentary person may be a little better than that of the active individual.

For those who choose to engage in more vigorous activity, the point at which the prognosis of the active person becomes less favorable than that of a sedentary individual is probably reached between 70 and 80 years of age (Linsted, Tonstad, and Kuzma 1991; Paffenbarger et al. 1994).

Such statistics might seem to suggest that the very old person should refrain from exercising. However, a simple statement of longevity ignores the critical issue of the quality of life. Enjoyment of the activity itself, enhancement of physical condition, and the resultant extension of independence do much to enhance the quality of survival for an active person. Thus, if we calculate a more appropriate statistic, the quality-adjusted life expectancy, it can be seen that there are substantial gains from maintaining a vigorous lifestyle, even in the oldest age categories (Shephard in press-a).

Table 4.5   All-cause mortality (deaths per 1000 person-years) among 9484 Seventh Day-Adventist men, classified by physical activity status at entry to the study.

Initial age	Inactive	Moderately active	Highly active
50-59	4.0	2.4	2.5
60-69	11.2	8.4	9.1
70-79	36.6	27.4	33.5
80-89	85.1	81.9	94.1
90-99	169.6	152.5	156.5

Reprinted from *Journal of Clinical Epidemiology*, Volume 44, K.D. Linsted, K. Tomstad, and J. Kuzma, "Self-report of physical activity and patterns of morality in Seventh-Day Adventist men," pages 355-364. Copyright 1991, with kind permission from Elsevier Science Ltd., The Boulevard, Langford Lane, Kidlington 0X5 1GB, UK.

Identifying the Vulnerable Individual

Attempts to identify high-risk individuals and thus to warn people who are likely to succumb to an exercise-induced cardiac emergency have been singularly unsuccessful (Franklin and Kahn 1995; Shephard 1984a; Thompson and Fahrenbach 1994).

A prior history of heart disease and/or the presence of major cardiac risk factors (cigarette smoking, a high cholesterol level, hypertension, infrequent or irregular bouts of physical activity, obesity, diabetes, and an adverse family history) are probably the clearest markers of a vulnerable person, although for each of these characteristics there is much overlap between those who develop a fatal heart attack and those who do not (Kannel, Gagnon, and Cupples 1990). Paradoxically, the individuals who are identified as being at increased risk should not be warned against exercising. Indeed, their prognosis will be substantially improved if they begin a moderate, progressive exercise program and take other measures to reduce their cardiac risk profile (Leon et al. 1987). However, people in the high-risk group require close supervision if they plan to undertake more than a program of light physical activity (American College of Sports Medicine 1995a).

One additional hazard is probably a Type A personality (Shephard 1981). Individuals with this characteristic sometimes assume that they can accomplish their intended fitness goals in a third of the time if they exceed the prescribed volume or intensity of exercise by a factor of three! In competitive games such as squash and tennis, they show an excessive desire to trounce an opponent, and in many demanding physical activities they are unwilling to admit when they are exhausted. Social and business problems are brought into the gym or onto the sports field, and the critical warm-up and warm-down phases of an exercise session are rushed because such individuals perceive that they have other more pressing time commitments (Shephard 1981).

Clinical and laboratory examinations are usually not particularly helpful in determining who is vulnerable to a heart attack (Franklin and Kahn 1995). Nevertheless, a few specific absolute and relative contraindications to exercise have been identified (see tables 4.6 and 4.7). A fever is one obvious warning sign, since a number of incidents of cardiac arrest have been provoked by a viral myocarditis (Chillag et al. 1990; Goodman 1995b). A high proportion of the elderly also show silent myocardial ischemia, disturbances of cardiac rhythm, and other abnormalities of the resting ECG (Sidney and Shephard 1977b). Again, there is at least a statistical association between such findings and an increased risk of sudden death, but this is not very helpful when one is advising the individual patient (Siscovick et al. 1991). The same is true of abnormal ambulatory ECG records (Hombach et al. 1990; Räihä et al. 1994). Because the overall risk of sudden death is greater in the elderly than in a younger person, there are somewhat fewer false-positive interpretations of the ECG record in an older person. Nevertheless, an abnormal exercise ECG is not usually an indication to avoid physical activity. Indeed, the optimal treatment for those individuals who have either myocardial ischemia (Balady 1992) or stable congestive heart failure (Kavanagh et al. 1996; Smith 1992) is a program of regular, moderate physical activity. The very old person should be allowed to undertake moderate exercise even if the exercise ECG has a very alarming appearance (Shephard 1984b, 1992b).

Table 4.6   Absolute contraindications to physical activity.

Acute infectious disease
Unstable metabolic disorder
Significant locomotor disturbance
Excessive anxiety
Recent or impending myocardial infarction
Manifest cardiac failure
Acute myocarditis
Aortic stenosis
Probability of recent pulmonary embolism

Reprinted, by permission, from R.J. Shephard, 1981, *Ischemic heart disease and exercise* (London: Croom Helm).

Table 4.7   Relative contraindications to physical activity.

Atrial fibrillation or flutter
Atrioventricular block
Left bundle branch block
Premature ventricular excitation

Reprinted, by permission, from R.J. Shephard, 1981, *Ischemic heart disease and exercise* (London: Croom Helm).

The sensitivity and specificity of a stress test can be increased if the results are combined with information from other sources such as echocardiography. However, most cardiologists are agreed that such testing is not a cost-effective method of detecting which person will succumb to an exercise-induced cardiac catastrophe (Franklin and Kahn 1995).

Immediate Warning Signs and Preventive Measures

Sometimes the individual who sustains a cardiac arrest has been aware of a vague sense of discomfort in the chest, frequent extrasystoles, or a general malaise during the previous 6 to 24 h (Shephard 1981; Thompson et al. 1979). Thus, it is wise to moderate the intensity of an exercise program in the face of such symptoms. A viral myocarditis is a possible precipitant of ventricular arrhythmia at any age, and coronary atherosclerosis may increase the vulnerability of the myocardium in an elderly person. Heavy exercise should thus be avoided in conjunction with a fever and during or immediately after an attack of influenza.

Many cardiac incidents occur when people are attempting to perform a physical feat for which they are ill prepared—for example, carrying a boat from their dock to a vehicle at the end of the summer. Regular physical activity of a consistent intensity is much less dangerous than the occasional performance of heavy, demanding tasks (Mittelman et al. 1993). It is particularly dangerous for elderly persons to allow pride or the desire to win a competition to dictate continuation of an activity when they feel physically exhausted.

Practical Implications

Precipitation of a cardiac crisis is indeed a catastrophe, and unfortunately, there seems no simple method of identifying the vulnerable individual. However, the risks of such an incident can be reduced by adoption of a moderate, progressive exercise program. Moreover, since the overall prognosis is better for an active than for a sedentary person, fears of a cardiac catastrophe are no reason to avoid regular, moderate physical activity.

Environmental Factors

The hazards of exercise are increased by abnormal environments (excessive heat, cold, high altitudes, and underwater environments, particularly if such factors exist in combination with psychological stress). These stressors increase risks at all ages, but especially in older individuals.

Heat

Hot weather increases the demand for skin blood flow, and heat waves are associated with an increase in the death rate among elderly individuals (Kenney 1995). Most older people have a poor tolerance of exercise in hot conditions, but it is unclear how far this is due to aging *per se* and how far it reflects a lack of physical conditioning, obesity, or cardiovascular disease. There has been only limited study of heat acclimation in the elderly; it does not appear to differ greatly from that observed in younger adults (Kenney 1995).

Cold

Cold weather causes cutaneous vasoconstriction, increasing both preloading and afterloading of the heart and thus augmenting cardiac work rate. The energy cost of many activities such as walking is also increased by deep snow. Tasks such as the shoveling of wet snow can impose a heavy isometric load upon the heart. Each winter brings new reports of cardiac deaths related to blizzards and snow shoveling (Emmett and Hodgson 1993; Shephard 1992c).

Exposure to extreme cold also brings risks of hypothermia, frostbite, and chilblains, the prevalence of these conditions being exacerbated by the poor peripheral circulation of the elderly person. Exposure to cold, dry air may finally provoke bronchospasm in the person who has developed chronic obstructive lung disease (Killian 1995).

High Altitude

Mountain climbing is sometimes pursued by quite elderly individuals. Surprisingly, the risk of high altitude illness seems less than in younger climbers, and not all of this advantage can be explained in terms of a slower rate of climbing (Balcomb and Sutton 1986). In theory, the risk of myocardial ischemia is increased by the low oxygen pressures found at high altitudes (Morgan et al. 1990), although in practice, Yaron, Hultgren, and Alexander (1995) found no new ST-wave abnormalities when a group of 97 sea level residents, 70 years old, spent several days at Vail, Colorado (elevation 2500 m); other reports have suggested an equally low morbidity at such altitudes (Halhuber and Humpeler 1985; Grover et al. 1990).

Underwater Exploration

Two important hazards of underwater activity in the elderly are the risk of a transient loss of consciousness due to a cardiac arrhythmia, and a sudden drop of systemic blood pressure on emerging from the water. The latter problem is particularly likely in the person whose age-related tendency to postural hypotension has been exacerbated by the use of antihypertensive medication.

Combination of Exercise and Psychological Stress

Psychological stress can increase the systemic blood pressure and thus the cardiac work rate at any given intensity of exercise. It may therefore be desirable to moderate the intensity of an exercise program at times when the individual feels under psychological pressure.

Injury

Musculoskeletal injuries have a strong negative impact on motivation to engage in a conditioning program. We will examine factors predisposing the elderly individual to injury and look at the risks associated with a moderate-intensity exercise program before suggesting some preventive measures.

Factors Predisposing to Injury

A number of factors increase the risk that a senior will be injured while exercising (Nevitt, Cummings, and Hudes 1991):

1. Advanced age and female gender
2. A history of previous falls or injury (Macera et al. 1989; Marti et al. 1988; Walter et al. 1989)
3. A history of postural hypotension or "drop attacks"
4. Hearing impairment, poor vision, and a slow reaction time
5. Clumsiness, associated with lack of recent practice of a skill, a deterioration of balance, unstable hip and knee joints, and a reduced foot lift
6. Obesity, increasing the strain per unit section of tendon (Pollock et al. 1977)
7. A low body mass, particularly if associated with the severe muscle wasting that some have termed sarcopenia (Marti et al. 1988)
8. Shortening of tendons associated with many years of inactivity (although the evidence of benefit from stretching exercises is equivocal [Pate and Macera 1994])
9. Failure to perform an adequate warm-up (Adrian 1981; Safran, Seaber, and Garrett 1989)
10. Violent bursts of movement (Fuller and Winters 1993; Pollock et al. 1991), especially rapid twisting and excessive stretching
11. Too rapid a progression of training, with exercise continuing when the subject is more than pleasantly fatigued (Fields, Delaney, and Hinckle 1990)—a problem that occurs typically in a person with Type A personality
12. Exercise on a hard or uneven surface (James, Bates, and Osternig 1978)
13. The use of shoes that provide poor ankle support (Bates 1982; Cavanagh 1980; Ting 1991)
14. Osteoporosis, which increases the likelihood of a fracture if a frail elderly person sustains a fall (Block and Genant 1989)

Risks of Moderate-Intensity Exercise Programs

It is not easy to determine the precise risk that physical activity will cause an injury, either for the average senior who is performing moderate exercise or for the Masters athlete. Most reports of injuries fail to define either the total population at risk, or the average duration of a given activity within that population (Pate and Macera 1994). Moreover, few studies have examined a sufficient number of subjects to allow one to form more than general impressions.

Cross-sectional analyses of relationships between patterns of physical activity or fitness and the risk of falls are further complicated by problems of self-selection. Fears created by a previous fall that in itself caused only minor trauma may lead to inactivity and/or a low level of fitness in a person who was initially vulnerable to falls (Svanstrom 1990). Again, those who are injured may abandon a vigorous sport in favor of some less demanding activity; for example, an injured runner may switch to walking, so that the incidence of injuries in those who continue running may even be lower than in younger cohorts (Nicholl and Williams 1983).

There have been four important longitudinal studies of seniors. MacRae, Feltner, and Reinsch (1994) took a typical group of sedentary, community-dwelling women of average age 72 years, allocating 42 subjects to an exercise group and 38 to an attention-control group. Over one year, the experimental group performed a circuit of four sets of five stand-ups from a chair and five step-ups onto a bench, with 10 repetitions of this routine three times per week. Only 36% of the experimental group experienced a fall over the year of observation, compared with 45% of the control subjects. Moreover, none of the experimental group sustained an injury of a severity that required medical attention, whereas 3 of 14 falls in the control group were treated by a physician. Reinsch et al. (1992) carried out a similar but less closely described and monitored program, also for one year; they found no change in the risk of falls or injury, but suggested that the intensity of exercise adopted in their program may not have been sufficient for benefit.

Carroll et al. (1992) enrolled 68 healthy but sedentary volunteers aged 60 to 79 years in a six-month program of uphill treadmill walking. Fourteen percent of the group sustained injuries, mainly in the early weeks of training when the intensity was low; this emphasizes the importance of adopting a slow progression rate when conditioning elderly subjects.

Pollock et al. (1991) compared the risks of a walk-jog program with those of a strength training program in subjects aged 70 to 79 years. One-repetition maximum strength testing injured 19% of participants, and jogging injured all women and 2 of 8 men. However, strength training injured only 2 people (9% of the group), and walking injured only 1 individual (5% of the sample).

Another study by Pollock (1988) compared the incidence of injuries in three groups of previously sedentary individuals who engaged in a six-month program of walking and jogging. The proportion of the sample who were injured increased from 18% in those aged 20 to 35 years to 41% in those aged 49 to 65 years and 57% in those aged 70 to 79 years. As in the study of Carroll et al. (1992), many of these injuries occurred during the first week of exercise, and it is thus likely that the risks of injury would be lower if a consistent, low-intensity exercise program were to be pursued on a regular basis.

Nevertheless, we must conclude that the risk of many types of musculo-skeletal injury increases with age, and that the dangers of rapid movements are appreciable, particularly if the person is untrained or is in the first few weeks of a conditioning program. Furthermore, when assessing the health significance of a given injury rate, it is important to note that the rate of recovery from a given lesion is slower in older age groups (Marti et al. 1988).

Preventive Measures

The surface on which exercise is to be performed should be even, well lighted, without shadows, and not slippery. The area should be cleared of loose carpets and other obstacles that might cause collisions or tripping (Livesley 1992; Pollock 1992).

Particular care is necessary in recommending exercise for someone who is obese, who has problems of balance, or who has a history of previous back, leg, or foot disorders. A walking stick, far from being a mark of invalidism, can provide useful exercise for the arms as well as offering a source of stability when walking. If there is joint pain or difficulty in supporting the body mass, pool (Shephard 1985a; White 1995) or chair exercises (McNamara, Otto, and Smith 1985) should be suggested as an initial measure.

Lessons From Older Athletes

A number of investigators have studied age-related changes in competitive performance in order to determine the rate of functional deterioration with aging. Such data have several attractions, including a high level of participant motivation and an accurate measurement of achievement in highly conditioned individuals. Others have seen the laboratory performance of the older athlete as a source of evidence concerning the maximum likely impact of many years of hard training on physiological characteristics and longevity. Finally, some authors have considered Masters competition as a possible mechanism for the delivery of physical activity to an aging population.

Age-Related Changes in Competitive Performance

The potential for a detailed physiological interpretation of performance curves in any event is limited by several factors:

1. There are large, constitutionally determined interindividual variations in both physiological endowment and the skill with which this endowment is converted into a world-class athletic performance. The world record at any given age is thus determined in part by the fraction of the

population of that age who participate in international competitions. In the oldest age categories, the pool of competitors is small, especially for women, and there is a corresponding decrease in the likelihood that candidates with an outstanding endowment will compete.

2. As a person becomes older, there is a tendency for both the intensity and the duration of training sessions to diminish, so performance is being compared between a well-prepared young competitor and an older individual who has been less well prepared.

3. Elderly competitors may be less willing than younger people to push themselves to extreme exertion during a race. Commonly, the stated goals of the Masters competitor are social, rather than winning at all costs (Kavanagh et al. 1989).

4. Gender bias and lack of social support for vigorous physical activity are other age-related factors limiting both the training and the competitive performance of older women.

Type of Event

The optimal age for athletic performance depends on the relative demands of an event in terms of physiological characteristics, skill, and tactical experience (Ericsson 1990; Schulz and Curnow 1988). In general, the performance in competitions that demands explosive muscular power (for example, sprinting) peaks at a younger age than in endurance races such as a marathon run. In some events such as female swimming competitions, world records have been established by adolescents. But in other types of competition in which acquired skills play a major role (for example, equestrian events or golf), the top performers have often been over 30 years of age. Economic factors also seem to influence the observed optimum age of competition; and the peak performances usually occur later in professional than in amateur players (see fig. 4.4). Finally, it is possible that as preparation for international competition becomes more "scientific" and technical, the optimal age of competition may increase (Spirduso 1995).

Limitations of Cross-Sectional Data

Several authors have plotted cross-sectional curves examining the relationship between age and the performance of athletic events demanding various combinations of aerobic function and strength (see figs. 4.5 and 4.6). The findings from such analyses necessarily differ from those obtained through longitudinal studies, since the pool of competitors from which the cross-sectional records emerge becomes smaller in the older age categories of contestants. When competitors are followed longitudinally, the losses in performance tend to be smaller than those seen in cross-sectional analyses during the early years of Masters competition, but larger in the final years, when many contestants are allowing the intensity of their training to wane.

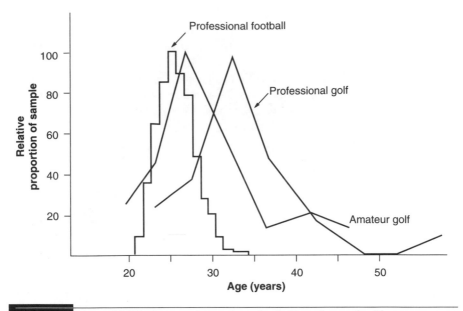

Age of 1630 players of American football, and age of golfers on winning amateur and professional golf championships.
Adapted, by permission, from H.C. Lehman, 1951, "Chronological age vs. proficiency in physical skills," *American Journal of Physiology* 44: 161-187.

Mathematical Modeling of Performance

Stones and Kozma (1986) fitted a variety of mathematical models to cross-sectional data. In aerobic events, for example, they suggested that world records could be represented by a generalized curve of the type:

$$\text{Log}_n \text{ (time, sec)} = \text{Log}_n (.049 \times [\text{distance, m}^{1.089}]) + .011 \text{ (age, yr)}.$$

The fit of this curve to the actual race times is no more than approximate. Thus, for a mile run (1609 m), the equation would predict times of 224.8 sec at age 35 and 368.7 sec at age 80 years. The corresponding Masters age records for male runners in 1990 were 235.0 sec and 403.3 sec. Despite the influence of a diminishing pool of competitors, Stones and Kozma (1986) noted that in the middle- and long-distance events, the slowing of running speed with aging closely matched the decline in aerobic power that was seen in laboratory measurements. Stones and Kozma (1986) argued that the age effect was greater for distance events than for sprints, although this is at variance with other information on the age of optimal performance, as discussed earlier, and is not very obvious from an inspection of Masters age records (see fig. 4.5). In swimming events (where such factors as flexibility and coordination are also

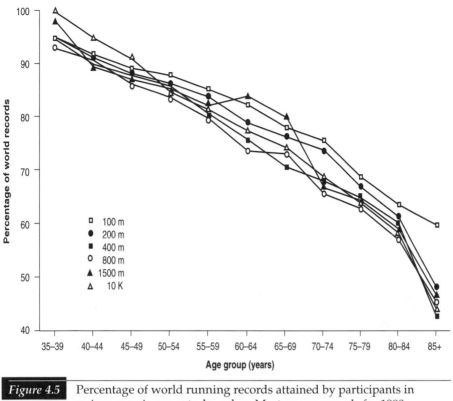

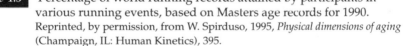

Figure 4.5   Percentage of world running records attained by participants in various running events, based on Masters age records for 1990.
Reprinted, by permission, from W. Spirduso, 1995, *Physical dimensions of aging* (Champaign, IL: Human Kinetics), 395.

important), Hartley and Hartley (1986) have observed just the opposite effect, youth being most important to success over short distances.

Intrinsic Aging of Body Functions

We have noted already that because a decline in habitual activity and an increase in obesity are frequent concomitants of aging, it is extremely difficult to determine the inherent rate of loss of either cardiovascular function or muscle strength.

The problem is further complicated because the performance of an initial set of physiological tests, or anticipation that testing will be repeated, often provokes an increase in habitual physical activity, thereby obscuring the intrinsic effects of aging. Such artifacts may account for studies that have found little deterioration of aerobic power over observation periods as long as 20 to 30 years (Åstrand 1986; Kasch et al. 1993).

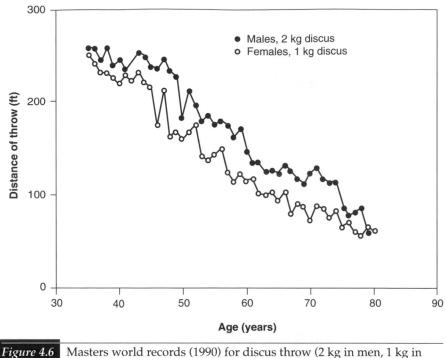

Figure 4.6 Masters world records (1990) for discus throw (2 kg in men, 1 kg in women).
Reprinted, by permission, from W. Spirduso, 1995, *Physical dimensions of aging* (Champaign, IL: Human Kinetics), 396.

Aerobic Power

If cross-sectional data are collected on athletes of various ages who all have similar training schedules (Kavanagh et al. 1989), the estimated rate of deterioration in aerobic power depends on the age span that has been studied. Between the ages of 30 and 59 years, a loss of about 3 ml/[kg · min] per decade seems typical, and if the span is broadened to 30 to 69 years, the value increases to about 4.2 ml/[kg · min] per decade (as discussed in an earlier section). In the eighth decade, when the training patterns of the Masters competitors are tending to relax, the losses of aerobic power increase further, to 5.8 ml/[kg · min] in men and 4.8 ml/[kg · min] in women (Kavanagh et al. 1989). Differences from the average rate of loss in a sedentary person are not very large; they could probably be explained by an age-related decrease of habitual physical activity and an accumulation of fat in the general sedentary population, rather than by any specific protective anti-aging effect derived from participation in Masters competition.

The substantial difference in current aerobic power between the well-trained Masters athlete and the general sedentary public has much greater practical significance. The aerobic power of most sedentary 65-year-olds has declined to around 20 to 30 ml/[kg · min]. However, the aerobic power of the 65-year-old Masters competitors examined by Kavanagh et al. (1989) averaged 36.1 ± 6.5 ml/[kg · min] in the men, and 31.7 ± 8.1 ml/[kg · min] in the women.

Lean Body Mass

In many categories of Masters athletes, lean body mass changes little between 30 and 65 years of age. Among the male competitors, Kavanagh et al. (1989) found average values of 61.3 ± 6.6 kg at age 35, and 62.2 ± 8.2 kg at age 65. In women, the corresponding values were 44.0 ± 5.9 and 45.2 ± 8.6 kg. Likewise, Sipilä et al. (1991) found that continuing athletes aged 70 to 81 years had a greater strength than their sedentary peers. Rogers, Hagberg, et al. (1990) also found no decrease of lean mass over eight years in a sample of runners who were first tested at an average age of 54 years. At first inspection, such figures might be thought to reflect a benefit of athletic competition, but in fact the Canada Fitness Survey obtained lean mass data rather similar to those of Kavanagh et al. (1989) in a representative sample of adults; in men of similar ages, values averaged 59.4 and 59.4 kg, respectively, and in the women the corresponding figures were 44.0 and 44.9 kg (Shephard 1986c).

Preservation of lean tissue seems to be particularly dependent on maintaining an adequate volume of resistance training. Concomitant with a relaxation of training schedules, average values for the lean mass of Masters competitors had slipped to 57.9 ± 7.2 kg in the men and 40.7 ± 2.8 kg in the women by the age of 75 years (Kavanagh et al. 1989). The limited extent of musculoskeletal benefit in younger age groups probably reflects the endurance nature of many Masters events (for example, distance running, swimming, and cycling).

Involvement in weight lifting seems to be more effective in sustaining both muscle bulk and muscle performance. Spirduso (1995) cites world record dead lifts (a lift that is purely strength-related) of 228 kg for 70- to 74-year-old male competitors and 100.2 kg for 75- to 79-year-old females. By 65 to 69 years of age, U.S. National lifting records are currently only about 50% of the values seen in a young adult. But as with aerobic power, the important advantage of the weight-lifting athletes over the general public is the continuing margin of abilities between the two groups.

Longevity

The longevity of athletes was originally studied because it was feared that prolonged training would shorten life. More recently, data have been examined with the opposite hope, that of demonstrating an increase of longevity with regular exercise or sport participation.

Given that an exercise program must be sustained over a very long period in order to induce many of its postulated benefits, an athlete might seem to provide a good model to test for any resulting changes in life expectancy. However, a number of factors have weakened or even invalidated comparisons of morbidity and mortality between athletes and the general public:

1. National- and international-class athletes are highly selected by factors ranging from socioeconomic status to body build. Thus, successful recruits to some sports such as North American football are mesomorphic (a body type associated with a short average life span), whereas other sports such as distance running attract the ectomorph (a body type that commands a prolonged life expectancy).

2. Some studies have compared those contestants who won athletic letters in college with their peers who were also members of the university athletic center.

3. Classification as an athlete has sometimes been based on the person's behavior while attending college or university. However, a long-term follow-up of athletic letter winners disclosed that by middle age, when chronic disease was becoming prevalent, those who had initially been classed as athletes were on average less active, more likely to be obese, and more likely to be regular cigarette smokers than those who had initially been classed as their sedentary peers.

4. Continuing athletes are distinguished from the general population by many features of personal lifestyle other than habitual physical activity. For example, many are lifelong nonsmokers, and some also adopt low fat diets with a high intake of antioxidants such as vitamin C and vitamin E (Kavanagh et al. 1989; Shephard, Kavanagh, and Mertens 1995).

5. The majority of athletes have a more competitive nature than the general population. Thus, an unusually large proportion die violent deaths—on the sports field, in battle, and in automobile accidents (Aggleton et al. 1994).

Recent studies have not added greatly to earlier knowledge of longevity in athletes. Beaglehole and Stewart (1983) found that New Zealand's international rugby players had the same life expectancy as New Zealanders in general. Waterbor et al. (1988) observed that major league baseball players in the United States had a standardized mortality ratio of 94, slightly less than that of the general United States population. Van Saase, Noteboom, and Vandenbroucke (1990) reported that participants in a Dutch long-distance ice-skating tour subsequently lived slightly longer than the general population of the Netherlands. Most recently, Sarna and Kaprio (1994) compared the longevity of Finnish male athletes with that of military conscripts. After statistical adjustment of the data for initial differences of socioeconomic status, marital status, and age, the mean life expectancy was 75.6 years for those involved in endurance sports (distance running and cross-country skiing), 73.9 years for those involved in team sports (soccer, ice hockey, and basketball), and 71.5 years for those involved in power sports (boxing, wrestling, and weight lifting); in contrast, a life expectancy of 69.9 years was estimated for the reference group. The endurance competitors lived longer mainly because they avoided premature cardiac deaths; there was no evidence that the maximum age at death was increased for any of the three athletic groups.

We may conclude that the calendar life expectancy of top athletes remains less than, equal to, or greater than that of the general population, depending upon the type of sport under evaluation. However, there remains scope for a thorough comparison of the quality-adjusted life span of athletes and sedentary individuals (Morgan 1986).

Competitive Sport as a Source of Healthy Physical Activity

From the viewpoint of health policy, two immediate questions arise: Are Masters competitions a safe form of exercise, and if so, do they provide an effective vehicle for the promotion of physical activity among an aging population?

Safety

As in the general population, there are concerns regarding the risks of cardiac catastrophe, musculoskeletal injury, and disturbances of immune function.

Cardiovascular risks.   There is no doubt that the risk of sudden cardiac death during athletic competition is increased relative to that anticipated during sedentary rest. But as in the general population, the overall mortality statistics suggest that this hazard is at least offset by a diminished risk of death between competitions (Sarna and Kaprio 1994).

Douglas and O'Toole (1992) examined ultra-endurance athletes of average age 58 years. They had substantially larger ventricular end-diastolic diameters than their sedentary peers, and the thickness of the posterior wall of the left ventricle was increased to an average of 1.1 cm. Likewise, Di Bello et al. (1993) noted an increased left ventricular mass in a group of 66-year-old athletes, but nevertheless two-dimensional echocardiography and Doppler analysis showed no deterioration of ventricular function; indeed, the athletes' ejection fraction during exercise (an average of 76%) was greater than that of control subjects.

Kabisch and Funk (1991) found roughly equal numbers of sport-related incidents of sudden death in each of the age decades 20 to 30, 30 to 40, 40 to 50, and at ages over 50 years, but in the absence of data on respective rates of sport participation, it is hard to draw any firm conclusion from such statistics. Again, anecdotes are heard about elderly people who develop angina or sustain a heart attack while trying to beat a younger partner at tennis or squash, but there is little evidence from either Masters competitions or overall mortality statistics (see table 4.4) to suggest that the oldest age categories are particularly vulnerable to cardiac complications while exercising. Shephard, Kavanagh, and Mertens (1995) completed a seven-year follow-up of 750 Masters competitors whose initial age averaged around 50 years. Only 10 subjects (1.4%) developed a nonfatal heart attack over the seven years. Detailed information was available for 4 of the 10 patients; 3 of the 4 were smokers, 2 of the 4 began the study with marked ST-segmental depression, and all had pushed themselves extremely hard during a direct measurement of maximal oxygen intake.

There are several probable reasons for the rarity of cardiac complications in Masters athletes. Cardiac incidents are much more likely to occur in the infrequent exerciser who undertakes a task for which she or he is ill-prepared (Mittelman et al. 1993; Shephard 1984a; Siscovick et al. 1984) than in a person who is training on a regular basis. Moreover, as age advances, an increasing proportion of Masters competitors participate in their sport for social reasons rather than from an overpowering desire to win (Kavanagh et al. 1989). The majority adopt a healthy lifestyle (Fogelholm, Kaprio, and Sarna 1994), and the proportion of smokers is much lower among Masters competitors than in the general population (2.9% of continuing smokers in the sample of Shephard, Kavanagh, and Mertens [1995]). Finally, elderly competitors tend to have more frequent medical examinations than the general population, and those who develop warning signs or symptoms of myocardial ischemia are likely to drop out of competitions.

Musculoskeletal injury.   There is little question that seniors who decide to exercise hard are at a high risk of sustaining an acute musculoskeletal injury (Kallinen and Markku 1995), but the influence of continued athletic activity on the risk of osteoarthritis is less certain.

Cross-linkage of collagen decreases the elasticity of both tendons and muscles, and bone strength decreases even in those who exercise regularly. As a competitor ages, an acute injury thus becomes more likely for a given applied force. However, it is less clear whether or not active individuals are protected against catastrophic injury because their bones are stronger and surrounded by a greater mass of lean tissue.

In the series of Masters athletes studied by Kavanagh et al. (1989), about half were injured in the course of a year. Moreover, although some of the problems were minor in nature, in a third of those injured the lesion was sufficiently severe to interrupt their training for a month or longer. Kallinen and Alén (1994) had a similar experience. They obtained a retrospective history from 97 Masters athletes aged 70 to 81 years; 81% had sustained at least one sport-related injury, and 38% of these injuries were related to overuse. In their survey, the upper limbs appeared particularly vulnerable to overuse whereas the lower limbs tended to be affected more by acute sprains. Endurance activities were associated with lower limb and joint injuries, whereas strength training led to sprains and muscle injuries. About 20% of problems persisted for several years.

Matheson et al. (1989) compared the distribution of injuries between older and younger individuals attending a sports injury clinic; the main differences

(Andrews and St. Pierre 1986) were a lower incidence of patellofemoral pain and stress fracture in the older group, with a greater incidence of meniscal injury, degenerative disk disease, and various inflammatory conditions. Jackson (1986) further noted that if degenerative changes had developed in an affected joint, the response to arthroscopic surgery was less favorable in the elderly than in a younger person.

A number of reports have suggested that many years of vigorous participation in such activities as ballet, soccer, football, boxing, and parachuting predispose to the onset of osteoarthritis (Panush 1994). Distance runners, in contrast, do not seem particularly susceptible to osteoarthritis unless the biomechanics of the knee joint is abnormal (Panush 1994). Lane et al. (1986) found that cartilage loss, crepitation, joint stability, and symptoms of osteoarthritis were no more prevalent in runners than in control subjects, although one difficulty in interpreting these data is that the onset of symptoms may have caused some individuals to stop running. A dissident report by Marti, Knobloch, et al. (1989) noted that the hip joints of Swiss long-distance runners showed more radiological evidence of osteoarthritis than those of either bobsledders or control subjects.

Immune function.   Although moderate exercise apparently has a favorable effect on immune function, as already discussed, there have been suggestions that an excessive volume of athletic training can impair immune responses, leaving an individual at increased risk of viral infection (Brenner, Shek, and Shephard 1994). However, the amount of training needed to induce such an effect is very large.

Shephard, Kavanagh, and Mertens (1995) noted that 15% of Masters athletes were conscious of a critical weekly training distance beyond which infections seemed to develop. Typically, problems were encountered with 72 km/week of jogging, 300 km/week of cycling, or 16 km/week of swimming. Nevertheless, 76% of Masters competitors considered themselves less vulnerable to influenza and colds than their sedentary peers of similar age.

Masters Competition as a Component of Health Policy

How effective is Masters competition as a means of promoting physical activity and general health among older members of the population? The typical volume of training that is undertaken (6 to 10 h/week) certainly does more than meet reasonable goals for aerobic fitness (American College of Sports Medicine 1995a), although it is less clear how well muscle strength is being conserved by the endurance athlete.

Other arguments for and against sport as a means of delivering physical activity seem much the same as for younger adults. For some of the population, particularly those with extroverted personalities, competition and the social aspects of sport are useful forces stimulating involvement and sustaining exercise participation. However, for the very competitive elderly person, there is a real danger that a contest may lead to overexertion. Moreover, an age-related waning of performance despite rigorous preparation may be a source of negative motivation for such people.

The majority of Masters athletes (91%) have a high interest in good health, and as already noted, few are currently smokers. Some 47% of former smokers indicated that their participation in Masters competition had helped in the process of cigarette withdrawal (Shephard, Kavanagh, and Mertens 1995). Among those over the age of 60 years, more than three-fourths also rated their quality of life as much higher than that of their age-matched peers.

When participation in competitive sport is compared with the typical active pursuits of other senior citizens, walking and gardening, it is seen to require a good deal more in terms of facilities, equipment, clothing, transportation, and disposable income. Shephard, Kavanagh, and Mertens (1995) estimated that many Masters competitors invested over $1000 a year in travel, accommodations, and other costs associated with their events.

Moreover, although the number of participants in Masters competitions is growing quite rapidly, such individuals still represent only a very small fraction of the total population of seniors, even in countries where the movement is well developed. For example, about 10,000 people attended the World Masters Games in Toronto in 1985, but only about 20% of the men and 9% of the women involved were over the age of 60 years; further, only 4.5% of the men and 1.7% of the women were over the age of 70 years (Kavanagh et al. 1989).

Almost all Masters competitors (95% of women and 93% of men) regard the opportunity to socialize with people who have similar interests as the main motivation for participation in Masters contests (Kavanagh et al. 1989). Most of the group enjoy competition, but 90% claim that they are not unduly disturbed if they do not win, and 20% admit that they are not serious competitors.

We may conclude that for a minority of seniors, Masters competition has become an extremely important part of their lives. However, it is unlikely that the numbers of people attracted to such events will grow to the point that they become a major instrument of health policy, at least for the foreseeable future. Contests involving elderly people are important mainly as a source of role models; they demonstrate that seniors do not need to accept a major decline of aerobic power and muscle strength as an inevitable feature of aging.

Age Limits to Functional Restoration

Several animal studies have suggested that whereas an exercise program extends the life span of young animals, if the onset of exercise is delayed, the intervention may actually reduce longevity.

Linsted, Tonstad, and Kuzma (1991) found some evidence of a similar trend in a 26-year follow-up of 9484 Seventh-Day Adventist men (see table 4.5), particularly in terms of the statistics for vigorous exercise. However, Langer et al. (1994) followed men and women who were initially aged 75 years or older for a period of five years; regular exercise at least three times per week was associated with a relative risk of death of 0.54 in men and 0.45 in women. Moreover, this advantage persisted when the data were adjusted for initial physical and emotional health, conventional cardiac risk factors, and changes in exercise level relative to 10 years previously.

In terms of restoring function, we earlier noted some evidence suggesting that the absolute gains in aerobic power over the duration of a typical training experiment are smaller in older subjects, although in percentage terms the response is similar to that of a younger individual (Shephard 1987a). A recent meta-analysis of 29 training studies by Green and Crouse (1995) concluded that over the age range 60 to 80 years, gains in aerobic power in response to training (delta ml/[kg · min]) were inversely related to age; among those aged 75 to 80 years, gains were no more than 1 to 2 ml/[kg · min]. Nevertheless, a major part of the problem in the attempt to train the frail elderly is in bringing them to a level of condition at which they can exercise effectively. Thus, if a modest intensity of training is continued over a longer period, larger gains of aerobic power are seen (Green and Crouse 1995).

Myofibrillar protein synthesis proceeds some 27% more slowly in subjects aged 62 to 72 years than in those aged 22 to 31 years (Welle et al. 1993). It remains unclear whether the young adult rate of protein synthesis can be restored by an increase of physical activity (Welle et al. 1993; Yarasheski, Zachwieja, and Bier 1993), but even the initial rate seems sufficient to allow muscle hypertrophy. There is no indication of an age ceiling beyond which functional gains can no longer be realized. Indeed, the observations of Fiatarone et al. (1990) suggest that a substantial increase of muscle strength and some gains of muscle bulk remain possible even in frail nonagenarians.

Conclusions

Excessive exercise can cause a cardiac catastrophe, musculoskeletal injury, and suppression of immune function. Nevertheless, seniors are able to participate safely in moderate physical training programs. Moreover, in many biological functions they show percentage improvements similar to those seen in younger adults. The adoption of an active lifestyle apparently does little to check the inherent process of aging, but training-induced gains of function are enough to have important consequences for the quality of life in an older person. Biological age is effectively reduced by as much as 10 to 20 years. A minority of seniors will gain the necessary activity through Masters competition, but because the initial level of fitness is usually low, many old people can make important functional gains through much more modest initiatives, including the vigorous pursuit of everyday activities.

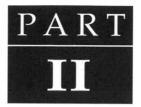

PART

II

Physical Activity and Health in Older People

For many people, physical activity, exercise, and sport carry intrinsic psychological rewards: self-actualization, or an increased sense of self-efficacy, for example. However, the most common motivation of older people who become involved in a program of regular exercise is a desire to improve personal fitness and health (Shephard 1994). Likewise, governments are interested in promoting physical activity during the "third age" mainly because they hope that the health of older citizens will be improved, their independence will be prolonged, and the economic costs of health and support services for seniors will be decreased. The second part of this volume considers interactions between physical activity, fitness, and health. Two consensus volumes (Bouchard et al. 1990; Bouchard, Shephard, and Stephens 1994) have previously reviewed important issues in the context of the general population, and a useful model has been proposed relating physical activity, fitness, and health. From the viewpoint of the senior citizen, physical activity usually becomes confined to leisure activity and domestic chores. Furthermore, the latter occupy an ever-increasing fraction of the individual's work capacity. Environmental factors also have an increasing impact on the model, as the proportions of the population with poor health and frank morbidity increase, and the ability to maintain the constancy of the *milieu intérieur* deteriorates.

The objective of this part of the book is to summarize available information on the relationships between physical activity, fitness, and health in the young-old, the very old, and the oldest-old. The source of physical activity in these age groups may still be a deliberate participation in sport, but other forms of

199

"active living" such as gardening and fast walking now demand a sufficient fraction of aerobic power that they also can make a substantial contribution to the development of personal fitness and thus an enhancement of health. Our discussion focuses specifically on diseases of the cardiorespiratory system, the musculoskeletal system, and metabolism for two reasons: these systems are very important both to overall function and to the individual's quality of life, and also there is good evidence that regular physical activity has a beneficial effect on many of the disorders affecting these systems. A final chapter in this section addresses interactions between function, overall well-being, and quality of life.

Chapter 5

Physical Activity and Diseases of the Cardiorespiratory System

The topics to be discussed in this chapter include ischemic heart disease, stroke, hypertension, peripheral vascular disease, congestive heart failure, end-stage renal disease, and chronic obstructive lung disease. For each of these conditions, we will consider first the prevalence and/or incidence of the disorder. We will then examine the role of physical activity in primary, secondary, tertiary, and quaternary prevention (see fig. 5.1). Taking ischemic heart disease as an example, primary prevention would seek to avoid clinically silent manifestations of disease (for example, the silent myocardial ischemia that can be detected by an exercise ECG). Secondary prevention would attempt to prevent clinical manifestations of myocardial ischemia in a person who already has ECG or laboratory evidence of subclinical cardiac disease. Tertiary prevention would aim at preventing a recurrence of myocardial infarction in a person who had already sustained a primary episode. Quaternary treatment would endeavor to optimize residual cardiac function and the quality of life in an elderly person for whom more active treatment was unwarranted because of advanced age and extensive disease.

Ischemic Heart Disease

Arteriosclerosis is a generic term, applied to any form of vascular degeneration that is associated with a thickening and loss of resilience in the arterial wall. Arteriosclerosis is a specific variety of such degeneration, associated with an accumulation of fat beneath the intimal lining of the vessels and an increase of connective tissue in the underlying subintima.

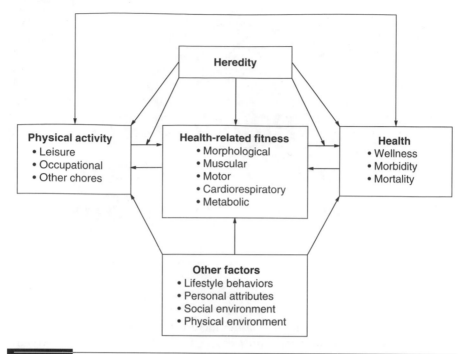

Figure 5.1   Model showing possible interactions between physical activity, fitness, and health.

Reprinted, by permission, from C. Bouchard and R.J. Shephard, 1994, Physical activity, fitness, and health: The model and key concepts. In *Physical activity, fitness and health*, edited by C. Bouchard, R.J. Shephard, and T. Stephens, (Champaign, IL: Human Kinetics), 78.

Prevalence and Incidence

Pathological consequences of arteriosclerosis vary with its site. If the lesion is located in the coronary vessels, then various manifestations of ischemic heart disease eventually appear, although vessel narrowing and the resulting ischemia may remain silent for many years, to be revealed only by such laboratory tests as exercise electrocardiography and echocardiography. Possible clinical presentations of myocardial ischemia include angina pectoris, a myocardial infarction, sudden death due to cardiac arrest or ventricular fibrillation, and (in the very old) progressive cardiac failure.

Silent Ischemia

Postmortem examination of traffic accident victims has provided unequivocal evidence that many young adults have some atheromatous plaques in their coronary vessels. However, the resistance to perfusion of the coronary arteries is proportional to the fourth power of vascular diameter, so that the atheromatous plaques do not usually have clinical significance until they occlude about 70% of a major coronary artery, a situation which does not usually arrive before the age of 40 or 50 years.

The prevalence of substantial but clinically silent atheromatous coronary vascular disease is usually inferred from the percentage of the population showing significant horizontal or down-sloping exercise-induced depression of the ST segment of the ECG (Shephard 1981; Siscovick et al. 1991). Interpretation of the exercise ECG becomes progressively more difficult in the elderly population, because a high proportion of most samples have abnormal resting records. The estimate of abnormal records is also distorted by various well-recognized causes of false-positive and false-negative tests (see table 5.1). Particular problems in the elderly patient are the use of diuretics and digitalis (false-positive records) and an inadequate exercise intensity (false-negative records). The proportion of false-positive results seems to be particularly high in elderly women (Sidney and Shephard 1978b).

In principle, other more direct methods of testing coronary blood flow, such as coronary angiography, could be used to clarify the prevalence of silent ischemia in the symptom-free population, but the financial costs and the clinical risks associated with the alternative procedures preclude their use in population surveys of disease prevalence.

The sensitivity and specificity of the exercise ECG are such that ST depression is not very helpful in distinguishing those individuals with silent myocardial ischemia. Nevertheless, the exercise ECG does give a useful indication of the prevalence of myocardial ischemia in the population as a whole. The percentage of individuals who develop significant ST-segmental

Table 5.1   Causes of false-positive and false-negative depression of the ST segment of the exercise ECG.

False-positive results	False-negative results
Resting ST depression	Insufficient exercise intensity
Hyperventilation	Resting ST elevation
Cigarette smoking	Use of nitroglycerin and other
Use of diuretics	vasodilators
Potassium ion loss	Abnormalities of interven-
Glucose and carbohydrate loading	tricular conduction
Abnormal stress on the left ventricle	
Abnormal conduction of the	
electrical impulse	
Anti-dysrhythmic drugs	
Digitalis therapy	

depression during an exercise test increases progressively with age (see fig. 5.2), and in terms of this indicator elderly women are affected somewhat more frequently than men. Aronow and Epstein (1988) used a Holter monitor to demonstrate that 34% of 185 nursing home residents (mean age 83 years) also had ECG evidence of myocardial ischemia when carrying out their normal daily activities.

Myocardial ischemia is particularly likely to remain silent in the elderly because often they take little exercise. Even if pain does occur, it tends to be

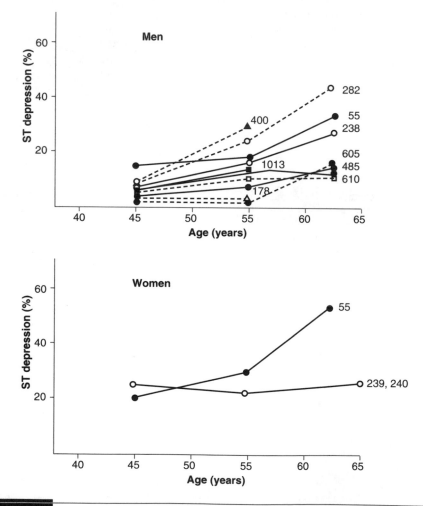

Figure 5.2   The percentage of subjects showing depression of the ST segment of the ECG at various ages (numbers refer to individual studies; for details, see Shephard 1977).

misdiagnosed as an arthritic shoulder or a peptic ulcer. Myocardial oxygen lack thus tends to present itself as congestive heart failure, acute pulmonary edema, stroke, or confusion.

Overall Prevalence

Some estimates of the prevalence of clinical disease have been based on simple indicators—for example, a history of angina or prior myocardial infarction or an abnormal Q/QS pattern on the resting ECG. In such terms, one early British survey found that the prevalence of ischemic heart disease in those over the age of 65 years who were living at home was about 20% in men and 12% in women (Kennedy, Andrews, and Caird 1977). However, these numbers would be greatly increased if silent ischemia were to be added to the total of those with coronary heart disease. There may currently be a secular trend to an increased prevalence of the disease because of the aging of a cohort who have had many of the major cardiac risk factors throughout much of their lives (Bild et al. 1993).

Morbidity

Available information on the prevalence of morbidity commonly refers to heart disease as a whole (International Classification of Diseases [ICD] 390-429). The prevalence rises from 153/1000 of men and 117/1000 women aged 45 to 64 years to 290/1000 men and 219/1000 women aged 65 to 74 years, and to 324/1000 men and 372/1000 women over 75 years; ischemic heart disease is the cause of death in some 58% of men and 26% of women over the age of 65 years (U.S. Department of Health and Human Services 1992). Heart disease is a frequent reason both for loss of independence and for hospital admission in the elderly (Gerstenblith 1980).

Anginal pain. Oxygen extraction in the coronary circulation is relatively complete, even at rest. If the work rate of the heart is increased by tachycardia, a rise of systolic pressure, or an increase of myocardial contractility, the coronary vessels must therefore dilate to increase the oxygen supply to the heart wall. In young adults, there is potential for a five- to sixfold increase of coronary blood flow, but this becomes impracticable in the rigid, arteriosclerotic vessels of an elderly person. Partly because vascular resistance is proportional to the fourth power of vessel radius, and partly because the main impedance to blood flow lies in the small arterioles, the onset of angina is almost always a portent of gross obstruction of the major coronary vessels (Ellestad 1985).

Typically, pain is precipitated by vigorous exercise such as hurrying uphill, but it is quickly relieved by resting. Symptoms are particularly likely if exercise is undertaken in cold weather, because of the associated vasoconstriction and increase of systolic blood pressure. It is also possible that the inhalation of cold, dry air may precipitate a reflex spasm of the coronary vessels. In many old people, vigorous physical effort is limited by other factors such as arthritis or chest disease, so that the full extent of myocardial ischemia may not be recognized.

However, anginal pain can severely limit all physical activity, causing a substantial reduction in the quality of life. Most medical treatments are palliative, and the patient is often glad to accept some form of surgery to open up or to bypass the atheromatous obstruction. However, it is also increasingly questioned whether prepaid medical budgets can afford to provide such a service to everyone, regardless of their age and general physical condition. Palliative measures include a moderation of the rise of blood pressure during physical effort (by the use of beta-blocking drugs and/or trinitrin tablets), where possible a lightening of exercise loads, and the introduction of extended rest pauses. During exercise outdoors, exposure to cold air can also be reduced by the use of a jogging mask that preheats inspired gas (Kavanagh 1983) and protects the skin of the face from the cold (Brown and Oldridge 1985).

Myocardial infarction.   Myocardial infarction reflects death of a segment of the ventricular wall. It usually follows total obstruction of a major coronary vessel, but it can also reflect the development of a severe relative oxygen deficiency. Several of the postulated mechanisms of vascular obstruction, including hemorrhage into an atheromatous plaque and impaction of an embolus from a fragmented plaque, could well be induced by a bout of vigorous physical activity. Other pathologies, such as the progressive accumulation of a thrombus on the surface of an ulcerated plaque, seem more likely to occur when a person is resting or asleep. In middle-aged adults, about a quarter of nonfatal episodes of myocardial infarction seem to arise during or immediately following vigorous physical activity (Shephard 1981). The risk of infarction during such activity relative to that while resting certainly does not rise as a person becomes older (Vuori 1995). Indeed, because the frail elderly are less likely to undertake violent bursts of physical activity, it is likely that more of them will sustain a myocardial infarct while they are resting.

Irrespective of the precipitating cause, much early and late morbidity and comorbidity are associated with myocardial infarction. Potential clinical problems include episodes of stroke, heart failure, and life-threatening ventricular arrhythmias (Wenger 1992). Although 75% of those over the age of 65 years survive a first heart attack, the majority live on with a greatly impaired quality of life (Castelli 1993). The probability of a late death in the years immediately following myocardial infarction also increases with age, whether the immediate cause be a ventricular arrhythmia or cardiac failure. Smith et al. (1990) found that 17.6% of myocardial infarct patients 75 years of age and older died in the year following hospital discharge, compared with 12.0% of those aged 65 to 75 years.

Myocardial Degeneration

The progressive decline in cardiac performance with age is well recognized (as discussed in chapter 3). Some authors have regarded the decrease in peak stroke volume of the exerciser as a normal manifestation of aging. Explanations have included a wasting of heart muscle, extensive amyloid infiltration of the myocardium, a slowing of ventricular relaxation, fibrotic changes in the heart valves, and a reduction in catecholamine sensitivity of the myocardium. Although many of these factors probably contribute to the age-related deterioration of cardiovascular function, chronic myocardial oxygen lack is also an important factor (Weisfeldt, Gerstenblith, and Lakatta 1985). Functional changes are much smaller in those elderly individuals who have retained a good myocardial oxygen supply. Oxygen lack has an immediate, direct effect in reducing the force of ventricular contraction. Further, small (and often undiagnosed) infarcts gradually destroy the ventricular wall in the frail elderly. The process may be exacerbated by an overt myocardial infarction, with death of a large segment of tissue and a paradoxical bulging movement of the scarred portion of the ventricular wall during systole. Eventually, a situation may be reached where the cardiac output remains adequate to meet resting needs, but attempts at exercise lead to persistent fatigue, severe breathlessness, and cardiac failure (Schuster and Bulkley 1980). In other patients, the heart has moved sufficiently close to failure that even the added venous return associated with lying down to sleep is enough to provoke pulmonary congestion and paroxysms of dyspnea.

Indications of an impaired cardiovascular response to exercise include a low resting cardiac ejection fraction that decreases rather than increases during exercise, an absence of the anticipated rise of systemic blood pressure with work rate, the accumulation of a substantial oxygen debt, and a slow recovery of heart rate and ventilation following a bout of exercise.

Overall Morbidity

A study from the Scottish Health Service (1981) found that on any given day, hospital bed occupancy by patients in the overall diagnostic band ICD 390-429 averaged 208 individuals aged 15 to 45 years, 2086 individuals aged 45 to 65 years, and 3536 individuals aged 65+ years. Moreover, those patients 65 years or older spent more than twice as long in the hospital as did the younger patients.

Mortality

Ischemic heart disease is responsible for about a third of all deaths in older men. In many hospitals, patients over the age of 75 years account for more than half of all fatal myocardial incidents (Wenger 1992). The proportion of deaths attributable to ischemic heart disease is similar at ages 45 to 49 years, 65 to 69 years, and over 80 years (Reeder 1991), but because of the increasing overall death rate, the disease-specific death rate also rises steeply with age (see table 5.2).

Table 5.2   Age-standardized mortality rates for cardiovascular diseases in Canada, 1988 and 1992 (all values, deaths per 10,000 population per year).

| | 35-54 yr | | | | 55-64 yr | | | |
| | M | | F | | M | | F | |
	'88	'92	'88	'92	'88	'92	'88	'92
IHD	67	50	13	10	402	310	113	90
AMI	44	33	9	6	262	191	75	56
Stroke	9	7	9	7	49	43	36	28
Other CV	12	14	7	7	77	80	36	37
Total CV	88	72	30	24	529	432	186	155

| | 65-74 yr | | | | 75-84 yr | | 85+ yr | |
| | M | | F | | M | F | M | F |
	'88	'92	'88	'92	'92	'92	'92	'92
IHD	1034	794	423	318	1947	1092	4241	3431
AMI	622	467	266	195	1069	598	1784	1281
Stroke	176	155	119	99	584	480	1631	1725
Other CV	251	250	123	135	735	470	2098	1983
Total CV	1461	1204	665	552	3265	2042	7970	7139

IHD = ischemic heart disease
AMI = acute myocardial infarction (heart attack)
CV = cardiovascular disease.
Adapted, by permission, from *Cardiovascular disease in Canada*, edited by R. Reeder, 1995 (Ottawa, ON: Laboratory Centre for Disease Control, Health Canada; Health Statistics Division, Statistics Canada), 9.

Prior to menopause, the incidence of deaths from ischemic heart disease is four to five times lower in women than in men. Much of this protection is lost in the postmenopausal years. Coronary vascular disease accounts for about a third of deaths in women aged 65 years and older. Beyond the age of 75 years, the number of cardiac deaths in women reaches about 70% of the male total.

The type of cardiac death changes with age. In the younger age categories, about two-thirds of incidents are due to cardiac arrest or ventricular fibrillation. But in those over the age of 75 years, sudden death is much less common. In this age group, about half of fatalities have other causes, usually a progressive cardiac failure secondary to massive infarction; probably because vigorous exercise is a rarity, it is uncommon to find cardiac deaths among people who are exercising (Vuori 1995).

Physical Activity in Primary and Secondary Prevention

It is now generally agreed that in the middle-aged adult, regular physical activity is helpful in correcting cardiac risk factors and in preventing the onset of clinically manifest ischemic heart disease (Berlin and Coldlitz 1990; Pate et al. 1995; Powell et al. 1987). Moreover, a longitudinal study in middle-aged individuals showed that beginning moderately vigorous activity, quitting cigarette smoking, maintaining a normal blood pressure, and avoiding obesity were each independently associated with a reduced risk of death from ischemic heart disease (Paffenbarger et al. 1993). However, two major meta-analyses (Berlin and Coldlitz 1990; Powell et al. 1987) did not consider either possible changes in the protective value of exercise as a person became older, or changes in habitual physical activity with aging (Lee, Paffenbarger, and Hsieh 1992b).

MacDonald et al. (1992) noted that the prevalence of two of the three traditional major cardiac risk factors (a high blood pressure and a high serum cholesterol) rose with age; in those aged 65 to 74 years, 80% of men and 89% of women had at least one of the three traditional cardiac risk factors. Thomsen, Larsen, and Schroll (1995) also noted an increase of serum triglycerides with aging. If one were to add a further recently recognized major risk factor, a sedentary lifestyle, then the elderly would be perceived as extremely vulnerable to ischemic heart disease, with a corresponding potential to reduce their risk by adoption of a better lifestyle. However, the exact magnitude of any benefit from altered habits is less clear, since the significance of the individual risk factors changes with aging. For example, an increase of serum cholesterol adds less to the relative risk of a heart attack as a person becomes older (although because of the greater overall prevalence of ischemic heart disease in elderly subjects, the attributable risk of a high serum cholesterol is also greater in seniors; Castelli 1993; Crepaldi and Manzato 1993; Shipley 1991). Cigarette smoking seems to be a somewhat less important cardiac risk factor for elderly than for younger men; in contrast, the adverse cardiac effects of smoking increase in women after menopause. Hypertension (particularly a high systolic pressure) has a more serious import in the elderly than in younger individuals (Castelli 1993), as does lack of regular exercise (Morris et al. 1980; Siscovick et al. 1984). Some studies have suggested that physical activity has less protective value in women than in men; nevertheless, this may merely be a criticism of the weakness of current instruments for assessing the habitual activity of women, since in terms of a fitness criterion (treadmill endurance time) women gain more protection from an improved physical condition than do men (Blair, Kohl, and Barlow 1993). In women, risks are changed by the sudden decrease in plasma estrogen levels; estrogen may not only have a favorable effect upon lipid profile, but it may also function as a peripheral or a coronary vasodilator (Rosano et al. 1993). Finally, the relative body weight has less influence on the chances of developing a fatal heart attack in the elderly than in a younger person (Hubert et al. 1983).

Possibly the loss of lean tissue has a confounding effect in many seniors who have a low relative weight.

A substantial minimum weekly energy expenditure (equivalent to a walking distance of 18-20 km/week) is needed to enhance the lipid profile of middle-aged adults (Kavanagh et al. 1983; Williams et al. 1982). Frail elderly individuals may not be able to achieve such an increase in energy expenditure, and moreover may not need to do so for optimization of serum lipids (Duncan, Gordon, and Scott 1991). Kohrt, Obert, and Holloszy (1992) described a favorable change in lipid profile when subjects aged 60 to 70 years participated in a 9- to 12-month program of aerobic exercise. Nevertheless, it might be argued that even if the lipid profile can be improved in an elderly person, there is little possibility of enhancing coronary perfusion, because the atheromatous plaques obstructing the myocardial blood supply have now become rigidly calcified.

Although existing silent coronary vascular disease is unlikely to be reversed if an elderly person increases his or her habitual physical activity, an improvement of lipid profile may yet limit the rate of progression of the disease process. This in turn delays the appearance of clinical manifestations of arteriosclerosis. The likelihood that myocardial ischemia will develop with any given degree of coronary arterial obstruction depends also upon the oxygen consumption of the heart. The myocardial oxygen demand is proportional to the product of blood pressure and heart rate, both factors that are reduced by an exercise program. We noted in chapter 3 that training increases the aerobic power and thus reduces the heart rate at any given work rate in elderly subjects. Webb, Poehlman, and Tonino (1993) have also demonstrated that systemic blood pressures are reduced with participation in a regular exercise program. They had a small group of men aged 55 to 77 years exercise at 60% to 75% of their maximum oxygen intake for 30 to 60 min per session, three times a week for eight weeks. At the end of this period, they reported a small (5%) reduction in blood pressure relative to control values, much as might be anticipated in younger individuals.

Empirical data on the benefits of exercise relate mainly to the secondary prevention of overall mortality; nevertheless, a substantial proportion of the total mortality is due to ischemic heart disease. There is strong evidence that regular physical activity enhances health and sustains longevity until a person reaches quite an advanced age. In a 17-year study of people over the age of 70 years, Kaplan et al. (1987) found an odds ratio of 1.73 for deaths in those who reported a low level of physical activity relative to those who were more active. Grand et al. (1990) also reported a lower risk of death in elderly French people who exercised regularly. Posner et al. (1990) carried out a two-year follow-up of subjects over 60 years of age; 2% of exercised subjects developed cardiovascular diagnoses, compared with 13% of controls. Over a 12-year follow-up of men initially aged 65 to 69 years, Donahue et al. (1988) again noted that the risk of coronary heart disease was lowest in those who reported a high level of habitual physical activity. Morris et al. (1990) found that over a nine-year follow-up, regular vigorous exercise protected against both fatal and nonfatal heart attacks in subjects who were 55 to 64 years at entry; in their study, the benefit was almost as great as had been observed in those who were initially 45 to 54 years of age. Blair et al. (1989) ranked fitness levels rather than reported physical activity; nevertheless, they also observed that in persons over 60 years of age, all-cause mortality was substantially lower among subjects whose initial treadmill scores fell in the upper four quintiles of their sample, relative to the least fit quintile.

Such data show that an increase of physical activity can improve the longevity of the average senior citizen. But there still remains a possibility that this is not true of the frail, very old patient. Linsted, Tonstad, and Kuzma (1991) provided some observations pointing toward an age-related ceiling intensity of effort; beyond this ceiling, exercise shortened rather than increased longevity. Nevertheless, their findings indicated that regular exercise protected against all-cause mortality through to at least 80 years of age (see table 4.5). Rakowski and Mor (1992) and Langer et al. (1994) had similar findings in their longitudinal studies of aging and habitual physical activity.

Physical Activity in Tertiary Prevention and Quaternary Treatment

Exercise is increasingly accepted as an important component in the tertiary treatment of angina, myocardial infarction, and even myocardial degeneration.

Angina

There are a number of reasons why an elderly person with angina pectoris might anticipate benefit from a progressive exercise program. There is little evidence that exercise can either alter the dimensions of the main coronary vessels or augment collateral flow in the frail elderly. Nevertheless, the oxygen demand of the myocardium can be reduced if the heart rate and blood pressure are decreased at a given level of physical activity. Moreover, the resultant lengthening of the diastolic phase of the cardiac cycle may facilitate perfusion of the ventricle (chapter 4; Balady 1992). Finally, a strengthening of the skeletal muscles may help to reduce the rise of blood pressure during exercise, thus bringing the rate-pressure product for many activities below the angina threshold (Franklin et al. 1991). Haslam et al. (1988) made direct arterial measurements during a program of resisted exercise; in their study, the mean arterial pressures reached a ceiling of no more than 139 ± 7 mmHg.

The likelihood that angina will progress from severe discomfort to frank myocardial infarction is increased in an elderly individual (Bugiardini, Borghi, and Pozzati 1993). Thus, any exercise program must be preceded by a careful assessment of the stability of the angina and the level of risk of disease progression. Stability of the resting ECG from day to day, Holter monitoring over a 24 h period (Bugiardini, Borghi, and Pozzati 1993), and the response to a treadmill stress test (Shaw and Miller 1994) are all useful methods of detecting vulnerable individuals. Standard programs of endurance training are not well tolerated by a person who is liable to develop anginal pain. However, substantial gains of aerobic power can be achieved using a modified interval training program that allows extended rest periods between individual exercise bouts (Shephard 1981).

Myocardial Infarction

In middle-aged adults, a number of meta-analyses (O'Connor et al. 1989; Oldridge et al. 1988; Shephard 1983c) have demonstrated that an exercise-centered program of cardiac rehabilitation reduces the number of fatal recurrences of myocardial infarction by 20% to 30%. The number of nonfatal recurrences is not altered among program participants, but fewer recurrences are fatal. Important functional and economic gains such as an earlier return to work are also associated with participation in an active rehabilitation program (Perk and Hedback 1988; Shephard 1992b). Unfortunately, experimental trials of postcoronary rehabilitation commonly excluded patients over the age of 60 years because it was feared that they would not survive long enough to permit an adequate follow-up.

As already noted, the mortality associated with myocardial infarction increases in older individuals. An early report from our laboratory also suggested that the physiological response to an exercise-centered rehabilitation program was less favorable in older patients (Kavanagh et al. 1973). When comparisons were made with middle-aged adults, the gains of aerobic power were found to be smaller in older patients, and the older subjects also showed less tendency to a reversal of ST-segmental depression as the rehabilitation program continued. However, investigators questioned whether the discrepancy in therapeutic response reflected an inability of the older postcoronary patients to undertake vigorous exercise, or whether the findings had a socioeconomic basis. In younger patients, the drive to repay a mortgage and provide for the education of children may have provided a strong motivation to compliance with prescribed exercise that would have been lacking in older individuals. A further factor is probably a smaller residual cardiac function and thus a diminished exercise tolerance in older individuals. Lavie and Milani (1994) found that in 60-year-old postcoronary patients, the likelihood of favorable changes in HDL/LDL-cholesterol ratio and in plasma triglyceride levels was greater in those with a peak aerobic power averaging 8.8 METs than in a second subgroup whose peak aerobic power averaged only 4.6 METs; nevertheless, another report from the same laboratory (Lavie, Milani, and Littman 1993) showed similar improvements in exercise capacity, obesity indexes, and lipid levels between patient groups with average ages of 54 and 70 years.

Most of the large trials that were included in meta-analyses of exercise-centered cardiac rehabilitation had an average patient age between 50 and 60 years. However, several smaller studies have suggested that cardiorespiratory function can be increased by a progressive exercise program, even in older individuals whose initial resting cardiac ejection fraction is no more than 25% (Squires et al. 1987) or 27% (Conn, Williams, and Wallace 1982). Froelicher et al. (1984) noted that older patients showed a slightly poorer response than younger individuals when a training program was begun some four months after a cardiac event, but Williams et al. (1985) found that the conditioning response was independent of age category. Shaw and Miller (1994) noted that in those over 70 years of age, a subgroup at high risk of a recurrence of their myocardial infarction could be detected by the short duration of their exercise test, a low peak exercise heart rate, and a poor coronary blood flow when thallium scintigraphy was performed after administration of a coronary vasodilator drug (dipyridamole).

Cardiac Failure

There is probably merit in persuading elderly patients with diffuse myocardial disease to preserve existing ventricular function through cautiously prescribed exercise, although the intensity of such activity must be kept below a level at which left ventricular failure begins to occur (see section on congestive heart failure later in this chapter). Once decompensated heart failure has developed, there is little alternative to a combination of traditional medical therapy and rest until the heart is again operating on the favorable (compensated) portion of the Frank-Starling pressure/volume diagram. Beta-blocking agents may worsen the tendency to cardiac failure, as may alcohol abuse (Wei 1994).

Need for Quaternary Treatment

There is now a growing discussion of the quantity of resources that should be allocated to active treatment of the frail elderly. It is probably inappropriate to apply costly, high-technology solutions such as coronary bypass surgery to the treatment of myocardial ischemia in this age group (Wenger 1992).

Even exercise rehabilitation programs can be much simpler than those recommended for younger adults, for whom an almost complete recovery of function is possible. The design of exercise-centered cardiac programs for the elderly patient must take due account of factors that influence recruitment and adherence to such programs. The initial motives of older exercisers are probably a fear that their illness will recur and a desire for better health, whereas subsequent involvement is sustained by perceptions of greater self-efficacy and well-being (Shephard 1993d).

When assessing the cost/effectiveness of cardiac rehabilitation during the retirement years (Shephard 1992a), several important items that are normally included in the balance sheet for a younger adult (such as an earlier return to work and a longer total period of employment) are no longer relevant. Moreover, economists argue that a prolongation of survival increases the elderly patient's charge against scarce pension funds. Nevertheless, the restoration of myocardial function can have a much greater bearing upon the quality of life for a senior than for a younger individual who enters a cardiac rehabilitation program with a substantial functional reserve.

Perhaps most importantly from the viewpoint of quality of life, Ben Ari et al. (1987) have claimed that exercise reduces the likelihood of developing anginal pain. Some authors have also found that an exercise-centered rehabilitation program enhances perceived energy and exercise tolerance, while reducing anxiety. But results have been inconsistent (Quaglietti and Froelicher 1994), and the findings are in any event complicated by the depressant nature of a number of the medications currently used in the treatment of cardiovascular disease.

Stroke

A stroke may be defined as a sudden and persistent loss of neural function having a focal distribution consistent with a vascular cause. In a young adult, many underlying pathologies such as cerebral vascular spasm and hemorrhage complicate the analysis of benefits from a physical activity program. However, in elderly individuals the issue is simpler; the great majority of incidents are attributable to an arteriosclerotic obstruction of the cerebral blood vessels, with resulting death of brain tissue.

Prevalence and Incidence

The risk factors for stroke are similar to those for ischemic heart disease, with hypertension playing a dominant role (Ostfeld 1980). Other predisposing factors include diabetes mellitus, cigarette smoking, a prior history of cardiovascular disease or atrial fibrillation, and left ventricular hypertrophy.

The usual presentation is as a major incident of unilateral muscular paralysis. About half of stroke victims die within the first four weeks after an attack, and about half of subsequent survivors have a recurrence within three years. In the frail elderly, occasional small strokes may pass undetected, causing a progressive deterioration in cerebral function.

Strokes are rare under the age of 50 years, but the incidence rises progressively in subsequent age quintiles (Reeder 1991). Thus, by the age of 85 years, the age-specific mortality rate for strokes is about 25% of that for ischemic heart disease. The prevalence of a history of stroke in the United States is 4.5% of men and 4.1% of women aged 65 to 69 years, and 5.7% of men and 5.5% of women over 70 years (White, Losonczy, and Wolf 1990). The overall incidence and mortality decreased by about 5% per annum between 1970 and 1990, reflecting in part decreases in cardiovascular risk factors (Bonita and

Beaglehole 1989), and in part more aggressive detection and treatment of hypertension (Wissler 1985). Current incidence data for Canada are shown in table 5.2. In Japan, the incidence remains much higher, probably because of the greater prevalence of hypertension.

Physical Activity in Primary and Secondary Prevention

Given the dominant role of hypertension in the causation of stroke, it is reasonable to suggest that exercise might have some role in primary prevention.

Shinton and Sagar (1993) carried out a case control study of patients who had sustained their first stroke. The authors estimated that the overall age and sex-adjusted risk ratio was 0.33 for those individuals who gave a history of vigorous exercise as young adults. Moreover, this protection was independent of other risk factors, and increased as the years of involvement in exercise were increased. Benefit diminished if exercise was not begun until middle age, and was somewhat smaller for those who sustained a stroke in old age (odds ratio for active subjects 0.20 for ages 35 to 54 years, compared with 0.36 for ages 65 to 74 years).

In a 9.5-year prospective study of 7735 men initially aged 40 to 59 years, Wannamethee and Shaper (1992) obtained similar findings. After adjustment of their data for age, social class, smoking, heavy drinking, and BMI, the relative risk ratio was 0.6 for those who were moderately active, and 0.3 for those who were vigorously active. Unfortunately, this study did not examine the influence of age upon relative risk.

Several other studies, reviewed by Kohl and McKenzie (1994), yielded conflicting results. Demonstration of benefit apparently depended on the investigators' success in measuring habitual physical activity, and on the extent of analytic control for other possible cardiovascular risk factors and confounding variables. Plainly, much of any benefit from exercise comes from the control of hypertension and hyperlipidemia. It is thus not very surprising that benefit is weakened if the variance attributable to such influences is extracted before testing for the benefits derived from exercise.

Tertiary and Quaternary Treatment

After recovery from the acute incident, there is much scope for exercise-centered rehabilitation of the person who has sustained a stroke. The main argument for such an approach is that the quality of the individual's remaining years of life will be enhanced. Because the systemic blood pressure is reduced, it also appears likely that the risk of a recurrence of the stroke and of complications such as falls (Forster and Young 1995) will be reduced in a patient who again becomes active. However, there are as yet little data available to test this hypothesis.

Immediately following the stroke, the affected body parts may be atonic. There is also an impairment of balance, due in part to a disruption of righting reflexes, and there may be a substantial loss of awareness in the affected limbs (anosognosia). The sensations of movement must be relearned through careful use of tactile and proprioceptive stimulation. If this precaution is not observed, muscle-strengthening exercises may merely reinforce abnormal, poorly coordinated movement patterns.

The usual goals of rehabilitation for an elderly stroke victim are independent ambulation and independence in the activities of daily living. Nerve cells killed in the initial incident will not regenerate, but the hope is that movement can be restored by exploiting the redundancy of neural connections within the brain. Problems may arise during rehabilitation because of associated losses of intellectual function and concentration, altered self-concept, and emotional stability. Successful adaptation is partly situational, and the ability to regain independent living may depend very much on changes that can be made in the living environment to reduce the requirement for powerful muscle movements. Unfortunately, the likelihood of successful rehabilitation also seems to be inversely related to the age of the patient (Granger, Hamilton, and Fiedler 1992).

Walking may be helped by a brace, particularly if weakness of dorsiflexion and eversion of the ankle are present (Lorentz 1985). Even if recovery is relatively complete, residual weakness of certain limb muscles can leave much asymmetry of movement. This increases the energy cost both of postural support and of body displacement. Continuing spasticity, joint stiffness, and a resort to trick movements foster an awkward and jerky task performance. Tremor may add further to the excessive energy expenditure associated with a given activity. At the same time, muscle wasting, an increase of body fat, and a progressive deterioration of cardiorespiratory fitness restrict the person's ability to deal with these handicaps. The increased cost of simple activities such as walking establishes a vicious cycle of fatigue, lack of physical activity, worsening mechanical inefficiency, and further fatigue.

Longmuir and Shephard (1994) have discussed possible simple test methods that will allow fitness appraisers with limited qualifications to evaluate people such as those with residual hemiplegia who are unable to perform the standard Canadian Aerobic Fitness Test. They have proposed an arm ergometer protocol that is closely analogous to the standard Canadian Home Fitness Test, with an equivalent system of scoring.

The net oxygen cost of walking, expressed in ml per kg per m traversed (ml/[kg · m]), is compared for able-bodied subjects and individuals with hemiplegia in figure 5.3. In the general population, the oxygen cost of walking conforms to a plateau of 0.110 to 0.120 ml/[kg · m] over a wide range of walking speeds, although the cost of walking unit distance increases steeply at speeds below 30 m/min. If a person with hemiplegia can attain the plateau speed of 40 to 50 m/min, then the cost of walking is only 10% to 20% higher

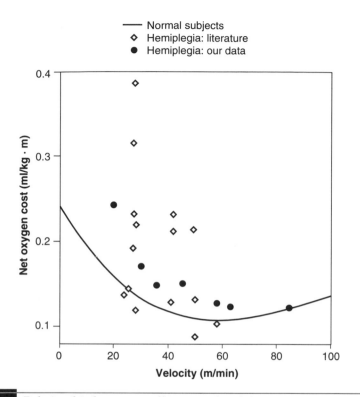

Figure 5.3 Relationship between walking speed and the net oxygen cost of walking a fixed distance (ml/[kg · m]). Data for subjects with hemiplegia are compared to curve for able-bodied subjects. The normal curve for normal subjects is a third-order polynomial fitted to published data.

Reprinted, by permission, from R.J. Shephard, T. Kavanagh, R. Campbell, and B. Lorenz, 1994, "Net energy cost of stair climbing and ambulation in subjects with hemiplegia," *Sports Medicine, Training and Rehabilitation* 5: 199-210.

than in a normal subject. However, many stroke victims cannot attain this pace, and the oxygen cost per meter of distance that they traverse is then greatly increased (Shephard et al. 1994). This is a serious problem for the oldest-old, many of whom have a very limited peak aerobic power.

Inefficiency of movement is particularly great if there is a partial paralysis of both lower limbs. The oxygen cost of walking can then rise to twice the normal value, and particularly in a frail elderly person with associated cardiovascular disease the required energy expenditure quickly exceeds the individual's maximal oxygen intake. The mechanical efficiency of movement can sometimes be improved by use of a brace, although many seniors have difficulty in learning to use any device that requires an alteration of established movement patterns.

It is particularly difficult for a person with hemiplegia to climb stairs. The net mechanical efficiency for the ascent and descent of a laboratory staircase is 6% to 8%, compared with the value of about 16% found in normal adults (Shephard et al. 1994).

Hypertension

Family physicians have a wide range of measurement methods and criteria for the diagnosis of hypertension (Fotherby, Harper, and Potter 1992). However, hypertension is commonly diagnosed if the systolic pressure exceeds 160 mmHg or the diastolic pressure exceeds 90 mmHg. In reaching the conclusion that blood pressure is abnormally increased, it is important to exclude the influence of any initial anxiety that may have arisen in the doctor's office by repetition of the measurements (Furberg and Black 1988). A substantial proportion of those who are said to have mild hypertension show normal readings if measurements are repeated in more relaxed surroundings. Although specific pathologies must be excluded, the elderly person who has a high blood pressure commonly suffers from "essential" hypertension (Forette, Henry, and Hervy 1982; Whelton 1985). This diagnosis merely implies that the cause is unknown.

The blood pressure distribution curve is unimodal, with no clear separation of "normal" and "abnormal" populations. Since aging also leads to some rise of the systolic blood pressure, it thus remains arguable that the essential hypertension of the older person is no more than an extreme form of normal aging. The preponderance of isolated systolic hypertension in older people (SHEP Cooperative Research Group 1991) adds weight to this argument.

Prevalence and Incidence

Hypertension may occasionally present itself to the clinician through some related symptom such as frequent or persistent headaches, but it is more commonly an incidental finding at a general medical examination.

The prevalence varies from one community to another—for example, in the Inuit community of Igloolik, where the population continue to consume a diet rich in marine-derived omega-3-fatty acids, there is almost no hypertension (Rode and Shephard 1995a; see fig. 3.6). In contrast, rates are extremely high in parts of Asia, probably due to a high dietary intake of salt. In the United States, at least, hypertension also seems to be more prevalent among African American than among white subjects. One study showed that as many as 40% of people over the age of 65 years in urban America had an elevation of the systolic reading, the diastolic reading, or both (Vokonas, Kannel, and Cupples 1988). Kannel (1994) put the overall prevalence of hypertension as high as 50%. The age-related increase of pressures seems to be greater in women than in men (Martin, Ogawa, et al. 1991), possibly because of the decline in estrogen production at menopause.

Some 65% of cases in the elderly are attributable to an excessive systolic pressure (Whelton 1985). In the Framingham study, Wilking et al. (1988) found that the prevalence of isolated systolic hypertension rose from 11% of men and 17% of women at age 65 years to 18% of men and 32% of women at age 80 years. The SHEP Cooperative Research Group (1991) also found prevalence to rise from around 10% at age 60 to 69 years to 20% in those over the age of 80 years. Some authors have argued that attention should be directed only to diastolic hypertension, but in seniors the cardiovascular risks (see table 5.3) seem to be at least as great for isolated systolic hypertension as for isolated diastolic hypertension (Berman 1982). The risk is particularly marked if there is associated ECG evidence of left ventricular hypertrophy (Kannel 1994).

Perhaps even more important than the increase of resting blood pressures is evidence that the rise of systolic pressure during exercise is greater in older than in younger individuals (Martin, Ogawa, et al. 1991; Michelsen and Otterstad 1990). Reasons apparently include a decrease in arterial elasticity, a decrease of lean muscle mass (and thus a greater risk of vascular occlusion during vigorous exercise), and an accumulation of body fat.

Primary and Secondary Prevention

The primary prevention of hypertension is an important goal. Klag, Whelton, and Appel (1990) suggested that between 60% and 70% of nonfatal and fatal cardiovascular events occur in patients with hypertension, and my colleagues and I also found that 40% of the deaths observed over a three-year program of postcoronary rehabilitation occurred in patients with a blood pressure exceeding 150/100 (Shephard 1981). In addition to ischemic heart disease, hypertension is an important risk factor for stroke, peripheral vascular disease,

Table 5.3 Risk ratios for various cardiovascular disorders in patients with hypertension.

Cardiovascular disorder	Risk ratio	
	Men	Women
Ischemic heart disease	1.6	1.9
Stroke	1.9	2.3
Peripheral arterial disease	1.6	2.0
Cardiac failure	1.9	1.9

Adapted, by permission, from W.B. Kannel, 1993, "Hypertension in the elderly: Epidemiologic appraisal from the Framingham study," *Cardiology in the Elderly* 1: 359-363. © 1993, Rapid Science Publishers.

and congestive heart failure (Kannel 1994; see table 5.3). It is assumed (but less clearly demonstrated for the elderly) that not only the prevention of hypertension, but also the reduction of pressures by a combination of exercise and other types of therapy, will reduce the likelihood of such problems.

Cross-sectional studies in general have suggested an association between physical inactivity and the development of hypertension. For example, Reaven, Barrett-Connor, and Edelstein (1991) categorized women aged 50 to 89 years on the basis of their habitual patterns of physical activity; the systolic pressure was approximately 20 mmHg lower in those who engaged in heavy activity relative to those who were inactive. Kasch et al. (1988) also claimed that regular participation in a physical activity program forestalled an increase of blood pressure, although it is difficult to eliminate from this study other complicating factors such as selective dropout and a reduction of body fat. Kasch et al. (1990) provided data for their control subjects in a subsequent report; as in other studies, the controls developed an increase of blood pressure as they became older. Others have noted that relative to untrained individuals of similar age, elderly athletes have a low blood pressure, both at rest and at a given level of work, (Kasch et al. 1990; Martin, Ogawa, et al. 1991; Rogers, Hagberg, et al. 1990). In contrast, Sedgwick et al. (1988) found only a weak relationship between age-related changes in blood pressure and the participation of women in a fitness program (retrospectively analyzed), and Gilders and Dudley (1992) pointed out that whereas the waking blood pressures might be reduced, the night-time readings often remained unchanged.

Tertiary and Quaternary Treatment

The majority of studies on the treatment of hypertension have concerned relatively young adults (Fagard and Tipton 1994; Tipton 1991). In such individuals, there is good evidence that prognosis is improved by the administration of drugs that lower systemic blood pressure. However, it is less certain whether there is similar benefit in the elderly (MRC Working Party 1985). Plainly, it is important to avoid drugs with side effects that increase morbidity (Pickering 1993). The use of beta-blocking agents may provoke cardiac failure (Wei 1994), and depressant drugs are likely to reduce physical activity levels that have already become inadequate for health. Other methods of treating hypertension are also more questionable in older patients. Reduction of plasma volume by the administration of diuretics may cause dangerous episodes of postural hypotension, and a reduction of salt intake is liable to exacerbate a lack of appetite (Applegate 1994).

Given that arteriosclerotic lesions become progressively calcified with age, one might suspect that an exercise program would be less effective in reducing blood pressures in the elderly than in younger individuals. Some authors have reported program-related decreases in systolic (Cononie et al. 1991;

Hagberg, Montain, et al. 1989; Singh et al. 1993; Steinhaus et al. 1990), diastolic (Howze, Smith, and DiGilio 1989; Singh et al. 1993), or mean resting pressure (Webb, Poehlman, and Tonino 1993), with decreases in pressures during submaximal exercise (Martin, Ogawa, et al. 1991). On the other hand, Spina et al. (1993) found no change of pressures in men and a decrease of diastolic pressures only in women when 64-year-old subjects participated in a 12-month endurance training program, and Hamdorf et al. (1993) found no change of resting pressures when 64-year-old women undertook a six-month program of endurance training. Possible artifacts in some of these studies included (1) a training-associated reduction of body mass, (2) an improved fit of the blood pressure cuff as subcutaneous fat was lost, and (3) a progressive habituation of program participants to the observer and the test laboratory. This last factor can lead to a substantial reduction of blood pressures, even in control subjects who are not exercised (Kukkonen et al. 1982).

Kavanagh and Shephard followed a total of 553 middle-aged and older postcoronary patients over three years of vigorous and progressive endurance exercise (Shephard 1981). During this time, there was a small but highly significant decrease of resting systolic pressure (see table 5.4), accompanied by a small but significant *increase* in the resting diastolic reading. At the maximum tolerated power output, the systolic pressure showed a small increase (because the subjects were able to exercise to a higher work rate), but the diastolic pressure remained relatively unchanged. Changes in a hypertensive subgroup were much as in other program participants. All subjects were initially well habituated to the testing laboratory, and many showed relatively little fat loss over the period of observation.

Table 5.4   Changes in systemic blood pressure with three years of vigorous endurance training.

Subject group	Resting Systolic	Resting Diastolic	Exercise Resting	Exercise Diastolic
All subjects (n = 553)				
Initial	133 ± 17	85 ± 9	169 ± 25	96 ± 13
Final	127 ± 15	87 ± 11	183 ± 29	96 ± 12
Difference	−6 ± 17	+2 ± 13	+15 ± 25	0 ± 14
Hypertensives (n = 141)				
Initial	161 ± 19	104 ± 9	172 ± 31	100 ± 12
Final	154 ± 12	103 ± 13	188 ± 30	99 ± 16
Difference	−7 ± 19	−1 ± 12	+15 ± 27	−1 ± 18

Data of Kavanagh and Shephard (Shephard 1981) for normotensive and hypertensive postcoronary patients at rest and when exercising to 75% of peak aerobic power.

The extent of any therapeutic response probably depends not only upon the extent of initial hypertension and the type of exercise program that is undertaken, but also on age and ancillary treatments such as a change of diet, control of obesity, a reduction of salt intake, and the administration of diuretics (Ehsani 1993). Thus, Weber, Barnard, and Roy (1983) observed substantial decreases in both resting blood pressure and exercise systolic readings in an uncontrolled group of men and women of average age 78.7 years who participated in the multifaceted Pritikin exercise and diet program. However, Suzuki et al. (1991) cautioned that in their sample of subjects aged 77 years, systolic function deteriorated during exercise, suggesting that the cardiac reserve was also limited in this group. Setaro et al. (1992) found that the mortality over a 48-month interval (64% vs. 36%) was substantially higher among those with hypertension who also showed impaired systolic function.

In general, people who are initially severely hypertensive are less able to comply with a vigorous training program, and the likelihood of a positive response is correspondingly reduced. Finally, it should be stressed that many of the drugs used in the treatment of hypertension, including alpha-adrenergic receptor agonists, beta-adrenergic receptor blockers, and Rauwolfia alkaloids, tend to impair cognition and lead to a depressed mood state (Bloomfield, Nivikov, and Ferrario 1994). This in turn can reduce habitual physical activity and complicate attempts to involve the hypertensive patient in an exercise program.

Peripheral Vascular Disease

Atherosclerosis and other forms of peripheral vascular disease can lead to partial or complete obstruction of the main arterial supply to the limbs. The practical consequences include intermittent claudication and (if gangrene develops) an above- or below-knee amputation. Intermittent claudication and amputation of a gangrenous limb have very important implications for the quality of life in the frail elderly.

Intermittent claudication is a severe muscular pain. Depending on the location of the obstruction (superficial femoral or iliac artery), the discomfort may be localized to the calf or it may also affect the thigh (Thiele and Strandness 1994). Like the analogous anginal pain in the heart, it reflects an acute oxygen lack in the affected muscle. Symptoms are provoked by modest exercise (such as walking up a slight incline). Although the pain is relieved by rest, the patient is strongly discouraged from taking exercise.

As the arterial obstruction becomes more complete, oxygen delivery becomes insufficient to sustain the life of the limb. Minor injuries and infections fail to heal, and gangrene develops. Amputation is then essential in order to preserve life. The elderly amputee rarely learns to use a prosthetic limb satisfactorily, and many of those who are treated by amputation subsequently become completely dependent.

Prevalence and Incidence

The prevalence of lower-extremity peripheral vascular disease is sometimes underestimated, because many of the affected individuals undertake too little physical activity to reveal their vascular incompetency. The true prevalence (including clinically silent cases) can be established by population surveys that use segmental arterial pulse volume determinations or Doppler waveform analysis to determine lower limb blood flows before and during exercise (Barnes et al. 1981). In a normal person, treadmill exercise tends to increase the systolic pressure at the ankle, but in the claudicant patient, the ankle pressure falls to a very low level during exercise and is slow to recover following a bout of physical activity (Thiele and Strandness 1994).

Some 25% of patients with ischemic heart disease have manifestations of arterial disease in the lower limbs. Given the progressive nature of arteriosclerosis, the condition is particularly common in older individuals. "Hardening of the arteries" was reported by 40.8/1000 men and 32.9/1000 women aged 65 to 74 years, and 54.6/1000 men and 50.7/1000 women aged 75 years and over. However, specific claudicant problems are restricted largely to males who have the dual risk factors of diabetes mellitus and a high cigarette consumption (Kannel and Brand 1985). Many patients in this group die of lung cancer, or are incapacitated by chronic bronchitis or angina before they have developed sufficient obstruction of the lower limb arteries to provoke symptoms of intermittent claudication.

Primary and Secondary Prevention

The primary prevention of peripheral vascular disease depends largely upon control of important risk factors such as hypertension, hyperlipidemia, diabetes mellitus, cigarette smoking, and a low level of habitual physical activity.

Once symptoms develop, the typical treatment has been surgical (excision of a thrombus, insertion of a vascular graft, luminal dilatation, or lumbar sympathectomy). However, the nature of the lesion rarely favors surgical intervention, and the friable nature of the affected artery leads to a considerable operative mortality (Fiessinger, Carmer, and Housset 1982).

A large number of studies (reviewed by Barnard 1994) have shown that exercise training can enhance performance and reduce or eliminate symptoms of intermittent claudication in the early stages of manifest clinical peripheral vascular disease. Some of the gains in performance may have a psychological basis, but in terms of blood lactate readings Sorlie and Myhre (1978) have demonstrated less ischemia after training. Others have shown an increase in maximal blood flow to the lower limbs (Hiatt et al. 1990). The suggested basis of such changes is the development of a collateral blood supply to that part of the limb beyond the site of arterial obstruction. The response to a training program is highly variable, depending in part upon the type of exercise that is adopted.

Prolonged walking to the point of severe pain seems the best method of enhancing performance in a claudicant patient (Hall et al. 1982).

Other practical suggestions for the person with intermittent claudication include (1) the wearing of adequate and well-insulated shoes, especially in cold weather (when blood flow to the periphery can be further restricted by a cold-induced vascular spasm); (2) correction of any anemia, so that oxygen transport is maximized per unit of limb blood flow; and (3) the taking of a peripheral vasodilator drug immediately prior to a bout of vigorous exercise. It may be wise to review the prescription of beta-blocking drugs in this class of patient. Although such treatment reduces central problems, particularly abnormalities of heart rhythm, the peripheral response to beta-adrenergic stimuli is already reduced in the elderly; and after beta blockade, uncontrolled peripheral alpha-adrenergic activity can exacerbate intermittent claudication (Berman 1982).

Clinicians have traditionally recommended Buerger's exercises. These require holding the legs elevated at 45° to 90° for 3 min, three or four times per day; each bout of exercise is followed by a 3-min period when the legs are held dependent. The rationale of such exercises is to improve collateral flow by provoking a reactive vasodilatation, but it is conceivable that any benefit arises from a strengthening of the affected muscles.

Tertiary and Quaternary Treatment

Irrespective of treatment, the mortality of the claudicant patient is high. A minor orthopedic anomaly such as a hammertoe can readily develop to a gangrenous lesion. Once the patient has become confined to bed, death frequently arises from coronary thrombosis, hemorrhage, or renal complications. It is usually preferable to attempt extremity revascularization (by arterial bypass surgery), even if the patient is no longer ambulatory. Where possible, such surgical intervention should precede the development of ischemic ulceration or gangrene. Amputations for ischemia or gangrene are further potential elements in the tertiary and quaternary treatment of the disease process. In patients who have both diabetes and peripheral vascular disease, the incidence of amputations is about 5% per year (Thiele and Strandness 1994).

Ambulation with a prosthetic limb has quite a high energy cost, particularly if the subject cannot attain the walking speed at which the oxygen cost per meter of distance traversed reaches its nadir (40-50 m/min; see fig. 5.4). The data shown in figure 5.4 are mainly for young adults who have adjusted well to their prosthesis, and costs are much higher in the elderly, particularly in the early phases of ambulation (Cruts et al. 1985). Energy expenditures can be as much as 268% above normal with newly fitted prostheses, and one study found that even after a year of rehabilitation the values for a thigh amputation still averaged 167% above normal, with lesser increments in those who

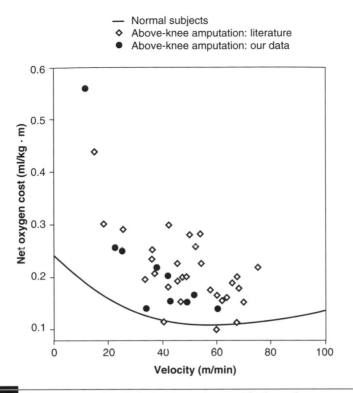

- — Normal subjects
- ◇ Above-knee amputation: literature
- ● Above-knee amputation: our data

Figure 5.4 Oxygen cost of ambulation in patients with above-knee amputations; values compared with curve for normal subjects. *Note*: The curve for normal subjects is a third-order polynomial fitted to data in the literature.

Reprinted, by permission, from R.J. Shephard, T. Kavanagh, R. Campbell, and B. Lorenz, 1994, "Net oxygen costs of ambulation in normal subjects and subjects with lower limb amputations," *Canadian Journal of Rehabilitation* 8: 97-107.

had received a below-knee amputation (Shephard et al. 1995; Tenette and Cuny 1982). Some economy of energy cost is possible if the patient moves at a slower speed, but in the frail elderly the oxygen consumption still quickly reaches its theoretical maximum. Attempts to use a prosthesis in individuals with impaired cardiac performance may cause a sufficient increase of oxygen consumption to precipitate cardiac failure.

Problems such as a very limited cardiovascular reserve, poor balance, reduced muscle strength, fragile skin and bones, impaired healing, a vulnerability to infection, myocardial ischemia and other cardiovascular abnormalities, slow learning of new skills, and altered responses to anxiolytic and narcotic medication all complicate rehabilitation of the elderly amputee (Lyon, Rivers, and Veith 1994). Kavanagh, Pandit, and Shephard (1973) used an arm ergometer to predict maximal oxygen intake in 27 elderly amputees (see table 5.5). All values for aerobic power were extremely low. Even allowing for the 28% to 30% difference between the working capacity of the legs and that of the arms, the peak oxygen intake was still only 50% to 60% of the values anticipated in normal adults of similar age. Because of tissue loss in the amputated limb, it is difficult to express results per kg of body mass; assuming that prior to amputation the patients had a body mass similar to that of the average senior in Toronto (77 kg in men, 64 kg in women), their aerobic power would have been only 10 to 11 ml/[kg · min]. In fact, many were somewhat lighter than the general population, even after the mass of amputated tissue was allowed for, suggesting that there had also been some wasting of muscles in other parts of the body subsequent to the amputation.

The actual working capacity of many amputees was even poorer than the submaximal predictions of maximal oxygen intake might suggest, since all-out tests were often halted for anginal pain or deep ST-segmental depression before the theoretical age-related maximal heart rate had been achieved. In their series of 62 elderly amputees, Kavanagh, Pandit, and Shephard (1973) noted a history of heart trouble in almost half of the patients, including such diagnoses as myocardial infarction (22 cases), digoxin therapy (18 cases), cardiac failure (3 cases), and angina (3 cases). In addition, 28 cases had resting ECG abnormalities, and 23 had a diastolic pressure of more than 100 mmHg. Other clinical complications included diabetes mellitus (10 cases), vascular emboli (3 cases), osteomyelitis (1 case), gangrene (1 case), and popliteal aneurysm (1 case). Additional factors that were considered to have hampered rehabilitation included cerebromuscular problems (4 cases), chronic alcoholism (4 cases), blindness (1 case), severe deafness (1 case), and gross obesity (1 case).

Given this litany of problems, it is not surprising that a wheelchair or crutches are often the preferred methods of ambulation for the frail elderly

Table 5.5   Predicted aerobic power of elderly amputees.

Age (years and gender)	Predicted aerobic power	
	l/min	ml/[kg · min]
Men		
50 ± 8	1.29 ± 0.37	16.8
67 ± 2	0.82 ± 0.18	10.6
75 ± 3	0.78 ± 0.25	10.1
Women		
66 (two subjects only)	0.81	12.7

Based on data of Kavanagh, Pandit, and Shephard 1973, and assuming a body mass of 77 kg in men and 64 kg in women.

amputee (see table 5.6). The likelihood that a prosthesis will be accepted can be increased by a suitable preliminary program of rehabilitation, aimed at improving cardiorespiratory performance and strengthening muscles in the patient's trunk and remaining limbs (Tenette and Cuny 1982). Where possible, the conditioning program should begin before surgery, and if walking is impossible because of intermittent claudication, ulceration, or gangrene, an arm ergometer should be used to provide the needed training stimulus. It is vital to avoid a further deterioration of cardiorespiratory condition in the immediate postoperative period.

Prosthetic ambulation is possible in some patients over the age of 70 years, but in the frail elderly individual, an amputation is often equivalent to permanent immobilization (Steinberg, Sunwoo, and Roettger 1985). If the patient's age is over 85 years, if the amputation is bilateral, or if there is severe cardiac impairment, false hopes are raised by the fitting of an artificial limb. There is little possibility that such a person will use a prosthesis successfully, and it is preferable to commence training in the operation of a wheelchair as soon as surgery is completed (Glaser 1985).

Congestive Heart Failure

Congestive heart failure may be defined as a pathophysiological state in which the heart fails to pump blood at a rate commensurate with tissue demand, or is able to meet this demand only by increasing filling pressure (Braunwald 1988). It is clear from such a definition that during vigorous exercise, the supposedly healthy elderly person often shows at least one manifestation of compensated cardiac failure (an elevated end-diastolic volume and/or pressure,

Table 5.6 Successful use of a prosthesis by elderly subjects (based on data of Clarke-Williams 1978).

Age at amputation (years)	Unilateral			Bilateral		
	Success %	Failure %	Death %	Success %	Failure %	Death %
60-69	56	44	—	67	33	—
70-79	55	27	18	40	40	20
Over 80	48	31	21	46	31	23

Success is defined as daily walking on the prosthesis for at least six months. Adapted, by permission, from M.J. Clarke-Williams, 1978, The management of aged amputees. In *Textbook of geriatric medicine and gerontology*, 2d ed., edited by J.C. Brocklehurst (Edinburgh: Churchill Livingstone), 556-559.

discussed in chapter 3). Congestive heart failure used to be seen largely as a late consequence of rheumatic heart disease, but is now most commonly the end stage of a massive myocardial infarction. Coronary disease is the underlying cause in about half of elderly patients (Lie and Hammond 1988; Wei 1994). Many such patients also suffer from hypertension (Kannel, Plehn, and Cupples 1988). The diagnosis of congestive heart failure is ominous, since 60% of the affected men and 40% of the women die within four years of the initial diagnosis (Kannel, Plehn, and Cupples 1988). A large fraction (35% to 45%) of the deaths are sudden. Usually the dysfunction is systolic (impaired cardiac ejection), although in some instances (mitral stenosis, the early stages of coronary disease, and infiltrative disorders such as amyloidosis), a diastolic dysfunction (impaired ventricular filling) is the primary feature (Smith 1992). In the usual systolic type of disorder, the performance of the cardiac pump is impaired by a combination of damage to the ventricular wall and a decreased response to adrenergic stimulation. At the same time, there are a variety of peripheral disturbances, some representing an attempt to sustain tissue perfusion. The vasodilatory response in the active limbs is reduced, and the individual's peak oxygen intake is closely related to the vascular conductance of the working tissues (Reading et al. 1993). There is also an increased secretion of pressor hormones (catecholamines, renin/angiotensin/aldosterone, antidiuretic, and natriuretic hormones). It is unclear whether the high catecholamine levels during exercise cause circulatory dysfunction (for instance, by increasing cardiac afterloading) or whether they are merely a marker of severe disease, but they are certainly linked with a high mortality rate (Goodman 1995a). Despite the increased activity of the renin/angiotensin/aldosterone system, the administration of angiotensin inhibitors often has little effect upon exercise tolerance. Finally, perhaps as a consequence of a decline in habitual physical activity, nuclear magnetic resonance studies usually show a wasting of the skeletal muscle (Mancini et al. 1992), and biopsies demonstrate a low activity of oxidative enzymes in the muscle fibers (Minotti et al. 1990; Stratton, Dunn, et al. 1994).

There is severe dyspnea on exertion. This was once attributed to pulmonary congestion, accumulation of interstitial fluid, and the stimulation of J-receptors, but pulmonary wedge pressures are poorly correlated with exercise tolerance (Sullivan, Higginbotham, and Cobb 1989). Alternatively, the ventilatory cost of a given activity is increased. Reasons could include a poor peripheral blood flow and thus an increased accumulation of lactate, an increase of ventilation due to a poor matching of ventilation and perfusion (with enlargement of the physiological dead space) (Sullivan et al. 1988; Sullivan, Higginbotham, and Cobb 1989), and an increase in the work of breathing. Exercise testing of the person with congestive heart failure is often halted before the patient has reached the usual limit of breathlessness (exploitation of 50% of his or her maximal voluntary ventilation) (Goodman 1995a). The dyspnea leads to a substantial restriction of physical activity and thus a deterioration in the patient's quality of life (Kavanagh et al. 1996).

Restriction of coronary blood flow to the ventricles may give rise to anginal pain, and an inadequate blood flow to the peripheral tissues may give the skin a bluish hue (peripheral cyanosis). The pulse rate of the patient with congestive heart failure typically rises over the course of the day, with a slow and incomplete recovery from exercise during rest pauses. There is usually ankle edema, although ankle swelling of cardiac origin must be distinguished from that due to problems of venous drainage. The edema of venous incompetence responds to raised leg exercises, but that associated with cardiac failure does not (Ciocon, Galindo-Ciocon, and Galindo 1995).

Prevalence and Incidence

Congestive heart failure currently occurs in about 1% of the population, although a high proportion of those affected are elderly individuals. Indeed, congestive heart failure is the most common cause of hospital admission for those over the age of 65 years. The annual incidence increases from an average of 3 per 1000 prior to the age of 65 years to 10 per 1000 in those over the age of 65 years (Smith 1992). In part because the population is aging, and in part because of success in resuscitating those with severe myocardial infarction, the overall incidence of congestive heart failure has doubled over the past two decades.

Primary and Secondary Prevention

Primary preventive measures are those associated with the control of etiological factors—a reduction of risk factors for hypertension and ischemic heart disease and the careful treatment of streptococcal infections.

The resting cardiac ejection fraction should be at least 45%, with a 5% increase during exercise (Goodman 1995a). However, cardiac function deteriorates with aging and disease, so that in many elderly people the ejection fraction either remains constant or even declines during exercise. Patients who show a low ejection fraction at rest and during exercise, plus a low peak aerobic power and a poorly maintained systolic pressure during exercise testing, are a vulnerable subgroup of elderly patients; they are at increased risk of progressing to clinical manifestations of congestive heart failure when confronted by (1) an acute infection, (2) an unexpectedly severe bout of physical activity, (3) an excessive intake of fluid, (4) the decline in myocardial function associated with normal aging, (5) a minor valvular malfunction, or (6) death of a substantial area of the myocardium through repeated small and undetected myocardial infarctions.

An exercise program plainly cannot reverse primary damage to the ventricular wall, but it can influence many of the other factors that would otherwise allow progression from a poor ejection fraction to frank cardiac failure.

In some studies, training has enhanced myocardial contractility (reviewed in chapter 4), with increases in blood flow to the active body parts, an increase of muscle capillarity, and a decreased peripheral resistance (Sullivan, Higginbotham, and Cobb 1989). Lactate accumulation decreases, with an associated reduction in ventilatory demand (Kavanagh et al. 1996; Davey et al. 1992). The blood pressure at any given external rate of working is also diminished, and the catecholamine secretion is reduced. Further, muscle strength is increased, and its oxidative enzyme activity is restored (Minotti et al. 1990; Stratton, Levy, et al. 1994).

Nevertheless, it is difficult to document the extent of the training response. Many patients with a limited ejection fraction fail to demonstrate an oxygen consumption plateau (Kavanagh et al. 1996). Oxygen consumption increases slowly (Coats 1993), and performance is often limited by dyspnea or muscle weakness rather than a true ceiling of cardiorespiratory performance. Further, it seems likely that the peak effort of individuals with a deteriorating myocardium will increase as they become habituated to the test protocol. Determination of the absolute ventilatory threshold is sometimes suggested as an alternative objective measurement of cardiorespiratory status in this class of patient, although in the experience of our group the gains of peak oxygen intake and ventilatory threshold are of a similar order (Kavanagh et al. 1996).

Tertiary and Quaternary Treatment

Patients who have developed congestive heart failure are usually classified according to the classic clinical categories proposed by the New York Heart Association. People in Class I show fatigue and dyspnea with extraordinary activity. Class II patients experience a slight limitation from shortness of breath or fatigue with normal physical activity. People in Class III show a marked limitation of physical performance even during ordinary daily activities, and those in Class IV have symptoms at rest, with inability to carry on any physical activity without shortness of breath or fatigue.

In many patients in Class I through Class III, cardiac compensation is possible by an increase of end-diastolic volume, left ventricular hypertrophy (if hypertension is a causative factor), or hormonal adaptations that increase blood pressures and redirect blood flow from the viscera to the heart and working muscles.

As with secondary rehabilitation, a progressive training program can enhance both physiological function and quality of life in patients whose congestive cardiac failure is well established but stable (Kavanagh et al. 1996). There seems little relationship between resting ejection fraction and either the immediate exercise response (Port et al. 1981) or the response to training (Sullivan, Higginbotham, and Cobb 1989). Nevertheless, a favorable response to exercise-centered rehabilitation has been described in patients where the resting ejection fraction is 25% or less (Arvan 1988; Coats et al. 1992; Kavanagh et al. 1996; Sullivan, Higginbotham, and Cobb 1989). In an eight-week cross-over trial involving Class III patients who were sufficiently free of ventricular arrhythmias to exercise effectively, Coats (1993) noted a 25% improvement in peak aerobic power and exercise duration. Kavanagh et al. (1996) found benefits of a similar order, and they were able to sustain these gains over a 52-week trial. The mechanisms of enhanced performance are similar to those suggested for secondary rehabilitation:

1. Resting left ventricular filling pressures and function show little change (Sullivan et al. 1988; Sullivan, Higginbotham, and Cobb 1989), although the peak oxygen pulse shows a small increase (Kavanagh et al. 1996).
2. There is a progressive habituation to exercise dyspnea.
3. A reversal of chronic deconditioning of the skeletal muscles (Mancini et al. 1992), increases in tissue enzyme activity (Minotti et al. 1990; Stratton, Dunn et al. 1994), and an increase of peripheral blood flow (Sullivan, Higginbotham, and Cobb 1989) lead to a lesser accumulation of lactate, with a reduced ventilation (Coats 1993; Davey et al. 1992) and a corresponding increase in the ventilatory threshold (Sullivan, Higginbotham, and Cobb 1989).
4. Substantial gains in the quality of life are associated with the physiological changes (Kavanagh et al. 1996).

However, close patient supervision is required when one is exercising patients with congestive heart failure because of frequent dysrhythmias and a risk that cardiac decompensation will develop suddenly.

About 85% of patients respond favorably to rehabilitation, but in two recent trials a minority of patients were obliged to withdraw from the program because of worsening cardiac failure (Kavanagh et al. 1996; Sullivan, Higginbotham, and Cobb 1989). Caution is particularly necessary if there is extensive anterior infarction, ST-segmental depression on exercise testing, and a low ejection fraction (Arvan 1988; Jugdutt, Mickorowski, and Kappadoga 1988). Jugdutt, Mickorowski, and Kappadoga (1988) warned that if there is an extensive area of akinetic left ventricular wall, excessive training can worsen structural damage, with an increase in wall motion abnormalities. On the other hand, Gianuzzi et al. (1993) noted that although patients with a poor left ventricular function were prone to further global and regional dilatation, long-term exercise conferred a significant improvement in physical work capacity without any additional negative effects on the ventricular muscle.

If the failure has become decompensated, as in most patients with Class IV disability, formal training is contraindicated until a compensated state can be restored by a combination of salt restriction, diuretics, and other drugs such as digitalis or angiotensin-converting enzyme inhibitors (Vitarelli et al. 1995).

In essence, the intensity of physical activity must be modified on a day-to-day basis, with the patient remaining as active as possible short of becoming symptomatic.

End-Stage Renal Disease

Renal disease is commonly the end result of hypertension or diabetes mellitus. Aerobic power and muscle strength become extremely limited in the affected individuals, and the quality of life is further reduced by the need for polypharmacy and repeated renal dialysis.

Prevalence and Incidence

Renal arterial occlusion is most commonly encountered in persons over the age of 60 years. It usually presents as severe hypertension. In addition to specific obstruction of the renal blood supply, aging leads to a more general deterioration of renal function (reviewed in chapter 3), marked by such changes as mesangial damage and severe obliteration of the renal capillary lumina. The risk of renal insufficiency is 17 times higher in those with diabetes mellitus when compared with the general population. Exercise-induced excretion of albumin is an early warning sign that diabetes is having such an effect. Conversely, 30% of patients with end-stage renal disease also have diabetes (Moore 1995). Other causes of chronic renal disease include hypertension, chronic infections of the kidneys, and autoimmune disease.

Primary and Secondary Prevention

Both primary and secondary prevention are directed mainly to the correction of a number of risk factors for chronic renal disease, particularly hypertension, arteriosclerosis, and diabetes mellitus. As noted elsewhere, a program of regular physical activity is beneficial in preventing and correcting each of these problems.

Tertiary and Quaternary Treatment

Elderly patients have commonly reached the end stages of the renal disease process when life must be sustained by repeated dialysis. There has been limited animal research on chronic renal disease, but experiments by Heifets et al. (1987) suggest that a training program may have some value in tertiary treatment, slowing the progress of the disease.

In humans, also, it seems logical that a regular program of moderate physical activity might be helpful in slowing the progressive deterioration in general condition of the patient, since end-stage renal disease is marked by an acceleration of arteriosclerosis and its various complications. Many such patients show hypertension, left ventricular hypertrophy, hyperlipidemia, glucose intolerance, and hyperinsulinemia (Goldberg and Harter 1994). Metabolic acidosis, hyperkalemia, hypercalcemia, hypermagnesmia, and autonomic dysfunction give the affected individual a poor exercise cardiac output and thus a poor aerobic power (Goldberg and Harter 1994). Often one sees anemia, left ventricular hypertrophy, and a poor chronotropic response to exercise, with a peak heart rate that is only 70% of the age-predicted maximal value (Moore et al. 1993). A variety of factors including reduced protein intake, metabolic acidosis, altered vitamin D and parathyroid metabolism, and insulin resistance also lead to protein catabolism, with resultant muscle wasting (uremic myopathy). Physical activity can therefore have some value in palliative treatment, sustaining cardiovascular and muscular performance and enhancing the patient's quality of life.

Aerobic training may increase peak aerobic power by as much as 20% to 25%, but this is due entirely to a greater arteriovenous oxygen difference. Stroke volume remains unchanged by physical conditioning, probably on account of the initial ventricular hypertrophy and the poor wall compliance associated with systemic hypertension. Oxygen transport can sometimes be enhanced if hemoglobin levels are boosted by the administration of erythropoietin (Robertson et al. 1990). However, the peak oxygen intake is usually more closely correlated with muscle strength than with hemoglobin concentration, suggesting that weakness of the limb musculature is restricting perfusion of the active body parts (Diesel et al. 1990; Kempeneers et al. 1990). Magnetic resonance spectroscopy shows that the muscles have an unimpaired intrinsic oxidative potential (Moore et al. 1993), but a further factor limiting oxygen uptake may be an increased capillary/myofiber diffusion distance.

The ideal exercise plan for such individuals combines a mixed program of aerobic and resistance training with modification of adverse lifestyle factors such as smoking and alcohol or substance abuse. Target heart rates do not provide a reliable method of regulating the exercise prescription, because dialysis causes large variations in plasma volume. The intensity of effort is best monitored in terms of ratings of perceived exertion. Resistance training may help to correct the myopathy, but such a program must be pursued cautiously, particularly if renal dysfunction has led to demineralization of bone; overvigorous muscle contractions can give rise to pathological fractures.

Unfortunately, only 60% of nondiabetic and 23% of diabetic patients with renal disease are capable of undertaking any physical activity beyond the needs of self-care (Evans et al. 1985). Several recent studies have nevertheless confirmed that when the patient has the ability to participate in an exercise program, this can lower risk factors, increase aerobic power, and enhance psychosocial functioning (Hagberg 1989; Painter 1988). The oldest group of patients to undertake such a training program was evaluated by Ross et al. (1989). Over 3.5 years of conditioning, these patients showed a 17% to 18% increase of aerobic power and physical work capacity.

In part because of muscle weakness and limitations of aerobic performance, the patient with renal dysfunction often has a very poor compliance with prescribed exercise (Shalom et al. 1984). It is thus helpful to organize at least some of the exercise sessions concomitantly with dialysis.

Chronic Obstructive Lung Disease

Chronic obstructive lung disease is another important reason for a pathological response to physical activity in the senior citizen. The underlying processes of bronchial hyperreactivity, chronic bronchitis, and emphysema are often coexistent and difficult to distinguish from one another.

Hyperreactivity

Hyperreactivity of vagal afferents leads to bronchospasm and an overproduction of mucus when the airways are exposed to irritants such as air pollution or even cold and dry air; exercise-induced bronchospasm (Killian 1995) is a common finding. Between 20% and 40% of patients also have an inherited allergic tendency, producing antibodies (IgE and IgG) to inhaled antigens (Crimi, Bartalucci, and Brusasco 1996).

Chronic Bronchitis

Chronic bronchitis is diagnosed if the patient has a chronic or productive cough on most days for a minimum of three months in a year in not less than two successive years. There is an increase in the secretion and expectoration of sputum, and episodes of superimposed infection occur frequently. Cigarette smoking, exposure to urban or occupational air pollutants, and a cold, damp climate are all predisposing factors. In the restrictive form of the disease, inspiratory capacity may be limited, but expiration is normal or even accelerated (Cooper 1995).

Emphysema

Emphysema is characterized by an abnormal enlargement of the terminal airways. In part, the condition is an expression of normal senescence, a loss of elastic tissue from the lungs leading to expiratory collapse of the larger air passages, hyperinflation of the chest, dilatation of the terminal airways, a decrease in the mechanical efficiency of the respiratory muscles, and difficulty in expiration (Cooper 1995). In the centrilobular form, where the disease is localized to the ends of the respiratory bronchioles, a vicious cycle of infection, destruction of the small airways, and increased vulnerability to further infection may be suspected.

"Fighters" vs. "Nonfighters"

During exercise, some patients (termed the "fighters" or "pink puffers") are able to maintain relatively normal partial pressures of oxygen and carbon dioxide in their arterial blood by a large increase of pulmonary ventilation, at the expense of a very heavy increase in respiratory work rate. But as chest disease advances, the ability to hyperventilate becomes progressively limited, and attempts at physical activity lead to a dramatic drop in arterial oxygen tension with a distressing dyspnea. Pulmonary arterial pressures rise, and the oxygen-starved myocardium progressively fails. Such patients have a cyanosed appearance, and they are described as "nonfighters" or "blue bloaters."

Prevalence and Incidence

Because of regional differences in climate, patterns of cigarette smoking, the type and extent of urban air pollution, and perhaps some biases in diagnosis, the prevalence of the obstructive group of chronic chest disorders has historically been much greater in Britain than in North America. Men also seem more susceptible to chronic obstructive lung disease than women, but it is not altogether clear whether this reflects merely a gender difference in exposure to cigarette smoke and industrial dusts among earlier generations.

By the age of 65 years, some 50% of unskilled laborers and 20% of professional men in Britain are affected by chronic bronchitis. Some 90% of heavy smokers report the warning sign of a chronic cough. Prospective measurements of dynamic lung volumes such as the 1 sec forced expiratory volume (Terry and Tockman 1985) show that the deterioration of function observed in the nonsmoker (perhaps 25 to 30 ml/year) is increased to as much as 60 to 80 ml/year by regular cigarette smoking. The problems of the smoker are exacerbated (1) if the airways show a hyperreactivity to methacholine or (2) if there is evidence that the person concerned has an abnormal alpha-antitrypsin phenotype. Antitrypsins normally limit proteolytic destruction of lung tissues following an intercurrent infection. The prognosis shows some worsening in a person who is a heterozygote, and the effect is much more serious in a patient who is a homozygote for the abnormal phenotype.

After the age of 60 years, about half of the population show some emphysema at postmortem, but this usually remains clinically silent. Only a small proportion of individuals progress to the point of developing symptoms. Cigarette smoking, gender, genetic predisposition, exposure to high concentrations of air pollutants, and a history of chronic respiratory infections are factors increasing the risk of overt disease.

Primary and Secondary Prevention

Both chronic bronchitis and emphysema usually have an insidious onset. Indeed, for practical purposes both disorders remain clinically silent for a number of years. There may be no more than a little expectoration of thick mucus on waking (a "smoker's cough"), or a slight breathlessness on hurrying, and the patient is inclined to dismiss the latter symptom as an inevitable expression of aging. As the obstruction of expiratory airflow becomes more severe, there is a progressive increase in the work of breathing. During bouts of exercise, expiratory pressures often reach the limiting value where further effort leads to airway collapse (Dempsey and Seals 1995), and the patient complains of increasingly severe dyspnea (Cooper 1995).

Exercise programs may have some value in primary prevention, since the active individual seems less likely to become or to remain a cigarette smoker (Shephard, Kavanagh, and Mertens 1995). However, the influence of physical activity upon personal lifestyle is not large (Shephard 1989a). The basis of any observed negative association between cigarette smoking and involvement in exercise may be an underlying interest in a healthy lifestyle, rather than a more specific effect of the exercise program; nevertheless, our recent questioning of Masters athletes (Shephard, Kavanagh, and Mertens 1995) suggested that in a proportion of them competition had been a factor contributing to smoking withdrawal. Any influence of exercise in reducing the prevalence of smoking seems greater for endurance activities than for social types of sport such as tennis (Shephard 1989a).

Even if it is accepted that program involvement has an effect on smoking behavior in younger adults, the potential for primary prevention is limited in the elderly population, since the most vulnerable group of smokers (the antitrypsin-deficient homozygotes) have already sustained extensive and irreversible damage to their pulmonary tissues.

Given that chest disease is usually far advanced before the patient seeks advice, it is probably appropriate to consider most therapeutic measures as tertiary and/or quaternary forms of treatment.

Tertiary and Quaternary Treatment

When tertiary treatment is being considered, the problems to be corrected include a very high oxygen cost of breathing, a poor distribution of inspired gas due to bronchospasm, an accumulation of mucus in the airway, expiratory collapse of the bronchi, and frank destruction of the alveolar spaces and associated pulmonary capillaries. In addition to these respiratory problems, the skeletal muscles often show weakness (Mertens, Kavanagh, and Shephard 1978; Schols et al. 1991), and a loss of oxidative capacity (Thompson et al. 1993), whether induced by chronic infection, chronic hypoxia, prolonged administration of steroids, poor nutrition, or electrolyte disturbances.

Exercise Response

During submaximal exercise, the heart rates of the patient with chronic obstructive lung disease are high, but the rise of pulmonary pressures and the reduced oxygen supply to the myocardium lead to a smaller maximal cardiac stroke volume than would be seen in a healthy person of comparable age. Severe breathlessness may arise from air-trapping and hyperinflation of the lungs. An increase of end-inspiratory volume places the respiratory muscles at a mechanical disadvantage, and it forces a stronger signal from the motor area of the cortex in order to meet the metabolic demands of effort. Because of the increased respiratory drive and muscle weakness, ratings of perceived exertion are increased, both at a given work rate and also at a given heart rate.

The meaning of peak oxygen intake is debatable in chronic obstructive lung disease, since exercise tests are often halted by breathlessness even though the cardiovascular and respiratory systems are far from fully stressed. Peak heart rates and lactate readings are lower than in a normal subject, and the peak ventilation may be a small fraction of the individual's maximal voluntary ventilation (O'Donnell and Webb 1995). Although the reason for halting a progressive exercise test is often dyspnea, leg weakness and muscle fatigue are also responsible for halting as many as a third of the tests conducted in patients with chronic chest disease (O'Donnell and Webb 1995).

Predictions of aerobic power thus cannot be based on submaximal heart rates. Possible alternative tactics are (1) to report a directly measured symptom-limited peak aerobic power, (2) to predict aerobic power from maximal voluntary ventilation and the ventilatory equivalent for oxygen, or (3) to report the physical working capacity at a fixed heart rate (for example, the PWC_{130}). Simple office and ward tests such as the distance walked in 6 min or the shuttle-walking speed are heavily dependent upon motivation, and they may thus overestimate the extent of disability in some patients (Singh et al. 1992).

Maximal exercise status and the extent of depression of mood state are together the best predictors of functional status (Weaver and Narsavage 1992).

Response to a Training Program

Exercise training induces a marked symptomatic improvement in many patients with chronic chest disease (Carter, Coast, and Idell 1992; Mahler and O'Donnell 1991; van Herwaarden 1984). Nevertheless, occasional patients fail to improve despite faithful program participation (Mertens, Kavanagh, and Shephard 1978). Unfortunately, the majority of studies of exercise rehabilitation have been uncontrolled, and in such circumstances it is difficult to be certain how much of the observed benefit should be attributed to ancillary forms of treatment. Helpful ancillary measures may include

1. breathing exercises or respiratory muscle training (Carter and Coast 1993; Weiner, Azgad, and Ganam 1992) (however, Guyatt et al. [1992] and Smith et al. [1992] both found such exercises to be ineffective in augmenting functional capacity);
2. postural drainage or stimulation of mucus clearance by the exercise itself (although Olseni, Midgren, and Wollmer [1992] found no increase in the pulmonary clearance of marker particles from rest to exercise);
3. prompt institution of chemotherapy for superimposed respiratory infections; and
4. habituation to the sensation of dyspnea, or even a placebo effect.

Other design problems in experimental studies of training programs have included small sample sizes; uncertainties regarding the intensity, frequency, and duration of exercise sessions; uncertainty regarding the clinical stability of patients at the outset of conditioning; the existence of comorbid conditions; and failure to quantify subjective responses, for example by the use of objective scales of breathlessness (O'Donnell and Webb 1995).

However, a large-scale controlled trial in patients of average age 66 years recently demonstrated a substantial increase of functional capacity that was sustained for six months (Goldstein et al. 1994). There remains little basis for disputing the fact that most patients with chronic obstructive lung disease perform physical activity with greater comfort after training. They attain greater independence, and the quality of their lives is enhanced (Folgering and van Herwaarden 1994; Reardon, Patel, and ZuWallack 1993; Wijkstra et al. 1994).

Following training, the sensation of breathlessness at the end of a test exercise is reduced, and there are often substantial gains in the distance that the patient can walk over a specified time (O'Donnell and Webb 1995; Swerts et al. 1990). Exercise is commonly carried to a larger respiratory minute volume, partly because the mechanical efficiency of ventilation has been increased by associated breathing exercises and partly because the patient now has gained the confidence to accept a greater shortness of breath. Direct measurements of peak oxygen intake thus show gains that range from 0% to 30%, although such gains are not necessarily correlated with improved scores on such measures as depression and self-efficacy scales (Toshima, Kaplan, and Ries 1990).

The arteriovenous oxygen difference is widened following training, perhaps because the muscles are stronger. However, there is usually no change of stroke volume or peak heart rate, unless the patient is encouraged to reach a greater peak effort when being retested. A training-induced increase of peak cardiac output seems particularly unlikely if the patient initially shows elevated pulmonary arterial pressures and other signs of left ventricular dysfunction. Nevertheless, a moderate training program does not usually precipitate cardiac failure, even if the ECG initially shows signs of right ventricular strain.

In some instances, a combination of a happier mood, greater physical activity, and improved appetite may also lead to gains in body mass, with related increases of muscular endurance (Mertens, Kavanagh, and Shephard 1978). On the other hand, the more severely affected patients show a continuing loss of lean tissue and deterioration of muscle strength despite program involvement.

Mechanisms of Benefit

Pulmonary tissue that has been destroyed cannot be restored by any form of exercise, and it is thus not surprising that measures of pulmonary function usually remain unchanged following participation in a training program. However, if conditioning has included supervised walking on a treadmill or in the gymnasium, there is often a substantial increase in the mechanical efficiency of ambulation, with a reduction in heart rate and ventilation at any given level of submaximal exercise (Casaburi et al. 1991).

Perhaps because the leg muscles are strengthened, there may also be less lactate formation at a given intensity of submaximal effort (Casaburi et al. 1991). Other commonly reported gains include a better coordination of both breathing and leg movements, a reduction in body fat content, a reversal of bronchospasm, and (if oxygen has been administered) a reduction of pulmonary arterial pressures (O'Donnell and Webb 1995). Perhaps most importantly, conditioning can break the vicious cycle of dyspnea, decreased physical activity, deterioration of physical condition, reduction of mechanical efficiency and exacerbation of dyspnea (Folgering and van Herwaarden 1994; Mertens, Kavanagh, and Shephard 1978).

Optimal Training Plan

The main objectives of a conditioning program for the patient with chronic obstructive pulmonary disease are to restore muscle strength and mechanical efficiency to the point that sensations of breathlessness and leg weakness are less readily attained and to make optimal use of residual cardiorespiratory function.

It is much more difficult to implement an effective training program for chest than for postcoronary patients. Initially, there is no critical incident that arouses the concern of a chest patient, and many of those with mild dyspnea consider this as normal for their age. Later, when dyspnea has become severe, conditioning can prove quite distressing, and patients find difficulty in progressing to a fitness level at which participation in the program is seen as pleasant and rewarding. Those patients whose arterial oxygen tensions increase during exercise are the most likely to respond favorably to exercise, but adverse features include a low forced expiratory volume and vital capacity, an increased hemoglobin level, advanced age, and a history of previous respiratory failure.

The first steps in rehabilitation are to optimize pharmacotherapy and to review techniques of avoiding respiratory panic attacks (counseling, relaxation sessions, pursed-lip breathing, or administration of anxiolytic drugs). If there is inspiratory muscle weakness, specific breathing exercises can be implemented (although as already noted, their functional value is still debated); and if breathlessness develops during arm work, then the exercise prescription should emphasize resistance exercises for the upper limbs (Dugan, Walker, and Monroe 1995; Ellis and Ries 1991; Weintraub, Dolan, and Stratmann 1993).

In the early phases of training, oxygen administration may help the patient to progress to the point where an aerobic conditioning response can begin (Wesmiller and Hoffmann 1994). As might be anticipated, those who show a drop of oxygen pressures, ST-segmental depression, and/or anginal pain during exercise benefit most from oxygen administration.

The response to a supervised program is superior to what can be accomplished by home-based exercise (Swerts et al. 1990). However, there are limits to what can be accomplished. Probably because the underlying chest disease is progressive in nature, exercise programs seem more effective in the young-old than in those over the age of 80 years (Emery 1994; Swerts et al. 1990; Toshima, Kaplan, and Ries 1990). Even a well-designed combination of aerobic training and resistance exercises cannot restore alveolar tissue that has been destroyed by years of exposure to cigarette smoke and other air pollutants.

Portable oxygen systems are sometimes provided for quaternary treatment of the patient with chronic obstructive lung disease, but their effectiveness is limited by the inherent conflict between the desired weight of the system (less than 2 kg) and a useful oxygen capacity (100 L minimum). Much of the supposed benefit of a portable domestic oxygen supply is probably psychological. Other therapeutic possibilities that may extend mobility and enhance the quality of life include a training of the inspiratory muscles (Carter and Coast 1993; Weiner, Azgad, and Ganam 1992), the use of codeine preparations (Terry and Tockman 1985), and provision of an ultra lightweight tricycle to encourage continued ambulation (Woodcock, Johnson, and Geddes 1983).

Conclusions

Regular, moderate physical activity has significant value in the primary and secondary prevention of a number of cardiovascular conditions, including ischemic heart disease, stroke, hypertension, peripheral vascular disease, and renal disease secondary to hypertension or diabetes. For individuals in whom such disease is established, both morbidity and mortality are favorably influenced by a moderate, progressive training program. Light exercise also enhances the quality of life in palliative, quaternary treatment. Congestive heart failure was traditionally treated by rest, but there is now growing evidence that light exercise can enhance both prognosis and the quality of life for those with stable congestive heart failure. In individuals with chronic obstructive lung disease, exercise cannot restore damaged lung tissue, and conditioning programs have little influence upon objective measures of pulmonary function. Nevertheless, regular physical activity is of considerable subjective benefit to such individuals.

Chapter 6

Physical Activity and Musculoskeletal Disease

The conditions to be considered in this chapter include extreme muscle wasting (sarcopenia), specific muscular dystrophies, rheumatoid arthritis and osteoarthritis, and osteoporosis.

Sarcopenia

Sarcopenia is a term that has been coined to denote the extreme muscle wasting that leaves the frail elderly unable to undertake many or all of the tasks of everyday living. It is not mentioned in many textbooks of gerontology or geriatric medicine, yet it is a major factor leading to a deterioration in the quality of life for the affected individuals. A combination of an inadequate diet and lack of strength creates a vicious cycle of progressive physical inactivity and accelerating muscle wasting (Bortz 1982). As the muscles become weaker, one sees a shortening of stride length (Fiatarone et al. 1990), a slowing of walking speed (Bassey, Bendall, and Pearson 1988), and a progressive decrease in the load that the muscles can lift (Jette and Branch 1981).

Prevalence and Incidence

The prevalence of sarcopenia can be gauged from a survey conducted in the United States in 1984 (Kovar and LaCroix 1987). By the age of 70 to 74 years, 23% of men and 27% of women had difficulty in walking 0.4 km, and 23% of men and 41% of women had difficulty in lifting or carrying a load of 11.4 kg (see table 6.1). Looking at even older samples, Coroni-Huntley et al. (1986) found that the majority of subjects were unable to undertake heavy housework, many were unable to climb a flight of stairs, and a growing minority had difficulty in walking across the room, getting from a bed to a chair, or even using the toilet without assistance (see table 6.2).

Primary and Secondary Prevention

Studies of Masters athletes (Kavanagh et al. 1989; Pollock et al. 1987) show that the lean tissue mass of an active person is well conserved through the seventh decade of life. But (perhaps because of some diminution of training schedules, or a neglect of resistance exercise), lean mass declines after the age of 70 years, as reviewed in chapter 3. The synthesis of protein proceeds more slowly in older adults (Welle et al. 1993), but at any given age, resistance training serves to maintain strength at a higher level than in a sedentary person. Thus, despite muscle aging, the active person remains much stronger than the sedentary individual even in the final years of life.

Factors that cause muscle weakness to pass from a physiologically measurable deficit to a clinically significant limitation of function include the local pain of rheumatoid arthritis and osteoarthritis, podiatric problems, musculoskeletal injuries, periods of general immobilization secondary to intercurrent infection or surgical treatment, and an inadequate dietary intake of protein. In these various situations, it is important to arrange appropriate corrective measures; these may include not only gently graded progressive exercise, but also nursing care and counseling, physiotherapy, occupational therapy, and/or electrical stimulation of immobilized muscles, so that as large a fraction of muscle strength as possible is conserved.

Tertiary and Quaternary Treatment

Fiatarone et al. (1994) have maintained that an appropriate combination of high-resistance exercises and nutritional supplements can enhance lost muscle

Table 6.1 Ability to walk 0.4 km and to lift or carry a load of 11.4 kg in relation to age.

Age (yr)	Walk 0.4 km				Lift/carry 11.4 kg			
	Difficult		Unable		Difficult		Unable	
	Men	Women	Men	Women	Men	Women	Men	Women
	%	%	%	%	%	%	%	%
55-59	12.3	12.6	5.0	5.8	11.6	22.9	3.5	9.1
60-64	17.0	15.8	7.9	8.0	15.4	31.0	3.8	8.7
65-69	20.1	19.9	9.4	7.9	16.8	33.8	5.6	9.3
70-74	23.3	26.6	8.7	10.2	23.1	40.8	7.5	10.7

Data for U.S. citizens collected in 1984.

Reprinted from M.G. Kovar and A.Z. LaCroix, 1987, *Aging in the eighties: Ability to perform work-related activities. Data from the supplement on aging to the National Health Interview Survey, United States, 1984*, Advanced Data from Vital and Health Statistics, No. 136, DHS Publication No. PHS 87-1250 (Hyattsville, MD).

Table 6.2 Inability to perform the activities of daily living in the frail elderly without assistance.

	East Boston				New Haven				Rural Iowa			
	80-84 yr		>85 yr		80-84 yr		>85 yr		80-84 yr		>85 yr	
	M	F	M	F	M	F	M	F	M	F	M	F
Walk across room	12	23	22	38	8	9	10	31	10	15	17	22
From bed to chair	4	14	11	22	1	8	5	14	8	9	8	9
Climb stairs	15	31	29	50	12	12	10	30	12	17	16	26
Heavy house-work	57	70	74	89	31	54	53	68	43	56	68	69
Use toilet	3	12	12	19	2	5	1	8	6	8	7	10

Data for three U.S. populations.
Reprinted from Coroni-Huntley et al., 1986, *Established populations for epidemiologic studies of the elderly: Resource data book;* NIH Publication 86-2443 (Washington, DC: National Institute on Aging).

function, even among nursing home residents who have reached the 10th decade of life (see table 6.3). Fisher, Pendergast, and Calkins (1991) also noted program-related gains of strength even in very frail institutionalized patients whose initial muscle force averaged only 50% of that found in age-matched peers. Mixed training (a combination of endurance exercise and low-intensity strength training) or low-resistance training usually yields only modest increases in strength (Hagberg, Montain, et al. 1989; Vitti et al. 1993), with little improvement of muscle morphology. In contrast, gains in peak force as large as 174% have been seen with a high-resistance, low-repetition approach to muscle conditioning (Fiatarone et al. 1994). Some of this large response probably reflects altered patterns of motor unit recruitment, but increases in muscle mass of 12% to 17% have also been demonstrated by objective techniques such as computed tomographic scanning (Brown, McCartney, and Sale 1990; Fiatarone et al. 1994; Nichols et al. 1993). In women who are already active in lower limb activities such as walking, the gains of strength are greatest in the upper half of the body, but this pattern of response is important in terms of their ability to undertake many of the activities of daily living (Nichols et al. 1993). Province et al. (1995) also reported that the frequency of falls was reduced by participation in an exercise program.

Elastic tubing can provide a simple but effective domestic source of resisted exercise for seniors who are living independently (Heislein, Harris, and Jette 1994; Mikesky et al. 1994). The total protein intake of the elderly person is

Table 6.3 Response of elderly patients to programs of resistance training.

Type of training	Age (yr)	Duration (wk)	Strength increase (%)	Author
Low resistance	71	12	9-22	Aniansson and Gustaffson (1981)
Low/moderate	70-79	26	18* 8•	Hagberg et al. (1989)
Moderate	74	6	64	Perkins and Kaiser (1961)
High resistance	90	8	174	Fiatarone et al. (1990)
	82	6	15	Fisher, Pendergast, and Calkins (1991)
	60-72	12	107, 227&	Frontera et al. (1988)
	69	6	72x	Kauffman (1985)
	61-70	6	17, 24&	Liemohn (1975)
	68	12	104	Meredith et al. (1992)
	70	8	23□	Moritani and DeVries (1980)
	68	24	5-64	Nicholls et al. (1993)
	74	6	57	Perkins and Kaiser (1961)

*upper body
•lower body
&knee
xfingers
□elbow

often inadequate, and muscle hypertrophy is seemingly facilitated by the provision of nutritional supplements. Thus, Meredith et al. (1992) found benefit from the daily ingestion of a mixture that added 0.33 g/kg of protein and 33.5 kJ/kg of food energy to the usual diet.

Specific Muscular Dystrophies

Most patients with congenital muscular dystrophies die before they reach old age. Amyloid usually accumulates in connective tissue rather than muscle, but on occasion it can cause an amyloid myopathy. Chronic alcoholism can also give rise to a myopathy, with associated muscle weakness, but perhaps the most common neuromuscular problem among seniors is motor neuron disease (ALS; Tandan and Bradley 1985). This last disorder attacks about 1 in 100,000 of the population; the prevalence increases with age, suggesting that the condition is a disease of aging. The mortality peaks at around 4 per 100,000 in women and 7 per 100,000 in men at an age of 70 years.

Management of ALS is based on the relief of symptoms and the maximization of residual function. The latter is accomplished in part by simple ergonomic measures such as the adaptation of cutlery to weak hands, and in part by regular range of motion and resistance exercises (McCartney et al. 1988); the latter are designed to improve coordination, eliminate unwanted movements, and increase the overall mechanical efficiency of limb movements (Chrétien, Simard, and Dorion 1987). An asymmetry of the muscular deficit may predispose to the development of contractures, and care must be taken to avoid movements that increase this tendency. Anxiety about falling is often greater than in the average senior of comparable age, and such individuals may be helped by programs of pool activities or other forms of weight-supported exercise. Tests of muscle strength and particularly of muscular endurance generally show severe weakness, but resting diastolic volume, stroke volume, and myocardial contractility may remain normal. Nevertheless, a very sedentary lifestyle leads progressively to severe functional deconditioning, with a low peak aerobic power (Ponichtera-Mulcare 1993). Mitral valve prolapse is also seen in a substantial minority of such patients during exercise (Logan et al. 1981).

Rheumatoid Arthritis

Rheumatoid arthritis is in essence a disorder of the immune system, a problem of autoimmunity. The serum shows a high titer of rheumatoid factor, and the erythrocyte sedimentation rate remains high even during periods when acute joint inflammation has subsided. The rheumatoid condition is sometimes generalized, but more commonly it is limited to one or more major joints. The main diagnostic criteria are morning stiffness, tenderness or pain on movement of the affected joint, a history or observation of joint swelling, the palpation of subcutaneous nodules, positive findings on laboratory tests, and the detection of characteristic radiographic or histologic changes in the affected joint.

The inflammatory process leads to a gradual destruction of the joint surface, together with the surrounding capsule and ligaments. The performance of simple activities such as walking and stepping may be impaired by as much as 50%, the peak aerobic power as measured on a cycle ergometer may be decreased by 30%, and the strength of the muscles acting on the affected joint may be reduced by up to 75% (Ekblöm 1982).

The American Rheumatoid Association has recognized four classes of disability:

* Class I—complete ability to carry out all usual duties
* Class II—adequate ability to carry out normal activities despite some handicap, discomfort, or limitation of motion

- Class III—limited ability to carry out usual occupation or self-care
- Class IV—largely or totally incapacitated

Prevalence and Incidence

Some people are affected by rheumatoid arthritis relatively early in life, but the disease becomes progressively more common as age increases. Estimates of prevalence depend upon the strictness of the diagnostic criteria applied. Some reports suggest that as many as 8% to 25% of senior citizens are affected (Linos et al. 1980), but only 1.8% of men and 4.9% of women over the age of 65 years have "definite" rheumatoid arthritis according to the criteria of the American Rheumatoid Association (Lawrence et al. 1989). Many patients are able to cope with the disease until they reach a relatively advanced age. Typically, they are forced to seek help because of either declining strength, or changed social circumstances such as loss of a spouse (Rivlin 1981).

Primary and Secondary Prevention

Little is known about the etiology of rheumatoid arthritis, and primary prevention is thus difficult. However, a genetic predisposition has been demonstrated; this involves two loci of the major histocompatibility complex that is involved in immune reactions (Harris 1990). The search continues for a precipitating microorganism and for pathological alterations in function of the various lymphocyte subsets. Polymorph infiltration of the joint contributes to inflammation through the release of prostaglandins, superoxide radicals, chemotactic factors, and proteinases.

Tertiary and Quaternary Treatment

Physician advice is typically sought when the condition is moderately advanced; it thus concerns tertiary and quaternary treatment. Even at this stage in the disease process, there is growing evidence that moderate progressive exercise is a helpful component of treatment.

Exercise Tolerance

Patients in functional Class I can perform most types of exercise provided that the disease is in remission. However, certain forms of hard exercise such as running or racquet sports place an excessive strain on the affected joint, exacerbating the condition.

Those in Classes II and III can often train by walking or use of a cycle ergometer, although ergometer loadings must be greatly reduced during exacerbations of the disease.

Class IV patients have only a very limited ability to participate in exercise programs, although conditioning is sometimes still possible provided that the body mass is supported by immersion in water.

Exercise Prescription

It is essential that people rest or at the most undertake only light activity during the acute stage of inflammation, in order to minimize further destruction of articular cartilage and underlying bone. However, an excessive period of bed rest can provoke severe muscle wasting, osteoporosis, bed sores, deep vein thromboses, and other complications of prolonged inactivity.

The primary functional deficit of the patient with rheumatoid arthritis is usually muscular rather than cardiovascular (Ekdahl and Broman 1992). It is thus important to insist on regular strengthening of key muscles such as the quadriceps during periods of enforced rest, and to begin light movements (exercise in warm water or loadless pedaling) as soon as the worst of a given attack has subsided. Both pool exercises and walking programs can enhance aerobic power (Minor et al. 1989), but the underlying disturbance of immune function is generally unchanged by a period of moderate aerobic training.

In a proportion of patients, pericarditis, peripheral arteritis, and polyneuritis may modify the ability to carry out specific exercises. Ekblöm (1985) maintained that after a few weeks of personalized instruction, 80% to 85% of those with rheumatic arthritis were able to undertake an effective home training program. However, he also recommended that if there was an exacerbation of the disease, the patient should return to the rehabilitation center for a few additional weeks of closely supervised and selective activity.

Swimming, rowing, and cycling are good exercises to enhance aerobic condition in the person with moderate disability, because such activities are weight-supported. In some instances, both peak aerobic power and muscle strength show a remarkable response to such programs, with associated psychosocial benefits (Ekblöm 1982, 1985). Assessments of habitual daily activity have shown related gains: a 14% improvement in level walking, a 25% increase in stair climbing, and a 23% to 73% increase of muscle strength. Moreover, a 5.5-year follow-up found radiographic benefit relative to controls, and the average duration of hospitalization for the follow-up period was 16 days, as compared with 36 days in the control subjects. Finally, social isolation was reported by only 20% of patients enrolled in the training program, in comparison to 36% of controls.

Palliative Treatment

Contractures are a frequent hazard in rheumatic patients with more severe disability, particularly during exacerbations of the disease. Sometimes it may be necessary to splint vulnerable joints such as the wrist or the knee, but mobility training is a preferable approach. Tension of the periarthritic muscles can create a vicious cycle of increased joint loading, worsening pain, and fear of movement. This cycle can be broken by a judicious combination of electrotherapy, cryotherapy, relaxation exercises, and analgesics. Nonsteroidal antiinflammatory drugs such as salicylate may be helpful in shortening acute exacerbations of the disease, although if they are given for prolonged periods there is a danger that they may provoke gastric irritation (with ulceration, hemorrhage, and anemia), together with tinnitus, giddiness, or both. The prolonged administration of corticosteroids is also undesirable, since these exacerbate the tendency to osteoporosis, skin atrophy, cataract, and peptic ulcer.

After any acute exacerbation of the disease process has been controlled, a careful blend of passive and active exercises is needed to increase the range of joint movements and restore muscle function (Suwalski 1982). Kirsteins, Dietz, and Hwang (1991) argued that tai chi chuan exercise is useful in strengthening bones and connective tissue weakened by the disease process. However, if movement continues to be painful or restricted, weight-supported exercises in a heated pool may be needed (White 1995). Other possible methods of conditioning applicable to such a situation include suspension exercises and the use of a pulley system.

In patients with residual joint deformities, occupational therapy may be needed to teach new approaches to the tasks of daily living. At this stage, the provision of aids for walking, toilet care, and the performance of household tasks is important to the preservation of function and enhancement of the quality of life.

Osteoarthritis

Osteoarthritis is the most common form of arthritis. It has also been termed degenerative joint disease, or osteoarthrosis. It is characterized by chemical changes in the affected articular cartilage, including a decrease in the content—but an aggregation—of proteoglycans. These abnormalities have been attributed to a stimulation followed by a failure of the chondrocytes, and by the associated action of various enzymes (cathepsin, hyaluronidase, and collagenase; Calkins and Challa 1985). Exostoses of bone develop at the sites of cartilaginous damage. The contribution of repeated trauma and autoimmune disorders to the etiology of these changes continues to be debated (Lane et al. 1986; Panush 1994).

The affected joints become painful and stiff, but there is no sign of current inflammation.

Prevalence and Incidence

More than 80% of 60-year-old subjects have some radiographic evidence of osteoarthrosis, but the findings from such investigations are poorly correlated with the incidence of symptoms. One survey conducted in the United States found that 57% of those over the age of 55 years complained of arthritis, and that in 24% of older adults this was sufficient to cause difficulty in carrying out everyday activities.

Primary and Secondary Prevention

Given the probable association between excessive trauma and subsequent osteoarthritis, it may be prudent to avoid power sports in which excessive forces are applied to the major joints (Kujala, Kaprio, and Sarna 1994). A variety of reports have claimed specific, sport-related sites of injury: lesions of the spine, knees, and elbows in wrestlers; of the patella in cyclists; of the fingers in cricketers; of the shoulders, elbows, and wrists in gymnasts; of the hips, knees, and ankles in soccer players; and of the knees and ankles in American football players. However, many of these studies had weaknesses of design: sport participation was poorly defined, diagnostic criteria were unclear, clinical examinations were not blinded, other possible etiological factors were not considered, and the follow-up period was uncertain (Panush and Brown 1987; Panush and Inzinna 1994). Moreover, it is difficult to circumvent the problem that involvement in a particular type of sport is self-selected and that where symptoms of arthritis begin to appear, the individual is likely either to become sedentary or to choose some alternative pursuit. Retrospective questioning of those who receive hip replacement surgery is less open to artifacts, and one study by Vingård et al. (1993) found a 4.5-fold increase in the risk of hip surgery among 50- to 70-year-old men who had been exposed to high physical loads through sport; track and field and racquet sports were the most common antecedents cited in this study.

A number of investigators have focused on long-distance runners. In general, they have concluded that running does not contribute to the development of osteoarthritis. Lane et al. (1987) compared 498 distance runners with 365 controls, finding that the runners had less physical disability than their peers; they also developed musculoskeletal problems at a slower rate, and sought medical advice less frequently than the control subjects. A five-year follow-up of this same population (Lane et al. 1993) found that some 12% of both runners and control subjects had developed osteoarthritis. Sohn and Micheli (1985) compared 504 runners with 287 swimmers at an average age of 57 years. The swimmers had a 2.4% incidence of severe arthritic pain affecting the hips and the knees, compared with only 2% in the runners. The corresponding figures were 19.5% and 15.5% for those reporting moderate pain, and 2.1% and 1.0% for those individuals who ultimately required surgical treatment. The runners had been averaging a weekly training distance of 40 km for 12 years. However, no correlation was found between the risk of developing arthritis and either the weekly distance run or the number of years that the person had been running.

Lane et al. (1993) made a five-year prospective comparison between runners and controls. The average age of subjects at entry was 50 to 72 years, and the incidence of osteoarthritis of the knees was no greater in the runners than in the control subjects. One report of an adverse response in runners came from Marti, Knobloch, et al. (1989); they found more radiological disease in the hips of former Swiss national champion runners than in bobsled participants. Likewise, although an earlier report from Finland had found no difference of radiologic joint deterioration between runners and nonrunners, Kujala, Kaprio, and Sarna (1994) concluded that participants in all types of competitive sports (including running) were at a slightly increased risk of developing osteoarthritis.

Various occupational stressors also predispose to an increased incidence of osteoarthritis relative to that observed in the general population. The hands are affected in garment, textile, cotton, and diamond workers; the shoulder and elbow in pneumatic drillers; and the knees in occupations that require knee bending, including mining (Panush and Brown 1987).

Tertiary and Quaternary Treatment

Much of the disability associated with osteoarthritis is probably secondary to deconditioning and muscle weakness (Ettinger and Fried 1991). However, there seems to be relatively little objective evidence concerning the value of either traditional modalities of physical therapy or more specific exercise programs for treatment of the person with established osteoarthritis (Basmajian 1987; Fisher et al. 1994; Semble, Loeser, and Wise 1990). Part of the problem is a reluctance to carry out functional testing, although Philbin, Ries, and French (1995) have suggested that most patients, even with severe arthritis, are capable of completing a maximal, symptom-limited exercise test.

The usual approach is to limit the strain on the joint by reducing body fat (many individuals with osteoarthritis substantially exceed the ideal body mass), to relieve pain by the use of analgesics, and to introduce active exercises that increase the range of motion and strengthen the muscles surrounding an injured joint. As with the chronic stage of rheumatoid arthritis, it is important to break the vicious cycle of a painful joint, muscle spasm or inhibition of muscle contraction, muscle atrophy, impaired joint stability, and further injury of the joint surface.

An uncontrolled study of 15 elderly men with osteoarthritis (Fisher, Pendergast, and Calkins 1991) claimed a 35% increase in both muscle strength and endurance in response to a four-month program of knee-strengthening exercises. Kovar et al. (1992) divided 102 patients with osteoarthritis of the knee into a standard treatment control group and an experimental group who began a progressive walking program. In the control group, the 6 min walking distance actually declined over eight weeks of observation, but in the experimental group there was an 18% improvement in the distance covered, sufficient to make an appreciable difference to the quality of life for the individuals concerned.

If the osteoarthritic disease is advanced, surgical treatment such as replacement of the hip joint by a metal femoral head and a plastic socket may be contemplated. The short-term results of arthroplasty are encouraging, but unfortunately the artificial joints have rather a limited life (10 to 15 years) relative to that of their natural counterparts. Where possible, it is thus desirable to delay replacement of a joint until it is reasonably certain that the replacement will outlive the patient.

Osteoporosis

We noted in chapter 3 that aging is associated with a progressive loss of both bone mineral and the underlying matrix. When a critical loss has developed, the bone becomes sufficiently brittle that minor trauma can cause a fracture. Osteoporosis may thus be defined objectively as a bone mineral density below which the incidence of fractures increases dramatically (Aloia 1989).

Some authors have distinguished this age-related condition from secondary osteoporosis, where the main cause is some factor outside of the skeletal system, such as an endocrine disorder, a drug-induced change in bone metabolism, a dietary deficiency or malabsorption of key nutrients, an inherited disorder, or a malignancy. Others describe the primary (silent) loss of bone mineral as osteopenia, and reserve the term osteoporosis for situations in which an overt pathological fracture has developed. A third possible classification is based on the site of the bone loss. Type I osteoporosis affects mainly the spongy bone, and it predisposes to vertebral fractures. It is seen predominantly in women, 5 to 20 years after menopause, and seems to be associated with an estrogen deficiency. Type II osteoporosis typically occurs in older individuals of both genders (those over 75 years of age). It affects mainly cortical bone and is associated with fractures of the hip and femoral neck.

Osteoporosis has considerable importance for both the quality of life and longevity. Some 50% of elderly women with a pathological fracture of the hip remain bedridden subsequent to their injury, and 6% to 20% die of complications such as pulmonary emboli or a urinary infection within 12 months of the acute episode (Drinkwater 1994; Phillips et al. 1988; Todd et al. 1995).

Prevalence and Incidence

The prevalence of osteoporosis increases progressively with age, but the condition is particularly common in those over 70 years. Some authors have suggested that in the United States as many as 10% of women over the age of 50 years will eventually sustain a pathological fracture (Fisher, Nelson, and Evans 1989), giving a total incidence of pathological fractures of 1.2 million per year (Smith, Raab, et al. 1989). Since the loss of bone mineral begins earlier and occurs somewhat faster in women than in men, the prevalence of the disorder among seniors is at least twice as great in women as in men. Incidents of pathological fracture are noted most frequently in the spine (type I osteoporosis; Ruegsegger et al. 1984) and in the hips, femoral neck, and the wrist (type II osteoporosis; Riggs et al. 1982).

Primary and Secondary Prevention

There is little question that the young adult who participates in regular weight-bearing or load-generating exercise develops a higher bone mineral content than the sedentary person. With aging, the bone mineral content of the active person diminishes, but at any given age he or she retains a substantial advantage over a sedentary individual. Thus, it takes many more years for the bone density of an active person to deteriorate to a level at which pathological fractures become likely. This trend is well shown by Michel et al. (1992). They carried out a five-year follow-up of Masters runners and matched control subjects; both groups were initially 55 to 77 years of age. Each group showed a substantial decrease of lumbar spinal density over the five-year interval, but at the end of the study the runners still maintained a large advantage over the controls. Moreover, the runners who showed the greatest decrease of bone density were those who had curtailed their weekly training over the five years of observation. On the other hand, Michel, Bloch, and Fries (1989) cautioned that bone densities were initially quite low in that minority of Masters runners who spent many hours per week in running, suggesting that an excessive volume of physical activity can have a detrimental effect on bone density, even in the elderly.

Benefits of Exercise in Late Middle Age

The ability to augment bone mineral content through a well-designed program of moderate physical activity certainly continues into late middle age.

For example, Chow, Harrison, and Notarius (1987) conducted a well-controlled and well-designed one-year prospective trial in postmenopausal women aged 50 to 62 years (see table 6.4). None of the subjects were receiving estrogens, calcium supplements, or vitamin D preparations, and to avoid problems from a regional specificity of exercise-induced changes in bone mineral content, the total body calcium was estimated by a neutron activation technique. As expected, an untreated cohort of subjects who had maintained their normal patterns of habitual physical activity showed a continuing decrease of 0.011 in their bone mineral index (the ratio of observed whole-body calcium to the value anticipated in a normal young adult of similar stature). However, the same index showed a covariance-adjusted gain of 0.044 in women who undertook supervised aerobic exercises three times per week;

Table 6.4 Change in bone mineral index (BMI) over one-year prospective trial in postmenopausal women (data covaried to allow for initial interindividual differences in BMI).

Variable	Group A	Group B	Group C
Delta BMI	−0.11	0.044	0.061
2 SEM delta	0.037	0.035	0.036
p versus Group A		0.038	0.008
p versus Group B			0.51

Group A maintained their normal pattern of habitual activity. Group B engaged in a supervised program of aerobic exercise, and Group C in a program of supervised resisted plus aerobic exercise three times per week.

Adapted, by permission, from R. Chow, J.E. Harrison, and C. Notarius, 1987, "Effect of two randomized exercise programmes on bone mass of healthy post-menopausal women," *British Medical Journal* 295: 1441-1444.

moreover, a trend (nonsignificant) to a larger gain of 0.061 was observed in those whose program combined aerobic activities with low-intensity strength training exercises.

Cross-sectional investigations. The correlation between bone density and reported habitual physical activity has often been quite weak in cross-sectional investigations (Smith and Gilligan 1989). This is due in part to the narrow range of habitual physical activity encountered among older North American women, and in part to problems in ascertaining their patterns of habitual physical activity using currently available questionnaires. Probably for the latter reason, associations have been weaker if movement patterns have been assessed by interview rather than through objective counters of physical activity (Black-Sandler et al. 1982). Associations have also been stronger for measurements of aerobic fitness than for assessments of physical activity (for example, Chow et al. 1986; Pocock et al. 1987).

Intertrial discrepancies. In studies relating bone density in late middle age and old age to habitual physical activity or participation in exercise programs, the benefit ascribed to exercise has varied widely from one trial to another. Some prospective studies have found an increase of bone mineral density, but other investigators have merely noted the maintenance of existing bone density in their active subjects while their controls continued to lose bone mineral. There are many possible reasons for the discordant results:

1. *Sample size.* Some investigations have lacked adequate statistical power. For example, Grove and Londeree (1992) distributed three treatments between a total sample of only 15 subjects.

2. *Site of the bone density determinations.* Measurements have often been localized to one or two conveniently measured sites such as the wrist or forearm, and these particular sites may not have been heavily involved in the exercise program. For example, Krølner et al. (1983) noted a 3.5% increase in the bone mineral content of the lumbar spine, but no change in the density of the forearm bones.

3. *Diet.* The postmenopausal woman may need a calcium intake as high as 1000 to 1500 mg/day to ensure calcium balance (American College of Sports Medicine 1995b), and many fall far short of this objective. However, regular exercise, by increasing appetite and thus total food intake, may help to augment calcium intake toward this target (Tiidus, Shephard, and Montelpare 1989).

4. *Provision of estrogen supplements.* Many postmenopausal women in the United States now receive hormone replacement therapy, and this can have an important influence on bone mineral density (Drinkwater 1994). Low-intensity aerobic exercise may have little influence on bone density in the absence of estrogen supplements, although more vigorous aerobic activity and muscle-building exercise continue to have a positive effect into the postmenopausal period (American College of Sports Medicine 1995b).

5. *Overall lifestyle.* Personal habits such as cigarette smoking or a high alcohol or caffeine consumption can adversely affect bone mineral content (Cummings et al. 1985). Moreover, lifestyle choices tend to be associated with patterns of habitual physical activity (Shephard 1989a).

6. *Type of exercise performed.* Not all exercise programs lead to increased mechanical loading of the bones. In particular, the pool exercises and swimming that are popular with the elderly lack the ability to increase mechanical loading of the skeleton.

7. *The pattern of exercise.* The frequency, intensity, duration, and supervision of the training have varied widely from one study to another. In some instances, the intensity was too light to have an effect on bone density, and in other studies much of the activity was unsupervised and possibly unperformed.

8. *Activities outside of the specified exercise program.* The extent of any activities performed outside of the specified exercise program has often been unknown. Thus, if a person with a high overall level of physical activity enrolls in a swimming program, an increase of bone density may be attributed to the swimming, when in reality some other component of the individual's daily schedule of physical activity is responsible.

9. *Body mass.* The loading of the spine and leg bones during walking and other daily activities depends on body mass. Thus, a positive effect from an exercise program could be offset by an associated decrease in body mass.

10. *Initial bone mineral content.* The potential for a favorable response is greater in subjects who enter a study with a low mineral content (Chow, Harrison, and Notarius 1987).

Late middle age. An early study by Sidney, Shephard, and Harrison (1977) followed 65-year-old men and women who carried out a program of aerobic exercise up to four times per week for one year. In contrast to the expected decline in bone density, whole-body calcium content was maintained over the year of observation. Other investigators found that total body calcium increased significantly in postmenopausal women in response to a year of exercise three times per week, although the bone mineral content of the radius remained unchanged. Smith, Gilligan, et al. (1989) included weight-bearing and arm-strengthening activities in their program for women aged 35 to 65 years, and they noted that with such a program the local loss of bone mineral from the radius was substantially reduced relative to that of controls.

Hatori et al. (1993) tested women aged 45 to 67 years, finding an increase in the density of the lumbar spine (L2 to L4) in response to seven months of high-intensity aerobic exercise (110% of the heart rate observed at the anaerobic threshold); in contrast, bone density decreased in controls and in subjects who exercised at only 80% of the anaerobic threshold.

The women in the study of Martin and Notelovitz (1993) had an average age of 58 years. Twelve months of treadmill training at 70% to 85% of maximal heart rate was insufficient to increase either lumbar or forearm bone density relative to control values, but it should be noted that the intensity of exercise in the experimental group was quite light, and that both experimental and control groups were receiving calcium supplements.

Grove and Londeree (1992) evaluated a small sample of women aged 49 to 64 years. The bone density of the lumbar spine showed a significant decline in control subjects, but it was maintained in exercisers. In part because the study had a low statistical power (three groups of five subjects), no significant difference in response was seen between high- and low-impact exercise.

Nelson et al. (1991) followed a group of women averaging 60 years of age. None of the subjects in their sample were taking estrogens. Over one year of observation, a supervised walk four times per week at 70% to 85% of maximal heart rate had a positive effect on both trabecular bone density in the spine and femoral bone density, but only when the exercise program was combined with a substantial daily calcium intake (average 1462 mg/day).

Other studies of postmenopausal women have been reviewed by Drinkwater (1994). She concluded that moderately paced walking alone might be insufficient to sustain bone health, but that more encouraging results were obtained from programs that included stair climbing, weight lifting, and dancing.

Benefits of Exercise in Old Age

Factors potentially modifying responses in the old and the very old include a limited ability to undertake significant amounts of physical activity, a declining intake of protein, minerals, and vitamins, a decreased exposure to sunlight, and a continuing decrease in the production of anabolic hormones.

Cross-sectional studies.   Despite these negative influences, several cross-sectional studies have suggested that elderly subjects who engage in regular physical activity have a continuing advantage of bone density over sedentary controls.

Krall and Dawson-Hughes (1994) found that women who walked at least 12 km/week had higher trunk and whole-body bone density than women who walked less than 1.6 km/week. Cheng et al. (1994) likewise found a significant correlation between current habitual physical activity and bone density in men born in Jyväskylä in 1914. Suominen and Rahkila (1991) tested bone densities in veteran Finnish athletes aged 70 to 81 years. Values were greater than in controls, significantly so for endurance and speed-trained competitors but not for strength-trained athletes.

Stillman et al. (1986) divided their sample of female subjects into pre- and postmenopausal groups. They found that whereas there was a correlation between habitual physical activity and bone density of the wrist in the premenopausal group, the difference was no longer significant in their postmenopausal sample.

Longitudinal studies.   Longitudinal studies of the elderly are summarized in table 6.5. Several of these investigations seem to support Stillman's viewpoint. Two of the studies detailed (Greendale, Hirsch, and Hahn 1993; Lau et al. 1992) found no significant effect from exercise alone, and Blumenthal et al. (1989) found an effect only when subjects entered the study with a very low bone mineral density.

One study with positive findings (Rikli and McManis 1990) was based on single photon bone densitometry of only a small group of subjects. More convincing evidence of benefit came from Dalsky et al. (1988). They compared an experimental group of 33 women aged 55 to 70 years with 16 controls. Training sessions were held three times a week, and these included 30 to 40 min of aerobic weight-bearing activity plus 15 to 20 min of upper body work. After 9 months, the bone mineral content of the lumbar vertebrae (L2 to L4) had increased 5.2% in the experimental subjects, compared with a loss of 1.4% in controls; at 22 months, the corresponding values were +6.1% and −1.1%. Rundgren et al. (1984) held a 1 h training program twice a week for 15 women of average age 72 years. At the end of 9 months, the bone mineral content of the heel was significantly greater in experimental than in control subjects, although the training group showed no significant increment relative to their initial values. The oldest subjects examined were those of Smith, Reddan, and Smith (1981); chair exercises three times per week yielded a nonsignificant 2.3% increment in the bone mineral content of the radius in the experimental group, whereas that of control subjects decreased by 3.3%.

Prophylactic value of physical activity.   A number of epidemiological studies have indicated the value of regular physical activity in preventing injuries (Åstrom et al. 1987; Cooper, Barker, and Wickham 1988; Wickham et al. 1989),

Table 6.5 Exercise in the development of bone mineral density in the elderly.

Subjects	Age (yr)	Training program	Pattern	Response	Author
51 F, 50 M	60-83	Aerobic exercise	3/week 4 months	Gains only if initial density low	Blumenthal et al. (1989)
49 F	55-70	Aerobic + upper body exercises	3/week 9 months 22 months	BMC L2-L4 +5.2% vs. −1.4% +6.1% vs. −1.1%	Dalsky et al. (1988)
30 F, 6 M	58-80	Exercise (weighted vests)	once/wk supervised 20 weeks	ns increase L2-L4 over control	Greendale, Hirsch, and Hahn (1993)
50 F	62-92	100 step-ups, 15 min submax	10 months	No response lumbar, hip, femur	Lau et al. (1992)
31 F	57-83	60-70% max HR	3/week 10 months	Sig. increase No added gain from wt. training	Rikli and McManis (1990)
30 F	72	Aerobic training	2/week	Heel BMC sig. diff. from controls	Rundgren et al. (1984)
30 F	81	Chair exercises	3/week 3 years	+2.3% (ns) −3.3% (sig. diff. radial BMC from controls)	Smith, Reddan, and Smith (1981)

although factors other than an increased bone density (for instance, larger muscles to protect the bones and initiate righting movements) probably contributed to the advantage of the active subjects; for example, Meyer, Tverdal, and Falch (1993) noted that lean body mass was an important predictor of hip fracture. Wickham et al. (1989) found that the risk ratio for hip fracture in the least active group of subjects was 3.9, relative to those with the largest score for outdoor activity.

Wyshak et al. (1987), in contrast, found no significant difference in the incidence of fractures between former university-class female athletes (29% injured) and other alumni who were classified as nonathletes. Not all of the subjects classed as athletes were still exercising regularly; a second problem with this type of comparison is that the athletic group may have undertaken more dangerous activities than the controls.

Tertiary and Quaternary Treatment

The administration of estrogen, calcium, or calcitonins helps to reduce the risk of hip fracture in the patient with established osteoporosis (Kanis et al. 1992).

Ayalon et al. (1987) treated subjects who had been diagnosed as osteoporotic on the basis of morphological changes in the spine. Exercise classes met three times per week for five months, subjects engaging in a program of warm-up, stretching, aerobic exercise, and dynamic loading of the forearm. The trabecular mass density, as assessed by Compton scattering, increased by 3.8% in experimental subjects, in contrast to a 1.9% decline in controls. However, the bone mineral content of the radius did not change significantly in either group of subjects.

Chow et al. (1987) evaluated a program that combined strength training and aerobic exercise in women with diagnosed osteoporosis who were receiving fluoride treatment. The subjects sorted themselves into adherents (exercising at least three times per week) and nonadherents, and there were substantial differences in the increase of calcium bone index between the two groups (+17% vs. +6%).

Once fracture has occurred, the main value of physical activity is in preventing the secondary complications of bed rest or immobilization. Calcium preparations, vitamin D, hormone replacement therapy, fluoride, calcitonin, and parathyroid hormone treatment have all been tried in an attempt to speed healing. Early mobilization is also important to the prevention of complications (Todd et al. 1995).

Krølner et al. (1983) examined the response to eight months of training, two times per week, in women aged 50 to 73 years who had recently sustained a Colles fracture of the wrist. The bone mineral content of the lumbar spine increased by 3.5% in the exercised group, compared with a loss of 2.7% in the control group.

We may thus conclude that exercise-induced mechanical loading of the skeleton is helpful at all stages from primary prevention to the quaternary treatment of osteoporosis.

Conclusions

Programs of moderate physical activity have been used successfully in the prevention and treatment of sarcopenia and osteoporosis; regular exercise can also maximize residual function in muscular dystrophies and in the chronic phase of rheumatoid arthritis. It remains debatable how far heavy exercise predisposes to osteoarthritis, but a strengthening of muscles around affected joints reduces functional loss.

Regular resisted exercise is particularly important to the avoidance of muscle wasting in the frail elderly. Such programs can yield a substantial increase of muscle mass even in the oldest-old, with a corresponding increase in the ability to undertake the activities of daily living. Osteoporosis and resulting fractures are a major cause of morbidity for the elderly. Prevention of osteoporosis requires an adequate calcium intake and a physical activity program that applies substantial force to the bones—either vigorous weight-bearing aerobic exercise or resisted muscle contractions. Estrogen supplements also increase the effectiveness of exercise in the postmenopausal woman.

Coventry University
Lanchester Library
Tel 02476 887575

Borrowed Items 04/02/2016 10:18
XXXXXX2204

Item Title	Due Date
38001002193781	25/02/2016
* Aging, physical activity, and health	
38001002629313	25/02/2016
* Physical activity and cardiovascular health : a national consensus	
38001005248376	15/02/2016
Anatomy and physiology for physiotherapists	
38001005584804	15/02/2016
Physiology of sport and exercise	

* Indicates items borrowed today
Thankyou for using this unit
www.coventry.ac.uk

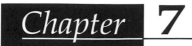

Chapter 7

Physical Activity and Metabolic Health

In this chapter we consider the influence of habitual physical activity on some of the common metabolic problems that affect the elderly subject, including malnutrition and obesity, diabetes mellitus, an adverse lipid profile, and various types of cancer.

Malnutrition

It is usually argued that obesity is the most common form of malnutrition among older people in developed societies. Nevertheless, there are also many theoretical reasons why a frail elderly person might develop serious deficiencies of key nutrients. Poverty sometimes restricts the types of food that can be bought, and it may deny the use of an efficient stove, refrigerator, and cooking utensils. Poor eyesight, gross tremor, muscle weakness, stroke, or crippling arthritis may further hamper both the purchase and the preparation of food. Appetite may be limited by a loss of the sense of taste or of smell (Minaker and Rowe 1982; Schiffman and Gatlin 1993), and the choice of foods may be restricted by a lack of teeth or poorly fitting dentures (Carlos and Wolfe 1989; Garry 1994). There may be difficulty in swallowing (dysphagia; Morris et al. 1991). A reduced gastric secretion of hydrochloric acid, enzymes, or both may restrict the absorption of iron. The resulting tendency to anemia may be exacerbated by internal hemorrhage or a decreased absorption of vitamin B_{12} (Johnson 1995). There may be delays in the emptying of both solids and liquids from the stomach (Moore et al. 1983). Psychological disturbances can add to these physiological problems. Refusal to take meals may become a means of protest against grievances, real or imaginary. Loneliness and social isolation do not encourage the preparation of appetizing or nourishing meals, and there may be a loss of morale, with little desire to stay alive. Many old people have never been taught the principles of good nutrition, and a lack of knowledge may be compounded by mental disturbances.

Further problems arise because the total daily volume of physical activity is so limited. The daily energy expenditure is commonly little more than 6 MJ, and in some of the frail elderly it drops to 4 MJ (Payette and Gray-Donald 1994). Particularly if the person drinks alcohol on a regular basis, the residual energy requirement leaves little scope to consume food that will provide adequate amounts of good quality protein, minerals, and vitamins. Often, a vicious cycle is established; those who are dissatisfied with their diet become increasingly frail, take less physical activity than their peers, and eat ever smaller amounts of food (Sem et al. 1988).

It remains unclear how far these various potential causes of malnutrition lead to actual deficiencies of key nutrients, and how far problems are exacerbated by a poor absorption of food or an increased requirement of proteins, minerals, and vitamins. Feibusch and Holt (1982) described a reduced absorption of carbohydrates among elderly individuals. Problems were particularly prevalent in those with diverticulitis; in this condition, distortions of the intestinal wall allow a colonization of the gut by unusual bacteria and a deconjugation of bile salts. The slowing of protein synthesis in the elderly may point to an increased protein need, and authors such as Fiatarone et al. (1994) have found it helpful to provide protein supplements when treating sarcopenia in the very old (reviewed in chapter 6).

Prevalence and Incidence

Information on obesity is given in a later part of this chapter. Here we examine the prevalence of deficiencies in protein, minerals, and vitamins.

Protein Deficiencies

Clinical markers of protein-deficiency malnutrition include a loss of 10% or more of body mass in six months or less and a current weight that is 90% or less than that of age-matched controls (Chernoff and Silver 1993). In addition to low serum albumin levels, other potential objective markers of protein/energy malnutrition include a low lymphocyte count and subnormal concentrations of hemoglobin, prealbumin, transferrin, and retinol-binding protein (Thomas 1994).

One recurrent problem when one is assessing nutrient intake is to establish the quality of the protein that is ingested. Sometimes the elderly eat an adequate total quantity of protein, but nevertheless they do not obtain a good balance of essential amino acids because their choice of food products has been limited by economic or other constraints (Shank 1985).

Early reports from Britain suggested that as many as 4% of elderly patients suffered from a sufficiently severe lack of protein to cause the development of tissue edema. An early study by the Department of Health and Social Security (1979) found that 12% of elderly subjects (mostly the very old) had serum albumin concentrations that fell below the usually accepted lower limit of normality (35 g/L). More recently, Sullivan et al. (1988) suggested that as many as 65% of elderly hospitalized patients were suffering from protein-calorie malnutrition. Harill and Kylen (1980) further reported that average blood levels of total protein and albumin declined by 1 g/L and 0.4 g/L per decade, respectively, between the ages of 62 and 99 years. Unfortunately, there is a wide dispersion of food and protein intakes within the elderly population, so an adequate or even an excessive intake of food by the majority of people at any given age can easily mask a substantial minority of seniors who are seriously undernourished (Debry 1982; see table 7.1). Guigoz, Vellas, and Garry (1994) noted that although three-fourths of the elderly population in Toulouse were well nourished, one-fourth were at risk of malnutrition and needed detailed evaluation.

In one sample of 879 British people over the age of 65 years, 27 individuals (3%) were excessively thin. These individuals were presumed to be undernourished. Of the 27 cases thus identified, 12 had major medical disorders, and socioeconomic problems were a factor in 7 instances, but in the remaining 8 cases there was no obvious explanation of malnutrition. In general, income had little influence upon nutritional status. The most important variables were biologically advanced age, limited mobility, and the onset of specific pathologies.

A study conducted in Albuquerque found that 11% of seniors had a serum albumin < 35 g/L (Guigoz, Vellas, and Garry 1994). In Sherbrooke, Québec, the situation of elderly people (age 60 to 94 years) who were receiving homecare services seemed even less favorable (Payette and Gray-Donald 1994); 40% of men and 47% of women in this sample were consuming less than the recommended minimum protein intake of 0.8 g/kg per day, and 38% of the group had developed an involuntary weight loss.

Mineral and Vitamin Deficiencies

Some 21% of the men and 32% of the women questioned by Payette and Gray-Donald (1994) were consuming less than two-thirds of the recommended quantities of vitamins A, D, and E and calcium. In 18% of these subjects, the total energy intake was less than 4.2 MJ/day.

Other Canadian surveys have suggested that seniors are vulnerable to deficiencies of calcium, the B vitamins, and vitamins C and D (Mongeau 1991; Tiidus, Shephard, and Montelpare 1989). Nevertheless, there are problems in basing assessments of nutritional status on the reported food intake relative to recommended dietary allowances, because (1) the recommendations include a substantial safety margin, (2) many old people are smaller and much less active than the individuals for whom the standards were designed (Hegsted 1989), and (3) food consumption is generally underreported.

Clinical deficiencies of the B vitamins have been rare except in alcoholics and in patients with pathological conditions affecting the gastrointestinal tract.

Table 7.1   Percentage of elderly subjects failing to meet arbitrary blood concentrations for selected nutrients.

Variable	Lower limit	Britain				Canada	
		M 65-74	M > 75	F 65-74	F > 75	M > 65	F > 65
Serum albumin	3.5 g/dl	10.7	15.3	10.2	13.6	0.3	0.1
Serum vitamin B$_{12}$	100 pg/ml	0.5	2.6	1.2	0.7		
Serum folate	3 ng/ml	14.8	14.5	10.6	18.0	25	23
Leucocyte ascorbic acid	7 µg/10^8 cell	6.3	15.9	2.6	5.7		
Serum iron	60 µg/dl	15.9	16.9	20.5	524.6	11.2	4.9
Hemoglobin	13 (M) or 12 (F) g/dl	5.5	9.6	8.1	5.3	5.7	4.0

Based on the data of the U.K. Department of Health and Social Security (1972) and Nutrition Canada (1976).

However, vitamin C deficiencies can arise in Canada and the northern United States during the winter months, particularly among seniors who lack the money to buy expensively priced imported vegetables.

During the winter months, any problems arising from a low intake of vitamin D are compounded by limited exposure of old people to sunlight; this decreases the endogenous synthesis of vitamin D. A lack of vitamin D, in turn, diminishes the absorption of calcium and exacerbates the tendency to osteoporosis (discussed in chapter 6).

The calcium intake of many older people falls substantially below the level recommended for the avoidance of osteoporosis (800 to 1500 mg/day in various reports; Tiidus, Shephard, and Montelpare 1989). Many old people seem prejudiced against drinking an adequate quantity of milk. Moreover, the prolonged administration of antacids may increase calcium loss in the stools (Albanese 1980), and currently popular cellulose-phytin diets can cause phytin binding, with a reduced absorption of both calcium and magnesium (Judge 1980).

Magnesium ions are important to the normal function of both cardiac and skeletal muscle, and problems associated with the drinking of soft water may be exacerbated in the elderly by the chelating action of hypertensive drugs, by the administration of diuretics, and by mineral loss from bed sores (Judge 1980; Smith 1995). An impairment of myocardial function and cardiac catastrophes is particularly likely to develop in warm weather, when there is a substantial magnesium loss in sweat (Verde et al. 1983). The great majority of elderly individuals do not suffer from anemia (see table 7.1), but absorption of iron can also be hampered by an excessive fiber intake.

Problems of electrolyte balance (particularly a decrease of potassium ions) can arise from the administration of diuretics, together with a decreased secretion of renin, aldosterone, and antidiuretic hormone (Beck 1994; Smith 1995).

Finally, it has been suggested that aging can lead to a deficiency in certain trace elements, particularly chromium (important to glucose tolerance) and zinc (important to twilight vision).

Primary and Secondary Prevention

Given the important role of an inadequate energy expenditure in creating specific forms of malnutrition (Payette and Gray-Donald 1994), an increase in habitual physical activity makes an important contribution to the prevention of malnutrition. Regular physical activity can also encourage protein synthesis and an enhanced intake of key nutrients once deficiencies have developed. Having company during meals is a second important measure that increases the individual's food intake.

Any dietary changes advocated by a health-care worker should be introduced gradually, with a full explanation of the new regimen in order to encourage compliance. Even if exercise is prescribed, the total energy intake of an elderly person is likely to remain relatively small, at least until strength has been restored. The intake of "empty" calories (pastry, confectionery, and alcohol) should thus be held to a minimum. Emphasis should be placed on such food items as green vegetables, milk, eggs, meat, and moderate amounts of whole wheat bread. If an elderly person is incapacitated, full use should be made of any special services that are available, such as "meals on wheels." Care should be taken to avoid salt depletion during hot weather, particularly if the intake of salt has been restricted for medical reasons. Fluid intake should be sufficient to sustain a urine flow of 1.5 L/day. At rest, this implies a daily intake of some 2 L of fluid, but if sweating is increased by exercising, several additional liters of water or diluted saline may be required to maintain fluid balance. Coffee or tea gives a useful stimulation of gastrointestinal motility, which may be decreased in an old person, but an excess intake of coffee late at night can exacerbate insomnia. Finally, if dentition is lacking or there are problems in swallowing, it may be necessary to mince food before it is served.

Tertiary and Quaternary Treatment

Severe malnutrition is associated with an increased incidence of infections, delays in wound healing, an increased liability to falls, and increased mortality; conversely, if body mass can be increased by at least 5%, then the risk of morbidity and early death is diminished (Keller 1995). If there is evidence of severe malnutrition, it is unwise to recommend more than light physical activity until a more normal energy balance has been restored through the provision of dietary supplements. Excessive and premature physical activity in a malnourished individual can exacerbate the tendency to protein catabolism.

Some authors have found that dietary supplements ranging from 2 to 8 MJ/day, and provided for as long as 12 weeks, are helpful in increasing nitrogen retention (Chiang and Huang 1988; Forbes et al. 1986). However, Fiatarone et al. (1994) have argued that multinutrient supplementation is not an effective method of correcting muscle weakness or physical frailty, unless it is accompanied by a vigorous program of resistance exercises.

Obesity

The essential pathology of obesity is an increase in the fat content of the body and thus the size of the adipose tissue cells. Lack of physical activity apparently slows the output of fat from the adipocytes, probably by altering the balance between adipocyte alpha-2- and beta-1-adrenergic receptors and thus reducing the lipoprotein lipase activity of adipose tissue (Després 1994).

Measuring Obesity

We will look at weight-for-height standards, body mass index, and alternative criteria of obesity.

Weight-for-Height Standards

Obesity is commonly diagnosed in the physician's office if a person's body mass exceeds the actuarial "ideal" value by some arbitrary margin such as 10 kg or 15 kg. The ideal value is specified in relation to height, and in some actuarial tables it is adjusted according to a visual estimate or a caliper measurement of body frame size. The U.S. National Nutrition and Health Examination Surveys set an alternative "ideal" value, based on a linear regression of weight upon height for subjects in the United States who were aged 20 to 29 years in 1960 to 1962 (Blair, Habicht, and Alekel 1989).

Body Mass Index

In recent years, the choice in large population surveys has been increasingly to base estimates of a healthy body weight on Quetelet's index (BMI, or the ratio body mass/height^2). The rationale for choosing this index is that it shows a good correlation with various measures of body fatness, but little correlation with standing height. There is little unanimity on possible cutoff points for the diagnosis of abnormality. The risk of ischemic heart disease seems to increase if readings exceed 25 kg/m^2 (see table 7.2). In the Canada Health

Table 7.2 Mortality of obese men in relation to body mass index.

Disease	Body mass index (kg/m²)						
	20	22	25	27	30	35	40
Diabetes mellitus	74	77	94	126	152	210	360
Digestive diseases	97	93	93	97	127	187	295
Nephritis	96	86	90	108	170	280	—
Vascular diseases of brain	114	106	104	106	114	152	200
Heart and circulation	87	89	93	100	120	155	206
Coronary heart disease	88	91	96	108	124	158	206
Hypertensive heart disease	134	128	134	157	230	345	—
Pneumonia and influenza	167	144	106	77	68	94	168
Malignant neoplasms	114	104	93	86	90	108	170
Accidents and homicides	92	91	90	93	110	145	200
Suicides	113	133	122	110	105	109	127

Data for subjects aged 40 to 69 years, expressed as a percentage of actual mortality.
Note: Values have been approximated.
Adapted, by permission, from R. Andres, 1990, Discussion: Assessment of health status. In
Exercise, fitness, and health, edited by C. Bouchard et al. (Champaign, IL: Human Kinetics), 135.

Promotion Survey (Health and Welfare, Canada 1985), a reported index of 20 to 25 kg/m² was judged "acceptable"; a value of less than 20 kg/m² was said to indicate "underweight"; values of 25 to 27 kg/m² were said to signify "possibly overweight"; and values above 27 kg/m² were said to denote "overweight." For the Royal College of Physicians in Britain (Truswell 1985), an index of 30 kg/m² denoted "obesity" and an index of 40 kg/m² "gross obesity." In the National Health and Nutrition Evaluation Survey (NHANES II) in the United States, the thresholds of "overweight" and "severely overweight" were defined by values of 27.8 and 31.1 kg/m² for men and 27.3 and 32.3 kg/m² for women, respectively (Kuczmarski et al. 1994). These figures were chosen arbitrarily to correspond with the 85th and 95th percentiles of data for the 20- to 29-year-old adults examined in 1960 to 1962. "Severe obesity" was normally diagnosed in the NHANES surveys when the BMI reached 40 kg/m², but a value of 35 kg/m² was adopted for a person in whom significant medical complications had developed.

Alternative Criteria

Specific problems that arise in the application of ratios of weight to height in an elderly population were discussed in chapter 3. Even in young adults, a BMI of 28 to 30 kg/m² can correspond to a body fat content ranging from 15% to 41%; moreover, the BMI accounts for only about half of the variance in fatness. An alternative approach is to base the diagnosis of obesity on a skinfold thickness or a body fat content that either exceeds the population norm for young adults by a specified percentage, or reaches an agreed percentile of the normal distribution. For example, Blair, Habicht, and Alekel (1989) reported the fractions of their population who exceeded the 85th, 90th, and 95th percentiles of summed average readings for triceps and subscapular skinfolds as observed at the age of 20 to 29 years, and Leon (1989) suggested that body fat should not exceed 20% of body mass in men and 25% of body mass in women.

However, the NHANES investigators concluded empirically that the Quetelet index was preferable to these alternative measures of fatness, in that it showed closer correlations with other known cardiac risk factors such as systemic blood pressure, serum cholesterol, and serum uric acid, at least when skinfold measurements were made under field conditions (Blair, Habicht, and Alekel 1989).

Health Consequences of Obesity

Data showing the influence of obesity on the risk of death from specific disorders are available only for the insured population, and then in broad age groupings (Andres 1994). For those aged 40 to 69 years, substantial obesity is associated with an increased mortality from a wide range of disorders including diabetes mellitus, digestive diseases, nephritis, hypertensive heart disease, vascular diseases of the brain, cardiovascular diseases in general, and certain types of neoplasm (endometrial cancer and postmenopausal cancer of the breast) (see table 7.2). Even a small increase in BMI leads to statistically measurable increases of mortality when data from large populations are examined. Nevertheless, it is worth emphasizing that for many of the disorders listed in table 7.2, there must be a substantial increase in BMI before there is a major deterioration of prognosis and thus an increase in population-attributable risk.

Regional Fat Distribution

In middle-aged adults, the adverse health significance of fat accumulation is greatest if the deposition of adipose tissue occurs intra-abdominally (as tested, for example, by the waist circumference [Lean, Han, and Morrison 1995] or the waist/hip circumference ratio [U.S. Surgeon General 1996]). The risk of morbid conditions and death relative to the risk for lean controls is approximately doubled by such a pattern of fat distribution (Bouchard and Després 1988). A waist circumference of > 94 cm in men or > 80 cm in women is associated with a Quetelet index > 25 kg/m² and a large waist/hip circumference ratio (> 0.95 in men, and 0.80 in women). Likewise, a waist circumference > 102 cm in men or > 88 cm in women is associated with a Quetelet index > 30 kg/m² (Lean, Han, and Morrison 1995). The female pattern of fat deposition, a subcutaneous accumulation around the hips and thighs, has less influence on cardiac risk and overall prognosis. It remains unclear to what extent the differential risk of intra-abdominal fat deposition that has been observed in middle-aged adults applies to older subjects (Bouchard and Després 1988).

Regional intra-abdominal and subcutaneous abdominal fat can be determined accurately by computed axial tomography (Ferland et al. 1989). Although subcutaneous fat measurements sometimes decrease in the elderly, there is a progressive increase of intra-abdominal fat. Computed tomography scans show that internal depots account for some 20% of total stores in young men, 38% in 46-year-old men, and 47% in 69-year-old men.

Variability of Body Mass

Blair et al. (1993) noted that in an analysis of data from the multiple risk factor intervention trial, month-to-month variability in body weight (presumably associated with repeated attempts at dieting) was associated with an increased risk of both cardiovascular disease and all-cause mortality.

Prevalence and Incidence

Many of the statistics on the prevalence of obesity are based upon population studies of height and mass, with calculations of Quetelet's index. In Canada (Health and Welfare, Canada 1985), information was sought by telephone interview. This immediately excluded those who did not have access to a telephone. Moreover, although there is a good correlation between reported and actual values in the elderly (Boutier and Payette 1994), telephone reports often tend to underestimate actual body weights. Nevertheless, some 20% of adults over the age of 65 years indicated heights and weights equivalent to a BMI of 27 kg/m^2 or greater (see table 7.3). The prevalence of very high indexes rose progressively with age. Thus, values of over 30 kg/m^2 were found in only 3% of Canadians aged 20 to 29 years, but in about 15% of those aged 50 to 70 years (Fitness Canada 1986). Furthermore, there was a parallel age-related increase in the percentage of individuals who showed an intra-abdominal accumulation of body fat.

In Britain, Lean, Han, and Morrison (1995) found that at an average age of 51 years, 48% of women and 38% of men exceeded the acceptable waist/hip ratios of 0.80 and 0.95, and slightly more than half of their sample had a BMI > 25 kg/m^2.

In the United States, Renold (1981) reported that 57% of elderly men and 68% of elderly women who were applying for life insurance had a body mass that was 10% or more above the actuarial ideal. Likewise, Blair, Habicht, and Alekel (1989) noted that a large percentage of older adults exceeded the weight and skinfold standards set by subjects aged 20 to 29 years (see table 7.4). More recently, the NHANES III estimate was that 58 million Americans (33.4% of the U.S. population) between the ages of 25 and 74 years were overweight in terms of the BMI criteria, African American women having a higher prevalence (48.7%) than white women (34.0%, Kuczmarski et al. 1994). The prevalence of overweight, paradoxically, was greatest in those living below the poverty line.

Table 7.3 Body mass index for Canadian population over the age of 65 years.

Body mass index	Percentage of population		
(kg/m²)	Men	Women	Men + women
< 20	7.7	14.6	11.6
20-25	51.1	49.8	50.4
25-27	21.1	14.8	17.5
> 27	19.9	19.6	19.7

Based on reported information for weight and height without shoes in a telephone survey; full-time residents of institutions excluded.

Adapted from *Canada's Health Promotion Survey*, Health Canada, 1985. With permission of the Minister of Public Works and Government Services Canada, 1997.

Table 7.4 Prevalence of obesity in U.S. citizens aged 65 to 74 years, based on excess body mass (relative to subjects aged 20-29 years) and skinfold percentile criteria.

Criterion	Men (%)	Women (%)
10% excess body mass	32.5	49.1
20% excess body mass	13.4	31.5
85th percentile	16.6	26.1
90th percentile	10.0	23.2
95th percentile	3.9	6.3

Reprinted from D. Blair, J.P. Habicht, and L. Alekel, 1989, "Assessments of body composition, dietary patterns, and nutritional status in the National Health Examination Surveys and National Health and Nutrition Examination Surveys." In *Assessing physical fitness and physical activity in population-based surveys*, edited by T.F. Drury, US PHS Publication No. 89-1253 (Hyattsville, MD: U.S. Department of Health and Human Services), 70-104.

There are few specific data on the elderly population. In part because of the age-related loss of lean tissue, the prevalence of excess body weight apparently falls in the oldest age categories. Thus, Debry (1982) suggested that in the United States, 30% of men and 40% of women aged 65 years showed moderate or severe obesity, and figures for the French population were similar (31.9% of men and 35.3% of women aged 60 to 64 years). However, by the age of 90 to 94 years, the body mass-based estimate of the prevalence of obesity in both the United States and France had dropped to 10%.

Primary and Secondary Prevention

Obesity seems much easier to prevent than to treat, both cross-sectional and longitudinal studies suggesting the value of regular physical activity in primary prevention.

Cross-Sectional Studies

Comparisons of active and sedentary groups of older people (DiPietro 1995; Kohrt et al. 1992) and studies of Masters athletes at various ages (Kavanagh et al. 1988) suggest that vigorous endurance activity can limit the commonly observed progressive accumulation of body fat with aging.

The preventive value of regular exercise seems greater in those reporting vigorous physical activity than in those indicating lower intensities. This could reflect a greater post-exercise stimulation of metabolism following bouts of vigorous activity, although it is also possible that reports of vigorous exercise are more accurate than are reports of light or moderate activity. Data from the 1989 Behavioral Risk Factor Surveillance System survey suggested that the association between body mass and participation in physical activities such as walking, running, and aerobics tended to be greater in older than in younger individuals (DiPietro 1995; DiPietro et al. 1993). However, other investigators have found little association between reported levels of habitual physical activity and body mass in the elderly (Caspersen et al. 1991; Marti, Pekkanen, et al. 1989).

Part of any advantage of leanness observed in the active groups could be attributable to genetic differences between those who are thin and those who are obese. It is certainly possible to breed animals with a strong genetic predisposition to obesity. Some humans also seem to carry "thrifty genes" that conserve body fat and thus predispose to obesity (Bouchard 1994; Lindpaintner 1995). Bouchard et al. (1992) have estimated that the age- and gender-adjusted transmissible variance is about 35% for the BMI and 50% for the body fat content as determined by underwater weighing. However, only about 5% and 25% of the respective variances have a true genetic origin; the residue of the transmitted variance is due to the strong familial influence of a shared lifestyle (for example, there are major interhousehold differences in patterns of habitual physical activity and eating behavior).

A further problem in interpreting cross-sectional surveys is that the development of obesity encourages adoption of a sedentary lifestyle (Williamson et al. 1993). Thus, Voorips, van Staeveren, and Hautvast (1991) compared obese and non-obese women > 70 years of age. They found no difference in reported physical activity earlier in adult life, although intergroup differences in body mass dated back to an age of 25 years. Nevertheless, those who were currently obese had become physically less active than their thinner peers.

Longitudinal Data

A longitudinal study of a large Finnish population assessed the determinants of significant weight gain over a five- to seven-year interval (Rissanen et al. 1991). After data were adjusted for smoking and intake of caffeine and alcohol, the risk ratio for an increase in body mass > 5 kg was 1.9 in men and 1.6 in women who rarely engaged in active leisure relative to those who were frequently active. In the National Health Examination and Fitness Survey (NHEFS), Williamson et al. (1993) also found that a low level of recreational activity was associated with a substantially increased risk of a large gain in body mass (see table 7.5).

Adverse Consequences of Obesity

The arguments for the treatment of obesity in the senior citizen are much as for a younger person (Garrow 1994). The skeleton is not well designed to carry an excess load, and many of the orthopedic problems of old age—flat feet, osteoarthritis of the knees, hips, and lumbar spine—are made worse by obesity (Silberberg 1979). The mechanical efficiency of the muscles is unchanged (Binkhorst, Heevel, and Nordeloos 1984), but the energy cost of movement is increased by the greater mass of the legs and an increase in the work of breathing (Binkhorst, Heevel, and Nordeloos 1984; Katch et al. 1984). The ungainly body of a fat person cannot move quickly, and is thus more vulnerable to accidents. Further, if a fall is sustained, the greater mass may increase the risk of a fracture (although the "padding" of the bones may also offer some protection against direct contact, and the added body mass may increase the density of weight-supporting bones).

Accumulation of fat around the chest and underneath the diaphragm interferes with breathing. This leads to a nonuniform distribution of ventilation,

Table 7.5   Odds ratio for weight gain (8-13 kg in men, > 13 kg in women) over 10-year interval in relation to level of recreational activity (low, moderate, or high).

	Odds ratio	
Pattern of activity	Men	Women
Low/low	3.9	7.1
Moderate/moderate	2.0	3.4
High/high	1.0	1.0
Decrease	3.3	6.2
Increase	2.4	3.4

Adapted, by permission, from D.F. Williamson, J. Madans, R.F. Auda, J.C. Kleinman, H.S. Kahn, and T. Byers, 1993, "Recreational physical activity and ten-year weight change in a U.S. national cohort," *International Journal of Obesity* 17: 279-286.

with a tendency to carbon dioxide retention, drowsiness, and an increased predisposition to respiratory disease. The cardiac work rate is increased by the physical load to be displaced and by any associated hypertension. In the young-old, a high BMI is thus associated with a poor ability to undertake the activities of daily living (Launer et al. 1994). The obese person also has an increased vulnerability to angina, cardiac failure, and sudden death, although if BMI is used as the index of obesity, the trend is less marked in those over the age of 65 years (Harris et al. 1988).

Furthermore, obesity is associated with maturity-onset diabetes, a high plasma cholesterol, and an increased risk of certain cancers, gallbladder disease, and biliary tract disease (Leon, 1989, 1992). Lastly, there are often psychological problems, although it may be hard to determine whether these are the cause or the consequence of the obesity.

A number of the adverse consequences of obesity, particularly the risk of atherosclerotic disease and an increased synthesis of carcinogens, are long-term hazards. The risk even of mild obesity thus increases the longer it is allowed to continue untreated (Bouchard and Després 1988; Feinleib 1985).

Treatment of Mild Obesity

There is some evidence that obese individuals show a decreased metabolic response to both feeding and exercise (Segal et al. 1987). However, they are also more prone to take the elevator rather than a staircase (Brownell 1984).

Studies of the mildly obese have shown that an improvement of body composition is possible through a well-designed physical activity program, even in old age (Ballor and Keesey 1991). Exercise has several important advantages over dieting alone. Mood is usually elevated by physical activity, and there is not necessarily any compensatory increase of food intake. Indeed, if physical activity is undertaken when a person begins to feel hungry, there may even be some short-term suppression of appetite. In contrast to strenuous dieting, moderate exercise helps to conserve lean tissue, although if physical activity is too vigorous it may create a large negative energy balance, with a loss of lean tissue (Pavlou et al. 1985; Tremblay, Després, and Bouchard 1985). Cardiac function is improved by an exercise program, and there is less risk of inducing ventricular fibrillation than with severe dieting. Above all, the exercise regimen is gradual, giving the patient time to accept the discipline of a new lifestyle. There is also opportunity for a readjustment of the metabolic set-point in the hypothalamus, and attendance at exercise classes establishes a new pattern of positive behavior. A well-designed exercise program provides a more effective long-term strategy for the control of obesity than dieting alone (Kayman, Bruvold, and Stern 1990). The one disappointment is that in few studies (only 4 of 17) has exercise countered the reduction of basal metabolism that frustrates attempts at inducing weight loss by dieting alone (Hill, Storandt, and Malley 1993).

The individual who wishes to reduce body fat must engage in a substantial volume of physical activity, preferably over an extended period. The best predictors of fat loss are initial obesity and the total increase in energy expenditure (Ballor and Keesey 1991). An early study from our laboratory demonstrated a 3.3 mm decrease in average skinfold readings over a 14-week training program in 65-year-old subjects who combined a high intensity of physical activity with regular program attendance (Sidney, Shephard, and Harrison 1977). No special dietary regimen was adopted in this study. Effects were smaller in those who attended less regularly or adopted a lower intensity of exercise (see table 7.6).

Physical activity has a favorable influence, not only on overall body fatness but also upon the distribution of body fat. Several large cross-sectional studies (Kaye et al. 1990; Seidell et al. 1991; Slattery et al. 1992; Tremblay et al. 1990; Triosi et al. 1993; Wing et al. 1991) have all reported favorable associations between estimates of habitual physical activity and such indicators of body fat distribution as waist/hip or waist/thigh circumference ratios. It appears that epinephrine, liberated by vigorous exercise, helps to mobilize abdominal fat in a selective fashion (Bouchard, Després, and Tremblay 1993; Wahrenberg, Bolinder, and Arner 1991). Mobilization seems to be achieved more easily in men than in women. For example, Kohrt, Obert, and Holloszy (1992) found that a 9- to 12-month program of aerobic exercise (performed for 30 to 50 min/session, three to five times a week for 9 to 12 months at 60% to 85% of the heart rate maximum) gave a selective loss of subcutaneous fat from central and upper body sites in male subjects. In contrast, women showed a roughly equal loss of subcutaneous fat at all of the body sites that were examined.

Table 7.6   Influence of self-selected intensity and frequency of training on decrease in averaged skinfold thickness in 65-year-old adults.

Type of program	Change in skinfold reading (mm)	
	7 weeks	14 weeks
Low frequency, low intensity	−0.8	−1.4
Low frequency, high intensity	−1.4	−1.9
High frequency, low intensity	−1.5	−2.9
High frequency, high intensity	−2.4	−3.1

Note: Low frequency = less than 2 sessions per week; high frequency = 2-4 sessions per week of aerobic exercise.

Low intensity = heart rate < 120 beats/min; high intensity = heart rate increasing progressively to 130-140 beats/min.

Adapted, by permission, from K.H. Sidney, R.J. Shephard, and J. Harrison, 1977, "Endurance training and body composition of the elderly," *American Journal of Clinical Nutrition* 30: 326-333, Table 3, © American Journal of Clinical Nutrition, American Society for Clinical Nutrition.

Tertiary and Quaternary Treatment

Efforts to achieve fat loss in those who have become very obese seem desirable, as such action continues to reduce the likelihood of developing complications such as maturity-onset diabetes mellitus and the various manifestations of atherosclerotic cardiovascular disease.

Light exercise such as progressively increasing volumes of walking can be an effective method of treatment for severely obese patients, particularly if it is combined with dietary restriction (Bouchard, Després, and Tremblay 1993; Leon 1989). However, fitness levels are typically very low in those who are grossly obese (Atkinson and Wallberg-Rankin 1994), and there may also be embarrassment about appearing lightly clothed in a gymnasium or a swimming pool (Brownell 1984). It may thus be difficult to persuade grossly obese individuals to take any substantial quantity of exercise. Foss et al. (1975) studied patients who initially weighed 133 to 238 kg; they found that sometimes eight weeks of slow but progressive training were needed to reach the point at which the patient could cover 1.6 km in 20 min. Walking is better tolerated than jogging, and often an obese person cannot continue exercising for long enough to produce a significant energy expenditure. The extent of body fat loss is increased if exercise is combined with moderate cold exposure (O'Hara, Allen, and Shephard 1977; Timmons, Araujo, and Thomas 1985).

Those treating obesity should note that there is a strong tendency for older people to conserve their energy balance (and thus to prevent fat loss) by reducing their habitual physical activity outside of any formal exercise program in which they are enrolled (Goran and Poehlman 1992b). Probably because of the preponderant gluteal and femoral deposition of fat in women, it seems more difficult to mobilize fat in female than in male subjects (Bouchard, Després, and Tremblay 1993).

During the period when body fatness is being reduced, the diet should remain varied and nourishing, although preferably there should be a small (400 to 800 kJ) reduction of daily energy intake. The emphasis should be on regular and not too widely spaced meals, without intervening "nibbling." In this way, peaks and troughs of blood sugar are avoided, and overeating is less likely. There is little evidence that the rate of fat loss is altered by qualitative variations in the diet, provided that a negative energy balance is achieved through a suitable combination of increased physical activity and dietary restriction. Proprietary "slimming" foods such as diet milk shakes are not recommended. Many old people find them too expensive, and some become confused, taking them in addition to their regular food. High protein diets may help to conserve lean tissue; they also induce some increase of resting metabolism through their "specific dynamic action," but they again may be too expensive for some older people.

Diabetes Mellitus

Diabetes mellitus is characterized by hyperglycemia and associated metabolic problems. In young adults, the disease can arise through an autoimmune process, with physical destruction of the pancreatic islet cells. This is known as type I, or insulin-dependent diabetes. In the elderly person, the problem more commonly stems from the development of cellular resistance to insulin. There is a decrease in the number or sensitivity of insulin receptors, or a failure of the second-messenger system that initiates intracellular glycogen synthesis. The etiology of the condition is very complex (Gudat, Berger, and Lefèbvre 1994), but potential contributing factors of interest to our present discussion include (1) increased amounts of adipose tissue, (2) decreased lean mass, (3) decreased habitual activity, and (4) increased sympathetic activity. Unfortunately, the loss of insulin sensitivity is usually greater in muscle than in adipose tissue, favoring the further accumulation of fat. A deficiency of trace minerals, particularly chromium, may contribute to these problems (Hughes and Meredith 1989). Islet cells that are still functioning relatively normally increase their output of insulin, but they are unable to produce sufficient quantities of this hormone to regulate the uptake of blood glucose by the peripheral tissues or to control the output of glucose by the liver. This is known as type II, or maturity-onset diabetes. The type II form of diabetes accounts for as much as 90% of all cases (Kral and Besser 1989) and it is particularly common in the elderly (Everhart, Knowler, and Bennett 1985).

Prevalence and Incidence

Diabetes mellitus is a major cause of both morbidity and premature death, accounting for as much as 10% of all days of acute hospitalization (Leon 1989). The diagnosis has traditionally been based upon the measurement of blood glucose 2 h after the administration of a glucose load, although the reported prevalence depends very much on the glucose loading chosen and the ceiling of blood glucose that is accepted as normal. The recent report of the U.S. Surgeon General (1996) endorses the diagnostic threshold of the World Health Organization (1980): a blood glucose concentration in excess of 11.1 mmol/L at 2 h after the oral administration of 75 g of glucose. Blood glucose readings between 7.8 and 11.1 mmol/L imply an impaired glucose tolerance. The individuals thus identified frequently (but not always) progress to overt diabetes (Keen, Jarrett, and McCartney 1982).

Some more recent investigations have examined the quantities of glucose infusion required to maintain a constant blood glucose when insulin levels are increased. Insulin responsiveness can be defined as the maximum glucose uptake observed when insulin levels are very high (for example, 1000 μU/ml).

From 3% to 5% of the urban North American population have physician-diagnosed diabetes (Leon 1992), with an annual incidence rate of 32 cases per 10,000 in adults aged 20 years and older (Everhart, Knowler, and Bennett 1985). However, there may be an almost equal number of undiagnosed cases. There is a striking increase in disease prevalence with age, and by 70 years of age some 20% of men and 30% of women show what would be regarded as a diabetic glucose tolerance curve in a younger person (Bennett 1984; Davidson 1982). The age of onset of type II diabetes is earlier and the incidence is even higher among many indigenous populations such as Pacific Islanders and Native American Indians, groups that until recently combined vigorous physical activity with a low carbohydrate intake (Joos et al. 1984; Szathmary and Holt 1983; Young et al. 1995).

Perhaps because of an impaired action of insulin and reduced intramuscular stores of glycogen, Goldfarb, Vaccaro, and Ostrove (1989) found that the oldest category of Masters swimmers showed a decrease rather than an increase in plasma glucose concentrations during a treadmill run to exhaustion.

Primary and Secondary Prevention

Depending on the definition of obesity, between 60% and 90% of cases of type II diabetes mellitus develop in those who are already obese (U.S. National Diabetes Data Group 1979). But even in the absence of obesity (Fink et al. 1983), the elderly population shows a rightward shift in the relationship between plasma insulin levels and glucose utilization (that is, a decrease in insulin response). The control over hepatic glucose release is also decreased (Fink et al. 1983).

It is not possible to avoid the influences of genetics and aging on the risk of developing diabetes, but studies of populations undergoing rapid acculturation to an urban lifestyle (Ravussin et al. 1992; Shephard and Rode 1996) suggest that regular physical activity and the avoidance of obesity are important preventive measures. Cross-sectional comparisons within developed societies have also shown an association between physical inactivity and clinically diagnosed type II diabetes mellitus (Kriska, Blair, and Pereira 1994; Ramaiya et al. 1991). Moreover, glucose readings were often significantly higher, and insulin secretion greater, in sedentary than in physically active individuals (Feskens, Loeber, and Kromhout 1994; Kriska, Blair, and Pereira 1994; Regensteiner 1991). Thus, Pratley et al. (1995) found that the insulin concentration producing a half-maximal increase in glucose disposal was 41% lower in 63-year-old Masters athletes than in sedentary individuals of similar age and overall body fatness. The advantage of the athletes was associated with a lower waist/hip circumference ratio, suggesting that they carried a smaller fraction of their total body fat intra-abdominally.

The preventive value of regular exercise has been confirmed in a number of prospective investigations. The incidence of type II diabetes mellitus among university alumni over a 14-year interval was inversely related to regular participation in physical activity as reported in an initial questionnaire (Helmrich et al. 1991). This association persisted after statistical control for current BMI, history of hypertension, and a parental history of diabetes. Exercise was of greatest benefit in those who entered the study with a BMI > 25 kg/m². In this study, vigorous sport conferred greater benefit than moderate activities such as walking. Likewise, women aged 55 to 69 years who had high levels of physical activity halved their relative risk of developing diabetes compared to those who were sedentary (Kaye et al. 1991). In contrast, the improvement of prognosis in an eight-year follow-up of nurses (Manson et al. 1991) and in a five-year follow-up of physicians (Manson et al. 1992) showed no obvious relationship to the frequency of physical activity, although overall benefit was obtained from exercising at least once a week.

Exercise is helpful in secondary prevention. Indeed, the correction of obesity and a modest increase in habitual physical activity may be sufficient to correct a mild case of maturity-onset diabetes without recourse to more drastic forms of treatment (Leon 1992). Exercise is particularly helpful in the elderly person with diabetes, since as many as a third of seniors have difficulty in understanding even a simple diet. A five-year follow-up of men with impaired glucose tolerance showed that those who were enrolled in a regular twice-weekly program of supervised physical activity reduced their body mass, improved their glucose tolerance, and greatly reduced their chances of developing diabetes relative to nonparticipants (10.6% of the exercisers affected vs. 28.6% of the control subjects; Eriksson and Lindgärde 1991).

In general, regular physical activity helps to normalize both glucose tolerance and tissue insulin sensitivity (Gudat, Berger, and Lefèbvre 1994; Hespel et al. 1995). There remains some uncertainty about how much of the benefit is a training response, and how much of it is due to replenishment of glycogen stores following the last session of programmed exercise. Certainly, one big difference between dieting alone and a combination of exercise and dietary control is that the exercise program enhances tissue glucose uptake (Bogardus et al. 1984). However, given that improvement is observed with as little as 30 min of exercise at 50% to 60% of maximal oxygen intake, a residual effect from the prescribed activity seems unlikely as the full explanation of benefit. Other possible mechanisms include enhanced insulin receptor activity in adipose tissue and other adaptations in skeletal muscle that augment glycogen storage (an increase of lean mass, an increased local blood flow, and an increase of muscle membrane glucose transporter proteins; Gudat, Berger, and Lefèbvre 1994; Horton 1991; Leon 1992).

Tertiary and Quaternary Treatment

In patients for whom medication is currently prescribed, the need for insulin may be substantially reduced and/or the diet simplified as a result of participation in a regular exercise program. Possibly of even greater consequence, regular endurance exercise may enhance the blood lipid profile and reduce systemic blood pressure, so that some of the common cardiovascular complications of diabetes become less likely.

Favorable effects of increased physical activity have now been demonstrated not only in sophisticated urban societies, but also in some of the more remote indigenous populations who are currently at high risk of diabetes (Heath et al. 1987). Benefit is greatest when an increase of physical activity is accompanied by some restriction of food intake (Lampman and Schteingart 1991; Wing et al. 1988). However, the benefits of exercise in established, clinical type II diabetes are sometimes less dramatic than for those individuals whose disease has not yet progressed to the point of requiring medication.

In the person with advanced diabetes, one must prescribe exercise with care, having regard for the danger from a number of specific complications. There is some risk that an exercise-induced acceleration of insulin absorption may provoke a hypoglycemic attack. In general, participation in an exercise program must be accompanied by a reduction in insulin dosage. Careful self-monitoring of blood glucose levels is also important, as is the timing of exercise in relation to meals and to insulin injections. An emergency supply of glucose should be readily available during and immediately after bouts of physical activity. Peripheral neuropathies predispose to both injuries and ulceration of the skin; because of impaired nerve function, the patient is unaware of the stress imposed on bones and tendons, and radiographs may often disclose one or more unsuspected fractures. Loss of vascular reflexes increases the risk of postural hypotension, and associated atherosclerosis may lead to myocardial infarction and sudden death. A proliferative retinopathy may allow hemorrhage and exudation into the retina, cataract, glaucoma, retinal detachment, and blindness. Ill-fitting shoes with protruding nails can cause slow-healing ulcers, and if there is also peripheral vascular disease, the ulcers may develop secondary infection or progress to gangrene (Leon 1992). Sweating should be avoided unless there is opportunity to shower and to dry the skin carefully with clean towels.

However, if these precautions are observed, people with even quite advanced cases of type II diabetes benefit from participation in a progressive exercise program.

Hypercholesterolemia and an Adverse Lipid Profile

Both total cholesterol and plasma triglyceride concentrations tend to increase from puberty through middle age, in part because of a decrease in physical activity and in part because of a decrease in the affinity of lipoprotein receptors (Arbetter and Schaefer 1989). As the individual becomes older, cholesterol and triglyceride concentrations plateau, and they may decline in the final years of life (Hazzard and Ettinger 1995). Many old people are taking diuretics, alpha-blockers, beta-blockers, or cortisol, and all these medications influence plasma lipoprotein levels (Ettinger et al. 1992; Henkin, Como, and Oberman 1992). Mancini, Lirato, and Pauciullo (1993) found that the respective average plasma cholesterol levels in men and women declined from 222 mg/dl and 238 mg/dl at an age of 60 to 64 years to 203 and 226 mg/dl at 75 to 79 years, and to 186 and 223 mg/dl in those over 80 years of age. Age-related changes in HDL- and LDL-cholesterol concentrations were less clear-cut; the ratio of total cholesterol to HDL-cholesterol of men declined from 5.3 at age 60 to 64 years to 4.5 in those over the age of 80 years, but there was no consistent age gradient in women. The classic Seven Countries Study (Keys 1980), the Baltimore Study on Aging (Shock et al. 1984), and the recent study of Thomsen, Larsen, and Schroll (1995) all showed similar trends toward a declining ratio of total cholesterol to HDL-cholesterol during the retirement years, in part because people with hypercholesterolemia were dying and in part because total cholesterol levels were falling.

Decreases in sex hormone levels with aging also influence the lipid profile (Arbetter and Schaefer 1989). Testosterone decreases and estrogen augments HDL-cholesterol levels. In keeping with these observations, the administration of exogenous estrogens to postmenopausal women increases HDL-cholesterol and lowers LDL-cholesterol (Applebaum-Bowden et al. 1989; Walsh et al. 1991), with associated reductions in the risk of ischemic heart disease (for more detailed discussion see chapter 5).

Lipid Profile and Cardiac Risk

In examining the influence of the lipid profile upon cardiac risk in the elderly, we will consider epidemiological data and the effect of deliberate manipulation of the lipid profile before suggesting a threshold for the diagnosis of abnormality.

Epidemiological Data

A meta-analysis of data from 25 studies found that total cholesterol, LDL-cholesterol, and triglyceride concentrations were each related to the risk of subsequent clinical manifestations of ischemic heart disease in older men. In women, plasma HDL-cholesterol concentrations were also inversely related to the risk of subsequent heart disease (Manolio et al. 1992).

In the Honolulu Heart Study, the relative risk of coronary heart disease in individuals with high plasma cholesterol levels was 1.7 in both middle-aged and elderly subjects (Mancini, Lirato, and Pauciullo 1993). Nevertheless, in many studies the adverse effects of an "abnormal" lipid profile on cardiac risk have diminished or even disappeared in advanced old age, partly because individuals with dyslipidemia die at a younger age and partly because of an association between a low serum cholesterol and general debility (Ives et al. 1993; Manolio et al. 1993). Lerner and Kannel (1986) reported that a high total cholesterol and a low HDL-cholesterol were independent risk factors for coronary artery disease in elderly members of the Framingham population; nevertheless, this risk disappeared after the age of 70 years (Kronmal et al. 1993). Serum triglycerides were an independent cardiac risk factor in elderly women, but not in men.

Estimated Effects of Modifications to Lipid Profile

Accepting the proposition that high lipid concentrations are associated with some increase in the risk of cardiac disease even in the elderly, is it advantageous to attempt to lower serum cholesterol by some combination of exercise, dietary modification, and medication?

A combined analysis of data from the Framingham and MRFIT trials estimated that a reduction of serum cholesterol from 285 to 200 mg/dl would reduce the relative risk of coronary disease by 77% in subjects aged 35 to 45 years, but by only 30% in those aged 75 to 85 years. Some investigators have even concluded that there is little potential benefit either in determining the lipid profile or in treating dyslipidemia in patients over the age of 60 years (Canadian Consensus Conference on Cholesterol 1988; Kronmal et al. 1993; Krumholz et al. 1994). However, others have argued in terms of attributable risk, noting that although the relative risk from a high serum cholesterol is smaller after the age of 65 or 70 years, the number of lives that would be saved by correcting the dyslipidemia may still be greater among the elderly because they have such a high prevalence of coronary vascular disease (Gordon and Rifkind 1989; Mancini, Lirato, and Pauciullo 1993; Rubin et al. 1990).

Thresholds of Abnormality

As with blood sugar readings, various thresholds have been suggested for the diagnosis of a clinical abnormality of lipid profile.

The U.S. National Cholesterol Education Program (1993) proposed a ceiling of 6.2 mmol/L (240 mg/dl) for total cholesterol, with limits of 0.9 mmol/L for HDL- and 4.1 mmol/L for LDL-cholesterol. As with body mass, there seems to be a J-shaped relationship between overall mortality and cholesterol levels (Hazzard and Ettinger 1995). Those with very low readings are also at an increased risk of death (Ives et al. 1993; Manolio et al. 1993), and in one survey of women aged 82 ± 9 years, the optimal five-year survival was associated with a serum cholesterol level as high as 7.0 mmol/L (Forette, Tortrat, and Wolmark 1989). However, a cholesterol level greater than 6.1 mmol/L reemerged as a significant risk factor if the analysis was restricted to subjects who were still living normally active lives (Harris et al. 1992).

There is no generally accepted ceiling of triglyceride concentrations, although Thomsen, Larsen, and Schroll (1995) have proposed 2.5 mmol/L, corresponding to the 90th percentile of the Danish population.

Prevalence and Incidence

The average levels of serum cholesterol vary substantially with the level of economic development of a country. Respective values for men and women average 4.2 and 4.3 mmol/L in Beijing, but 6.5 and 6.4 mmol/L in Lille, France (Sans 1993).

The determinations of lipid profile are subject to considerable methodological errors and day-to-day intraindividual variability. Estimates of the proportion of any population with abnormal values are thus greater for single observations than for multipoint surveys (Feinleib et al. 1993). Thomsen, Larsen, and Schroll (1995) noted that 29% of Danish adults had levels of total cholesterol and lipoprotein that were elevated relative to the standards cited earlier, but among the 70-year-old segment of this population, 53% of women and 31% of men demonstrated abnormal values.

Likewise, using NHANES III data, Sempos et al. (1993) estimated that 50% of men and women in the United States had levels of dyslipidemia that required treatment. The prevalence of an abnormal lipid profile was increased by a sedentary lifestyle, obesity, a low socioeconomic status, and clinical disorders such as diabetes mellitus, hypothyroidism, and renal impairment (Hazzard and Ettinger 1995).

Primary and Secondary Prevention

A dramatic program to control hyperlipidemia and other coronary risk factors has been undertaken in eastern Finland over the past 20 years. A series of public health and educational initiatives has focused on a decrease in the consumption of saturated fat, an increased use of vegetable oils, and an increased consumption of vegetables.

As a consequence of these measures, the average cholesterol level in that population has declined by some 30% (Vartiainen et al. 1994). The age-standardized mortality from ischemic heart disease has also decreased dramatically: in men, from 647 per 100,000 during 1969 to 1972 to 289 per 100,000 in 1992, and in women from 114 per 100,000 to 36 per 100,000.

Weight Loss as a Cause of Exercise Benefits

Programs of sustained exercise can make a useful contribution to the improvement of lipid profile, but it remains unclear how far the benefit is mediated through an associated change in body fat stores (Tran and Weltman 1985).

A meta-analysis of 27 longitudinal studies (Lokey and Tran 1989) concluded that exercise reduced both total cholesterol and serum triglyceride concentrations, but if data were statistically adjusted for changes in body mass, there was no residual effect of exercise. Likewise, Kohrt, Obert, and Holloszy (1992) noted that improvements in the lipid profile over a 9- to 12-month program of aerobic exercise were linked with changes in body composition, and Wood et al. (1988) achieved rather similar benefits whether body mass was reduced by exercise or by dieting.

Despite these statistics, there remain at least two important arguments for including exercise in any plan for the treatment of dyslipidemia: (1) exercise is more effective than many other techniques for the reduction of body fat content, and (2) exercise brings other important health benefits that are not achieved by dieting alone.

Cross-Sectional Studies

A cross-sectional study by Reaven et al. (1990) found a positive association between participation in regular, strenuous exercise and age-adjusted plasma HDL-cholesterol concentrations. Likewise, Nieman, Warren et al. (1993) found that a high level of physical activity (1.6 h/day for five years) was associated with a high HDL-cholesterol, although it was unrelated to total cholesterol or LDL-cholesterol concentrations. In a second sample of female subjects aged 67 to 92 years, no difference in lipid profile was seen between those classed as active and those regarded as inactive (Nieman, Warren et al. 1993). Likewise, Danielson, Cauley, and Rohay (1993) found no association between reported habitual physical activity and lipid profile in subjects of average age 71 years. Presumably, self-selected activities did not reach the threshold required for a modification of lipid levels in these last two studies.

Longitudinal Studies

The acute effect of exercise is a transient improvement in lipid profile, which persists for a few hours (Durstine and Haskell 1994).

In longitudinal investigations of exercise programs, the improvement in resting lipid profile seems greatest when lipid values are initially high. Possible mechanisms whereby exercise could influence the lipid profile include not only a decrease in body fat content, but also changes in the activities of hormones and enzymes that control the rates of synthesis, transport, and clearance of lipids and lipoproteins from the blood (Young and Steinhardt 1993). However, controlled investigations often show little change after due allowance has been made for exercise-induced changes in plasma volume, diet, and body composition (Durstine and Haskell 1994).

Lindheim et al. (1994) had a group of postmenopausal women walk on a treadmill for 30 min three times per week. At the end of the training period, they found a 5.2% decrease in total plasma cholesterol, a 2% decrease in triglyceride concentrations, and a 10% diminution in LDL-cholesterol, but no increase in HDL-cholesterol. Schwartz et al. (1992) had 67-year-old men engage in a six-month endurance training program that included 45 min sessions of supervised exercise five days per week at up to 85% of heart rate reserve. This regimen induced a 15% increase in plasma concentrations of HDL-cholesterol, and a 63% increase in the important HDL-2-cholesterol fraction, along with a 21% decrease in plasma triglycerides and a 13% decrease in LDL-cholesterol.

In contrast to these positive findings, Coon et al. (1990) saw no change in lipid profile over a six-month training program that increased the aerobic power of 60-year-old men by 32%. Seals et al. (1984a) also found no benefit from a low-intensity exercise program, but there was a 14% increase of HDL-cholesterol in response to high-intensity exercise that caused a substantial decrease in body fat.

Some authors have argued that the total volume of physical activity required to enhance the lipid profile is substantial (corresponding to a minimum energy expenditure of 4 to 6 MJ/week, or 16 km/week of jogging in a person of average body mass; Stefanick and Wood 1994; Superko 1991). This is a volume of activity that exceeds the tolerance of many frail elderly populations, explaining some of the negative results already noted.

Tertiary and Quaternary Treatment

It is technically possible to correct severe hypercholesterolemia by a combination of an active lifestyle, dietary modification, and the administration of cholesterol-reducing drugs, at least in the young-old, but it remains debatable whether this has any beneficial effect on prognosis (Hazzard and Ettinger 1995). In particular, there remains a need to examine whether a reduction of serum cholesterol decreases nonfatal as well as fatal heart attacks; there is some evidence that although the cardiac fatality rate has been falling, the number of nonfatal attacks (which may subsequently progress to cardiac failure) has been increasing in the elderly population (Bonneux et al. 1994).

Cancers

Cancer is a multistage molecular and cellular process. Often a long silent period covering precancerous change and the initiation of metaplasia precedes the onset of metastasis. The likelihood of developing many types of tumor is also influenced by cumulative exposure to noxious physical and chemical agents in the environment. Thus, it is not surprising that the prevalence and particularly the incidence of most types of neoplasm increase with age.

Moderate occupational or leisure activity is thought to have a beneficial influence on both the overall cancer rate and the risks of developing certain specific types of tumors: carcinoma of the colon, carcinoma of the breast, and possibly cancers of the reproductive tract. On the other hand, some types of outdoor activity are associated with an increased risk of skin cancers (Greenwald et al. 1995; Kohl, Laporte, and Blair 1988; Lee 1994; Shephard 1993e, 1996; Shephard and Shek 1995a).

Prevalence and Incidence

Cancer accounts for about 20% of all deaths in the United States. In 1994, there were 1.21 million new cases and 0.54 million deaths (Boring et al. 1994). In England and Wales, people over the age of 60 years accounted for 67% of 155,000 cases registered in 1970; in 1982, this figure increased further to 75% of 197,000 cases (Wilkins 1991).

The growing number of cases that are registered reflects in part more accurate diagnosis, and in part a progressive lengthening of the average person's life span. Tumors commonly seen among those over the age of 60 years are for men, cancers of the lung, prostate, skin, stomach, and colon, and for women, cancers of the breast, skin, colon, lung, and stomach.

Lung Cancer

The prevalence of lung cancer has increased progressively, as a cohort of lifetime cigarette smokers has reached old age. The incidence of the disease currently peaks around the age of 65 years. In the United States, each year now brings about 100,000 new cases in men, and 70,000 cases in women (Perry 1994), and in the United Kingdom this form of cancer accounts for some 30,000 deaths per year (Davies 1991).

In England and Wales, respiratory deaths account for some 23% of all male and 14% of all female deaths among people over the age of 65 years (Cullinan 1988). In men, about half of these deaths are due to respiratory neoplasms (631/100,000). In women, the proportion of neoplastic deaths is as yet smaller (150/100,000), but it is moving rapidly up toward the male level as a cohort of female smokers become older.

Prostate

About 8500 cases of prostate cancer are diagnosed in Britain each year. Tumors at this site account for about 10% of all cancer deaths in men. In the United States, prostatic cancer is the second most common malignancy, and is the third most common cause of cancer death in men over the age of 55 years, with 14 deaths per 100,000 in white Americans and 22 per 100,000 in African Americans (Brendler 1994).

The prevalence of the disease among frail elderly men is much greater than these figures might suggest. As many as 50% of men over the age of 80 years have the earliest form of the condition, cancer *in situ*. Prostatic cancer is 200 times more common in the age range 60 to 80 years than it is in men aged 20 to 30 years (Green 1991).

Skin Cancers

Excessive exposure to sunlight causes solar keratoses, warty or scaly grey or pink patches on exposed skin. As many as 25% of people over the age of 65 years have lesions of this sort (Harvey et al. 1989), but fortunately only a small fraction progress to squamous cell carcinomas of the skin.

People who work outdoors, or who engage in sports in which exposure to ultraviolet light is combined with cooling from wind or water (e.g., sailors and competitors in other types of water sports), are particularly vulnerable to skin cancers.

Cancer of the Colon

Malignant tumors of the colon are often preceded by adenomas, polyps, or papillomas. Some 50% of large polyps eventually undergo a carcinomatous change. The incidence of colorectal tumors shows much geographic variation, cases being frequent in developed societies and rare in the third world. People in the United States have about a 6% lifetime chance of developing a colorectal cancer, tumors of the large intestine accounting for about 50,000 deaths per year. The incidence of the disease doubles with each decade over the age of 50 years (Cheskin and Schuster 1994).

Cancer of the Breast

The incidence of breast cancer has been increasing over the past 30 years, and it is now the most common form of cancer in women. Some 12% of women develop malignant breast tumors, and the condition now accounts for almost 50,000 deaths per year (Muss 1994). The risk rises steeply in the postmenopausal years, and approximately 60% of cases occur in those over 60 years of age.

Primary and Secondary Prevention

Evidence linking habitual physical activity and the primary prevention of tumors is almost entirely epidemiological. Both occupational and leisure activity have been examined in large-scale population surveys (Kohl, Laporte, and Blair 1988; Lee 1994; Shephard 1993e, 1996; Shephard and Shek 1995a; Sternfeld 1992). The data have been hard to interpret, because physical activity has generally been self-selected, and many other important factors (often unmeasured) have been associated with the levels of both occupational and leisure activity—for instance, socioeconomic status, cigarette smoking, alcohol consumption, obesity, diet, and overall interest in health. Moreover, it has been unclear whether these variables were important in their own right, or whether they were serving merely as surrogate markers of physical activity.

Occupational Studies

The main advantage of using occupation as an indicator of habitual physical activity is that the energy expenditure thus defined has usually been maintained over many years. This is an important issue in a process such as cancer, which has a very slow onset. However, mechanization in North America has now reduced the energy cost of most occupations to very low levels, so that except in a few specific instances, domestic chores (in women) and leisure pursuits (in men) account for a large fraction of the interindividual variation in daily energy expenditures. Moreover, job category is closely linked to socioeconomic status, involvement in active leisure pursuits, and exposure to carcinogens both at work and (because of differences in area of residence) at home. Finally, the very old have been retired for many years.

Occupational studies have often been based on job classifications, although these provide only a crude index of an individual's physical activity at work, usually at only one point early in a career. Often, the onset of illness may cause a recorded or a *de facto* change in job category. A few authors have noted the amount of time spent walking or sitting at work, or the resting heart rate of employees. A high heart rate may unfortunately reflect either a low level of physical activity (and thus a lack of fitness) or recent cigarette smoking.

Leisure Studies

Some early studies of leisure pursuits compared former athletes with nonathletes, although there was then great uncertainty as to how far university-age exercise behavior had been maintained over the adult life span. More commonly, reliance was placed on either prospective or retrospective physical questionnaires. These ranged from a single question on habitual physical activity to a detailed physical activity inventory covering many pages. In some surveys (for example the NHANES and Framingham studies) the data were not initially collected with a view to looking at linkages between habitual physical activity and the incidence of cancer, and in consequence quite limited information was obtained on leisure activity patterns.

Nevertheless, investigators are increasingly recognizing that even lengthy physical activity questionnaires provide only a very approximate indication of an individual's patterns of habitual physical activity (Shephard 1994). In particular, most questionnaires fail to elicit information about the physically demanding household tasks that have traditionally been performed by women, and many instruments also neglect the traditional active pursuits of the elderly. In a few instances (for example, Blair, Kohl, et al. 1989), inferences about activity patterns have been based on one- or two-point measurements of aerobic fitness. These are in some respects more objective than the questionnaires, but they also reflect the individual's genetic endowment and are influenced negatively by body fat content.

All-Cancer Mortality

The influence of physical activity on all-cancer death rates has been examined in at least 5 occupational and 10 leisure studies.

Occupational studies.   Only two of the five occupational studies have demonstrated an advantage to the active group, but the benefit seen in one of the positive studies (NHANES I; Albanes, Blair, and Taylor 1989) was particularly convincing, since the authors had used only a simple questionnaire classification of activity patterns, but had used multivariate techniques to control for the effects of age, race, smoking history, socioeconomic status, BMI, reproductive history, and family history. The risk ratio for sedentary work in this study was 1.8 (95% CI 1.4 to 2.4) in men and 1.3 (95% CI 1.0 to 1.8) in women.

Leisure activities.   Two studies of former athletes showed no significant association between involvement in university sport teams and subsequent protection against cancer. This apparently negative result could reflect the "athletic" subjects' loss of interest in physical activity after leaving a university, the pursuit of noncompetitive physical activities by the supposedly inactive controls, or an unfavorable influence of certain athletic builds on the risk of developing cancer.

The remaining eight studies made a more global assessment of physically active leisure. Five of the eight investigations showed varying degrees of protection against all forms of cancer. The largest effect was in a study by Blair, Kohl, et al. (1989), in which habitual physical activity was assessed by an initial treadmill test of aerobic fitness. In this eight-year prospective study, the risk ratio for the least fit quintile relative to the most fit quintile was 16.3, with benefit in both men and women. Unfortunately, 55% of deaths were untraced, and perhaps because of a small number of cancer deaths, the data were covaried only for age. A retrospective reanalysis of the data, making a correction for the likely association between fitness and smoking behavior (Shephard 1992a), did not eliminate the benefit previously ascribed to the fit members of the group.

The NHANES I study included many covariates, but had only a limited assessment of leisure activity patterns (Albanes, Blair, and Taylor 1989). This study found a marginal trend to a greater risk of cancer in inactive men (risk ratio 1.2, 95% CI 1.0 to 1.6), but no activity-related gradient of all-cancer risk in women.

Wannamethee, Shaper, and MacFarlane (1993) found that the risk ratio for all forms of cancer among patients consulting general practitioners in the United Kingdom decreased from 1.00 in those who reported no more than occasional leisure activity to 0.59 (95% CI 0.38 to 0.92) in those who reported moderate or vigorous physical activity. In the same study, the risk ratio increased from 1.00 in persons whose resting heart rate was less than 60 beats/min to 2.25 (95% CI 1.34 to 2.28) in patients with resting heart rates in the range 80 to 90 beats/min. The data were covaried for age, smoking behavior, cholesterol, and BMI, so high resting heart rates were presumably attributable to a lack of habitual physical activity.

Conclusions.   We may conclude that both occupational and leisure activity are associated with a general trend toward protection against all-cancer deaths. Moreover, this association persists even after adjustment of the data for BMI, so it is likely that exercise is exerting a part of its benefit through mechanisms other than the control of body fatness.

These other mechanisms of primary prevention could be relatively direct—for example, a stimulating effect of regular moderate activity on such aspects of immune function as natural killer cell activity (Shephard 1996; Shephard and Shek 1995a). Alternatively, benefit might come through a change of lifestyle induced by exercise (for example, a cessation of cigarette smoking), or through an indirect association between habitual physical activity and an overall interest in health.

Colon Cancers

The evidence of benefit from habitual physical activity is perhaps most convincing in terms of tumors of the transverse and descending colons. Protection does not seem to extend to rectal tumors (Shephard 1993e, 1996). The relative risk of colonic tumors has been analyzed in at least 18 occupational studies and in 15 studies of leisure-time or total physical activity.

Occupational activity. The occupational studies have been remarkably consistent, with 15 of the 18 investigations showing a significant advantage to active individuals (see table 7.7). However, the interpretation of some of these studies is difficult, because only a limited number of covariates were included in the analyses.

In the well-controlled NHANES I study (Albanes, Blair, and Taylor 1989), the average risk ratio for males with a job demanding little physical activity was substantial (1.6), but not statistically significant.

A case control study by Peters et al. (1989) found that a low level of job activity was associated with a risk ratio of 3.0 (95% CI 1.2 to 7.2) for cancer of the transverse or descending colon, even after control of the data for age, race, BMI, diet, and occupational exposure to carcinogens. Gerhardsson et al. (1986) followed 1.1 million Swedes for 19 years; they found a risk ratio of 1.3 (95% CI 1.2 to 1.5) for a sedentary job after control of results for age, population density, marital status, socioeconomic status, and religion.

The one study in which physical activity apparently showed a nonsignificant adverse effect (male San Francisco dock workers) was for a job category in which the intensity of occupational activity had decreased dramatically over the course of the study. The originally assigned job classifications thus had only limited relevance to the recent physical activity patterns of the subjects (Paffenbarger, Hyde, and Wing 1987).

Leisure activity. The majority of studies of active leisure also point to benefit from exercise, with 10 of 15 investigations showing a significant inverse association between reported habitual physical activity and the risk of colon cancers. Four of the five studies in which no association was seen relied on either university involvement in sport or a single question to classify habitual activity. In many instances, the number of covariates was less than optimal, but benefit apparently persisted in those studies that adjusted for interindividual differences in diet, body build, or both.

Table 7.7   Association between lack of physical activity and deaths from colon cancers.

Author	Subjects	Activity index	Risk ratio (95% CI)	Covariates
Occupational activity				
Albanese et al. (1989)	12,554 NHANES 10-12 yr incidence	*Nonrecreational activity*		Age
		Highly active	1.0	
		Moderately active	1.2 (0.7-2.2) (M)	
		Low activity	1.6 (0.7-3.5) (M)	
		Moderately active	1.3 (0.8-2.2) (F)	
		Low activity	1.3 (0.3-2.0) (F)	
Brownson et al. (1991)	1838 M cases 14,309 controls	*Job classification*		Age
		Highly active	1.0	
		Moderately active	1.1 (1.0-1.3)	
		Low activity	1.2 (1.0-1.5)	
Fredriksson et al. (1989)	370 cases 658 controls (incidence)	*Self-reported job*		Age, sex
		Highly active	0.49 (.25-.93)	
		Moderately active	0.73 (.48-1.2)	
		Low activity	1.00	
Garabrant et al. (1984)	3779 M (all colon cancers LA county 1972/81	*Job classification*		Age, race, SES
		Highly active	1.00	
		Moderately active	1.61	
		Low activity	1.84 (1.62-2.2)	
Gerhardsson et al. (1986)	1.1 million M Swedes, 19 yr incidence	*Job classification*		Age, population density, SES, marital status, religion
		Active	1.0	
		Sedentary	1.3 (1.2-1.5)	

Study	Description	Activity measure	Result	Adjustments
Gerhardsson et al. (1988)	Swedish twins 14 yr colon cancer incidence	*Self-reported job* Highly active Moderately active	1.0 1.6 (1.0-2.7)	Age, sex, meat and coffee intake
Marti and Minder (1989)	1995 M cases	*Job classification* Active Inactive	1.0 1.35	Age
Paffenbarger et al. (1987)	6351 M dockers (22 yr deaths)	*Job classification* Highly active Moderately active Low activity	1.00 0.43 0.85 (ns)	Age, BP, "heavy" smoking
Peters et al. (1989)	147 cases < 45 yr 147 controls	*Job classification* Highly active Moderately active Low activity	0.8 (0.2-2.7) 1.0 3.0 (1.2-7.2)	Age, race, BMI, diet, occupational exposure
Vena et al. (1985)	486 M cases 1431 controls (incidence)	*Years sedentary work* None 1-20 yr > 20 yr	1.00 1.49 1.97 (p < .001)	Age
Vena et al. (1987)	455,000 M,F (proportional mortality)	*Usual occupation* Highly active Moderately high activity Moderately low activity Low activity	89 (M), 80 (F) 95 (M), 106 (F) 113 (M), — 120 (M), 113 (F)	Age

(continued)

Table 7.7   *(continued)*

Author	Subjects	Activity index	Risk ratio (95% CI)	Covariates
Whittemore et al. (1990)	905 cases 2448 controls (Chinese)	*Self-reported job* Active Inactive (M) Inactive (F)	1.0 1.4 (0.6-3.5) 1.7 (0.6-5.2)	Age, sex, body size, diet, time since migration
Leisure activity				
Albanes et al. (1989)	12,554 NHANES 10-11 yr incidence	*Self-reported activity* Highly active Moderately active Low activity Moderately active (F) Low activity (F)	1.00 1.0 (0.5-1.9) (M) 1.0 (0.5-0.9) (M) 1.2 (0.7-1.3) (F) 1.2 (0.6-2.8) (F)	Age, race, SES
Ballard-Barbash et al. (1990)	4214 M and F 28 yr incidence	*Self-reported activity* Highly active Moderately active (M) Low activity (M) Moderately active (F) Low activity (F)	1.00 1.4 (0.8-2.6) 1.8 (1.0-3.2) 1.2 (0.7-2.1) 1.1 (0.6-1.8)	Age, BMI, smoking, education, cholesterol, alcohol
Gerhardsson et al. (1988)	16,447 twins 14 yr incidence	*Self reported activity* Highly active Light activity Low/ no activity	1.00 1.7 (1.0-2.8) 1.3 (0.6-2.6)	Age, sex, meat and coffee intake, region
Gerhardsson et al. (1990)	569 cases 512 controls	*Self-reported activity* Highly active Moderately active Inactive	1.00 1.4 (0.9-2.2) 1.8 (1.0-3.4)	Age, sex, BMI

Kune et al. (1990)	202 M, 190 F; 398, 329 controls	Total physical activity reported; ns effect		
Lee et al. (1991)	17,148 alumnae; 11-15 yr incidence	Self-reported activity: >10.5 MJ/week; >4.2 MJ/week; <4.2 MJ/week	0.50 (0.27-0.93); 0.52 (0.28-0.92); 1.00	Age
Markowitz et al. (1992)	440 M; 1156 controls	Self-reported activity: Active; Inactive	1.00; 1.4 (1.1-2.0)	22-44 yr
Paffenbarger et al. (1987)	56,683 M	College athletics: Active; Inactive	1.10; 1.00	
Persky et al. (1981)	1233 M, 1899 M; 5784 M	Resting heart rate; ns effect		
Polednak (1976)	8393 alumnae	College athletics; ns effect		
Severson et al. (1989)	8066 Hawaiian M (incidence)	Self-reported activity: Highly active; Moderate activity; Low activity	0.71 (0.51-0.99); 0.56 (0.39-0.80); 1.00	Age, BMI, smoking

(continued)

Table 7.7 *(continued)*

Author	Subjects	Activity index	Risk ratio (95% CI)	Covariates
Slattery et al. (1988)	229 cases 384 controls	*Self-reported activity* Highly active Light activity Highly active Moderately active Light activity Inactive	0.27 (0.11-0.65) (M) 0.83 (0.4-1.75) (M) 0.48 (0.27-0.87) (F) 0.91 (0.56-1.60) (F) 0.97 (0.56-1.69) (F) 1.00 (M and F)	Age, BMI
Whittemore et al. (1990)	905 cases 2488 controls N.A. N.A. China China	*Self-reported activity* Active Inactive (M) Inactive (F) Inactive (M) Inactive (F)	1.0 1.6 (1.1-2.4) 2.0 (1.2-3.3) 0.85 (0.39-1.9) 2.5 (1.0-6.3)	Fat intake, weight for height, time in North
Wu et al. (1987)	11,888 M and F	*Self-reported activity* Active (M) Active (F) Inactive	0.4 (0.2-0.8) 0.89 (0.5-1.6) 1.0	Smoking, BMI, alcohol

Note: For details of references not discussed in text, see Shephard (1993e and 1996).

Conclusions.   There seems to be good evidence of an association between regular physical activity and protection against colon cancers. The most commonly suggested mechanism of prevention has been that exercise stimulates a faster passage of food through the large intestine, thus allowing less time for carcinogens to provoke a carcinoma. Other possibilities include differences in diet between active and inactive individuals, a greater consumption of aspirin by those who are vigorously active, and exercise-induced changes of immune function.

Breast Cancers

At least 3 occupational and 10 leisure studies have looked at habitual activity and malignant tumors of the breast. One other study looked at benign tumors of the breast (see table 7.8).

Occupational activity.   Two of the three occupational studies showed a favorable effect of physical activity at work. In the third, which involved teachers, activity was inferred from the type of class taught; language teachers had a risk ratio that did not depart significantly from the population average, but in the case of the physical education teachers the risk was less than anticipated.

Leisure activities.   The data from leisure studies are somewhat confusing; in three studies, the benefit was statistically significant, but in two other well-designed studies (Dorgan et al. 1994; Sternfeld et al. 1995), the risk of breast cancer was greater for exercisers than for nonexercisers. Part of the discrepancy might be age-related, since the two negative studies were on older subjects.

Other well-controlled studies suggested some benefit of physical activity at work (Albanes, Blair, and Taylor 1989; Frisch et al. 1987; Giglia 1992), with respective risk ratios of 1.8 (not significant), 1.5 (not significant), and 1.35 (just significant).

Conclusions.   Although there is some suggestion that regular physical activity reduces the risk of breast cancer, further study is necessary to reach a definite conclusion. One possible protective mechanism would be a reduction of body fat content in those who exercise regularly, although in the three studies in which exercisers demonstrated favorable risk ratios, statistical allowance was made for body size or BMI.

Other Tumors of the Female Reproductive Tract

Frisch et al. (1987) carried out a well-controlled study of other female reproductive tract tumors (ovary, uterus, cervix, and vagina), comparing the prevalence in former university athletes with that seen in their nonathletic peers. Evidence was offered that both groups had sustained their respective patterns of habitual physical activity into later adult life, and a substantially in-

Table 7.8   Association between habitual physical activity and deaths from breast cancer.

Author	Subjects	Activity index	Risk ratio (95% CI)	Covariates
Occupational activity				
Vena et al. (1987)	25,000 women	*Usual occupation* Moderate to high Light activity Sedentary	1.00 0.97 1.35	Age
Vihko et al. (1992)	3447 PE teachers 997 language teachers	*Teaching category* Physical education Languages	1.3 (ns)[+] 1.6 (p < .001)	Age
Zheng et al. (1993)			Significant inverse association	
Leisure activity				
Albanes et al. (1989)	7408 women	*Self-report* Premenopausal Inactive Postmenopausal Inactive	1.0 0.4 (0.1-1.8) 1.0 1.5 (0.7-2.8)	Age, race, smoking, SES, BMI, diet, reproductive history
Bernstein et al. (1994)	545 cases 545 controls	*Self-report* Highly active Inactive	1.00 2.38 (1.56-3.70)	
Dorgan et al. (1994)	2307 women	*Physician questionnaire*	1.6 (active, ns) 1.0	Reproductve history

Frisch et al. (1987)*	5398 alumnae	*College activity*		Age at menarche, age, body size, no. of pregnancies, family history
		Active	1.0	
		Inactive	1.8 (1.0-3.5)	
Giglia (1992)	89,935 women (prospective case control study)	*Self-report*		Smoking, obesity, reproductive history, family history
		Vigorous activity	0.74 (.56-.99)	
		Moderate activity	0.87 (.78-.99)	
		Inactive	1.00	
		Active	0.88 (.78-.99)	
		Inactive	1.00	
Paffenbarger et al. (1987)	4706 alumnae	*College activity*		Age
		Active	1.00	
		Inactive	1.04 (ns)	
Sternfeld et al. (1995)	301 cases	*Self-report*		
	248 controls	Active	1.00	
		Inactive	0.53 (0.27-1.02)	

*Prevalence study; ⁺standardized incidence ratio.
Note: For details of references not listed in text, see Shephard (1993e and 1996).

creased risk ratio (2.5, 95% CI 1.2 to 5.5) was found in the nonathletes. Albanes, Blair, and Taylor (1989) applied a simple activity classification to the NHANES data; they also found a high risk of cervical cancer in women who were classed as inactive (5.2), although in their study the increase of risk was not statistically significant. These two studies were adjusted for body size and BMI, respectively.

Levi et al. (1993) found that a low total physical activity was associated with a 2.4- to 8.6-fold increase in the incidence of uterine cancer. In contrast, Zheng et al. (1993) found no association between occupational activity and uterine or ovarian cancer, and Mink et al. (in press) found a twofold *increase* of risk of ovarian cancer in the most active women.

Plainly, further studies are needed before a firm conclusion can be reached regarding the influence of physical activity on cancer of the female reproductive tract.

Male Reproductive Tract Tumors

Five of six occupational studies have suggested some association between a sedentary job and an increased risk of prostate cancer (Shephard 1996), with the trend reaching statistical significance in three of these reports. However, LeMarchand, Kolonel, and Yoshizawa (1991) found a trend in the opposite direction, significant in men > 70 years of age. In the best-controlled investigation (Albanes, Blair, and Taylor 1989), the benefit from active employment was not statistically significant (risk ratio 1.3, 95% CI 0.7 to 2.4).

In terms of leisure activity, seven major studies have looked at prostate cancer and two at testicular cancer. Three studies showed a significant inverse relationship between prostatic cancer and active leisure pursuits (Albanes, Blair, and Taylor 1989; Lee, Paffenbarger, and Hsieh 1992a; Severson et al. 1989), and a fourth (Thune and Lund 1994) showed a similar tendency. Against these results must be set two studies of former athletes (Paffenbarger, Hyde, and Wing 1987; Polednak 1976), each of which found increased risks of prostate cancer among men who had been active during their college days. One study (U.K. Testicular Cancer Study Group 1994) found that regular physical inactivity was associated with a twofold increase in the risk of testicular carcinomas. A second study, by Thune and Lund (1994), found that occupational (but not leisure) activity was associated with an *increased* risk of testicular cancer.

As in the female, more research is needed before firm conclusions can be reached about physical activity and the prevention of tumors of the male reproductive tract.

Tumors at Other Sites

There is no strong evidence that exercise is helpful in preventing tumors at other body sites.

Tertiary and Quaternary Treatment

Most investigations of physical activity during the later stages of cancer have been based on animal models. In general, physical activity has retarded the growth of implanted tumors, although the effect has commonly been greatest at moderate intensities of exercise, with a lessening of benefit if animals were exercised more intensely (Shephard 1993e, 1996; Thompson et al. 1988). Hoffman-Goetz and Husted (1995) also noted that if a tumor is metastasizing, vigorous physical activity may promote the adhesion of tumor cells to the walls of blood vessels and their subsequent penetration of the endothelium, thus exacerbating the disease process.

Research in humans has involved only small numbers of subjects, and it has been difficult to control for such variables as tumor size, the short-term effects of recent irradiation or chemotherapy, and overall debility. In general, the high metabolic demand of the tumor, the production of tumor necrosis factor, a depression of mood state, and a poor appetite lead to a vicious cycle of wasting of lean tissue, lack of physical activity, and generalized weakness (Bruera et al. 1984, 1987; Dewys and Kisner 1982). Often the initial exercise capacity of the cancer patient is in the range 3 to 6 METs (10.5-21.0 ml/[kg · min]), with a hemoglobin level of less than 10 g/dl and a platelet count of less than $50,000/mm^3$ (American College of Sports Medicine 1995a).

Moderate physical activity helps in elevating mood, stimulating appetite, and maintaining lean tissue mass, at least in the early stages of tumor development (Dietz 1981; Whittaker et al. 1991). By enhancing the patient's general physical condition, it also increases the quality of the remaining months or years of life.

However, the prescribed activity program must take account of possible electrolyte imbalances, dehydration, and an increased risk of hemorrhage and pathological bone fractures. If there are actual or potential bone metastases, non-weight-bearing exercises should be recommended. Severe anemia and a low platelet count are other indications for a cautious approach to exercise (Winningham, MacVicar, and Burke 1986). It is important to adopt a flexible attitude to the filling of an exercise prescription, since on some days the patient may be badly affected by the nausea and malaise that follow chemotherapy and irradiation. Nevertheless, MacVicar, Winningham, and Nickel (1989) noted a decrease of nausea and a 40% increase of symptom-limited aerobic power when women with stage II breast cancer undertook 10 weeks of exercise three times a week at 60% to 85% of the heart rate reserve.

In cases where a tumor has been "cured," low levels of fitness may persist because of fear on the part of the patient or the supervising physician. However, both physiological and psychological condition can generally be enhanced by a program of progressive exercise (Turchetta et al. 1990).

Conclusions

In essence, metabolic health depends on striking an appropriate balance between the intake and the expenditure of food energy. Problems such as obesity, diabetes, and hypercholesterolemia can thus be addressed by drugs that reduce appetite or in other ways restrict the intake of food, by voluntary restriction of eating, or by an increase of daily physical activity. The recommendation of exercise has the virtue of being positive advice that allows the continued intake of adequate amounts of important vitamins and minerals. Further, exercise is a natural form of activity that has the potential to enhance rather than depress mood state. Finally, it carries many additional benefits that are not obtained from dieting or drug treatment, including not only the well-recognized cardiovascular and musculoskeletal effects discussed in chapters 5 and 6, but also a reduction in the risk of a number of types of malignancy, particularly cancers of the colon, and in women cancers of the breast and reproductive tract.

Chapter 8

Physical Activity, Function, and Well-Being

Aging is associated with a variety of physical and psychological impairments. Often this makes it difficult for individuals to undertake certain actions (they suffer a disability); depending on their motivation, environmental circumstances, and reactions to the disability, those who are so affected may also be handicapped (unable to carry out desired activities). The consequence of such a handicap is a deterioration in the quality of life.

The average senior citizen spends a substantial period with some type of disability: about 10.8 years for men and 14.0 years for women (Spirduso 1995). During the final year of life, he or she may be almost totally disabled. The resulting handicap is a progressive loss of independence (Health and Welfare, Canada 1982). Many of the very old face a substantial and growing deterioration in the quality of life and thus a substantial discrepancy between their calendar longevity and their quality-adjusted life expectancy (Shephard in press-a). One very important objective of an exercise program for the senior citizen is thus to increase the quality-adjusted life expectancy of the participant; this is a much more significant goal than the mere extension of total life span (which has frequently been the focus of attention). In the present chapter, the issues of disability and quality of life are discussed further.

Physical Disability

Studies of physical disability among the frail elderly typically examine an individual's ability to undertake the basic activities of daily living (see table 8.1)—items such as eating, dressing, bathing, and moving around independently. However, from the viewpoint of the quality of life, what have been termed intermediate and advanced activities of daily living are of at least equal significance. Intermediate activities include items such as housekeeping, shopping, and transportation; advanced activities reflect voluntary pursuits such as travel,

Table 8.1 Fourteen groups of items rating ability to perform the basic activities of daily living (modified Barthel Index, based in part on Granger et al. 1979).

Drinking from a cup
Able to drink from cup, pour liquids, and open a carton

Eating from a plate
Able to cut meat, butter bread, and eat from a standard plate

Clothing upper body
Able to take clothes from a drawer or closet, put on a waistcoat or blouse opening at the front, and do up the buttons

Clothing lower body
Able to take clothes from a drawer or closet, put on trousers and socks or stockings

Capable of fitting a prosthesis
Capable of fitting a prosthesis without help

Personal hygiene
Capable of brushing teeth, combing hair, and shaving or applying makeup; capable of bathing without assistance, including washing and drying

Bladder control
Complete voluntary control

Rectal control
Complete voluntary control without laxatives, suppositories, colonic lavage, or rectal stimulation

Transfer to and from chair
Able to move to and from chair safely without aid

Transfer to and from toilet seat
Able to move to and from toilet seat safely without aid

Transfer to and from bath
Able to get into and out of bath safely without aid

Walking ability
Able to get up, sit down, and walk 50 m with or without a walking aid

Stair-climbing ability
Able to go up and down stairs without aid or means of support

Ability to operate manual wheelchair
In those unable to walk, ability to maneuver wheelchair around tables, to toilet, and up or down ramps with a limited slope

Note: A score is assigned for each activity, depending on the individual's ability to perform the task, ranging from 7 units (total ability to perform the task), through need of some assistance, task modification, or a longer performance time (4 units) to totally dependent (1 unit).

hobbies or recreational exercise, employment (if desired), and participation in social and religious groups (Reuben et al. 1990).

There is a wide range of pathological causes of physical impairment, for example, specific neurological conditions such as a stroke or a myopathy, deafness, and a progressive failure or a sudden loss of vision. However, often the impairment has a simpler physiological basis; muscle strength, cardiorespiratory power, or flexibility has decreased to below the critical minimum value needed to perform the desired activity. The extent of the resulting handicap depends greatly on the assistance that can be provided by a spouse or relative and on the ability to accommodate the impairment by making appropriate changes in the immediate living environment (Svänborg 1985).

Prevalence of Disability

Some 20% of U.S. seniors were functionally disabled in 1985, with about a third of these being confined to their homes; moreover, projections suggested that the proportion of disabled individuals would rise progressively to 30% by the year 2060, to a total approaching 10 million people (Kunkel and Appelbaum 1992; Manton 1989). More than 1.5 million U.S. citizens reside in nursing homes; a similar number have accepted other sheltered living arrangements, or receive home-care or day-care services (Ouslander 1994). Some authors have suggested that a further 5 million receive informal care from family and friends, and as many as another million do not receive such care but are in need of it.

The Canada Health Survey (1982) found that during the final 8 to 10 years of life, most people developed some type of disability that reduced their quality of life. Problems included not only general frailty, but also pathological conditions ranging from occasional arthritis to a stroke or poorly compensated congestive cardiac failure. The Health and Activity Limitation Survey (Statistics Canada 1986) reported that 83% of adults aged 75 to 84 years, and 89% of those over the age of 85 years, had disabilities that limited their agility and mobility. In a more recent survey, 25% of Canadians over the age of 85 years classed themselves as having moderate disability, but 64% considered that they were severely disabled (Health and Welfare, Canada 1993). As early as 55 years of age, some 10% of Canadian women and 2% of Canadian men were unable to carry their groceries alone, but in those over the age of 80 years, the prevalence of this particular handicap had risen to 30% of women and 20% of men (Statistics Canada 1985).

In Britain, a total of 2.1 million men and 5.2 million women were unable to walk on a level surface at a pace of 4.8 km/h. When presented with a moderate slope, the numbers who could not maintain this speed increased to 5.6 million men and 11.7 million women. Furthermore, this total included 81% of all men and 92% of all women aged 65 to 74 years (Sports Council and the Health Education Authority 1992).

Coroni-Huntley et al. (1986) provided more detailed information on the extent of specific disabilities in the middle-old and the very old (see table 8.2). In each of three United States populations, the combined effects of aging and disease had brought aerobic power, muscle strength, flexibility, or some combination of these three variables down to a level that prevented many of those questioned from performing various common daily activities without assistance. The process may be envisaged most easily for aerobic power, where function declines by approximately 5 ml/[kg · min] per decade. The critical level that permits performance of many of the tasks of daily living (Shephard 1987a) is probably in the range of 12 to 14 ml/[kg · min], and for the senior who begins retirement with an aerobic power of 25 ml/[kg · min], the threshold of functional incompetence is likely to be broached somewhere between 80 and 85 years of age (Guralnik et al. 1993). Likewise, a progressive deterioration in muscle strength causes problems with such daily activities as opening jars, carrying parcels, and lifting the body mass from a chair, toilet seat, or bed (Bassey et al. 1992).

Primary and Secondary Prevention

Regular involvement in physical activity plainly can delay the time when functional capacity declines to the critical threshold for a loss of independence. Indeed, given that habitual physical activity has little influence upon the longevity of the middle-old and very old, it is quite possible that the active senior will die of some intercurrent disease before function has decreased to the critical level at which independent living can no longer be sustained (Shephard 1987a).

This point can again be illustrated in terms of aerobic power, although similar calculations are possible for muscle strength and flexibility. Let us suppose that the difference in aerobic power between an active and a sedentary person at any given age is 10 ml/[kg · min]. It will then take 20 years longer for the aerobic power of an active individual to decrease to the critical level of 12 to 14 ml/[kg · min]; this person would be 100 to 105 rather than 80 to 85 years of age when institutionalization was required, and the likelihood of his or her survival to this age would be quite small.

Cross-Sectional Studies

Kohl, Moorefield, and Blair (1987) noted an association between aerobic fitness and the prevalence of chronic fatigue, even in middle-aged individuals. Likewise, Avlund et al. (1994) reported that in 75-year-old Danish subjects a poor performance on a stepping task (the highest step the subject could climb without a handrail) was associated with dependence in mobility and other activities of daily living for men and with tiredness for women. A poor performance on a walking test was also associated with tiredness in both sexes. Moreover, the findings of Avlund et al. (1994) showed a dose-response rela-

Table 8.2 Percentages of three populations showing specific limitations of ability in the ninth decade of life.

	East Boston				New Haven				Rural Iowa			
	80-84 yr		>85 yr		80-84 yr		>85 yr		80-84 yr		>85 yr	
	M	F	M	F	M	F	M	F	M	F	M	F
Walk across room	12	23	22	38	8	9	10	31	10	15	17	22
From bed to chair	4	14	11	22	1	8	5	14	8	9	8	9
Climb stairs	15	31	29	50	12	12	10	30	12	17	16	26
Heavy house-work	57	70	74	89	31	54	53	68	43	56	68	69
Use toilet	3	12	12	19	2	5	1	8	6	8	7	10

Data for three U.S. populations.
Based on data of Coroni-Huntley et al. (1986).

tionship, protection from a loss of the activities of daily living being greater among those who habitually engaged in the heavier physical activities.

The findings from these various cross-sectional surveys could be explained if habitual physical activity conserved or improved functional ability (Manton 1989). However, it is also quite possible that physical activity acts indirectly, by preventing chronic disease or by enhancing mood state. A third possibility is that because function has been preserved or disease avoided, the individuals concerned are able to sustain a greater habitual physical activity than their peers. Hawkins and Duncan (1991) attempted to disentangle the various possible causes of an enhanced life quality by applying a structural equation (the Lisrel VII statistical model) to their data. They concluded that regular physical activity was associated with greater life satisfaction, less depression, fewer physical disabilities, greater self-esteem, and a more internal locus of control. Further information about these various benefits of an active lifestyle is given in later sections of this chapter.

Longitudinal Studies

Strawbridge et al. (1992) noted that over a six-year follow-up, about a fourth of seniors who were initially independent became dependent. However, both retrospective (Shephard and Montelpare 1988) and prospective data (Bokovy and Blair 1994; Morey et al. 1991) suggest that people who are active and fit in later middle age are less likely to develop disability as they become older.

Shephard and Montelpare (1988) made a retrospective evaluation of senior citizens. Those who reported a high level of habitual physical activity at the age of 50 years had an increased likelihood of continuing to live without disability as a senior (see table 8.3).

Kaplan, Feeny, and Revicki (1993) made a longitudinal study of seniors living in Alameda County, California. The loss of functional ability over a six-year interval was associated with initial responses to a five-item habitual physical activity inventory. LaCroix et al. (1993) conducted a four-year prospective study of subjects who were initially aged 65 years and older. Those who reported such activities as frequent walks, gardening, or vigorous exercise when first examined had an increased likelihood of maintaining their ability to walk 800 m or to go up and down a flight of stairs without assistance. Lifestyle factors associated with a loss of functional ability included cigarette smoking, a substantial alcohol consumption, and a large BMI.

The longitudinal studies provide stronger evidence that the onset of disability is prevented by regular physical activity, although it remains arguable that the performance of those who initially were less active may have been limited by subclinical disease. It is also unclear how far any exercise-related reduction in disability reflects greater aerobic power, muscle strength, and flexibility and how far it is due to a change of mood state or a reduction in chronic disease. Robine and Ritchie (1991) attributed all of the normally observed loss of disability-free life expectancy to specific diseases (see table 8.4), although the main causes of disability in their study were cardiovascular, locomotor, and respiratory problems.

Secondary Prevention

Analogous theoretical arguments may be advanced to justify the secondary prevention of disability by exercise programs. A senior who begins an exercise program to enhance aerobic fitness is likely to improve his or her maximal oxygen intake by at least 5 ml/[kg · min] (see chapter 4), with parallel

Table 8.3   Relationship between retrospectively reported level of physical activity at age 50 years and level of current disability as a senior citizen.

Activity at age 50 years (Arbitrary units, mean ± SD)	Level of disability
9.3 ± 9.8 (n = 286)	None
8.1 ± 8.9 (n = 126)	Minor
7.7 ± 9.4 (n = 173)	Major
4.1 ± 6.6 (n = 25)	Institutionalized

Adapted, by permission, from R.J. Shephard and W.M. Montelpare, 1988, "Geriatric benefits of exercise as an adult," *Journal of Gerontology* 43: M86-90. © The Gerontological Society of America.

Table 8.4   Anticipated gain of life expectancy and of disability-free years if different causes of ill health were to be eliminated.

Cause	Life expectancy (years)	Disability-free life expectancy (years)	Total (years)
Circulatory diseases	4.1	4.2	8.3
Locomotor disorders	0.2	5.1	5.3
Respiratory disorders	0.5	2.2	2.7
Malignant neoplasms	1.7	0.3	2.0
Injuries	1.5	0.4	1.9
Vision and hearing		1.1	1.1
Mental disorders	0.4	0.6	1.0
Diabetes	0.2	0.7	0.9
Perinatal mortality	0.7		0.7
Infectious diseases	0.1	0.2	0.3

Adapted, by permission, from J-M. Robine and K. Ritchie, 1991, "Healthy-life expectancy: Evaluation of a global indicator of change in population health," *British Medical Journal* 302: 457-460.

gains in muscle strength and flexibility. Moreover, such gains should delay the onset of disability and institutionalization by around 10 years.

Tertiary and Quaternary Treatment

Relatively little is known about the feasibility of restoring independence once disability has appeared.

At first inspection, it seems unlikely that measures such as chair exercises will be of sufficient intensity and duration to restore a useful walking ability. Nevertheless, available data are encouraging. Sulman and Wilkinson (1989) made uncontrolled observations on hospital patients over the age of 70 years; 45 min sessions of seated exercise five times per week for six months substantially improved the performance of such activities as eating and dressing. Fiatarone et al. (1994) also demonstrated valuable gains of muscular strength among institutionalized residents of a nursing home in response to a program of heavy weight-lifting resistance exercise.

O'Hagan, Smith, and Pileggi (1994) carried out a one-year controlled trial on a small group of frail nursing home residents. The average age of their sample was 83 years. Exercise classes for 1 h once a week and for 10 min twice a week enhanced the function of the experimental group, reducing the time needed for an individual to move from a sitting to a standing position and also diminishing the need for hand assistance during the process. McMurdo and Rennie (1993) studied 81-year-old residents of nursing homes in Dundee. Their activity group undertook seven months of seated exercises designed to increase the range of motion at major joints and to strengthen both upper and lower limbs. Scores improved on the Barthel Index (a method of scoring the activities of daily living), the sit-and-reach test (an index of spinal flexibility), and the chair to stand test. In contrast, a deterioration of performance was observed in a control reminiscence group who had received equal social contact and interaction with project staff.

Quality of Life

Perhaps because death is an easily measured endpoint, many epidemiologists have focused on overall longevity as a measure of the benefit that can be achieved from the adoption of an active lifestyle. However, such an assessment is unsatisfactory whether examined from the viewpoint of young or of elderly individuals. Because of time discounting, many young adults are not impressed by the possibility that exercise might delay a death that is in any event some 50 or 60 years distant. In the case of the frail elderly, the mere prolongation of life—whether by rigorous exercise or by high-technology medicine—again may not in itself be a particularly enticing or pleasant prospect.

The World Health Organization (1948) recognized some 50 years ago that health was not simply the absence of disease: it implied a state of complete physical, social, and mental well-being. This broader definition of health has been accepted increasingly by the medical and scientific communities. Interest has thus shifted from a simple maximization of survival and associated measures of life expectancy to such statistics as healthy life expectancy (Robine and Ritchie 1991), active life expectancy (Kinsella 1992), and quality-adjusted life expectancy (Butler 1992; Fitzpatrick et al. 1992; Kaplan 1985; Shephard 1982a; Wood-Dauphinee and Küchler 1992).

Quality-Adjusted Life Years

The concept of quality-adjusted life years (QALY) is best illustrated by a simple example. The overall quality of life for any given person can be envisaged as lying on a continuum. At one end of the scale is an optimal quality of life. This can be assigned a value of 1.00, so that for each calendar year of survival, the individual gains one QALY. At the other end of the scale, the quality of life drops to near zero, as a person presses for euthanasia, refuses to eat, or in some other manner expresses a loss of the will to survive. Such a state can be assigned a multiplier of zero. In other words, an added calendar year of survival has no influence on QALY. The quality of life at various points throughout the life span having been rated, the total of QALY can be calculated by integrating the (calendar year × quality of life) product over the individual's life course.

The life of the average adult is not Utopian, so the quality multiplier for the period 30 through 65 years of age might be 0.9 rather than 1.0. During the next 10 years, the quality of survival might drop to a coefficient of 0.5 to 0.8 as a variety of chronic disabilities develop. In the final year of life, when dependency becomes progressively more complete, the calendar survival might need to be multiplied by a quality coefficient of no more than 0.2 to 0.5. The potential to increase QALY by exercise and other health and lifestyle measures could then be summarized as shown in table 8.5. In this example, the individual who exercises regularly would have a total potential for a gain in QALY of 6.0 to 10.3 years, without any change in calendar longevity. This is a large figure relative to the one- to two-year extension of calendar life span that can be achieved by beginning regular exercise in middle age (as discussed in chapter 4).

For most people, the major deterioration in the quality of life occurs during the retirement years, as the effects of diminishing functional capacity and chronic disease become sufficient to limit the performance of normal daily activities. The issue of quality-adjusted life expectancy is thus of particular importance to our consideration of physical activity and aging.

Measuring Quality of Life

Early investigators represented the quality of life by a single number. More recently it has been recognized that the perceived quality of life at any given instant is a Gestalt that the individual forms by integrating current personal status with respect to a wide range of perceptions of health, function, and mood state. The QALY reflects an integration of this instantaneous perception over the person's entire life span. During the final years of a person's life, there is a strong interaction between the perceived quality of life and the environment in which the person must live. The availability of adapted housing and simple aids to daily living can make a substantial difference to the quality of this life stage (Hart et al. 1990).

Table 8.5 Hypothetical calculation illustrating the potential to increase a person's quality-adjusted life years by adoption of an exercise program.

Age range (years)	Potential change (quality coefficient)	Gain in QALY (years)
30-65	$0.9 \rightarrow 1.0$	$(0.1) \times 35 = 3.5$
65-75	$(0.5\text{-}0.8) \rightarrow 1.0$	$([0.2\text{-}0.5]) \times 10 = 2.0\text{-}5.0$
75-76	$(0.2\text{-}0.5) \rightarrow 1.0$	$([0.5\text{-}0.8]) \times 1 = 0.5\text{-}0.8$

Kaplan's Technique

Kaplan (1985) was one of the first to make a more detailed assessment of the quality of life. He suggested that the perceived quality reflected an appropriately weighted combination of both functional status and perceived symptoms.

Among functional concerns, Kaplan listed the following:

- Mobility (a five-point scale, ranging from ability to drive a car or board a bus to a chronic need for specialized hospital care)
- Physical activity (a four-level scale, ranging from the ability to walk without problems to confinement to a bed or chair)
- Social activity (a five-point scale extending from participation in employment, housework, and other activities to a need for help with the most elementary aspects of personal care)

Perceived symptoms were listed in the form of 35 symptom complexes, such as pain, stiffness, numbness or discomfort of neck, hands, feet, arms, legs, or several joints.

Kaplan then used a random sample of citizens to assign desirability weightings to each of the combinations of mobility, physical activity, and social activity on a scale ranging from zero (death) to 1.00 (optimal function); he adjusted the resulting scores by a constant corresponding to any reported symptom complex. The integral of this score over time (both as observed in the past and as anticipated in the future) was then used to calculate the likely quality-adjusted life span for a given person.

Generic Questionnaires

Some instruments, such as the Sickness Impact Profile (Bergner et al. 1981) and the Nottingham Scale (Hunt, McEwen, and McKenna 1986), ask subjects to respond to a generic questionnaire. Such questionnaires rate a wide range of elements of health (physical, social, and emotional function), role performance, and pain and other symptoms.

The questionnaire responses are generally reliable, but in order to cover a wide range of possible clinical problems, subjects are asked many questions that may be perceived as irrelevant to their personal condition. This reduces cooperation and weakens the sensitivity of the instrument (Patrick and Deyo 1989). Moreover, because the questionnaire is lengthy, subjects are reluctant to accept repeated evaluations. This makes it difficult to integrate the quality of life over a number of years of survival.

With the exception of the Quality of Life Index (Spitzer et al. 1981), the scores for the separate domains of response to these questionnaires are not intended to be combined. Indeed, it can be argued that the investigator is unlikely to find a single weighting system appropriate to all ages, socioeconomic groups, and disease conditions (Fletcher et al. 1992). It becomes particularly difficult to assess the overall quality of life if individual subscales of a test show contradictory trends.

Finally, some aspects of a quality of life assessment, such as those bearing on function, seem likely to be influenced by an increase of habitual physical activity; but for others (such as social relationships), benefit from a change of lifestyle seems less probable (Fitzpatrick et al. 1992).

Disease-Specific Instruments

Disease-specific instruments such as the Back-Pain Disability Questionnaire (Roland and Morris 1983) or the Arthritis Impact Scale (Meenan et al. 1982) are useful for comparing various methods of treating a particular pathology, but are less helpful for evaluating the general influence of physical activity upon population health.

Function-Specific Instruments

Another approach is to use a series of function-specific questionnaires, such as the Profile of Mood States, a Psychological General Well-Being Index, or a Symptom-Rating Test. Such tests are useful in demonstrating gains of mood state from an exercise program, but it is difficult to translate the findings into an overall increase in QALY.

Gestalt Approach

A final option is to use a Gestalt approach, for example a utility measure, a time trade-off, or a "standard gamble" (Guyatt et al. 1989; Spiegelhalter et al. 1992; Torrance 1987). In one example of this approach, the individual is offered the choice between the current state of health and a wonder treatment that may result in either an optimal quality of life or death, with respective probabilities of P and (1–P). A colored disk is then used to vary the values of P until the person rates the wonder treatment and the current status as equally attractive.

Critique of Existing Measurements

One major problem in making any external judgment about a person's quality of life is that these responses are intensely individualistic. The reported score depends on the attitude of the individual to any physical or psychological impairment, on the extent to which a positive attitude allows disability to be avoided, and on whether adjustments in the immediate living environment have been sufficient to avoid any potential handicap.

For any given level of impairment, a well-educated person with a high socioeconomic status will in general suffer less handicap and will show less deterioration in the quality of life than a person with limited education and economic resources. However, many variables enter into the observed response.

Any treatment (including an exercise program) may enhance one dimension of life quality, but lead to no change, or even a deterioration, in other components of the overall appraisal of life quality. Options to overcome the difficulty created by the multivariate nature of the assessment include the use of a multidimensional measurement scheme and the use of a "standard gamble," in which the subject makes an overall assessment of current quality-adjusted life expectancy relative to a life of ideal quality (Stewart, King, and Haskell 1993). Stewart, King, and Haskell (1993) reported that healthy seniors who participated in an endurance exercise program had better ratings of physical functioning and health and lesser perceptions of pain than their sedentary peers, but the active individuals showed less evidence of gains in physical well-being, energy, and physical or psychological well-being. In some circumstances, there may even be a conflict between an expected increase in QALY and an anticipated shortening of calendar life span (for instance, in the 90-year-old who enjoys vigorous participation in Masters athletic competitions). One objection to the use of Gestalt measures is that conflicting outcomes are obscured by scores that combine the quality and the duration of life (Fletcher et al. 1992).

Ceiling effects present a further problem. Thus, the gains in QALY from a graded exercise program are larger among those who enter the program with a low quality of life due to chronic disease than among those who initially have few complaints and thus little scope for an increase in QALY (Lennox, Bedell, and Stone 1990).

Whichever method of assessment is chosen, scoring is relatively crude, and if an exercise program yields no response, it remains possible that the treatment has produced functional gains important to the individual, but that these cannot be detected because of the crudity of the measuring tool.

Factors Influencing Quality of Life

Factors such as physical, social, cognitive, and emotional functioning, personal productivity, and intimacy can all influence the overall quality of an individual's life.

Plainly, regular physical activity has a positive impact in many of these domains (Rejeski, Brawley, and Shumaker 1996): physical well-being (dyspnea, fatigue, level of energy, pain, symptom perception, appetite, and sleep patterns), psychological well-being (self-concept, self-esteem, mood, and affect), perceived levels of physical function, social function, and (to a limited extent) cognitive function.

Physical Well-Being

Current physical well-being can be considered as the individual's standing on a continuum that ranges from optimal health to clinical illness. The position of the individual along this continuum depends upon functional status, the presence or absence of organic pathology, and mood state.

Fatigue is likely in subjects who use more than 40% of their aerobic power for a substantial part of the day. Such a situation is likely to occur in many of the frail elderly who have allowed their aerobic power to deteriorate to an extremely low level. Likewise, dyspnea may be anticipated if exercise-induced hyperventilation demands more than 50% of the vital capacity range. Regular physical activity has value in increasing functional capacity, thus preventing and/or correcting such problems. As a consequence of conditioning, the individual's sense of energy is increased and physical well-being is augmented. In many disease conditions, regular physical activity is also able to maximize residual function (as seen in chapters 5-7); this response, again, is usually accompanied by a reduction of symptoms and an increase of physical well-being.

Some years ago, the influence of a 12-month program of aerobic exercise on the perceptions of health in 65-year-old subjects was assessed (Sidney and Shephard 1977a). There was little change of overall score during the course of the experiment, but there was a significant reduction in the number of miscellaneous diseases reported (section K of the questionnaire). Subjects who elected a high-frequency, low-intensity training program also made fewer responses to section O (on anxiety) when they were retested at the end of the 12-month period (Sidney and Shephard 1977a).

Caspersen, Powell, and Merritt (1994) concluded that the positive influence of physical activity on the bodily well-being of the elderly was well established. McAuley and Rudolph (1995) reviewed findings in 38 studies of older adults (average age 57 years) who had participated in 10- to 20-week programs of physical activity. In general, reports of physical well-being were enhanced, and this change was independent of either gender or age. However, as in the early study of Sidney and Shephard (1977a), individual gains of well-being were not always closely correlated with gains in fitness, suggesting that the health benefit may have arisen from the positive psychological effects of participation, independent of any physiological conditioning response to the exercise program.

Regular physical activity may have beneficial effects on appetite and bowel movements, often concerns of the frail elderly (Shephard 1986d). A number of authors have noted that regular exercise increased the quantity, but not necessarily the quality, of ingested food (Butterworth et al. 1993; Pomrehn, Wallace, and Burmeister 1982). Much depends on the reason for exercising. Masters athletes and members of some fitness facilities tend to be health-conscious groups, and for this reason they may choose a "prudent" diet that is optimal from the viewpoint of disease prevention (Blair, Kohl, and Brill 1990; Nieman et al. 1989; Pate et al. 1990). However, in the frail elderly with a very low food intake, any stimulation of appetite is likely to enhance nutrition (reviewed in chapter 7).

Difficulty in sleeping is a common reason for impaired well-being in the elderly, and if exercise is performed early in the day, it may help to correct this difficulty (Hawkins and Duncan 1991; Horne and Minard 1985). However, if exercise sessions are organized too late at night, their arousing effect may increase the participant's difficulty in getting to sleep.

Perhaps more important than these findings of physical changes is evidence that exercise generally induces at least a transient enhancement of mood state. We will examine this issue further in the present chapter. Indeed, many people indicate that the main reason they exercise is in order to "feel better."

Psychological Well-Being

Measurements of psychological well-being have included not only tests of anxiety, depression, and mood state, but also assessments of positive affect, life satisfaction, negative affect, stress, affect balance, coping, and enjoyment. Unfortunately, many of the tests that have been employed were intended for clinical assessment, rather than for study of the normal elderly. Scores on some tests are unlikely to change greatly, because they explore psychological states rather than traits. Positive affect has shown the most consistent relationship to habitual physical activity (McCauley 1994).

Much of the evidence relating habitual physical activity to overall psychological well-being has been derived from studies conducted in children and young adults. Here, there is fairly strong evidence that regular physical activity induces a number of psychological benefits: it enhances positive affect, boosting body image and increasing self-esteem, self-efficacy, and life satisfaction. At the same time, it reduces psychological distress, correcting "stress," anger, anxiety, and depression; it gives the person involved a more internal locus of control and encourages a reduction in the consumption of alcohol as well as other mood-altering drugs.

McCauley (1994) suggested that some 69% of published studies indicated a positive association between physical activity and psychological well-being. Caspersen, Powell, and Merritt (1994) further concluded that the influence of physical activity upon the self-concept and emotional well-being of elderly individuals was well established. Two studies of Masters athletes (Morris et al. 1982; Shephard, Kavanagh, and Mertens 1995) noted that such individuals perceived an above-average quality of life. In a cross-sectional analysis of four major studies, Stephens (1988) concluded that the association between physical activity and psychological health was particularly strong for women and for older age groups.

Body Image

Body image continues to command the interest of those who exercise, even in the retirement years. Hallinan and Schuler (1993) found that in women aged 60 to 88 years, there was a larger discrepancy between perceived and desired body shape among those who had elected to enroll in an adult fitness program than among controls who were involved in local service groups.

Studies of middle-aged adults have shown that enrollment in an exercise program enhances body image, but information of this type is very limited with respect to the elderly. Sidney and Shephard (1977a) reported gains in body image among 65-year-old exercisers who attended classes regularly and attained a high level of physical activity. Those who exercised less had small and statistically insignificant improvements, and those who exercised the least showed a statistically insignificant widening of the gap between perceived and desired body image. Similarly, on Barry D. McPherson's The Real Me Test, subjects who achieved little or no gain of aerobic power had a decline of score, whereas subjects with moderate or large gains of maximal oxygen intake improved their rating (McPherson and Yuhasz 1968). Another report from this same era claimed that eight weeks of rhythmic breathing, slow stretching, and upright exercises significantly improved the body image of nursing home residents.

Sidney and Shephard (1977a) thus cautioned that if an overenthusiastic instructor made excessive demands of an exercise class, this could induce a deterioration in self-concept and body image. Enjoyment seems to be the most important component of programs designed to enhance psychological well-being in the senior age group (Berger and Owen 1986; Wankel and Kreisel 1985).

Self-Esteem and Self-Efficacy

In adolescents and young adults, quite strong associations have been shown between such measures as self-confidence during exercise (the sense of self-efficacy in this domain) and physical well-being. However, a part of this relationship stems from the high value that many young people attach to an outstanding sport performance, and the praise that such performance attracts from their peers.

In older adults, there is less expectation of achieving an outstanding athletic performance. Nevertheless, many seniors continue to find satisfaction in their ability to undertake vigorous activities competently, and they value the independence that this ability gives them relative to peers who have done less to sustain their physical condition. Volden et al. (1990) found that there were no age-related differences in self-acceptance.

Self-esteem.   Self-esteem may be defined as the extent of the favorable perceptions that one has of the self, or as the evaluative component of self-concept (McCauley 1994). Some 60% of published studies show a positive association between habitual physical activity and self-esteem, although many of these investigations have been poorly designed and controlled. As might be expected, benefit is greatest in those who enter an exercise trial with low self-esteem (Sonstroem 1984). One meta-analysis further noted that the effect size was greater for aerobic activities than for participation in other types of physical activity (Gruber 1986).

A number of cross-sectional studies have shown associations between self-esteem and the functional status of seniors (Duffy and MacDonald 1990; Weaver and Narsavage 1992). Blumenthal et al. (1989) compared findings between subjects who were enrolled in aerobic exercise, yoga, and wait-list control groups; ages ranged from 60 to 83 years. As the program continued, 55% of aerobic exercisers and 68% of participants in the yoga classes reported increased self-confidence, and 61% of aerobic exercisers and 38% of the yoga group also noted an improvement in personal appearance. Controls showed no significant change in either variable.

Perri and Templar (1984/1985) had 65-year-old volunteers participate in 30 min sessions of aerobic exercise three times per week for 14 weeks. The extent of any gains in fitness unfortunately was not ascertained. The investigators observed significant increases in the self-concept of experimental subjects, whereas there was no change in a non-randomly assigned control group who had maintained their normal lifestyle. Valliant and Asu (1985) examined four groups of subjects aged 50 to 80 years; no significant changes in the Coopersmith self-esteem inventory were seen in response to 12 weeks of structured exercise (two 1 h sessions per week), although again the study did not include any assessment of the functional effectiveness of the exercise program.

Self-efficacy.   Self-efficacy reflects the individual's beliefs in his or her ability to undertake the optimal course of action demanded by a particular situation. It seems to be a critical determinant of both physical and psychological functioning. Older people frequently underestimate their physical abilities, in part because of the ageism endemic in North American society, and this is one likely reason for their decreasing involvement in physical activity.

Many studies of exercise and self-efficacy have used middle-aged rather than elderly subjects. Exercise seems to enhance the self-efficacy of middle-aged groups, and this in turn encourages their greater involvement in exercise (McCauley 1994).

One early study (Hogan and Santomier 1984) had 65-year-old subjects learn to swim; the experimental group reported significant gains in self-efficacy relative to non-randomized control subjects. The data are somewhat difficult to generalize, since the primary question answered by the subjects referred to swimming skills rather than to the standard concept of self-efficacy. Nevertheless, 78% of the experimental subjects claimed to have developed not only swimming skills, but also more generalized feelings of competency. Atkins et al. (1984) assigned subjects with chronic obstructive pulmonary disease to one of three patterns of aerobic exercise or to an attention control group. At the end of three months, all three exercised groups had increased expectations with regard to their walking ability, whereas the status of the control group remained unchanged. In confirmation of these findings, Toshima, Kaplan, and Ries (1990) randomly assigned patients with chronic obstructive pulmonary disease to a control group or to an eight-week program of exercise. Self-efficacy increased in the latter group, and the initial eight-week gain was maintained when a further evaluation was made after a four-month follow-up.

Life Satisfaction

Almost all the studies of life satisfaction and physical activity in the elderly have been cross-sectional.

Loomis and Thomas (1991) compared 25 women aged 80 years who were living in a Windsor, Ontario, nursing home and 28 women of average age 69 years who were living at home. The women living independently apparently had more opportunities to engage in physical activity, and were more satisfied with their level of activity than were the nursing home residents (although it should be emphasized that those who lived at home were also substantially younger, and their satisfaction may have related as much to their independent situation as to their greater physical activity).

Kelly, Steinkamp, and Kelly (1987) examined the influence of physical activity on subjective integration (the feeling of belonging to society) and objective integration (as assessed by the number of visits from family and friends). Involvement in leisure activity was associated with both types of integration, although in those over the age of 65 years it seemed particularly important to subjective integration.

Riddick and Daniel (1984) also found a strong association between participation in active leisure pursuits and life satisfaction among older women. In their study, income was shown to have a strong indirect influence on life satisfaction, because it controlled the ability to participate in many types of leisure activity.

Ragheb and Griffith (1982) noted that the higher the frequency of participation in leisure activities, the higher the level of life satisfaction. The meaning of leisure, attitude toward leisure, and quality of leisure were more closely associated with life satisfaction than was mere participation, with sports and outdoor activities showing the strongest linkages to life satisfaction.

Concerning all these studies, it could be argued that because seniors were satisfied with life, they had an enhanced mood state and thus engaged in a greater amount of physical activity (rather than the converse). In partial support of this contention, Sidney and Shephard (1977a) used Neugarten's Life Satisfaction Index to assess whether or not life satisfaction was changed by a year of participation in a program of vigorous endurance exercise. No changes of score were observed.

Stress

The elderly face many stressful life events: retirement, a decrease in physical abilities, chronic illness, the death of friends and life partners, financial problems, and undesirable changes in physical appearance. Various authors have suggested that exercise might provide a useful mechanism for reducing stress, whether through the biochemical changes induced by vigorous physical activity (for instance, an increased secretion of beta-endorphins), through the development of a social support network, or by providing an outlet for the individual's frustrations and anger.

If exercise does indeed have a useful therapeutic effect, then psychotropic drugs (with all their side effects) may be avoided; further, there are many other important health benefits to be derived from regular physical activity. However, the only available data on exercise programs and stress reduction relate to people in late middle age rather than the elderly.

The response probably depends greatly on the ambiance of exercise and on the intensity of the effort undertaken. Athletic competition is generally undesirable for people who are already experiencing stress in some other domain of life. If the intensity of the required activity is perceived as heavy relative to the capacity of an elderly person, then the exercise program itself can become a significant source of stress. Self-paced, predictable, and rhythmic activities are the optimal recommendation for individuals who are under stress, since they allow the participant to "tune out" (Berger 1989).

Long (1985) claimed that a walk-jog program reduced stress in subjects aged 20 through 65 years. However, benefits were unrelated to individual improvements in fitness, and thus seemed attributable to the psychological rather than the physiological or biochemical effects of the exercise program. Norvell, Martin, and Salamon (1991) found no reduction in perceived stress when postmenopausal women participated in a 12-week structured program of moderate aerobic exercise (30 min sessions at 70% to 85% of maximal heart rate, twice per week). King, Taylor, and Haskell (1993) compared home- and group-based programs; they found that whether the exercise was of high or low intensity, the reduction of stress was greater with a home-based than with a group program.

Anxiety

There have been various cross-sectional studies examining associations between regular physical activity and anxiety levels. Perhaps the most comprehensive investigation is that of Stephens (1988). Looking at four national studies in Canada and the United States, he found that the reported level of habitual physical activity was inversely associated with the individual's level of anxiety.

As with stress, we may presume that the reduction in anxiety depends very much on the ambiance of the program, including the intensity of the exercise demanded relative to the capacity of the participants. Among longitudinal studies, the reduction of anxiety seems to be greater if high initial levels of anxiety have been induced (for example, by various types of chronic disease). Thus, Emery (1994), Emery and Blumenthal (1991), and Gayle et al. (1988) all found a significant decrease in anxiety when seniors with chronic obstructive pulmonary disease participated in a program that involved both respiratory therapy and aerobic exercise, the latter practiced in small groups. Minor et al. (1989), likewise, showed a significant decrease in scores on the anxiety subscales of the Arthritis Impact Measurement Scale when subjects participated in a 12-week program of walking and aerobic pool exercises for 1 h three times per week.

At least three longitudinal studies of healthy subjects have reported some decrease in anxiety scores after exercising. Sidney, Niinimaa, and Shephard (1983) noted a modest overall decline in scores on the Taylor Scale of Manifest Anxiety when 65-year-old subjects participated in a one-year program of vigorous aerobic exercise. However, the gains were unrelated to changes in aerobic power, and were largest in the group who attended frequently but exercised at a low intensity, suggesting that much of the observed benefit was due to group support. King, Taylor, and Haskell (1993) continued their study for 12 months at a relatively high intensity, but again responses did not differ between high- and low-intensity programs. Perri and Templar (1984/1985) made a non-random allocation of their subjects to experimental and control groups; anticipation may have contributed to the positive outcome of their study.

A number of other investigations of elderly subjects have shown no change of anxiety over three-month exercise conditioning programs (Blumenthal, Emery, Madden, Schniebolk, et al. 1991; Emery and Gatz 1990; Gitlin et al. 1992), although some of these studies did not assess the efficacy of the exercise program in terms of changes in fitness.

In summary, 159 studies of anxiety and exercise have covered subjects of all ages; Landers and Petruzello (1994) concluded that there was a small to moderate relationship showing that physically fit individuals had less trait anxiety than those who were unfit, and that an exercise training program appeared to induce a small reduction in state anxiety relative to that of untreated controls. Moreover, any benefit was largest for aerobic-type activity and increased in longer trials, with the greatest response being observed in those who were initially anxious.

Depression

Declining physical capacity is one of many problems faced by the elderly that contribute to a depression of mood; clinically significant depression becomes increasingly prevalent in old age. Kaplan, Feeny, and Revicki (1993) demonstrated a significant association between the functional deterioration of seniors and a deterioration in their mood state. Likewise, Weaver and Narsavage (1992) found that measurements of exercise capacity and depression together gave a good prediction of the individual's functional status.

Even in young adults (Morgan 1994), the evidence that regular physical activity relieves depression is quite weak. In part, this is attributable to a ceiling effect, with benefit seemingly greater if the person initially shows a substantial amount of depression. The cross-sectional analysis of Stephens (1988) found that the reported level of habitual physical activity was inversely related to the depression of mood, the association being particularly strong in women over the age of 40 years.

Uson and Larrosa (1982) conducted a nine-month exercise program in subjects aged 60 to 80 years; 70% of those who exercised reported reductions in depression. Bennett, Carmack, and Gardner (1982) arranged a mild program of balance and flexibility exercises for clinically depressed nursing home residents aged 50 to 98 years. After eight weeks, depression was again reported as significantly reduced.

King, Taylor, and Haskell (1993) completed a well-designed 12-month prospective study; this showed that exercisers developed fewer depressive symptoms, although the strength of their conclusion was weakened by a lack of correlation between changes in psychological test scores and gains in objective measures of fitness.

Part of the response in many trials is due to the attention received, rather than to the exercise itself. Thus, McMurdo and Rennie (1993) found decreases of depression score in elderly people, whether they participated in an exercise program or in a reminiscence group that provided equivalent opportunities for social interaction. However, the changes in depression score were significantly larger in the exercised subjects. McNeil, LeBlanc, and Joyner (1991) examined a group of depressed elderly patients; depression was decreased by both exercise and social contact programs relative to values for a wait-list control group, although the exercised group also showed a decrease in the somatic symptom score of the Beck depression inventory.

Minor et al. (1989) noted changes in the depression subscale of the Arthritis Impact Measurement Scale. A substantial sample of elderly patients with rheumatoid arthritis or osteoarthrosis showed significant decreases in scores over a 12-week program of walking and pool exercises.

Blumenthal et al. (1989) also observed a decrease of depression in men (but not in women) in response to a four-month program of aerobic exercise. Blumenthal, Emery, Madden, Schniebolk, et al. (1991), in a further study of the same pool of subjects, found a continuing trend to reduced depression over 14 months of observation, but this no longer reached statistical significance despite a relatively large sample size. Mood seemed to improve in the men, but to deteriorate in the women. Gitlin et al. (1992) also found no significant changes of mood over a four-month cycle ergometer training program; their subjects exercised for 40 min, three times per week, at 70% of their maximal heart rates. Emery and Gatz (1990) observed no change in depression scores with exercise, but they noted that their sample initially had a very normal mood state, and they questioned whether their physical activity program was of adequate intensity to induce either physiological or psychological gains.

Locus of Control

Well-adjusted individuals have an internal locus of control. In other words, they perceive that they are in control rather than at the mercy of events.

Not surprisingly, Kaplan et al. (1993) demonstrated that an external locus of control was associated with a low functional capacity. Speake, Cowart, and Stephens (1991) also reported that those with an external locus of control were less likely to participate in health-related behaviors (including exercise).

A 20-week program in which subjects aged 58 to 80 years wore weighted vests as a means of increasing their habitual physical activity led to a significant shift of perceptions toward an internal locus of control (Greendale, Hirsch, and Hahn 1993). Perri and Templar (1984/1985) also found an increase in internal locus of control in response to 14 weeks of walking and jogging.

In contrast, Emery and Gatz (1990) saw no changes in locus of control over a 12-week program, but the level of exercise selected (70% of maximal heart rate) failed to induce any changes in fitness scores. Valliant and Asu (1985) also saw no change in locus of control when their subjects participated in a 12-week program of calisthenics and flexibility exercises, but they failed to test whether the program had been effective in enhancing fitness.

Physical Function

Currently the effects of regular physical activity on perceptions of physical function are quite limited, at least in the middle-aged and young-old, since in the automated world of the late 20th century, relatively modest levels of strength and cardiorespiratory function suffice to accomplish most of the tasks of daily living. However, this aspect of life quality becomes increasingly important as attention is focused on the middle-old, the very old, and people in whom the consequences of aging have been accelerated by chronic disease, particularly heart disease (Ewart 1989) and arthritis (Fisher et al. 1993).

Social Function

There is relatively little information on interactions between physical activity and social functioning. However, it is widely recognized that many old people live very lonely and isolated lives. One reason for this social isolation is that the frail elderly lack the necessary physical strength to move out into the community, meet other people, and participate in events. An enhancement of physical condition could plainly help in filling this need, and if the activity takes the form of a group program, it also provides a more direct source of social interaction and support.

Rosenberg (1986) found an association between seniors' membership in sports organizations and their level of happiness. However, there was no direct evidence that membership in the association led to any significant increase of physical activity, and in any event the observed social benefits were no greater than would have been obtained from membership in other types of social organizations.

Cognitive Function

Cognitive function does not deteriorate in healthy adults until they reach middle or late old age. At this stage, there is limited evidence from both cross-sectional and longitudinal studies (Dustman, Emmerson, and Shearer 1994; Landers and Petruzello 1994; Rikli and Edwards 1991; Shephard and Leith 1990; Stones and Kozma 1988; Thomas et al. 1994) that regular physical activity enhances a number of objective measures of cognitive function. However, the intensities of activity associated with such gains have been quite high, immediately biasing the available sample, and it has been less clear how far the benefit seen in specialized laboratory tests of psychomotor function generalizes to an enhanced cognitive performance and satisfaction with everyday life (Patrick and Erickson 1993).

Alcohol Consumption and the Use of Other Drugs

There is limited evidence that regular exercise can make a useful contribution to treatment of the alcoholic, decreasing depression and anxiety, elevating mood state, and enhancing sleep (Dupree, Broskowski, and Schonfeld 1984).

O'Brien-Cousins (1993) has also noted a significant inverse association between the use of prescription medication and habitual physical activity. She found that a self-reported lack of involvement in physical activity as a child was a significant predictor of the use of medication during the retirement years.

Conclusions

In part because of its impact upon various aspects of physical health, regular physical activity has an important influence on the functional abilities, quality of life, and mental health of the senior citizen. The average senior spends 10 or more years suffering from an increasing degree of physical impairment, and there is a corresponding decrease in the ability to live independently. There are many causes for this disability, but both normal age-related declines in the function of various physiological systems (chapter 3) and the effects of a number of debilitating diseases (chapters 5-7) can be countered by an appropriate training program. Although the habit of regular physical activity can extend a person's life span by one to two years, a much more important benefit of exercise is a 6- to 10-year increase in quality-adjusted life expectancy. Immediate practical consequences of the increased quality of life include reports of greater well-being, an enhanced self-esteem, and sense of self-efficacy, as well as a reduced risk of anxiety and depression.

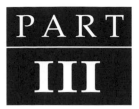

PART
III

Economic and Social Consequences of an Aging Society

Many countries, both developed and developing, are becoming concerned about the economic and social consequences that stem from the increasing average age of their populations. Fears have been expressed that an aging labor force could lead to a diminished national productivity, an increased number of accidents, and extensive loss of working time due to poor health. In this part of the book, we examine the reality of these fears and explore the extent to which any shortcomings of the aging worker can be corrected by appropriate exercise and lifestyle programs. We also consider the broader social implications of population aging, including such topics as job equity in hiring, promotion, and retirement; the job performance assessments that are needed to support such decisions; increasing dependency ratios and their implications for the stability of pension funds; the likely growth in demand for medical services and institutional support; and the costs and benefits of encouraging older people to a greater level of habitual physical activity.

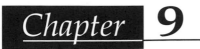

Chapter 9

The Aging Labor Force

This chapter explores the constraints on the composition and effectiveness of the labor force that are imposed by current changes in demographics. It also critiques the current myth that elderly workers have a low productivity, a high accident rate, and a high absenteeism rate. Specific issues to be reviewed include the influence of aging upon employment prospects, productivity and aging, and the ability to extend the span of productive working life. Potential ergonomic initiatives include modifications of general working conditions (including the introduction of part-time work [Taeuber 1985] and phased retirement), retraining programs, and improvements in personal fitness and health.

Labor Force Demographics

The demographics of the labor force in any given country depend on the age characteristics of the national population and also on the proportion of the population of various ages who choose to work or who are allowed to work (the labor force participation rate).

Population Demographics

The demographic structure of a nation depends on its fertility, the net migration rate, and the mortality rate. Future projections are somewhat tenuous, since each of these variables is subject to unpredictable change. Fertility rates have declined dramatically in developed societies in response to a wider access to contraception, the feminist movement, and the involvement of women in the wage-earning sector of the economy. There has also been a steady legal and illegal migration of young families and single adults from India, Africa, and Central and South America to developed countries, and the death of middle-aged and older workers has been greatly diminished by the conquest of infectious diseases.

327

In recent years, the end result of these various trends in North America and other developed societies has been a steady decrease in the percentage of the population who are of working age (Ilmarinen 1991, 1993; ILO 1992; Robinson, Livingston, and Birren 1985). Both in Europe and in North America, a large proportion of the population are now over the age of 55 years and the number who have reached retirement is growing.

To compare current figures with the situation in 1950, many countries have seen a 20% to 50% decrease in the number of workers under the age of 65 years in relation to that segment of the population who are over the age of 65 years (see table 9.1). By the year 2025, it is estimated that individuals over the age of 55 years will account for 31.9% of the population in Europe, 29.6% in North America, 21.1% in Asia, and 17.1% in Latin America (ILO 1992).

The increasing proportion of older workers concerns not only economists, but also sociologists and health-care workers. In particular, the ILO Older Workers Recommendation of 1980 (#162) highlighted the need to avoid discrimination against elderly employees. The ILO has also advocated measures both to increase the social protection of older workers, and to prepare them for a smooth and healthy transition into the retirement years.

Table 9.1   Number of persons in the labor force under the age of 65 years* for each person 65 years of age and over.

Country	1950	1960	1970	1980	1990	1995	2000	2010
Austria	4.6	3.9	2.9	2.9	3.1	3.1	3.2	2.9
Belgium	3.6	3.1	2.8	2.8	2.7	2.6	2.5	2.4
Canada	4.9	4.8	5.0	5.2	4.6	4.4	4.2	3.7
France	3.8	3.6	3.2	3.1	3.1	2.9	2.8	2.6
Germany	4.7	4.1	3.2	3.0	3.3	3.3	3.1	2.7
Japan	8.5	7.9	6.9	5.1	4.1	3.5	3.0	2.3
Netherlands	4.9	3.9	3.6	3.4	3.6	3.5	3.4	2.9
Sweden	4.1	3.5	3.3	3.0	3.0	3.1	3.2	2.9
United Kingdom	4.1	3.8	3.5	3.1	3.1	3.1	3.1	3.0
United States	4.9	4.2	4.2	4.2	4.0	3.9	4.0	3.9

Data for selected developed countries in 1950-1990 with corresponding estimates for 1995, 2000, and 2010.
*As in the previous editions, the ILO Bureau of Statistics had fixed a lower age limit of the labor force of 10 years.
Source: ILO Bureau of Statistics estimates based on economically active population, 1950-2010, fourth edition, International Labour Office, Geneva, Dec. 1996. Copyright © International Labour Organization 1996.

Labor Force Participation Rates

The demographic effects of an aging society have been exacerbated by a decline in labor force participation rates, particularly among older male workers. This trend has continued steadily throughout the 20th century. From the worker's perspective, it reflects the wider availability of adequate pension plans; from the viewpoint of government it highlights the perceived problem that older workers must be displaced in order to provide employment opportunities for the youth of the community (Casey 1984).

During the 1930s, about half of American men over the age of 65 years were still working. By 1950, male participation rates in the United States were 95.8% in the age range 45 to 54 years, 86.9% in those aged 55 to 64 years, and 45.8% in those over the age of 65 years (U.S. Bureau of Labor Statistics 1982). However, by 1995, the corresponding figures had decreased to 91%, 64%, and 13%.

Until recently, the decrease in male participation rates was offset by an increased participation of women in the paid labor force, so that the total number of employed people continued to grow. In the United States, only 36.8% of women aged 25 to 54 years were working outside of the home in 1950 (Fullerton 1984), but by 1995 the projected proportion of employed women for this same age group was 79%. Even if the female labor force participation rate continues to increase, reaching the same level as that for men over the next few years, the reserve pool of women who could compensate for a further decrease in male participation is now quite limited.

People with high incomes tend to retire later than those of low socioeconomic status. On the other hand, most studies suggest that the average number of years worked by any given cohort of the labor force has been inversely related to their average lifetime earnings (Clark 1984). The progressive decrease in labor force participation rates of males during the 20th century has reflected their greater earnings. Future changes in labor force participation rates may thus depend not only on such governmental and corporate policies as the age of enforced retirement, the date of its commencement, and the extent of social security payments (Easterlin, Crimmins, and Ohanian 1984), but also on whether the lifetime earnings of the average worker continue to increase as they have over the past 40 years.

The Decision to Retire

Is the decision to retire made by the worker, the employer, or the government? The answer to this question remains unclear, as there are many subtle and not-so-subtle tactics for encouraging an older person to retire.

It has been widely assumed by sociologists that workers resent enforced retirement, and that termination of a career creates a sense of "rolelessness" and social isolation (Sheppard 1985). However, this may be a myth created by intellectuals who have jobs that they enjoy. The average employee who is consigned to the noisy monotony of an automobile production line, or indeed the person who must meet the demanding targets expected of junior management, may well show no loss of life satisfaction at retirement (Vallery-Masson et al. 1981). Deterrents to retirement include a loss of money (and sometimes of health benefits), together with a separation from the less tangible social and psychological rewards of the workplace.

Nevertheless, at all ages, the number of workers who take voluntary early retirement exceeds those who are compelled to retire (Poitrenaud et al. 1982; U.S. National Council on Aging 1981). Investigators in one early study questioned Norwegian workers and found that 90% claimed to be satisfied with their current jobs. Nevertheless, 51% also stated that they were looking forward to retirement, and only 26% admitted that they dreaded this turning point in their lives. A positive anticipation of retirement was more common in women than in men and more common in the sick than in those who were healthy. By the normal age of retirement, 40% of those who wanted to continue working and 60% of those who wanted to retire were medically incapable of continued effective employment in their current occupation (Beverfeldt 1971).

More recently, Kilbom et al. (1993) suggested that about a half of Nordic workers left the labor force prior to the age of compulsory retirement through a combination of personal choice, unemployment, and illness. In some European countries, the problem was that too many healthy workers elected to retire at an early age. For instance, in Finland more than half of those aged 55 to 64 years had already retired, and two-thirds of the remainder were planning on drawing an early pension (Gould and Takala 1993). Tuomi, Järvinen, et al. (1991) estimated that some 50% of male and 70% of female pensioners in Finland still had a good working ability. They thus argued that such individuals could and should continue to make a productive contribution to society through part-time if not full-time employment.

One useful objective measure of worker attitudes is the percentage of employees who elect to remain in full- or part-time employment after they have reached pensionable age. In Finland, about 18% of retirees stated that they would like to continue working (Piispa and Huuhtanen 1993). Prerequisites of a desire for continued employment were adequate health and strong financial incentives. Although anticipated pension payments are the dominant issue when retirement is first contemplated, ill health and difficulty with strenuous work become more important concerns as the actual retirement date approaches (Huuhtanen and Piispa 1993).

Perhaps because physical demands of work are lower and pension rights less secure in North America, the U.S. National Council on Aging (1981) noted that nearly 80% of those over the age of 55 years wanted to continue at least part-time work after formal retirement, although 40% also indicated that they wished to find a different kind of job. Those who were aged 55 to 64 years indicated that they planned to retire at a median age of 65.5 years, but among workers who were already older than 65, the median planned retirement age was nearly 75 years; 84% of those over 70 years of age said that they were not looking forward to complete retirement.

Factors likely to induce workers to delay retirement include an improvement of the working environment, reductions in the speed of working, flexible working hours, provision of rehabilitation services, and substantial financial incentives.

Aging and Employment

The employment prospects of older people who wish to continue working are influenced in part by their human capital (the attained level of education and any acquired technical skills), and in part by employer perceptions of their current health status and functional capacity. In many countries, governments have tacitly accepted that older people who lose their jobs (for example, through technological change) are unlikely to find alternative employment, and unemployment benefits and pension plans have sometimes been modified to allow such individuals to take a *de facto* early retirement (Casey 1984).

Although the influence of health on working ability has been the subject of extensive discussion, there has been less examination of the possible influence of work cessation on the individual's health.

Technical Skills

In part because of greater societal wealth and in part because of a decrease in demand for young workers, the formal qualifications of labor force entrants have increased dramatically over the past 50 years. From the norm of an eighth-grade education at the end of World War II, a large proportion of North American students now attend either a technical college or a university, and many are obtaining doctorates or even postdoctoral experience.

At the same time, there is a rapid depreciation in some components of human capital. Much of the formal learning that was acquired by older segments of the labor force has now become obsolete. Nevertheless, the informal experience that has been gained through working in a specific job probably enhances the corporate value of most employees, at least until they reach an age of around 50 years (Andrisani and Sandell 1984).

Debate continues on the ability of older workers to learn new skills and on the most effective methods of teaching them modern techniques (Shephard 1987a). But perhaps the most important handicap faced by the person nearing retirement is that irrespective of the ability to learn, a combination of a high current salary and a short period to retirement make it uneconomic for employers to invest in extensive retraining. As the pace of technological change accelerates, this places an increasing limitation on the employment prospects of people over the age of 50 years. Until recently, most older workers with limited technical skills who were displaced by the automation of factories could find employment in the service sector. Currently, service industries employ the majority of North American workers. However, further growth of service work seems likely mainly in such low-paying areas as the fast-food industry. Future generations of older workers who lose their present jobs will find that any alternative employment is low-paying and that it offers only very limited fringe benefits.

Employer Perceptions of Health and Functional Capacity

The labor market and governmental policies are shaped not by the actual abilities of the individual worker, but by stereotypical perceptions of average status at any given age. Employers thus tend to view aging as a progressive loss of the physiological capacity and cognitive skills needed for job performance, exacerbated by the effects of an accumulating burden of chronic ill health.

Stereotypic Metaphors of Aging

Several of the metaphors of aging presented in chapter 2, particularly the *Abnutzungstheorie* of "wear and tear," have placed a strongly negative evaluation upon the aging process. Such perceptions suggest that older workers are nearly ready for the scrap heap and should be discarded at an early opportunity. Inevitably, acceptance of the stereotype leads to a loss of self-esteem among older employees, with a self-fulfilling prophecy of deteriorating physical and mental performance in the workplace. There is a need for both employers and gerontologists to affirm the positive attributes of older workers, particularly the knowledge and experience that they can bring to a company.

Employers should not accept that a decline in physical or mental ability is an inevitable argument for dismissal. Rather, employers should recognize their ability to compensate for any age-related decline of working capacity; options include the introduction of ergonomic measures to reduce either task demands or hours of work, and the development of employee lifestyle programs that maximize the individual's residual functional capacity (Shephard 1986b).

Erroneous Cross-Sectional Perceptions

Most perceptions of the aging process have been formed on the basis of cross-sectional analyses. However, such information can be quite misleading when one is assessing the working potential of the present generation of older workers, since a variety of secular trends have led to large intercohort differences in health and biological function.

For instance, in previous cohorts of older workers, heavy cigarette smoking doubled the average period of absence following an upper respiratory infection from 10 to 20 days, and it also shortened the average life span by as much as eight years. However, smoking behavior has changed dramatically over the past three decades, and in North America only a small minority of well-educated people now smoke. This secular change has potentially extended the span of healthy working life by five or more years.

Changing female social roles equally complicate comparisons between young and older women. The productivity, fatigue, and absenteeism rates of the current cohort of young female employees are often adversely influenced by the competing needs of young children, so that their work-site performance may be poorer than that of older women.

Finally, the content and physical demands of work have changed rapidly over the past 20 to 30 years. Tasks that until recently were beyond the physical capacity of the average 60-year-old have now been automated and present little physical problem.

Health Prospects

Despite a progressive squaring of the mortality curve (Fries 1980a), morbidity remains greater in older than in younger members of the labor force. Certain occupations have played their own part in generating chronic illness and premature death, whether through physical problems such as an excessive exposure to air pollutants, or through excessive mental stress and resulting psychosomatic complaints. Thus, Marin (1986) noted a high mortality rate among housepainters, presumably because they had suffered repeated exposure to hepatotoxic fumes, and Vinni and Hakama (1980) reported a low mortality rate but poor health among the administrative segment of municipal workers. Future cohorts of older workers are less likely to show a deterioration of health due to a poor working environment, since occupational health standards have become progressively more rigorous over the 20th century.

Interindividual Differences

Averaged cross-sectional data admittedly show a progressive deterioration in the function of most body systems as a person becomes older (discussed in chapter 3). Moreover, illness-related absences from work and the premature death of older workers together have a substantial influence on overall national productivity (Shephard 1986b).

However, the averaged data mask large interindividual differences. The best-preserved 65-year-old worker has a greater functional capacity than a poorly endowed person of 25 years, and if employment decisions are based simply on calendar age, then an unsatisfactory (and often inappropriate) assessment is made of the person's productive potential. Equitable treatment of the individual employee ideally requires a consideration of biological age. Unfortunately, a valid method of combining physiological, biochemical, and psychological data to yield an effective index of biological age has so far proved elusive, as seen in chapter 2.

Health Consequences of Retirement

Until recently, the immediate health impact of retirement has had little formal study. Our own observations (Sidney and Shephard 1977a) suggested that (particularly in men) there was an increase of physical activity in the year immediately following retirement, probably in an attempt to fill empty hours of enforced leisure. On ceasing regular employment, a heavy-manual worker may notice physiological effects from the decrease in daily energy expenditure. However, psychological problems are generally more serious: a loss of social integration, feelings of loneliness and uselessness, a lack of behavioral norms, and obsessive thoughts of old age and death. In some instances, the act of retiring may actually serve to trigger perceptions of impaired work ability (Bazzoli 1985).

Once the immediate shock of retirement has passed, the perceived advantages that have been reported include a greater opportunity for leisure activities and rest. The negative aspects most commonly noted are a lack of money and difficulty in passing the time. Perhaps as many as half of workers currently enjoy their retirement, but this proportion could probably be increased through a combination of lateral movement of older workers to more appropriate jobs, provision of part-time employment where desired, retirement preparation classes, and improved pension plans (Shephard 1987a; Taeuber 1985).

Repeated studies have failed to clarify whether retirement improves or worsens an individual's health (Colsher, Dorfman, and Wallace 1988; Palmore, Fillenbaum, and George 1984). Some observers have found an association between retirement and a decrease in the number of complaints requiring medical attention, but Cascells et al. (1980) claimed that there was also a significant increase in the incidence of cardiac deaths in the period immediately surrounding retirement.

The proportion of those who enjoy retirement can be increased through preparatory programs that explore both the problems and the opportunities of old age. The U.S. National Council on Aging (1981) found that 48% of those aged 55 to 64 years and 28% of those over 65 years were interested in learning new skills. Possible topics for such classes include income management, coping with ill health in a relative or in oneself, and new activities and hobbies suited to the retirement years. The latter can usefully include supervised exercise, social activities such as old-time dancing, and physically demanding crafts (such as the manufacture of toys for grandchildren).

Personal Productivity and Aging

Prospects for the continued employment of the older worker are influenced not only by the perceptions of employers, as just discussed, but also by the individual's innate physical and mental endowment, the attained level of training and experience, socioeconomic status, physical health, and the influence of these several variables upon productivity.

Definition of Productivity

Productivity is not simply a maximization of output. In any given situation, there is a hyperbolic relationship between the quantity and the quality of production achieved by a given individual. Productivity is best defined as an optimization of this hyperbolic function for a minimum investment of human or material resources, or both.

Unfortunately, the investment side of the equation is critical, and accumulated salary and vacation benefits make older employees less productive per dollar, even if they are still able to work as hard as younger workers. As the age of the labor force rises, there may thus be a need to reexamine the current supposition that salary and fringe benefits should rise automatically with years of employment in a company.

The average young worker may have the superficial attraction of a high volume of production. However, the older employee often counterbalances a somewhat slower speed of working by a greater quality of output, based on many years of accumulated experience. Thus, the potential productivity and even the attained output in many jobs show little decline up to and beyond the normal age of retirement.

In recognition of these trends, the ILO (1992) has recommended that industrial remuneration should reflect not only the quantity of goods produced but also accumulated experience and "know-how." Another of the ILO's suggestions is that older workers should be paid by the time spent at the work site rather than by results or piecework.

Measuring Productivity

Given a physical end product, productivity can be measured directly, as the number of items of acceptable quality produced per hour of work, or per dollar of total investment. Indirect inferences about the productive potential of the individual can also be drawn from aerobic work capacity and muscle strength, since the use of more than a fixed fraction of either peak oxygen transport or maximal voluntary force is fatiguing. Other options for assessing the person engaged in a physically demanding task are to make ratings of muscle weakness, to measure changes in hand or limb steadiness over the working day, or to record self-perceptions of fatigue at the end of a shift.

The productivity of the office worker depends on occupancy (whether the individual actively seeks fresh work or sits passively awaiting instructions), effectiveness (selection of an appropriate task), and efficiency (adoption of an optimum task approach). Performance can be compared with the standard time allotted for completion of a given task such as the typing of a page of correspondence, the answering of an inquiry by a telephone operator, or the sale of an airline ticket. Computer terminals are sometimes equipped to monitor the speed and rhythm of working, although this approach has been widely criticized as an invasion of personal privacy. Even if such measurements are accepted by the employees, it remains difficult to assess the quality of the service that has been provided to the consumer in many practical situations. Alternative approaches include self-ratings of productivity, supervisor ratings of worker performance, and counts of commendations, merit pay, and error scores.

Worker Performance and Aging

Many industrialists believe that the performance of the older worker is threatened by such factors as a loss of cardiovascular function or muscular strength, a deterioration of the special senses, loss of brainpower, poor health, or a risk of ischemic heart disease that endangers the safety of either the employee or the general public (Shephard 1992d). There have been suggestions that if demanding physical work is unpaced, problems of fatigue begin to appear in the late 50s or early 60s and that difficulties are encountered at an even earlier age in paced work. How real are such fears and negative stereotypes?

Cardiorespiratory Function

Fatigue is likely if a worker uses an excessive fraction of maximal oxygen intake throughout an 8 h day. Estimates of the limiting percentage range from 33% to 50%, depending on the duration of rest pauses (Rutenfranz et al. 1990), the peak loads that must be sustained, environmental temperatures, and any added postural demands imposed by unfavorable working conditions (for example, in crawl space or overhead work).

Currently, few occupations have an energy requirement that exceeds the aerobic threshold for a young male employee. However, in an average 65 year-old man or woman, the peak aerobic power has shrunk from 12 to 14 METs to around 7 METs (25 ml/[kg · min]), so that 40% of this figure would allow an energy expenditure of only 2.8 METs (10 ml/[kg · min]). This would seem to limit the oldest employees to very light physical work. Leino and Hänninen (1993) found an association between the self-perceived physical ability of construction workers and measurements of their physical fitness. However, age-related complaints of fatigue are less common than might be inferred from the decline in physical working capacity. There is a considerable self-selection of well-endowed individuals into physically demanding work and of poorly endowed individuals out of such work. Moreover, daily task demands help to maintain physical condition in heavy work, and because of acquired mechanical skills the older and more experienced worker can reduce the energy cost of many work-site tasks. Finally, seniority allows many older individuals to adopt a supervisory role, or to depute the more arduous tasks to younger employees.

Despite the theoretical effects of aging, Suurnakki, Nygard, and Ilmarinen (1991) saw no change in the rate of performance of physically demanding self-paced work by older employees. Presumably because of reduced cardiorespiratory function, some older individuals reached heart rates corresponding to as much as 91% of peak aerobic effort. Fallentin, Nielsen, and Sogaard (1993) also found that older female office cleaners developed heart rates corresponding to 50% rather than 40% of aerobic power (although their working day was generally less than 8 h). However, heart rate data must be interpreted with caution, since such measurements can overestimate the intensity of aerobic loads, especially if a task has an isometric element, or the working environment is hot and humid.

Current employment standards, set by the U.S. National Institute for Occupational Safety and Health (NIOSH) in 1981, indicate an "Action Limit" that calls for implementation of ergonomic measures—either task redesign or the special selection and training of workers—when the average energy expenditure exceeds 14.6 kJ/min. The NIOSH standard corresponds to an oxygen consumption of about 10 ml/[kg · min], which represents perhaps 80% of the fatigue threshold for a 45-year-old man but around 100% of this same ceiling in the average 65-year-old. The ILO (1992), likewise, has proposed a threshold limit, recommending that energy expenditures be limited to 33% of the individual's maximal oxygen intake.

Currently, some 20% to 25% of work in Europe and North America remains physically strenuous, because the task cannot conveniently be either automated or eliminated (Rutenfranz et al. 1990). Recommendation #150 of the ILO (1992) calls for the development of improved work methods, tools, and equipment to meet the particular needs of an elderly employee in such situations. Corrective action by an ergonomist could probably allow average 65-year-olds to cope with an 8 h working day at many of the work sites where strenuous activity is still required. Such action would not only sustain output as the labor force ages but would also help to preserve health and avoid accidents. However, if attempts are made to extend a physically demanding career beyond the age of 65 years (in order to ease the pressure on pension funds, for example), the proportion of the labor force who can meet the physical requirements of the task falls rapidly. If sociodemographic trends require the employment of older workers, it will thus be necessary to adjust working conditions. Possible changes include an increase in the length of rest pauses, a reduction in daily or weekly hours of work, and the introduction of part-time or flexible hours of working.

Limitations of aerobic working capacity are particularly likely to be seen in elderly women, since at all ages they average only about two-thirds of the absolute maximal oxygen intake of male workers (discussed in chapter 3). Some ergonomists have suggested that older women should be excluded from heavy physical work (Rutenfranz, Klimmer, and Ilmarinen 1982). However, such a decision is unfair to that minority of women who can match or even exceed the physical performance of their male peers.

Muscular Strength

Industrial performance is quite commonly limited by the ability to lift heavy objects repeatedly. Nottrodt and Celentano (1984) found a high incidence of problems even in young military recruits; 9% of men and 99% of women were unable to meet the minimum lifting requirements of the Canadian army. Again, NIOSH (1981) has specified an Action Limit, and the ILO (1992) a threshold limit at which task modification is required. The current NIOSH standard is reached if fewer than 75% of women and 99% of men can meet the job requirements safely, whereas the ILO specifies that the median load must be less than 10% of the individual's maximal voluntary force and the peak load less than 50% of maximal force.

Given that the average person's strength decreases 25% over the course of working life (as reviewed in chapter 3), it seems almost inevitable that the typical employee will have difficulty in meeting the lifting demands of heavy work by the usual age of retirement. However, ergonomic measures (provision of lifting platforms, instruction in lifting techniques, lightening of the load, and sharing of the task) can again help. For instance, Hopsu and Louhevaara (1993) found that a simple redesign of industrial cleaning tasks reduced the average heart rates of older female workers from 110 to 99 beats/min.

Other Changes in Physiological Function

Other physiological consequences of aging with an adverse influence on the performance of certain categories of older worker include a deterioration of balance, poorer thermoregulation, and difficulties in adjusting circadian rhythms after a change of shift (Härmä and Hakola 1993).

Cognitive Function

Many aspects of cognitive function depend on the extent of interneuronal connections (which increases with age) rather than the total neuron count (which diminishes). Loss of cerebral function before the age of 70 years usually reflects a specific disease such as Alzheimer's disease or multi-infarct cerebral vascular disease, rather than constituting a more general manifestation of aging. Chronic disorders such as a back injury or coronary vascular disease may sometimes exert a general adverse influence on somatic function (Eskelinen et al. 1991), but if a person remains in good health, it is difficult to demonstrate any loss of cognitive function prior to the eighth decade of life (Berg 1993).

Sensory loss, a deterioration in the signal/noise ratio, and a slower tracing of information in the long-term memory slow the rate of central processing of information (Spirduso 1995). Complex choice reaction times are thus increased. Recent memory is also poorer than in a younger worker (Suvanto et al. 1991), and the elderly employee often shows an increased rigidity of response. No deficit of work performance is usually seen under normal, routine operating conditions, but the solving of unfamiliar problems is slowed (Chown 1983). The older person may thus be at a substantial disadvantage if a rapid decision is required (as, for example, in a novel, emergency situation; Molander and Backman 1993). But in contrast to such limitations, writing speed and vocabulary commonly do not peak until a person has reached 40 to 50 years of age. Accumulated wisdom and experience are other assets of the older worker, although some of this potential advantage is now being eroded by the rapid introduction of new technology and the displacement of traditional occupations to the third world.

Too often, technological change leaves the elderly worker redundant, with well-honed skills that are no longer relevant. Recognizing this problem, ILO conventions #142 and #150 (ILO 1992) have suggested that vocational guidance and training policies and programs should help workers throughout life. Such training needs to be age-adapted, and older people should be involved in the development of training and retraining manuals. Training may include not only an updating of specific knowledge and skills, but also an upgrading of general education. Older workers need encouragement to attend such classes, and management must be educated as to their economic and practical value.

Job Satisfaction

Older workers sometimes complain of quantitative overload and a lack of support (Goedhard 1993). However, Torgen, Nygard, and Wahlstedt (1993) found that older postal workers had a higher level of job satisfaction than their younger peers, and Nielsen (1993) obtained similar findings in a study of municipal cleaners. Presumably, successful psychosocial coping depends on the nature of the job, the extent of turnover among those who are dissatisfied, and age-related opportunities for the selection of tasks that appeal to the individual.

Accidents

A rigidity of response in the face of novel situations (Molander and Backman 1993), the slowing of complex reactions, and progressive decreases in acuity of the special senses (Chown 1983) do surprisingly little to increase the risk of accidents among older workers. This generalization seems true even in occupations such as bus driving, where public safety is a major concern and a deterioration of psychomotor function might be thought critical to job performance (Shephard, Prien, and Hughes 1988).

One reason the accident record of elderly employees remains good is that they develop methods of coping with and compensating for inevitable physiological changes, at least over the usual period of employment. Perhaps more importantly, most accidents do not arise from any defect in cognition or the special senses. Rather, they are attributable to a small segment of the population who are "accident prone" because of inattention, poor judgment, failure to acquire the skills needed in their job, or the abuse of alcohol and other drugs. Such individuals are usually detected and dismissed from sensitive jobs at a relatively early point in their careers.

Experience of Vehicle Operators

Detailed statistics are available showing the demographics and accident experience of bus drivers in a number of transit companies. In one survey of a medium-sized North American transit authority (Shephard, Prien, and Hughes 1988), only 3.5% of drivers were over the age of 60 years, but in the London Transport system, a minority of individuals elect to drive until they reach the age of 70 years.

The incidence of accidents (when matched for the employee's number of years of operating experience) is lowest in workers over the age of 45 years (see table 9.2). If the data are not adjusted for years of employment, account is taken of accumulated experience; the older drivers then far outperform their younger peers. It may be that older drivers are more cautious, and that if they are hired in middle age they begin transit employment with much greater overall driving experience than young recruits. A further factor is that most incidents are attributable to a small subgroup of accident-prone bus drivers, and many of these have their worst experience during their first few years of employment. Subsequently, many of this subgroup are disabled, killed, dismissed, or leave the transit company voluntarily. Finally, drivers with many years of service are able to select routes that avoid the worst traffic hazards,

Table 9.2   Chargeable accidents in medium-sized urban bus company in the United States (expressed per driver-year).

Age (years)	Length of service (years)				
	0-5	6-15	16-25	26+	Total
25-35	3.02	3.18			3.05
36-45	2.35	1.90			2.17
46-55	1.90	1.91	0.92	0.20	1.65
56-60	3.00	3.00	2.00	0.39	1.18
60+		4.33	0.00	0.88	1.43

Adapted, by permission, from R.J. Shephard, E.P. Prien, and G.L. Hughes, 1988, "Age restriction on bus driver selection," *Journal of Human Ergology* 17: 119-138.

and they usually do not have to operate the split shifts that would involve younger employees in working during two periods of rush hour per day.

Perhaps the greatest difficulties of the elderly driver arise at dusk and nighttime, when lens opacities and a resultant scattering of light lead to a substantial decrease of both visual acuity and glare tolerance. Visual acuity is correlated with accident rates among truck drivers, and some jurisdictions restrict nighttime driving for the very old. Nevertheless, accidents among bus drivers rarely occur at night (Pokorny, Blom, and Van Leeuwen 1987).

Because they are more cautious, older drivers tend to have less serious accidents than younger ones (Shephard, Prien, and Hughes 1988). Problems sometimes arise from "load-shedding" as the driver discards signals which he or she no longer has time to process; but the slowing of reaction time remains of questionable safety significance to vehicle operators until they have reached a very advanced age. A restriction of the visual field and limitations of spinal movement sometimes reduce the effective range of vision, making shoulder checks of road conditions more difficult to carry out; however, this difficulty can be largely overcome by an effective positioning of rearview mirrors. Slow accommodation of vision also tends to hamper the reading of road signs during fast driving.

Despite the theoretical handicaps of the elderly vehicle operator, the American Automobile Association (1985) noted that total license revocations decreased with age. Moreover, car drivers between the ages of 50 and 59 years were the group with the lowest incidence of accidents.

Other Occupational Accidents

In many other occupations, the decline in physical and cognitive performance with aging might be thought to increase the risk of accidents. In the final decade of work, accidents are sometimes caused by a failure to avoid moving vehicles, as well as from difficulty in slowing the pace of machine-paced work to match the diminishing reaction speeds of older employees. However, for many workers, the main problem is not injury itself, but rather the fear of being injured by machinery that they cannot control.

Again, the physiological handicaps of aging are usually countered by the greater caution and experience of the older worker. Thus, Salminen (1993) reported that work-site accidents from all causes were actually fewer in older than in younger workers.

General Health

The incidence of major health problems undoubtedly increases with aging. However, as in younger individuals, there is a strong influence of environmental and psychological factors. Complaints of poor health are most frequent in jobs with a high physical demand, exposure to extremes of heat or cold, lack of freedom in decision making, few possibilities for career advancement, and role conflicts (Tuomi, Eskelinen, et al. 1991). In part for these reasons, the physical health of the elderly shows a strong relationship to social class (Black 1980).

As early as 45 to 50 years of age, the labor force becomes polarized into those who regard their health as good and those who report it as poor (Tuomi, Ilmarinen, et al. 1991). The most common complaints are of musculoskeletal problems, cardiovascular disease, and mental disorders. In some jobs (for example, teaching), the ability to cope with high levels of stress seems to decrease with age (Kinnunen, Rasku, and Parkatti 1993), and this has been blamed for more frequent reports of physical tiredness, stress, and absenteeism among older employees.

Specific health concerns include the side effects of medication and the safety hazards presented by sudden catastrophic illness such as a heart attack or stroke.

Absenteeism Rates

Industrial economists have commonly speculated that aging of the labor force might increase absenteeism rates and thus reduce productivity.

However, analyses of the overall impact of aging that are based simply upon health status ignore important personal and organizational causes of poor productivity other than chronic illness. Up to one-half of industrial absenteeism has no medical basis. Current statistics show a four- to fivefold difference in absenteeism rates between nonunionized workers in North American companies (4 to 5 days absence per year) and unionized companies in Europe (20 to 30 days absence per year) (Shephard 1995b). For the past five to six years, many North American companies have also operated at no more than 70% of capacity because of a poor demand for the goods and services that they produce. In Canada, 9% to 10% of the labor force have been unemployed for much of this same period. Often, employees could have achieved a greater output if their personal efforts had not been frustrated by poor management, union regulations, the absence of a key colleague, a lack of necessary materials, or a lack of investment in modern machinery, research, and development (Shephard 1986b). Production is increasingly a team effort between good and bad workers and between younger and older employees. So it becomes quite difficult to assess the productivity of the individual worker, and it is simplistic to claim that absenteeism could be reduced and productivity enhanced by decreasing the average age of the labor force.

In fact, older employees seem to take few of the disruptive one- to two-day absences that impair the performance of a substantial minority of younger employees. On the other hand, if absence is enforced by an exacerbation of chronic ill health (for example, an attack of chronic bronchitis or a recurrent back injury), the older worker may be absent for a substantial period (Shephard 1986c).

Side Effects of Medication

A substantial proportion of older workers are taking prescribed drugs that have at least a potential impact upon their productivity and risk of accidents. For instance, Ilmarinen (1991) noted that the majority of older workers in physically demanding jobs were receiving beta-blocking medication, which can limit cardiovascular performance and increase the likelihood of muscular fatigue. Again, the use of antihypertensive medications may cause depression and drowsiness.

Unfortunately, as yet there is little specific information on the impact of this problem on organizational effectiveness.

Ischemic Heart Disease

Since age is a major risk factor for myocardial infarction, cardiac arrest, cerebrovascular catastrophe, and stroke (chapter 5), it has been argued that a fixed age of retirement should be adopted in order to avoid accidents caused by a loss of consciousness or death during work in occupations that involve public safety (for instance, airline pilots, train and bus drivers, and police officers).

An acute manifestation of cardiovascular disease presents the largest potential problem. Nevertheless, the public safety hazard arising from heart attacks at work is surprisingly small. First, the proportion of disabling heart attacks that occur on the job is much smaller than would be anticipated from the length of the normal working day (see table 9.3). Secondly, in most jobs only a small fraction of a typical 8 h working day is occupied by tasks where public safety is at risk (Shephard 1992d). Many of the paid hours are occupied by paperwork and rest pauses. Finally, in many critical situations, a co-worker or an automated override system is available. Even a solo driver of a truck or bus usually has sufficient warning of an impending heart attack to stop a vehicle safely (Shephard 1986a).

Table 9.3   Relative incidence of nonfatal heart attacks over the course of the day.

Activity	Duration (min)	Expected number of attacks	Observed number of attacks
Sleep	460	75	48
Work	400	55	30
Sports	30	5	30
Walking	20	3	13
Odd jobs	30	5	21

Reprinted from R.J. Shephard, 1981, *Ischemic heart disease and exercise* (London: Croom Helm).

Illness and Voluntary Retirement

From the viewpoints of both productivity and safety, key questions are whether employees recognize when their physical health is inadequate to continue in a particular type of occupation and whether they then choose to retire voluntarily.

Eskelinen et al. (1991) argued that most workers made realistic appraisals of their working ability. Tuomi (Tuomi, Järvinen, et al. 1991; Tuomi, Toikkanen, et al. 1991) also found that many of those reporting ill health took early retirement. Changes of occupation and early retirement were seen most frequently in jobs that required strong muscles, tolerance of poor posture, and acceptance of an unfavorable physical environment, although it is less clear from these studies how far the turnover was voluntary and how often it was initiated by the employer.

Enhancing the Productivity of the Older Worker

Genetic endowment, personal lifestyle, and habitual physical activity all have a substantial impact on biological age and thus potential productivity at any given age. The negative effects of aging can be minimized if the employer recruits workers with appropriate initial characteristics, develops a work-site fitness and lifestyle program, and encourages employees to participate in this program. Despite such measures, the older worker may still show residual deficiencies of biological function. Nevertheless, compensation is often possible by appropriate ergonomic measures, including optimizing the layout of the work site. Using a combination of these various approaches, a company can substantially extend the age range of employee productivity, effectiveness, and safety.

Genetic Endowment

Recent estimates suggest that genetic factors account for 30% to 40% of an employee's initial aerobic power and muscle strength. Constitutional factors also have a substantial influence on the individual's response to either a deliberate training program or a career of heavy physical work (Bouchard 1994). If a high physical demand cannot be avoided by the mechanization of a given job, it is thus helpful to use physical screening tests at the time of hiring; this allows the selection of individuals who are likely to be productive employees, not only immediately, but also in the latter part of their careers.

Hiring decisions are sometimes made, consciously or unconsciously, in terms of physique. However, current data offer surprisingly little objective evidence that those engaged in physically demanding jobs have been either self- or employer-selected in terms of matching their physical abilities to task demands (Ilmarinen 1991).

Training Response

In some jobs, the task itself may serve to maintain and even to develop the individual employee's physical condition. But in many occupations, a heavy physical demand arises only occasionally, the normal load is insufficient to have any substantial training effect, or the demand is too localized, too one-sided, or too static to enhance the worker's physical condition (Ilmarinen 1988, 1989).

As automation becomes more widespread, physical condition will depend increasingly on leisure pursuits rather than on physical activity associated with performing the job. Suurnakki, Nygard, and Ilmarinen (1991) found no difference of aerobic work capacity between people employed in physically demanding jobs and those engaged in mentally demanding employment. Others (Huuhtanen and Piispa 1993; Nygard et al. 1987) also have observed no unusual muscular development in "heavy" workers.

In principle, employees with a deficient physical working capacity could be identified either by physiological tests or more simply by observations of performance on the job. The introduction of training programs to enhance the capacity of such individuals seems desirable in order to reduce fatigue and resultant risks of musculoskeletal injury (Cady, Thomas, and Karwaski 1985; Tuomi, Ilmarinen, et al. 1991). An appropriate fitness program for the middle-aged or older worker can boost their maximal oxygen intake by 5 to 10 ml/[kg · min] and their muscular strength by 10% to 20% (as discussed in chapter 4). Such gains are equivalent to a 10- to 20-year reversal of the normal aging process, and should have a corresponding impact on both the subjective tolerance of daily work and productivity in physically demanding jobs.

Suurnakki, Nygard, and Ilmarinen (1991) measured heart rates on the job, noting that workers with a good cardiorespiratory capacity showed 10% less cardiorespiratory strain than those who had only a moderate to low physical work capacity. Also, because they were able to complete their work assignments more rapidly, the fit workers enjoyed longer rest pauses than their poorly conditioned colleagues.

Indirect Benefits of Training Programs

Some reports have suggested that exercise training programs have benefits that extend beyond increases in aerobic power, strength, and control of obesity. Observers have noted improvements in such measures of psychomotor performance as color recognition and reaction and movement times (Rikli and Edwards 1991; Spirduso 1995; Tomporowski and Ellis 1986).

Lifestyle Changes

Involvement in a regular fitness and lifestyle program can enhance many facets of general health.

The small immediate decrease of absenteeism seen among regular program participants is probably related to an improvement of perceived health (chapter 8; Shephard 1986b). Employees "feel better" and are thus better able to face a day of work. As participation in a conditioning program continues, there are more long-term gains. Improvements of personal lifestyle may include a cessation of smoking (Shephard 1989a), the control of obesity (with a lesser risk of developing maturity-onset diabetes and other forms of chronic disease), and a reduction of cardiac risk factors (Leon et al. 1987).

The cessation of smoking influences not only general health, as discussed earlier, but also physiological function. A heavy smoker diverts 5% to 10% of maximal oxygen intake to the chest muscles, and as the bronchial obstruction is reversed, part or all of this aerobic power can be redirected to the performance of external work. Likewise, the obese employee who carries an additional 20 kg of body fat faces a 25% increase in the energy cost of tasks that require the displacement of body mass; if the body fat content can be reduced by an appropriate combination of dieting and exercise, there is a corresponding improvement in physical working capacity. The cessation of smoking and the correction of obesity together can indeed yield an improvement in aerobic performance that matches all the anticipated age-related deterioration of function that occurs over an entire working career!

Ergonomic Measures

When a company is contemplating the introduction of ergonomic measures to aid the performance of older employees, the first requirement is a task analysis to determine which particular facets of a task limit job performance. The process can then be redesigned to modify critical, rate-limiting, or hazardous steps.

Aerobic Power

Court hearings have sometimes suggested that employees must meet an arbitrary standard, such as a maximal oxygen intake of 3 L/min, or 42 ml/[kg · min] (12 METs), in order to carry out heavy physical work.

Data supporting such a requirement have been based on the steady state oxygen consumption observed during performance of each of a battery of work-related tasks. However, there is little evidence of voluntary early retirement from jobs in which task simulation implies such high metabolic demands. One possible explanation is that many work assignments are completed in 1 to 2 min. A substantial part of the oxygen consumption theoretically required to undertake the task can then be accumulated as an oxygen debt, rather than being met as a steady rate of oxygen transport (Shephard 1991d).

Nevertheless, the heaviest components of a job should be automated, where possible. Alternatively, older workers can be promoted to a supervisory role in which use is made of their accumulated experience rather than their physical working capacity. Even if such an accommodation is for some reason impossible, the ergonomist still has the option of adding or extending a rest pause, or of shortening the average workday, in order to bring the job within the theoretical fatigue threshold for an older employee (40% of that person's aerobic power for an 8-hour day).

Strength

Where a task currently exceeds the strength of an older employee, the preferred ergonomic solution is again automation. However, many other options can also bring a muscular task within acceptable limits for an elderly worker.

The ergonomist can teach the adoption of a better posture (Suurnakki, Nygard, and Ilmarinen 1991) and other improvements in individual lifting technique; the task can be shared between two or more workers, the contents of a heavy box can be lightened, loading platforms can be built to reduce the height of a lift, the rate of lifting can be reduced, or longer rest pauses can be allowed.

Special Senses

Brighter lighting of the workplace and the use of corrective lenses, control of extraneous noise, and the use of hearing aids help many older workers with a moderate impairment of sensory function. One task very commonly performed in modern office buildings is the operation of a visual display terminal. Here, problems of vision can lead to poor posture with resultant back problems (Sundstrom 1986). Nevertheless, difficulties can be at least partially alleviated by such simple ergonomic measures as a change of chair design or varying the size of type displayed on the screen.

There remain a few specialized tasks for which productivity is impaired by a deterioration of vision or hearing; these will be discussed in the next chapter. Careful testing is needed to identify, reassign, and retrain vulnerable individuals in such trades.

Cognitive Function

Older people bring to their jobs attributes of emotional stability and seasoned judgment that can help with difficult personal or social situations. Relative to younger employees, they are also less inclined to take risks, some of which may be dangerous or unwarranted. The productivity, effectiveness, and safety of older workers are thus maximized if advantage is taken of their assets through appropriate job placement.

Older workers are often intimidated by technological advances and are correspondingly reluctant to master new processes. Any necessary retraining takes somewhat longer than in a younger person, owing in part to loss of recent memory. However, the supposed additional cost of retraining an older person is in part illusory, since young workers are more apt to change their place of employment after retraining has been completed. Moreover, the slower learning of an old person may be offset by greater diligence and accuracy once a task has been mastered.

Conclusions

Although aging leads to decreases in both physical and mental function, these processes are relatively late manifestations of aging, and a critical loss of performance can be delayed by the adoption of an active lifestyle. An employer may have concerns that older workers endanger public safety or lack the necessary working capacity to achieve a high level of productivity; however, this should be an incentive to take all available countermeasures. The workstation should be well designed, with automation of heavy tasks where possible. Employees should be carefully selected and should also be encouraged to attend an effective work-site fitness and lifestyle program.

In general, differences of productivity between a young and an older worker are small. But even if differences can be shown, it may also be appropriate to critique the concept of maximizing worker productivity. In a world of shrinking nonrenewable resources, does it make sense to seek to manufacture and to sell an ever-growing quantity of consumer products? Automation is rapidly bringing us to an era when workers do not need to work at maximal speed for 8 h/day in order to produce all of the goods and services that society needs, even if some argue that only frenetic activity can provide all that society wants. Automation may soon offer society a unique opportunity to accommodate the special requirements of the older employee with respect and dignity.

Chapter 10

Implications of Aging for Society

Ageism seems inherent in North American society. This is particularly true in the sector of industrial employment, where unscrupulous employers have attempted to obtain a competitive edge over their rivals by age discrimination in hiring, promotion, and retirement policies. Equal opportunity and human rights commissions have thus found it necessary to examine whether restricted opportunities for employment were legitimately demanded by the nature of the task to be performed. Likewise, exercise physiologists and ergonomists have been required to assess the physical demands of a variety of occupations, correlating this information with the physical capacities of older potential employees.

The growing proportion of senior citizens among the populations of most developed countries has posed a number of economic problems. Changing dependency ratios have created uncertainties about the solvency of pension funds. There has been a rapid growth in the demand for costly, high-technology medical services and related institutional support, particularly in the final few months of life. Further, policy makers have questioned whether the encouragement of regular physical activity, either in young adult life or during the retirement years, could help to contain the burgeoning health-care costs associated with an aging society.

These are the issues to be considered in this final chapter.

Job Equity in Hiring, Promotion, and Retirement

Equal employment opportunity and human rights commissions in North America are frequently asked to investigate complaints of discrimination against job applicants or employees. The alleged basis of discrimination may include age, gender, or some type of physical or mental disability. An employer may have refused to hire workers who exceed a specific age. For example, until recent rulings from the Canadian Federal Court of Appeal and the U.S. Equal Employment Opportunity Commission, a number of North American bus companies were unwilling to hire bus drivers over 40 or 45 years of age. Occasionally, there may be evidence suggesting that because of their age, older workers have been denied promotions for which they appeared to be well qualified, a desired transfer of employment has been refused, or an opportunity for retraining has been withheld. Most commonly, the complaint is that retirement has been enforced before the individual wished to leave the full-time employment of a company.

In general, these various forms of age discrimination are forbidden by federal, state, or provincial law (for instance, the U.S. Federal Age Discrimination in Employment Act). But in some jurisdictions, there have been rulings that a "reasonable" age ceiling can be imposed for paid employment (for example, 65 years in the case of university professors in Ontario). Discrimination in both hiring and retirement practices is also allowed in certain jobs with a *bona fide* occupational qualification (Leon 1987): that is, an occupation for which it can be proven that a person's age, gender, or disability makes it impossible for that individual to perform one or more essential elements of the job. Such rulings are particularly likely in instances when a single employee, such as an airline pilot or a train driver, has responsibility for the safety of many members of the general public (Bruce and Fisher 1987).

In some jobs, difficulties may arise from a deterioration in the special senses: a watchmaker may lose the visual acuity needed to repair a small mechanism, a train driver may no longer be able to distinguish a red from a green signal, a vacuum cleaner inspector on a production line may miss the telltale noises emitted by a faulty motor, or a construction worker may lose the sense of balance needed when walking on a tall building in a high wind. Often, the difficulty arises from the real or the perceived obsolescence of the older worker. But in the context of this monograph, the most important impact of aging is still on some facet of physical working capacity: aerobic power, anaerobic capacity, or muscular strength.

Recruitment Restrictions

The nature of the arguments advanced to support a restriction on the age of hiring can be illustrated by the specific case of the bus driver.

Safety Concerns

The main reason offered by transit companies in defense of their existing policy of a 40- or a 45-year ceiling age at entry was that older recruits had difficulty in mastering various aspects of the bus driver's job (including safe operating procedures). Plainly, the accident statistics from various companies (summarized by Shephard, Prien, and Hughes 1988) argue strongly against this position. Indeed, in part because of greater experience in the operation of motor vehicles, the oldest drivers are involved in the smallest number of accidents (as shown in table 9.2).

Adaptation to Unusual Working Hours

New recruits to a transit company are usually assigned to the "extra board," that is, they are required to work arduous and unpredictable split shifts. However, aging is associated with a decreased ability to withstand fatigue and to adapt to sleep deprivation or shift work (Morgan 1987; Webb 1981). Older employees are thus likely to have somewhat greater difficulty in adapting to the required work schedule.

Physical Demands

The driver's job sometimes demands moderate to substantial physical strength (for example, when loading passengers in wheelchairs or maneuvering a bus that lacks power steering). Company representatives have argued that it is unrealistic to thrust such responsibilities suddenly upon a frail, postmenopausal female driver. However, the fact that drivers hired at a younger age are able to continue working through to an age of 70 years (as has been allowed in central London) makes it unlikely that a person recruited at 40 or 45 years of age would lack the physical strength needed for the job.

Back Problems

There is an age-related increase in the prevalence of back problems in many occupations. Transit authorities have suggested that such disorders might be exacerbated if older people were recruited to drive buses over bumpy city streets. Any problem is likely to be cumulative in nature, and difficulty thus seems less likely in older recruits than in those who have been driving buses since young adulthood. Moreover, a study of Israeli bus drivers (Barak and Djerassi 1987) found no evidence of pathological vertebral changes that could be attributed to vibration. In their experience, slips, falls, and incorrect handling of baggage were the most frequent causes of back injuries among bus drivers.

Sensory Limitations

An age-related deterioration in auditory acuity and discrimination might lead to difficulties in meeting the requests of passengers, in detecting mechanical problems in the vehicle, and in hearing sounds that give warning of a dangerous situation within or outside the vehicle. The testing of hearing might well be a useful component of an annual medical examination for bus drivers, but again considering their demonstrated ability to continue operating public service vehicles safely through to an age of 70 years, loss of hearing cannot be accepted as a reason justifying a blanket restriction on the hiring of 40- to 45-year-old drivers.

Cognitive Function

Transit authorities have argued that the process of learning to operate a public service vehicle safely is prolonged. Thus, older recruits may not master the demands of their task fully until they are close to the age of retirement (Shephard, Prien, and Hughes 1988). This argument is quickly countered by reference to the accident statistics already cited (shown in table 9.2).

Covert Reasoning

In addition to these overt reasons for not hiring older people, transit companies undoubtedly had covert fears that older drivers would be perceived as unsafe by the traveling public and would suffer more frequent and/or more prolonged bouts of illness, with resultant increases in the costs of absenteeism, health insurance, and long-term disability and pension benefits.

Ability to Meet Task Demands

A detailed task analysis counters most of the overt arguments in favor of age discrimination (Shephard, Prien, and Hughes 1988), as will be seen later in this chapter. Such analysis demonstrates that the job requirements can be met quite readily by a person who is recruited at as late an age as 45 years. Indeed, in terms of the primary criterion, accident experience, there is strong suggestive evidence that 45 years is close to the optimum recruitment age for bus drivers (see table 9.2).

There is thus no *bona fide* occupational reason for imposing an age restriction on the recruitment of older drivers, and the U.S. Equal Employment Opportunity Commission ruled that such restrictions must be lifted.

Compulsory Retirement

Discussions of a compulsory retirement age have usually had as their overt basis the argument of employers that a waning of aerobic power, strength, or heat tolerance leaves older people with too narrow a functional margin to fulfill the physical requirements of their job. In a few instances, concerns have also been expressed that an increasing risk of incapacitating illness and sudden death might endanger the safety of the individual worker or the general public (Leon 1987; Shephard 1991d).

Covert reasons for attempting to rid the labor force of older workers are in general similar to those noted in connection with restrictions on the age of employee recruitment.

If a lack of functional capacity is advanced as a *bona fide* reason for enforced retirement at a fixed age, it is first necessary to carry out a careful assessment of job demands. Such an analysis may establish that the limiting component of the overall task demands a large aerobic power—for example, in the case of the postal carrier who must walk many kilometers each day carrying a heavy bag of mail (Shephard 1982b), or the marine surveyor who must climb many long ladders into and out of cargo holds before a vessel is allowed to sail (Shephard 1983b). Alternatively, the job may call for anaerobic power and capacity as well as agility (for the police officer who must chase offenders, jumping fences and other obstacles; Davis and Dotson 1987), or it may demand a substantial muscle strength and endurance (for the firefighter who must carry unconscious victims out of burning buildings while wearing a portable oxygen system).

If a *bona fide* occupational qualification is demonstrated, practical options are to relate this demand to either the ability of the average older worker or the capacity of a specific employee. It is often difficult to develop a field measurement of functional capacity that is reliable, valid, and appropriate to the individual's work (Davis and Dotson 1987). In part because of assessment problems, and in part because failure of a test is an unsatisfactory way to end a career, some have argued that where functional capacity can limit performance, it is best to apply a fixed age limit based on the average characteristics of the labor force. Others have argued that this approach is unfair to workers who have maintained a high level of personal fitness and health throughout their careers, and still have as good a functional capacity as those many years their junior.

Inadequate Aerobic Power

The many contentious issues involved in establishing a minimum aerobic power requirement for a particular job can be illustrated by the specific case of the mail carriers. In this occupation, union regulations specify both the maximum load that can be carried (17 kg) and the maximum allowable pace of walking (a speed of around 5 km/h, designed to permit the carrier to sort the mail and complete deliveries on the longest likely route within an 8 h shift). Two to three hours of a typical shift are allocated to the preliminary sorting of parcels and uncoded mail, and the remaining time is spent on door-to-door delivery of the mail.

Calculating energy costs. On first inspection, it seems quite a simple matter to calculate the energy cost of carrying a 17 kg shoulder satchel at 5 km/h, and then to relate this figure to both the likely aerobic power of the employee (Shephard 1993a) and the portion of this aerobic power (about 40%) that can reasonably be expended over 5 to 6 h without causing excessive fatigue (see table 10.1).

Bonjer (1968) maintained that the allowable load, expressed as a percentage of aerobic power, was a function of task duration. He suggested calculating it from the equation:

$$\text{Allowable load } (\%) = 32.3 \, (\log 5700 - \log t)$$

where t is the task duration, in minutes.

Table 10.1   The allowable intensity of occupational work in relation to the duration of effort and the voluntary choice of workers engaged in self-paced activities (both values expressed as a percentage of the individual's peak aerobic power).

Duration of aerobic task (hours)	Recommendation of Bonjer (1968)	Voluntary choice (Bonjer 1968; Hughes and Goldman 1970)
1	63%	76%
2	53	—
4	47	—
8	33	40

Based, in part, on data collected by F.H. Bonjer, 1968, "Relationship between working time, physical working capacity, and allowable calorie expenditure." In *Muskelarbeit und Muskeltraining*, edited by W. Rohmert (Stuttgart: Gentner Verlag).

Variables modifying energy cost.   The initial cost of carrying a laden mailbag is a little higher than might be inferred from most physiological reports, since the bag is slung from the left shoulder rather than carried centrally on the back (where the weight would be optimally distributed). This arrangement allows the carrier to reach for letters with the right hand while walking. The load does not remain at 17 kg, as has been assumed in most military studies of load carriage. Indeed, the weight of the carrier's bag rarely reaches the agreed ceiling, except on days when there are large bulk deliveries of mail (for example, the day welfare checks are distributed). Moreover, the weight of the bag diminishes progressively as mail is delivered.

The cost of the task is increased somewhat relative to that observed during level walking at the same pace, since the carrier must climb and descend a number of hills while covering the typical postal route. However, with a little advance planning, it is possible to be carrying a full bag of mail downhill and a nearly empty bag back uphill. The energy cost of a given walking pace is increased by snow, but extra time is usually allowed for deliveries under adverse weather conditions.

Variables modifying task duration.   The distance to be walked is determined by a supervisor, who follows official footpaths, but by crossing lawns and pushing through hedges it may be possible for a carrier to shorten the supposed walking distance substantially. Moreover, individual postal routes vary substantially in both their length and the number of house doorsteps that must be climbed. Thus, only the longest routes require the full shift to complete.

All these variables affecting both the intensity and the duration of effort make it very difficult to calculate an average energy expenditure for the postal carrier. Plainly, there is much scope for older workers (by virtue of seniority) to opt for an easier route than their younger colleagues.

Relation to aerobic power.   If the required daily energy expenditure can be established, it is then necessary to relate this to an allowable fraction of the individual's aerobic power. Accepting a 47% ceiling of effort as appropriate to a task performed for 4 h/day (Bonjer 1968), the requisite maximal oxygen intake can be established (see table 10.2). Such calculations suggest that many older women and some older men would find difficulty in sustaining more than light work for 4 h/day. The most taxing of the mail routes probably demands that the carrier sustain an average energy expenditure of at least 21 kJ/min for 4 to 5 h, and (applying the 47% ceiling) the maximal oxygen intake must be at least 2.13 L/min.

Nevertheless, before concluding that this puts the task beyond the tolerance of older workers, we would need a population-specific age distribution curve of likely aerobic power values. We do not currently have such information for mail carriers, nor indeed are such figures available for many other occupations. However, it is likely that a task such as mail carrying attracts the fit individual because of its high aerobic demands. Such fitness also tends to be conserved by a substantial daily aerobic energy expenditure. It is not permissible to base calculations on general population data; employee-specific measurements of aerobic power are needed.

Extension of Working Life

In terms of extending the age range of potential employees, several possible tactics can supplement a seniority-based selection of "easy" routes: smoking cessation and weight control programs can each materially increase the effective aerobic power of many employees, and part-time employment could allow older people to walk only a part of the mail route.

Automation is perhaps more important than any personal initiatives. The energy cost of a number of other aerobically demanding tasks is summarized

Table 10.2 Relationship between energy cost of task (as defined by Brown and Crowden 1963) and maximal oxygen intake needed to sustain this activity for 4 h (limiting task to 47% of aerobic power).

Task	Energy cost (kJ/min)	Maximal oxygen intake (l/min)
Light work	< 14	< 1.42
Moderate work	14-23	1.42-2.33
Heavy work	23-38	2.23-3.85
Very heavy work	> 38	> 3.85

in table 10.3. This table illustrates how mechanization has progressively extended the ability of companies to employ older people: the transition from a pick and shovel to a mechanical grader, from the binding and shucking of corn to use of a combined harvester, and from hay making by scythe to the use of a tractor, as well as the introduction of milking machines, power saws, and tree-planting machines. All these developments have greatly reduced the energy demands on employees. Further, the trend is continuing, as machines become ever more sophisticated and less dependent upon human effort.

Inadequate Muscular Strength

In a survey of the Canadian Armed Forces, where age and gender discrimination had been contentious issues, Nottrodt and Celentano (1984) found that 95% of tasks that were physically demanding and also performed frequently by a substantial proportion of personnel involved the lifting or the carrying of heavy objects, rather than a bout of sustained aerobic work.

The most demanding task of the military recruit involved lifting a load of 36 kg, and some categories of personnel had to lift loads of 18 kg frequently. Most lifts were made from ground level to a level between waist and shoulder height, but in 15% of instances it was necessary to lift the load above shoulder level. Plainly, many older people would be unable to meet such demands (as discussed in chapter 8). Indeed, 99% of young women and 9% of young men who were recruited to the armed forces could not meet this challenge even after they had completed their basic military training (Nottrodt and Celentano 1984).

Lifting can be a problem for older employees in other jobs. However, the need for unassisted lifting is in part peculiar to the military situation, since the working environment of the front-line soldier is highly varied and unpredictable. In contrast, an industrial lifting task can often be facilitated by the construction of a loading platform. It may also be possible to reduce the rate of working, to modify the task (perhaps interspersing the lifting of boxes with

Table 10.3   A comparison of the energy cost of selected tasks using traditional and mechanized methods (selected largely from data collected by Durnin and Passmore 1967).

Task	Traditional	Mechanized
Digging	20-42 kJ/min	15.5-30.5 kJ/min
Grain harvesting	21-36	8.3-13.0
Hay making	23-43	7.5-18.8
Milking	9.2-21.3	6.3
Sawing wood	30	22.6
Tree planting	27	11.7

their labeling), to reduce the load to be lifted, or to install some mechanical device that can undertake much of the physical work.

Heat Tolerance

We have noted earlier that the older person has an impaired tolerance of hot environments. The productivity of even a young worker falls, and the risk of accidents increases, if the wet-bulb temperature rises above 32 °C; physical work becomes progressively more difficult at rectal temperatures in excess of 38 °C, and there is a danger of heat fatalities if rectal readings exceed 39.2 °C.

Factors contributing to the poor heat tolerance of the older worker include a deterioration of physical condition, an accumulation of subcutaneous fat that impedes the elimination of body heat, and a poorer regulation of peripheral blood flow. In the later stages of a normal working career, fat accumulation is the most obvious handicap. A 4 mm increase in average skinfold readings can increase the thermal gradient between the body core and the environment by 0.8 °C in light work, 1.2 °C in moderate work, and 2.0 °C in heavy work. Assuming near-limiting environmental conditions, with a total temperature gradient of 7 °C from the deep body tissues to the surrounding air, the thermal equilibrium of a person with a 4 mm increase in skinfold thicknesses could be restored at the respective expense of an 11%, 17%, or 28% reduction in the rate of working for the three intensities of effort.

Standard Rates of Working

In many unionized operations, standard rates of working have been established. The employee who achieves a rate of working above the accepted standard then qualifies for bonus payments. The standard rate has typically been set so that it is acceptable to 80% of the employed male population.

The median age of the labor force varies from one industry to another. Usually, it is higher in older industries where the demand for physical effort remains substantial. To a first approximation, the standard rate of working for a given task may be set at 1 SD below the level appropriate for an average 45-year-old worker; traditionally, male subjects have been used in setting this standard.

If we deduct 1 SD from the aerobic power of the average 45-year-old man, we obtain an absolute standard of 1.62 L/min, roughly sufficient to permit the performance of light work (see table 10.2) throughout an 8 h day; notice that although this figure corresponds to a maximal oxygen intake of 23.1 ml/[kg · min] in a 70 kg man, it is equivalent to 29.4 ml/[kg · min] in a woman weighing only 55 kg. Such calculations illustrate one reason why more than half of 65-year-old men can still meet the standard rate of working, whereas it becomes impossible for all except a minority of 65-year-old women.

Applying the same concepts to tasks that demand substantial strength, we may assume that men have lost some 5% of their young adult strength by the age of 45 years (discussed in chapter 3). There is also a coefficient of variation of some 18% about the average scores, so that an acceptable standard loading would be 240 N if developed at a height of 1.8 m above the ground, and 335 N at 1.1 m above the ground. Given a further 20% loss of strength through the age of 65 years, about one-half of 65-year-old men would still be able to lift the standard load. However, given an average gender differential in strength of 25% (Shephard 1982c), most elderly women would be unable to meet this same requirement.

Influence of Training

Although a number of jobs occasionally make heavy physical demands, in most occupations the challenge arises too infrequently to sustain physical condition. Thus, effort tolerance can be enhanced by an employee fitness program, even in supposedly heavy physical work.

But whether fitness is developed through the normal demands of employment, or through deliberate participation in work-site and leisure-time exercise programs, regular vigorous physical activity can counter many of the physical problems that otherwise might limit the productivity of the older worker. The resultant training can induce a 20% improvement of both aerobic power and muscle strength (reviewed in chapter 4). This is equivalent to a 10- to 20-year reduction in biological age, and it is sufficient to bring most older workers within the range at which they are still able to function as effective members of the labor force.

Risk of Catastrophic Illness

The risk of developing a catastrophic or incapacitating illness has been invoked to justify enforced retirement for several classes of vehicle operators (airplane pilots, bus drivers, and drivers of articulated trucks), and for public safety officers (for example, police, where a heart attack might allow the escape of a dangerous criminal, and firefighters, where a rescue effort might be aborted for a similar reason; Shephard 1992d).

Vehicle operators.   Aging is associated with a progressive increase in the risk of a heart attack (chapter 5; Leon 1987). In theory, such an episode could cause a vehicle accident. However, in practice, there is a margin of useful consciousness (always more than 5 sec, and often as long as 20 min); this is almost always sufficient to allow the operator to park the vehicle safely (Fox 1986; Robinson and Mulcahy 1986; Shephard 1986a).

One early British study found only 992 road accidents with a medical cause over the course of a year (Norman 1960). Commercial drivers accounted for a disproportionate number of such incidents, but this was so mainly because they operated their vehicles for 8 h/day or more. A periodic medical examination of 2130 London bus drivers aged 50 to 70 years judged that 73 operators were medically unfit to drive during the year under investigation; 51 had cardiovascular problems, 7 had a deterioration of vision, 2 had diabetes mellitus, 2 had arthritis, and 11 had other medical conditions. Over a total of

220,000 bus driver-years, there were 46 incidents in which the vehicle operator had lost consciousness; 26 of these events had led to an accident (8 cases of epilepsy, 5 "faints," and 3 "heart attacks"). Twelve coronary attacks had occurred while a bus was moving, but the driver had been able to stop the vehicle completely in seven instances, and in only three cases was minor vehicle damage reported.

Likewise, in a sample of 1031 professional drivers, Robinson and Mulcahy (1986) were unable to find any examples of men who had died at the wheel of their vehicles, even though a substantial minority of this group had been allowed to return to work following a first heart attack. Shephard, Prien, and Hughes (1988) again found no examples of moving vehicle accidents attributable to coronary disease in their study of a medium-sized transit company.

It is clear from the foregoing data that accidents attributable to cardiac disease are not a *bona fide* reason for insisting on the retirement of commercial vehicle operators.

Public safety officers. It has been argued that in an emergency situation, the problems of an aging myocardium are compounded by the release of catecholamines. If the emergency also requires heavy physical effort, then catecholamine release is likely to increase with age, because older people generally have a lower strength and aerobic power than younger individuals.

Some studies of firefighters have shown a relatively high incidence of heart attacks (Shephard 1991d), although this is probably due to a combination of carbon monoxide exposure, heavy smoking, and the development of obesity from inactivity between emergencies rather than the physical demands imposed during an occasional rescue attempt. Certainly, the overall experience of sudden death among public safety officers is not greatly out of line with that for the general public of comparable age.

Both in police work and in firefighting, older employees tend to transfer from front-line to administrative jobs, so that the number of workers who are exposed to the postulated risks of an emergency situation diminishes progressively with age. The risk of a critical incident may well be augmented 5- or even 10-fold during an emergency response as compared to seated rest (Shephard 1981; Vuori 1995). However, the average firefighter sees active service for no more than 3% of employed time (Davis and Dotson 1987). Because the frequency of solo operation in a life-threatening situation is rare even for front-line officers, the possibility that an employee will develop a heart attack during an emergency presents a negligible threat to the safety of the general public.

Leon (1987) has emphasized that modifiable risk factors (smoking, hypertension, a high serum cholesterol, and a lack of exercise) make a much greater contribution to the risk of a cardiac fatality than does age. Thus, employers who have concerns that a cardiac catastrophe may jeopardize public safety should direct their efforts to health promotion programs, rather than insisting upon the dismissal of older workers.

Assessment of Job Demands and Worker Performance

Given the quasi-legal nature of the Equal Employment Opportunity and Human Rights Commissions, thorough documentation of both job demands and worker performance is important to successful prosecution of a case.

Job Demands

The techniques used to analyze the nature and severity of job demands may be illustrated by the investigation of an urban transit company (Shephard, Prien, and Hughes 1988). Job analysts first reviewed published literature (including previous court proceedings), U.S. Department of Transportation manuals, proprietary reports, and documents from various transit authorities. They then rode with operator trainers and interviewed supervisory personnel. On the basis of this information, a job analysis questionnaire was developed to explore the various tasks and job skills required of the bus operator.

Three expert witnesses spent a total of 80 h riding representative bus routes, recording the frequency of occurrence of the individual tasks that had been identified, and rating the skills or physical abilities that were needed to perform each of the various tasks. The importance of each item to performance of the job as a whole was also rated on a six-point scale. Items given a rating of 3 or higher were included in the final job description of the vehicle operator. Activities given the highest ratings included estimation of bus position in relation to the road and other vehicles, the rapid reading of route signs, the recognition of obstacles and hazards, and the judging of distances and speeds when merging into moving traffic.

Specific requirements of physical strength and psychomotor abilities were rated using Fleishman's *Abilities Analysis Manual* (Hogan, Ogden, and Fleishman 1978). Here, the speed of limb movement (reflected in use of the brake for emergency stops and in steering through narrow streets), with a score of 6.67/7.0, was scored highly (intermediate between the estimated requirements for a police officer and a firefighter). However, the need for dynamic strength (score 1.73) was quite modest, lying between scores for an accountant and a social worker, and the need for stamina (4.40) was also only moderate, similar to that of a painter or a custodian.

Worker Performance

Because of the wide interindividual range in biological ages (discussed in chapter 2), age alone is a poor predictor of work performance across the full range of a working career (Davis and Dotson 1987). One alternative is to make an objective assessment of performance on all employees at recruitment, and periodically thereafter.

The ideal test of worker performance is reliable and valid relative to frequently encountered job demands, and is independent of skill or test learning. It identifies, on an objective basis, both persons with a high probability of successful job performance and those with deficiencies that are critical to job performance. It also excludes those who are vulnerable to injury (Brownlie et al. 1982; Shephard 1990). If possible, the test should indicate the type of appointment for which a person is best qualified. The assessment should also be safe, easy to perform by those with limited testing skills, economical, and robust against legal challenge. Unfortunately, such a test does not exist!

Laboratory Tests

Laboratory tests include a treadmill measurement of maximal oxygen intake, isotonic lifting tests, and stress ECGs. But such tests are costly, require skilled personnel, and can usually be carried out on only a small subsample of the labor force. Moreover, despite the cost of such tests, the results lack precision; accuracy is limited, even in the laboratory, and deteriorates still further if an attempt is made to make annual work-site measurements on the entire labor force over the age of, say, 50 years (Louhevaara and Lusa 1993).

Aerobic power.   If maximal oxygen intake is measured on a treadmill, a combination of day-to-day variations in physical condition, the effects of any intercurrent acute illness, and technical errors can cause 1 test in 40 to underestimate a worker's true aerobic power by as much as 10 ml/[kg · min]. This is equivalent to a 20-year error in the determination of biological age, and would lead to a grave injustice in the supposed objective determination of retirement age! If simpler, submaximal predictions of aerobic power are made from a cycle ergometer or a step test, interindividual differences in peak heart rates and the mechanical efficiency of exercise lead to even larger errors in the assessment of physical status.

If the accuracy of the laboratory tests could be improved, the information obtained would still be specific to the type of exercise performed (for instance, uphill treadmill walking, or pedaling a cycle ergometer). The correlation between scores on such laboratory tests and the performance of different types of activity on the job remains quite limited.

Muscle strength.   In many occupations, difficulty in carrying heavy loads and resulting back injuries are larger causes of concern than a lack of aerobic power and thus a slow running speed. However, laboratory assessments of muscle strength are no more successful than measurements of aerobic power when they are used to predict performance in the field. Nottrodt and Celentano (1984) found that scores on an isotonic lifting test gave only a marginally better classification of worker performance than a simple determination of body mass. Either type of assessment accounted for only about 25% of the variance in performance on the job.

Cardiac abnormalities.   The exercise stress ECG is often used to identify employees such as airline pilots or truck drivers who are at risk of developing a heart attack while working. However, as with the other procedures of the physiologist, ECG tests have only a limited prognostic value when applied to the individual subject. In essence, the stress ECG is being applied to diagnosis in a symptom-free population, and as would be predicted from Bayes theorem, as many as two-thirds of apparent electrocardiographic abnormalities are false-positive test results (Shephard 1981). The precision of evaluation can be increased if account is taken of the presence of standard cardiac risk factors (Leon 1987) and if other tests such as echocardiography, scintigraphy, or angiography are undertaken subsequently. However, the detection of the vulnerable employee then becomes a very complex and costly matter.

Field Test Procedures

Field simulations of a job are sometimes easier to defend before a jury than are sophisticated laboratory tests; the field measurements have construct, content, and face validity (Davis and Dotson 1987; Wilson and Bracci 1982), particularly if the items included in the test battery have been identified by task analysis and subsequently validated against performance on the job. One proposed test circuit for police officers involved getting out of their car, running 6 m, climbing a 1.5 m wall, running 30 m, climbing a 1.8 m fence, making a simulated arrest, and dragging a 75 kg dummy over a distance of 46 m.

Scores on a performance test of this type are heavily dependent on body size, and thus penalize women. Such discriminatory tests are inappropriate unless their predictive value can be demonstrated by professionally acceptable methods, or they correlate highly with conditions that prevail at the anticipated place of work (Bard et al. 1985). There is also a large day-to-day variation in field test scores due to such factors as differences in ground and weather conditions and learning of the required test procedures.

Determination of Body Mass

Given the problems inherent in assessing aerobic power and muscle strength under either laboratory or field conditions, one simple alternative might be simply to look at body mass.

Body mass shows a substantial association with the performance of firefighters (Davis, Dotson, and Santa-Maria 1982), and body mass is almost as helpful a criterion as laboratory measurements of muscle strength in the selection of personnel for the armed services (Nottrodt and Celentano 1984). On the other hand, there is little relationship between body mass and the successful performance of active police duties, probably because body mass is influenced by muscularity as well as by obesity.

Body mass is highly correlated with lean mass, and in young adults it can be a useful indicator of the potential to perform a task that requires great strength. In older adults, however, body mass is highly correlated with body fat, and this greatly weakens its predictive value, particularly when one is attempting to evaluate the physical potential of elderly workers in affluent and obese North America.

Job Performance

Given the limited success of either laboratory or field assessments of working capacity, the employer is often forced back to the tactic of rating productivity at the work site. Care must then be taken to exclude ageism on the part of appraisers. Sometimes it is useful to compare assessments made by young and older evaluators (Mehrotra 1985). The development of objective procedures to assess performance on the job should help to determine when an individual employee should retire; also, it should suggest ways of enhancing performance and/or extending the length of the average working career.

Dependency Ratios and the Solvency of Pension Funds

A number of health economists have warned that if regular physical activity were to increase life expectancy, this would hasten the insolvency of pension plans that are already sorely taxed by the growing numbers of old and very old people (Warner 1987; Warner et al. 1988). Even if this scenario were true, it hardly seems a good reason not to maximize the health and life expectancy of seniors! However, as we shall see further on, fears about the negative economic effects of enhanced fitness are at worst exaggerated, and are probably groundless.

Dependency Costs

If A is the number of adults of working age, P is their participation in the labor force, W is the fraction of the labor force that is currently employed, C is the number of children, and E is the number of elderly individuals, then the overall dependency ratio (D) for any given population can be calculated as:

$$D = ([1 - APW] + C + E)/APW.$$

Data are sometimes cited for the aged dependency ratio (E/APW). It is also helpful to calculate the dependency ratio for the very old (E'/APW), since this group is the most costly segment of the total senior population.

The overall dependency ratio is influenced by the birth rate during the previous 20 years, the time when education is completed (an average age of about 14 years before World War II, but currently extending to an age of 30 years and more for doctoral and postdoctoral students), the average employment rate (which presently seems to be decreasing progressively with each recessionary cycle), the number of senior citizens, and the age of retirement (assumed to be 65 years in many calculations, but *de facto* showing a progressive decrease throughout the present century).

The overall dependency ratio for the United States was 0.64 in 1950. It had increased to 0.82 by 1960 (because of the baby boom), but by 1976 it had dropped back to 0.69 (Decker 1980). In contrast, the old age dependency ratio increased steadily, from 0.13 in 1950 to 0.18 in 1976, with a predicted value of 0.32 in the year 2030. The Canadian figures for the old age dependency ratio are rather similar—0.18 in 1976, with a projected value of 0.33 for the year 2031 (Denton and Spencer 1980). More refined economic calculations take account of the differing economic needs of children, working adults, and seniors; the costs of supporting children and seniors are about 70% of expenditures on working adults.

Costs are particularly high for university-age students and for the very old. In recent years, some of the increase in costs imposed by the burgeoning population of very old people has been accommodated by reduced expenditures on higher education, but soon this buffer will have been exhausted. It then will be necessary for governments to meet the full economic costs associated with an increase in the old age dependency ratio.

Actuarial Considerations

The ever-increasing proportion of seniors who make no formal contribution to national economies has raised serious actuarial problems. In countries that rely mainly on private pension plans, high premiums are becoming a major factor in dissuading employers from hiring workers over the age of 45 years (Sheppard 1985). Where pensions are met from government sources, the combination of a relatively static gross national product and a rising money supply due to increased health-care and pension payments has inevitably led to inflation, and (except in countries where pensions have been indexed to the cost of living) to an increase in poverty of the elderly.

The proportion (P) of earnings that must be contributed to ensure the solvency of a pension fund that provides a fraction (F) of employed earnings to the elderly (E) can be calculated according to the formula:

$$P = \frac{F(E)}{F(C + E) + A}.$$

Note that the symbols are as in the dependency equation, with A signifying all adults of working age (whether in the salaried economy, seeking work, working at home, or not participating in the labor force).

A study of Western Europe conducted in 1970 found that pension provisions ranged from 28% to 37% of working salaries, with a corresponding P value of 5.4 to 9.0%. Provision of a 50% pension would have required an increase of P to 11.2%, and if seniors were to be given a 75% pension, the P value would have become 16.8%.

The extent of destabilization in pension funds in subsequent years can be judged from the fact that an increase in the average school-leaving age from 15 to 20 years, and a decrease in the retirement age from 65 to 60 years, would almost double the dependency ratio even if there were no change in the proportion of elderly people. Potential solutions to the increased social costs imposed by an aging population include the following:

1. An increase in the gross national product through automation
2. More effective training of the labor force
3. A decrease in unemployment and underemployment
4. A continued increase in the use of female workers
5. The admission of young, well-trained immigrants from developing countries

During the past 20 years, North American governments have exploited many of these remedies, so that a substantial segment of the senior population has enjoyed an increasing standard of living. However, it is less clear that such gains can be sustained in the face of current demographics and the exhaustion of nonrenewable resources.

An alternative approach is to make a detailed review of national expenditures. Money may then be diverted from nonproductive areas of the economy (such as national defense), or (as is currently happening in a number of western democracies) there may be an erosion of other social services.

A third and even less palatable option is to increase the economic burden carried by some segment of society—for example, to impose a special levy on the rich, or to reduce the effective value of pensions through inflation. The last "remedy" is becoming ever less practicable, since the elderly now form a powerful, well-organized, and growing block of the electorate who are particularly prone to exercise their franchise.

Exercise and the Actuarial Dilemma

If regular exercise were to increase life expectancy by two years (as seems to be the case if it is begun at an age of 35 years, Paffenbarger 1988), will this not worsen the actuarial and health insurance dilemma by a factor of 15% to 20%, as Warner (1987) seems to suggest?

There are several possible fallacies in such an argument. The first is that payments to seniors represent the sole charge on pension plans. In Canada, major components of the total "pension" cost include (1) disability payments received by those suffering from chronic disease, (2) death benefits, and (3) payments made to orphans and to the children of disabled contributors (see

Table 10.4   Disbursements under the Canada and Québec Pension Plans during 1986 (values expressed in 1995 U.S. dollars).

Source of expense	Amount	Percentage of total disbursements
Survivors' pensions	1.336B	50.4
Disability pensions		
Musculoskeletal	0.275	10.4
Cardiovascular	0.247	9.3
Other diseases	0.427	16.1
Death benefits	0.160	6.0
Orphans' pensions	0.131	4.9
Children of disabled	0.077	2.9
Total	2.652	100.0

Adapted from *Economic Burden of Illness in Canada*, Supplement to *Chronic Diseases in Canada*, Volume 12, No. 3, Health Canada, 1991. With permission of the Minister of Public Works and Government Services Canada, 1997.

table 10.4). Many of these payments involve young and middle-aged adults, and such costs would likely be reduced if the population were to adopt a healthier and more active lifestyle.

Secondly, most calculations have made the simplifying assumption that the age of retirement is the same for active and sedentary individuals. However, poor health is a major factor influencing the decision to retire (as seen in chapter 9), and since regular exercise not only increases life span but also reduces morbidity, the active person is likely to continue working for a longer period than a sedentary individual.

Thirdly, a large fraction of the total costs involved in supporting seniors is incurred during terminal care for the very old. It is thus important to stress that although exercise prevents premature death, it does little to extend years of life among the very old (Paffenbarger 1988; Pekkanen et al. 1987)—indeed, beyond the age of 80 years, it may have just the effect that actuaries have been seeking, a shortening of calendar life span (Linsted, Tonstad, and Kuzma 1991; Paffenbarger et al. 1994).

Finally, the actuarial calculations assume that seniors make no contribution to society. Again, the contribution from sedentary, totally dependent frail elderly persons may be very limited, but the fit elderly do much for their communities through part-time employment, volunteer work, and caring for grandchildren.

It remains unlikely that involvement of the elderly population in exercise programs will solve of all our current actuarial and health insurance problems. On the other hand, there is no good evidence that the encouragement of regular physical activity will exacerbate current fiscal difficulties.

Demand for Medical Services and Institutional Support

The costs of providing medical services and institutional support for the elderly are often assumed to be vast. Old people are affected less often by acute illnesses, but the likelihood of disability and thus a continuing need for medical services is greater than in younger adults (Davidson and Marmor 1980).

The prevalence of chronic disease, and thus the demand for medical care, increase progressively with age. According to the U.S. National Center for Health Statistics (1991), physician visits averaged 3.1 per person per year in those aged 45 to 64, 4.6 per year in those aged 65 to 74, and 5.4 per year in those over 75 years. Hospital bed days per 1000 of the population in the three age groups were 903, 2115, and 4087/1000 per year.

The per capita cost of providing medical and hospital care for the elderly is increasing with time, not only because of a medical inflation rate that exceeds increases in the consumer price index and an increased sophistication of available services, but also in many instances because inappropriate or unnecessary treatments are provided (Chassin et al. 1987). The respective costs of Medicare and Medicaid for those over 65 years in 1975, 1980, and 1985 were $20, $42, and $87 billion (Pawlson 1994). Expressing all values in 1995 U.S. dollars, the average figure per senior in the United States in 1970 was $3077, 2.67 times the expense of $1148 for adults aged 19 to 64 years (U.S. Senate Special Committee on Aging 1972). Some $2077 of this total was met from various health insurance plans, leaving an average of $1000 to be taken from the individual's meager resources. Gibson and Fisher (1979) estimated that by 1979 the per capita personal health-care expenditures of those over 65 years had increased to $3630 per year, some 3.3 times the average for the remainder of the population.

New technologies such as coronary revascularization, heart, lung, and liver transplantations, and renal dialysis have caused the gap in medical costs between the young and the old to widen still further in recent years. Some authors estimate that medical costs for those over the age of 65 years are now four to five times higher than for younger people. Much of the expense associated with old age is concentrated in the final year of life. This reflects at least three influences. Irrespective of age group, a fourth of the population are hospitalized during the two months that precede death, and as many as half of the population are hospitalized in the final month of life (Fries 1980b). Older people also have a greater morbidity and are affected by different types of illness than younger people. The prevalent problems of the elderly—cardiovascular disease and cancer—are now open to complex and expensive methods of diagnosis and treatment (Collishaw and Myers 1984). Moreover, many of the procedures adopted are not cost-effective. It is instructive to compare expenditures on the elderly between the United States, where high technology *in extremis* is too often the norm, and the United Kingdom (see table 10.5), where a careful cost-effectiveness assessment is undertaken before expensive treatments are applied.

The conclusion of Fries (1980b) still holds: the high cost of providing hospital-based medical services to the elderly in the United States is due almost entirely to painful, undignified, and agonizing interventions that prolong the final year of life. If due allowance is made for the large fraction of the very old who are in their final year of life, then there is little evidence that the provision of medical services to the remainder of the elderly population is any more costly than for younger individuals.

Expressing expenditures in 1995 U.S. dollars, the estimated total cost of illness in Canada in 1986 (Health and Welfare, Canada 1986) was approximately $97 billion. Distributed over a population of some 29 million, this amounted to $3345 per head (see table 10.6). However, almost half of the total was attributable to indirect costs: premature mortality and loss of work from short-term and chronic disability. It is unclear how far such indirect costs should be excluded from the calculations for seniors, since (as noted in the previous section) many older people do make substantial part-time and voluntary contributions to society. Direct costs (the value of resources that could have been directed to other uses in the absence of disease; Rice, Hodgson, and Kopstein 1985) were $50.17 billion, or $1730 per head. Assuming a 4.5-fold increase in this component of the total for those over the age of 65 years, direct costs for this age group would have amounted to $7266 per person per year. Much of the difference between Canada and the United States is due to the later date of the Canadian figures, since medical costs have been rising much faster than the general rate of inflation. In the United States, annual expenditures on health care, expressed in 1995 dollars, increased from $766 to $1645 per head between 1970 and 1995; again applying a 4.5-fold multiplier to the cost for seniors, this implies a 1995 figure of $7403 per person.

Table 10.5   Medical costs of services for the elderly in the United Kingdom.

Hospital costs	$2.703B
Professional services	0.667B
Residential care	2.131B
Day care and home help	1.110B
Medical aids	0.088B
TOTAL	6.484B

Notes: Population = 6.58M over the age of 65 years; cost of NHS hospital bed $84/day, nursing home $52/day, residential home $38.50/day, domiciliary care $27.80/day.

Adapted, by permission, from the Report from Social Services committee, Session 1985-86, 1985-1986, (London: Her Majesty's Stationery Office). Crown copyright is reproduced with the permission of the Controller of Her Majesty's Stationery Office.

Table 10.6   Total costs of illness in Canada during 1986 (values expressed in 1995 U.S. dollars).

Direct costs	
Hospital care	$17.097B
Professional services	9.978
Pensions and benefits	6.856
Non-hospital institutions	4.550
Drugs	3.584
Health research	453
Other*	7.655
Subtotal	50.172
Indirect costs	
Premature mortality	25.566
Chronic disability	19.007
Short-term disability	2.447
Subtotal	47.020
Grand Total	97.192

*Other health expenditures include ambulance services, home care, medical appliances, capital expenditures on hospitals and related institutions, public health measures, medical and dental schools, administrative costs of health insurance plans, and miscellaneous costs.

Adapted from *Economic Burden of Illness in Canada*, Supplement to *Chronic Diseases in Canada*, Volume 12, No. 3, Health Canada, 1991. With permission of the Minister of Public Works and Government Services Canada, 1997.

Excluding pensions, benefits, health research, and miscellaneous items, the direct medical costs in Canada total $35.19 billion per year. Respective percentages of the total are 48.6% (hospital costs), 28.4% (professional services), 12.9% (nursing homes), and 10.2% (drugs). The distribution of costs is somewhat similar in the United States. One survey found that for those aged 65 years and older, respective percentages were 49.4% (hospital costs), 22.3% (professional services), 17.1% (nursing homes), and 11.2% (drugs). Both in the United States and Canada, the largest single component of the direct costs is hospital care. The Canadian figure amounts to $17.1 billion per year. Two conditions susceptible to exercise (cardiovascular diseases, $3.5 billion, and cancer, $1.5 billion) account for almost 30% of these hospital expenditures.

Another substantial element in national costs (Health and Welfare, Canada 1986) is care in institutions other than hospitals. Here, a large fraction of the total expenditure is undoubtedly attributable to the frail elderly (see table 10.7). Many of those who are institutionalized have no access to relatives. The need for institutional support of the elderly is increasing, as families become more widely dispersed geographically and an ever-larger fraction of middle-aged women enter the ranks of full-time employed workers.

Table 10.7   Types and costs of institutional care for the elderly in Canada in 1975.

Type of care	Percentage of elderly	Total population	Daily cost (per person[a])	Annual total
Active treatment	1.47	24,990	$223	$2.036B
Chronic treatment	0.89	15,130	61	0.337
Mental care	0.32	5,440	61	0.122
Extended care	4.17	70,890	34.5	0.893
Other residential	2.37	39,100	32.5[b]	0.463

Notes: All values expressed in 1995 U.S. dollars. Capital costs of facilities are not included.

[a]Estimates for the City of London, Ontario, in 1975; the subsequent costs of hospital and institutional care have approximately doubled relative to the standard consumer price index.

[b]Includes a $20/day charge for the occupation of ambulatory care facilities, plus a surcharge that varies with the amount of nursing care required by the individual.

Reprinted, by permission, from K.H. Sidney, 1975 (Ph.D. dissertation, University of Toronto).

Costs and Benefits of Greater Physical Activity

Unfortunately, there is very little direct information on either the costs or the benefits of exercise for seniors.

Likely Costs

The costs depend very much upon the intensity of the program that is contemplated. Light chair exercises, for example, could easily be conducted by volunteers, using a minimum of equipment. Moreover, such activities might have some beneficial outcomes for the frail elderly, including increased flexibility and an improved mood state.

On the other hand, a more rigorous group program is needed to increase aerobic fitness, to restore muscle strength, to reduce body fatness, serum cholesterol, and high blood pressure, and to enhance bone density. This will probably require regular evaluations of fitness (perhaps as many as four per year), and the supervision of classes by a well-trained fitness instructor (perhaps a 1 h commitment, at least three times per week). Sometimes suitable space for exercising may be available in a nursing home, but for seniors who are living in the community, it may be necessary to hire a hall and arrange transportation to and from the facility. The costs per class will depend on the size of the group, but are unlikely to be less than $4 to $5 per session, plus transportation. Although many middle-aged adults would not find this a large cost for an enjoyable activity, the expense can be a serious disincentive to someone who is living on a restricted income.

There are two main arguments in favor of group programming. Safety is likely to be greater than when exercise is pursued individually. Moreover, the combination of social involvement and perceived safety/efficacy of the program may stimulate more regular participation than an alternative, self-directed option such as brisk walking in an air-conditioned shopping mall. Against these two advantages must be set the costs of group programming, and (for seniors living in the community) the logistic difficulties of arranging appropriate transportation to and from a facility.

Likely Benefits

Savings from an increase of habitual activity are likely to be less in seniors than in younger adults, since many of the pathological changes that cause a deterioration of health now require tertiary and quaternary care.

Acute and Chronic Hospital Care

An active lifestyle continues to have some influence on the number of acute and chronic hospital admissions (Shephard 1986b). Common causes of both acute and chronic admissions for elderly patients are summarized in table 10.8. If we assume that the cardiovascular benefit of regular exercise is half as great as in a younger person, we might anticipate a 25% reduction in admissions for cardiovascular disease; likewise, if regular physical activity still has some benefit in reducing blood pressure and in preventing or reversing muscle

Table 10.8 Admission diagnoses of elderly patients receiving acute and chronic care.

Diagnosis	Acute treatment	Chronic treatment
Cardiovascular disease	42%	34*
Stroke	22	18
Chronic respiratory disease	8	22
Acute infection	11	15
Coma	0	4
Other	17	7

*Data recalculated, assuming that all 28% of admissions with chronic brain syndrome were treated in mental hospitals.

Adapted, by permission, from J.C. Brocklehurst, 1973, Geriatric services and the day hospital. In *Textbook of geriatric medicine and gerontology*, edited by J.C. Brocklehurst (Edinburgh: Churchill Livingstone), 676.

wasting, there might be at least a 10% reduction in strokes and chronic respiratory disease, for an overall reduction in acute hospital admissions of perhaps 13.5%. Applying similar reasoning to the causes of chronic admission, a 12.5% reduction in costs might be anticipated.

Chronic Mental Disorders

There is no reliable information on how the incidence of senile dementia might be affected by regular physical activity. Mental problems arise from a combination of degenerative neuropathies cerebral atherosclerosis and hypertensive hemorrhage. It thus seems acceptable to impute some advantage to the regular exerciser: atherosclerosis is lessened, resting blood pressure is reduced by about 5 mmHg, and the exercise blood pressure is also less at any given rate of working (discussed in chapter 5). For the purpose of the present calculation, an arbitrary 10% reduction in new admissions will be assumed.

Extended and Residential Care

Perhaps the most intriguing item in the calculation is a possible reduction in the demand for extended and residential care. One analysis of the causes of impaired mobility and the need for residential care is given in table 10.9. General frailty is assigned a relatively minor role in this analysis. This is probably correct if the overall population of seniors is considered, but if attention is focused upon the very old, a progressive loss of aerobic power, muscle strength, and flexibility may have a large influence on the need for institutionalization (reviewed in chapter 8).

Table 10.9   Causes of loss of mobility and of being house-bound or bed-fast.

Cause of disability	Percentage of sample
Arthritis, rheumatism	36.2
Pulmonary disease	17.2
Strokes, paralysis	14.9
Blindness, failing sight	14.4
Circulatory conditions	13.8
Cardiac conditions, blood pressure	13.2
Effects of accidents	9.8
Old age	6.9
Nervous conditions	4.6
Other illnesses	29.9

Note: Some individuals named more than one disorder, so the total of citations is substantially more than 100%.

Adapted, by permission, from A. Hunt, 1978, *The elderly at home* (London: Her Majesty's Stationery Office). Crown copyright is reproduced with the permission of the Controller of Her Majesty's Stationery Office.

Regular exercise could play a useful role in lessening the impact of many of the specific conditions that cause a loss of mobility (chapters 5-8). It also has a major impact on the age of onset of general frailty. A decline in aerobic power is likely to limit the daily activities of a typical senior by the age of 79 years, because peak oxygen transport has fallen below the critical threshold value of 1 L/min (14 ml/[kg · min]) needed to perform daily tasks without fatigue and breathlessness. However, if a training program were to augment aerobic power by 3.6 ml/[kg · min], as was observed by Sidney and Shephard (1978a) in seniors who undertook a vigorous training program (reviewed in chapter 4), then aerobic power would remain above the critical threshold for a further eight to nine years. Assuming that the exercise program had little effect upon longevity (discussed in chapter 4), the proportion of survivors might drop from around 30% of the population at an age of 79 years to only 10% at an age of 88 years. The cost of providing extended care for active seniors who had ultimately become frail would thus be only a third of that for a sedentary group.

True gains are probably somewhat smaller than these calculations might suggest, because organic pathologies still have some bearing on admission to extended-care homes, even at an advanced age.

Empirical Investigations

There have been few empirical investigations of the influence of physical activity and health education programs on the medical costs incurred by seniors. Perhaps not surprisingly, available investigations have also been relatively limited in scope and duration.

Schauffler, Agostino, and Kannel (1993) found that elderly members of the Framingham cohort (age 63-93 years) with risk factors for cardiovascular disease had 19% higher medical claims than those who did not have such risk factors. The added cost amounted to $371 per subject-year. Smoking increased claims by 16%, a systolic blood pressure of over 160 mmHg augmented expenses by 11%, and a serum cholesterol in excess of 260 mg/dl boosted costs by 9%. However, no data were reported for the effects of a sedentary lifestyle. Fries et al. (1993) initiated a low-cost health education program for retirees of the Bank of America; this included an initial risk appraisal and mailed reinforcement and management materials. The estimated health costs of experimental subjects were reduced by some 20% relative to those for controls; moreover, reductions in health risks and costs were similar among cohorts initially aged 55 to 65, 65 to 75, and over 75 years. A second report by the same authors (Fries et al. 1994) examined medical claims in a sample of 12,102 public employees and former employees. The experimental intervention comprised a health-risk appraisal every six months and a mailed educational program aimed at improving overall lifestyle (including habitual activity). There were small but significant increases in weekly exercise times for those in the full treatment group (from 185 to 200 min in those still employed, from 213 to 222 min in retirees, and from 184 to 192 min in seniors). The experimental subjects also showed reductions in the annual cost of medical visits, hospital days, and sick days relative to control subjects (see table 10.10). These benefits were significant in current employees (average age 50 years) and retirees (average age 63 years), but not in seniors (average age 73 years). Bell and Blanke (1992) compared hospital days, medical costs, and medical claims between participants and nonparticipants in an employee fitness program. None of the differences in their study reached statistical significance, but there was a trend for benefit in men under 40 years of age that was not seen in those over the age of 40 years.

We have already noted the retrospective observations of Shephard and Montelpare (1988), suggesting a relationship between the level of habitual physical activity at an age of 50 years and the likelihood that an individual would require extended care as a senior (see table 8.3).

Ascribed Benefit

Potential reductions in the costs of geriatric institutional care are summarized in table 10.11. The estimates are relatively crude, but they suggest a potential to save some 30% of the overall cost, much larger than the likely expense of even a highly supervised exercise program.

Table 10.10 Change in annual per capita medical expenditures over an 18-month program of health education.

Group	Initial cost	Final cost	Increase
Current employees			
Active participants	1604	2074	470
Passive participants	1295	1727	432
Controls	1206	1836	630
Retirees			
Active participants	1645	1948	303
Passive participants	1624	1989	365
Controls	1854	3060	1206
Seniors			
Active participants	609	702	93
Passive participants	614	748	134
Controls	Data not provided		

Adapted, by permission, from J.F. Fries et al., 1994, "Randomized controlled trial of cost reductions from a health education program: The California Public Employees' Retirement Scheme (PERS) Study," *American Journal of Health Promotion* 8: 216-223.

Table 10.11   Potential savings in costs of institutional care if elderly population were to adopt a physically active lifestyle.

Type of care	Cost	Saving factor	Total saving
Acute and chronic care	$2.373B	0.13	$0.309B
Mental care	0.122B	0.10	0.012B
Extended and residential care	1.356B	0.67	0.909B
Total	3.851B		1.230B

All data expressed in 1995 U.S. dollars.

Conclusions

Recent years have seen some progress in assuring equity for older individuals in occupational hiring, promotion, and retirement. Nevertheless, there remain many stereotypes to overcome. In fact, most older individuals are good employees in terms of their safety and productivity. Procedures established by equal employment opportunity and human rights commissions are now being used to assess specific occupations in which declining performance or issues of safety may impose a *bona fide* age criterion upon employees.

The solvency of pension funds is becoming a major social issue. Dependency ratios arc increasing not only because of the growing proportion of senior citizens, but also because training periods have increased for adolescents and the age of retirement has been progressively reduced. The supposed high cost of providing medical services for the elderly is largely a myth, created by excessive and inappropriate treatment administered in the final few weeks of life. Available cost-benefit analyses suggest that the expense of simple exercise programs for seniors can be more than met through savings in both medical expenses and the demands for institutional support.

In short, a regular program of moderate exercise is a very appropriate recommendation for almost all senior citizens. Moreover, there is no known pharmacological remedy that can so safely and effectively reduce a person's biological age and enhance his or her quality-adjusted life expectancy.

References

Abbas, A.K., Lichtman, A.H., and Pober, J.S. (1995). *Cellular and molecular immunology* (2nd ed.). Toronto, ON: Saunders.

Abourezk, T. (1989). The effects of regular aerobic exercise on short-term memory efficiency in the older adult. In A.C. Ostrow (Ed.), *Aging and motor behavior* (pp. 105-113). Indianapolis: Benchmark Press.

Abrams, M. (1977). *Three score years and ten*. London: Age Concerns.

Achenbaum, W.A. (1991). "Time is the messenger of the Gods." A gerontological metaphor. In G.M. Kenyon, J.E. Birren, and J.J.F. Schroots (Eds.), *Metaphors of aging in science and the humanities* (pp. 83-102). New York: Springer.

Adair, N. (1994). Chronic airflow obstruction and respiratory failure. In W.R. Hazzard, E.L. Bierman, J.P. Bass, W.H. Ettinger, and J.B. Halter (Eds.), *Principles of geriatrics and gerontology* (3rd ed., pp. 583-595). New York: McGraw-Hill.

Ades, P.A., Waldmann, M.L., Poehlman, E.T., Gray, P., Horton, E.D., Horton, E.S., and LeWinter, M.M. (1993). Exercise conditioning in older coronary patients. Submaximal lactate response and endurance capacity. *Circulation* 88: 572-577.

Adler, W.H., and Nagel, J.E. (1994). Clinical immunology and aging. In W.R. Hazzard, E.L. Bierman, J.P. Blass, W.H. Ettinger, and J.E. Halter (Eds.), *Principles of geriatric medicine and gerontology* (pp. 61-76). New York: McGraw-Hill.

Adrian, M.J. (1981). Flexibility in the aging adult. In E.L. Smith and R.C. Serfass (Eds.), *Exercise and aging. The scientific basis* (pp. 45-58). Hillside, NJ: Enslow.

Aggleton, J.P., Bland, J.M., Kentridge, R.W., and Neave, N.J. (1994). Handedness and longevity: Archival study of cricketers. *British Medical Journal* 309: 1681-1684.

Albanes, D., Blair, A., and Taylor, P.R. (1989). Physical activity and risk of cancer in NHANES I population. *American Journal of Public Health* 79: 744-750.

Albanese, A.A. (1980). *Nutrition for the elderly*. New York: Liss.

Allen, S.J., Benton, J.S., Goodhardt, M.J., Haan, E.A., Sims, N.R., Smith, C.C.T., Spillane, J.A., Bowen, D.M., and Davison, A.M. (1983). Biochemical evidence of selective nerve cell changes in the normal aging human and rat brain. *Journal of Neurochemistry* 41: 256-265.

Alnaqeeb, M.A., Zaid, N.S., and Goldspink, G. (1984). Connective tissue changes and physical properties of developing and ageing skeletal muscle. *Journal of Anatomy* 139: 677-689.

Aloia, J.F. (1989). *Osteoporosis: A guide to prevention and treatment*. Champaign, IL: Leisure Press.

Aloia, J.F., Vaswani, A.N., Yeh, J., and Cohn, S.H. (1988). Premenopausal bone mass is related to physical activity. *Archives of Internal Medicine* 148: 121-123.

American Automobile Association. (1985). *Safe driving for mature operators*. Falls Church, VA: Traffic Safety Department.

American College of Sports Medicine. (1990). The recommended quantity and quality of exercise for developing and maintaining fitness in healthy adults. *Medicine and Science in Sports and Exercise* 22: 265-274.

American College of Sports Medicine. (1995a). *Guidelines for graded exercise testing and exercise prescription* (5th ed.). Philadelphia: Lea & Febiger.

American College of Sports Medicine. (1995b). Position stand on osteoporosis and exercise. *Medicine and Science in Sports and Exercise* 27: i-vii.

Amiel, D., Kuiper, S.D., Wallace, C.D., Harwood, F.L., and VandeBerg, J.S. (1991). Age-related properties of medial collateral ligament and anterior cruciate ligament: A morphologic and collagen maturation study in the rabbit. *Journals of Gerontology* 46: B159-B166.

Anacker, S.L., and Di Fabio, R.P. (1992). Influence of sensory inputs on standing balance in community-dwelling elders with a recent history of falling. *Physical Therapy* 72: 575-582.

Anderson, T.W., Brown, J.R., Hall, J.W., and Shephard, R.J. (1968). The limitations of linear regressions for the prediction of vital capacity and forced expiratory volume. *Respiration* 25: 465-484.

Andreotti, L., Bussotti, A., Cammelli, D., Aiello, E., and Sampognaro, S. (1983). Connective tissue in aging lung. *Gerontology* 29: 377-387.

Andres, R. (1985). Normal aging versus disease in the elderly. In R. Andres, E.L. Bierman, and W.R. Hazzard (Eds.), *Principles of geriatric medicine* (pp. 38-41). New York: McGraw-Hill.

Andres, R. (1994). Mortality and obesity: The rationale for age-specific height-weight tables. In W.R. Hazzard, E.L. Bierman, J.P. Blass, W.E. Ettinger, and J.B. Halter (Eds.), *Principles of geriatric medicine and gerontology* (pp. 847-853). New York: McGraw-Hill.

Andrews, J.R., and St. Pierre, R.K. (1986). Osteoarthritis, athletes and arthroscopic management. In J.R. Sutton and R.M. Brock (Eds.), *Sports medicine for the mature athlete* (pp. 279-286). Indianapolis: Benchmark Press.

Andrisani, P.J., and Sandell, S.H. (1985). Technological change and the labor market situation of older workers. In P.K. Robinson, J. Livingston, and J.E. Birren (Eds.), *Aging and technological advances* (pp. 99-112). New York: Plenum Press.

Aniansson, A., and Gustafsson, E. (1981). Physical training in elderly man with special reference to quadriceps muscle strength and morphology. *Clinical Physiology* 1: 87-98.

Aniansson, A., Hedberg, M., Henning, G.B., and Grimby, G. (1986). Muscle morphology, enzyme activity and muscle strength in elderly men: A follow up study. *Muscle and Nerve* 9: 585-591.

Aniansson, A., Sperling, L., Rundgren, A., and Lehnberg, E. (1983). Muscle function in 75 year-old men and women. A longitudinal study. *Scandinavian Journal of Rehabilitation Medicine* 9 (Suppl.): 92-102.

Aoyagi, Y., and Shephard, R.J. (1992). Aging and muscle function. *Sports Medicine* 14: 376-396.

Applebaum-Bowden, D., McLean, P., Steinmetz, A., Fontana, D., Matthys, C., Warnick, G.R., Cheung, M., Albers, J.J., and Hazzard, W.R. (1989). Lipoprotein, apolipoprotein, and lipolytic enzyme changes following estrogen administration in postmenopausal women. *Journal of Lipid Research* 30: 1895-1906.

Applegate, W.B. (1994). Hypertension. In W.R. Hazzard, E.L. Bierman, J.P. Blass, W.H. Ettinger, and J.E. Halter (Eds.), *Principles of geriatric medicine and gerontology* (3rd ed., pp. 541-554). New York: McGraw-Hill.

Araujo, D.M., Lapchak, P.A., Meaney, M.J., Collier, B., and Quirion, R. (1990). Effects of aging on nicotinic and muscarinic autoreceptor function in the rat brain: Relationship to presynaptic cholinergic markers and binding sites. *Journal of Neurosciences* 10: 3069-3078.

Arbetter, J.A., and Schaefer, E.J. (1989). Lipoproteins, nutrition, exercise and aging. In R. Harris and S. Harris (Eds.), *Physical activity, aging and sports* (pp. 239-250). Albany, NY: Center for Studies of Aging.

Arking, R. (1987). Successful selection for increased longevity in Drosophila: Analysis of the survival data and presentation of a hypothesis on the genetic regulation of longevity. *Experimental Gerontology* 22: 199-220.

Arking, R., Buck, S., Wells, R.A., and Pretzlaff, R. (1988). Metabolic rates in genetically based long-lived strains of Drosophila. *Experimental Gerontology* 23: 59-76.

Armbrecht, H.J., Perry, H.M., and Martin, K.J. (1993). Changes in mineral and bone metabolism with age. In H.M. Perry, J.E. Morley, and R.M. Coe (Eds.), *Aging and musculoskeletal disorders* (pp. 68-77). New York: Springer.

Armstrong, D. (1991). Ceroid-lipofuscinosis: A natural model for studying lipopigments and the ageing process. In M.S.J. Pathy (Ed.), *Principles and practice of geriatric medicine* (2nd ed., pp. 55-68). Chichester: Wiley.

Aronow, W.S., and Epstein, S. (1988). Usefulness of silent myocardial ischemia detected by ambulatory electrocardiographic monitoring in predicting new coronary events in elderly patients. *American Journal of Cardiology* 62: 1295-1296.

Arvan, S. (1988). Exercise performance of the high risk acute myocardial infarction patient after cardiac rehabilitation. *American Journal of Cardiology* 62: 197-201.

Asano, K., Ogawa, S., and Furuta, Y. (1978). Aerobic work capacity in middle- and old-aged runners. In F. Landry and W.R. Orban (Eds.), *Exercise physiology* (pp. 465-471). Miami, FL: Symposia Specialists.

Åstrand, P.O. (1986). Exercise physiology of the mature athlete. In J.R. Sutton and R.M. Brock (Eds.), *Sports medicine for the mature athlete* (pp. 3-13). Indianapolis: Benchmark Press.

Åstrom, J., Ahnqvist, S., Beertema, J., and Jonsson, B. (1987). Physical activity in women sustaining fractures of the neck of the femur. *Journal of Bone and Joint Surgery* 69B: 381-383.

Atkins, C.J., Kaplan, R.M., Timms, R.M., Reinsch, S., and Lofback, K. (1984). Behavioral exercise programs in the management of chronic obstructive pulmonary disease. *Journal of Consulting and Clinical Psychology* 52: 591-603.

Atkinson, R., and Wallberg-Rankin, J. (1994). Physical activity, fitness and severe obesity. In C. Bouchard, R.J. Shephard, and T. Stephens (Eds.), *Physical activity, fitness and health* (pp. 696-771). Champaign, IL: Human Kinetics.

Avlund, K., Schroll, M., Davidsen, M., Levborg, B., and Rantanen, T. (1994). Maximal isometric muscle strength and functional ability in daily activities among 75-year-old men and women. *Scandinavian Journal of Medicine, Science and Sports* 4: 32-40.

Ayalon, J., Simkin, A., Leichter, I., and Raifmann, S. (1987). Dynamic bone loading exercises for postmenopausal women: Effect on the density of the distal radius. *Archives of Physical Medicine and Rehabilitation* 68: 280-283.

Babcock, M.A., Paterson, D.H., Cunningham, D.A., and Dickinson, J.R. (1994). Exercise on-transient gas exchange kinetics are slowed as a function of age. *Medicine and Science in Sports and Exercise* 26: 440-446.

Baber, R.J., and Studd, J.W.W. (1989). Hormone replacement therapy and cancer. *British Journal of Hospital Medicine* 41: 142-149.

Bäckman, L., and Molander, B. (1989). The relationship between level of arousal and cognitive operations during motor behavior in young and older adults. In A. C. Ostrow (Ed.), *Aging and motor behavior* (pp. 3-33). Indianapolis: Benchmark Press.

Badenhop, D.T., Cleary, P.A., Schaal, S.F., Fox, E.L., and Bartels, R.L. (1983). Physiological adjustments to higher- or lower-intensity exercise in elders. *Medicine and Science in Sports and Exercise* 15: 496-502.

Bagge, E., Bjelle, A., Eden, S., and Svänborg, A. (1991). Osteoarthritis in the elderly. Clinical and radiographic osteoarthritis in two elderly European populations. *Annals of the Rheumatic Diseases* (London) 50: 535-539.

Bagge, E., Bjelle, A., and Svänborg, A. (1992). Radiographic osteoarthritis in the elderly: A cohort comparison and longitudinal study of the 70-year old people in Göteborg. *Clinical Rheumatology* (Brussels) 11: 486-491.

Balady, G.J. (1992). Exercise therapy in patients with angina and silent ischemia. In R.J. Shephard and H.J. Miller (Eds.), *Exercise and the heart in health and disease* (pp. 369-396). New York: Marcel Dekker.

Balcomb, A.C., and Sutton, J.R. (1986). Advanced age and altitude illness. In J.R. Sutton and R.M. Brock (Eds.), *Sports medicine for the mature athlete* (pp. 213-224). Indianapolis: Benchmark Press.

Ballard, J.E., McKeown, B.C., Graham, H.M., and Zinkgraf, S.A. (1990). The effect of high level physical activity (8.5 METS or greater) and estrogen replacement therapy upon bone mass in postmenopausal females, aged 50-68 years. *International Journal of Sports Medicine* 11: 208-214.

Ballor, D.L., and Keesey, R.E. (1991). A meta-analysis of the factors affecting exercise-induced changes in body mass, fat mass and fat-free mass in males and females. *International Journal of Obesity* 15: 717-726.

Barak, D., and Djerassi, L. (1987). Musculo-skeletal injuries among bus drivers due to motor vehicle accidents and hazardous environmental conditions. *Ergonomics* 30: 335-342.

Bard, C., Fleury, M., Jobin, J., Lagassé, P., and Roy, B. (1985). Elaboration des normes physiques d'admission aux corps d'agents de la paix [Development of physical entry norms for peace officers]. Laval University Faculty of Physical Education, unpublished manuscript.

Barnard, R.J. (1994). Physical activity, fitness and claudication. In C. Bouchard, R.J. Shephard, and T. Stephens (Eds.), *Physical activity, fitness and health* (pp. 622-632). Champaign, IL: Human Kinetics.

Barnes, C.A., Forster, M.J., Fleshner, M., Ahanotu, E.N., Laudenslager, M.L., Mazzeo, R.S., Maier, S.F., and Lal, H. (1991). Exercise does not modify spatial memory, brain auto-immunity, or antibody response in aged F-344 rats. *Neurobiology of Aging* 12: 47-53.

Barnes, R.F., Raskind, M., Gumbrecht, G., and Halter, J.B. (1982). The effects of age on the plasma catecholamine response to mental stress in man. *Journal of Clinical Endocrinology and Metabolism* 54: 64-69.

Barnes, R.W., Thornhill, B., Nix, L., Rittgers, S.E., and Turley, G. (1981). Prediction of amputation wound healing. Roles of Doppler ultra-sound and digit plethysmography. *Archives of Surgery* 116: 80-83.

Baron, D.T., Bergfeld, M.A., Teitelbaum, S.L., and Avioli, L.V. (1978). Effect of testosterone therapy on bone formation in an osteoporotic hypogonadal male. *Calcified Tissue International* 26: 103-106.

Barrett-Connor, E. (1995). The economic and human costs of osteoporotic fracture. *American Journal of Medicine* 98 (2A): 35-85.

Barrett-Connor, E., and Palinkas, L.A. (1994). Low blood pressure and depression in older men: A population based study. *British Medical Journal* 308: 446-449.

Baslund, B., Lyngberg, K., Andersen, V., Kristensen, J.H., Hansen, M., Klokker, M., and Pedersen, B.K. (1993). Effect of 8 wk of bicycle training on the immune system of patients with rheumatoid arthritis. *Journal of Applied Physiology* 75: 1691-1695.

Basmajian, J.V. (1987). Therapeutic exercise in the management of rheumatic diseases. *Journal of Rheumatology* 14 (Suppl. 15): 22-25.

Bass, A., Gutmann, E., and Hanzlikova, V. (1975). Biochemical changes in energy supply pattern of muscle of the rat during old age. *Gerontologia* 21: 31-45.

Bassey, E.J., Bendall, M.J., and Pearson, M. (1988). Muscle strength in the triceps surae and objectively measured customary walking activity in men and women over 65 years of age. *Clinical Science* 74: 85-89.

Bassey, E.J., Fiatarone, M.A., O'Neill, E.F., Kelly, M., Evans, W.J., and Lipsitz, L.A. (1992). Leg extensor power and functional performance in very old men and women. *Clinical Science* 82: 321-327.

Bassey, E.J., and Harries, U.J. (1993). Normal values for handgrip strength in 920 men and women over 65 years, and longitudinal changes over four years in 620 survivors. *Clinical Science* 84: 331-337.

Bates, W.T. (1982). Selecting a running shoe. *Physician and Sportsmedicine* 10 (3): 154-155.

Baylink, D.J., and Jennings, J.C. (1994). Calcium and bone homeostasis and changes with aging. In W.R. Hazzard, E.L. Bierman, J.P. Blass, W.H. Ettinger, and J.B. Halter (Eds.), *Principles of geriatric medicine and gerontology* (pp. 879-896). New York: McGraw-Hill.

Bazzoli, G.J. (1985). The early retirement decision: New empirical evidence on the influence of health. *Journal of Human Resources* 20: 315-330.

Beaglehole, R., and Stewart, A. (1983). The longevity of international rugby players. *New Zealand Medical Journal* 96: 513-515.

Beck, L.H. (1994). Aging changes in renal function. In W.R. Hazzard, E.L. Bierman, J.P. Blass, W.H. Ettinger, and J.B. Halter (Eds.), *Principles of geriatric medicine and gerontology* (3rd ed., pp. 615-624). New York: McGraw-Hill.

Belchetz, P.E. (1985). Idiopathic hypopituitarism in patients over 65. *British Medical Journal* 291: 247-248.

Bell, B.C., and Blanke, D.J. (1992). The effects of an employee fitness program on health care costs and utilization. *Health Values* 16: 3-13.

Bell, N.H., Godsen, R.H., Henry, D.P., Shary, J., and Epstein, S. (1988). The effects of muscle building exercise on vitamin D and mineral metabolism. *Journal of Bone and Mineral Research* 3: 369-373.

Bellamy, D. (1991). Mechanisms of ageing. In M.S.J. Pathy (Ed.), *Principles and practice of geriatric medicine* (2nd ed., pp. 13-30). Chichester: Wiley.

Belman, M.J., and Gaesser, G.A. (1991). Exercise training below and above the lactate threshold in the elderly. *Medicine and Science in Sports and Exercise* 23: 562-568.

Bemben, M.G., Massey, B.H., Bemben, D.A., Boileau, R.A., and Misner, J.E. (1995). Age-related patterns in body composition for men aged 20-79 yr. *Medicine and Science in Sports and Exercise* 27: 264-269.

Bemben, M.G., Massey, B.H., Bemben, D.A., Misner, J.E., and Boileau, R.A. (1991). Isometric muscle force production as a function of age in healthy 20- to 74-yr-old men. *Medicine and Science in Sports and Exercise* 23: 1302-1310.

Bemben, D.A., Massey, B.H., Boileau, R.A., and Misner, J.E. (1992). Reliability of isometric force-time curve parameters for men aged 20- to 79 years. *Journal of Applied Sport Science Research* 6: 158-164.

Ben Ari, E., Rothbaum, D.A., Linnemeier, T.J., Landin, R.J., Steinmetz, E.F., Hilles, S.J., Noble, J.R., Hallam, C.C., See, M.R., and Shiner, R. (1987). Benefits of a monitored rehabilitation program versus physician care after percutaneous transluminal coronary angioplasty. Follow-up of risk factors and rate of restenosis. *Journal of Cardiopulmonary Rehabilitation* 9: 281-285.

Benestad, A.M. (1965). Trainability of old men. *Acta Medica Scandinavica* 178: 321-327.

Bengele, H.H., Mathias, R.S., Perkins, J.H., and Alexander, E.A. (1981). Urinary concentrating defect in the aged rat. *Clinical Journal of Physiology* 240: 147-150.

Benham, T., and Heston, M. (1989). Memory retrieval in the adult population. In A.C. Ostrow, *Aging and motor behavior* (pp. 87-104). Indianapolis: Benchmark Press.

Bennett, J., Carmack, M.A., and Gardner, V.J. (1982). Effect of a program of physical exercise on depression in older adults. *Physical Educator* 39 (1): 21-24.

Bennett, P.H. (1984). Diabetes in the elderly: Diagnosis and epidemiology. *Geriatrics* 39: 37-41.

Ben-Yehuda, A., and Weksler, M.E. (1992). Immune senescence—mechanisms and clinical implications. *Cancer Investigations* 10: 525-531.

Berg, S. (1993). Psychological indicators of healthy aging. In E. Heikkinen and S. Harris (Eds.), *Physical activity and sports for healthy aging*. Albany, NY: Center for Studies of Aging.

Berger, B.G. (1989). The role of physical activity in the life quality of older adults. In W. Spirduso and H.M. Eckert (Eds.), *Physical activity and aging* (pp. 42-58). Champaign, IL: Human Kinetics.

Berger, B.G., and Owen, R.D. (1986). Mood alteration with swimming: A re-evaluation. In L. Vander Velden and J.H. Humphrey (Eds.), *Current selected research in the psychology and sociology of sport: Vol. 1* (pp. 97-114). New York: AMS Press.

Bergner, M., Bobbitt, R., Carter, W., and Gilson, B. (1981). The sickness impact profile: Development and final revision of a health status measure. *Medical Care* 19: 787-805.

Bergstrom, G., Bjelle, A., Sorensen, L.B., Sundh, V., and Svänborg, A. (1986). Prevalence of rheumatoid arthritis, osteoarthritis, chondrocalcinosis and gouty arthritis at age 79. *Journal of Rheumatology* 13: 527-534.

Berlin, J.A., and Coldlitz, G.A. (1990). A meta-analysis of physical activity in the prevention of coronary heart disease. *American Journal of Epidemiology* 132: 612-628.

Berman, N.D. (1982). *Geriatric cardiology*. Lexington, MA: Collamore Press.

Beverfeldt, E. (1971). Psychic behavior of the worker facing old age. In J.A. Huet (Ed.), *Work and aging* (pp. 135-146). Paris: International Center for Social Gerontology.

Bidlack, W.R., and Wang, W. (1995). Nutrition requirements of the elderly. In J.E. Morley, Z. Glick, and L.Z. Rubenstein (Eds.), *Geriatric nutrition: A comprehensive review* (pp. 25-50). New York: Raven Press.

Biewener, A.A. (1993). Safety factors in bone strength. *Calcified Tissue International* 53 (Suppl. 1): S68-S74.

Biggemann, M., Hilweg, D., Seidel, S., Horst, M., and Brinckmann, P. (1991). Risk of vertebral insufficiency fractures in relation to compressive strength predicted by quantitative computed tomography. *European Journal of Radiology* 13: 6-10.

Bild, J.E., Fitzpatrick, A., Fried, L.P., Wong, N.D., Haan, M.N., Lyles, M., Bovill, E., Polak, J.F., and Schulz, R. (1993). Age-related trends in cardiovascular morbidity and physical functioning in the elderly: The Cardiovascular Health Study. *Journal of the American Geriatric Society* 41: 1047-1056.

Binder, E.F., Brown, M., Craft, S., Schechtman, K.B., and Birge, S.J. (1994). Effects of a group exercise program on risk factors for falls in frail older adults. *Journal of Aging and Physical Activity* 2: 25-37.

Binkhorst, R.A., Heevel, J., and Nordeloos, A.M. (1984). Energy expenditure of (severe) obese subjects during submaximal and maximal exercise. *International Journal of Sports Medicine* 5: 71-73.

Birge, S.J. (1993). Factors contributing to falls and fractures. In H.M. Perry, J.E. Morley, and R.M. Coe (Eds.), *Aging and musculoskeletal disorders* (pp. 101-122). New York: Springer.

Birren, J.E., and Lanum, J.C. (1991). Metaphors of psychology and aging. In G.M. Kenyon, J.E. Birren, and J.J.F. Schroots (Eds.), *Metaphors of aging in science and the humanities* (pp. 103-130). New York: Springer.

Birren, J.E., Woods, A.M., and Williams, M.V. (1980). Behavioral slowing with age. Causes, organization and consequences. In L.W. Poon (Ed.), *Aging in the 1980s* (pp. 293-308). Washington, DC: American Psychological Association.

Bjorksten, J. (1974). Cross linkage and the aging process. In M. Rockstein (Ed.), *Theoretical aspects of aging*. New York: Academic Press.

Björntorp, P., Smith, U., and Lönnroth, P. (1988). Health implications of obesity. *Acta Medica Scandinavica* 223 (Suppl. 723): 121-134.

Black, D. (1980). *Inequalities in health: Report of a research working group*. London: Department of Health and Social Services.

Black, J.E., Polinsky, M., and Greenough, W.T. (1989). Progressive failure of cerebral angiogenesis supporting neural plasticity in aging rats. *Neurobiology of Aging* 10: 353-358.

Black, M. (1979). More about metaphor. In A. Ortony (Ed.), *Metaphor and thought* (pp. 19-43). London: Cambridge University Press.

Blackman, M.R., Kowatch, M.A., Wehmann, R.E., and Harman, S.M. (1986). Basal serum prolactin levels and prolactin responses to constant infusions of thyrotropin release in old and young male rats. *Journal of Gerontology* 41: 699-705.

Black-Sandler, R., LaPorte, R.E., Sashin, D., Kuller, L.H., Sternglass, E., Cauley, J.A., and Link, M.M. (1982). Determinants of bone mass in menopause. *Preventive Medicine* 11: 269-280.

Blair, D., Habicht, J-P., and Alekel, L. (1989). Assessment of body composition, dietary patterns, and nutritional status in the National Health Examination Surveys and National Health and Nutrition Examination Surveys. In T. Drury (Ed.), *Assessing physical fitness and physical activity in population-based surveys* (Publication No. US

PHS 89-1253, pp. 79-104). Hyattsville, MD: U.S. Department of Health and Human Services.

Blair, S.N., Brill, P.A., and Kohl, H.W. (1988). Physical activity patterns in older individuals. In W.W. Spirduso and H. Eckert (Eds.), *Physical activity and aging* (pp. 120-139). Champaign, IL: Human Kinetics.

Blair, S.N., Kohl, H., and Brill, P. (1990). Behavioral adaptation to physical activity. In C. Bouchard, R.J. Shephard, T. Stephens, J. Sutton, and B. McPherson (Eds.), *Exercise, fitness and health* (pp. 385-398). Champaign, IL: Human Kinetics.

Blair, S.N., Kohl, H.W., and Barlow, C.E. (1993). Physical activity, physical fitness, and all-cause mortality in women: Do women need to be active? *Journal of the American College of Nutrition* 12: 368-371.

Blair, S.N., Kohl, H.W., Paffenbarger, R.S., Clark, D.G., Cooper, K.H., and Gibbons, L.W. (1989). Physical fitness and all-cause mortality: A prospective study of healthy men and women. *Journal of the American Medical Association* 262: 2395-2401.

Blair, S.N., Shaten, J., Brownell, K., Collins, G., and Lissner, L. (1993). Body weight change, all-cause mortality, and cause-specific mortality in the multiple risk factor intervention trial. *Annals of Internal Medicine* 119: 749-757.

Blaxter, M. (1990). *Health and lifestyles*. London: Tavistock Routledge.

Block, J.E., and Genant, H.K. (1989). Strategies and risk identification for the prevention of osteoporotic fractures. In R. Harris and S. Harris (Eds.), *Physical Activity, aging and sports* (pp. 295-300). Albany, NY: Center for Studies of Aging.

Bloomfield, R.L., Nivikov, S.V., and Ferrario, C.M. (1994). Hypertension in the elderly. *American Journal of Geriatric Cardiology* 3: 39-44.

Bloomfield, S.A. (1995). Bone, ligament and tendon. In D.R. Lamb, C.V. Gisolfi, and E. Nadel (Eds.), *Exercise in older adults* (pp. 175-236). Carmel, IN: Cooper.

Bloomfield, S.A., Williams, N.I., Lamb, D.R., and Jackson, R.D. (1993). Non-weight-bearing exercise may increase lumbar spine bone mineral density in healthy postmenopausal women. *American Journal of Physical Medicine and Rehabilitation* 72: 204-209.

Blumberg, J.B., and Meydani, M. (1995). The relationship between nutrition and exercise in older adults. In C.V. Gisolfi, D.R. Lamb, and E. Nadel (Eds.), *Exercise in older adults* (pp. 353-394). Carmel, IN: Cooper.

Blumenthal, J.A., Emery, C.F., Madden, D.J., Coleman, R.E., Riddle, M.W., Schniebolk, S., Cobb, F.R., Sullivan, M.J., and Higginbotham, M.B. (1991). Effects of exercise training on cardiorespiratory function in men and women >60 years of age. *American Journal of Cardiology* 67: 633-639.

Blumenthal, J.A., Emery, C.F., Madden. D.J., George, L.K., Coleman, R.E., Riddle, M.W., McKee, D.C., Reasoner, J., and Williams, R.S. (1989). Cardiovascular and behavioral effects of aerobic exercise training in healthy older men and women. *Journals of Gerontology* 44: M147-M157.

Blumenthal, J.A., Emery, C.F., Madden, D.J., Schniebolk, S., Walsh-Riddle, M., George, L.K., McKee, D.C., Higginbotham, M.B., Cobb, F.R., and Coleman, R.E. (1991). Long-term effects of exercise on psychological functioning in older men and women. *Journals of Gerontology* 46: P352-P361.

Bogardus, C., Ravussin, E., Robbins, D.C., Wolfe, R.R., Horton, E.S., and Sims, E.A.H. (1984). Effects of physical training and diet therapy on carbohydrate metabolism in patients with glucose intolerance and non-insulin dependent diabetes mellitus. *Diabetes* 33: 311-318.

Böhm, M., Dorner, H., Htun, P., Lensche, H., Platt, D., and Erdmann, E. (1993). Effects of exercise on myocardial adenylate cyclase and G$_i$alpha expression in senescence. *American Journal of Physiology* 264: H805-H814.

Böhm, M., and Erdmann, E. (1989). Regulation of force of contraction in the aged and diseased myocardium. In D. Platt (Ed.), *Gerontology* (pp. 107-120). Berlin: Springer-Verlag.

Bokovoy, J.L., and Blair, S.N. (1994). Aging and exercise: A health perspective. *Journal of Aging and Physical Activity* 2: 243-260.

Bonita, R., and Beaglehole, R. (1989). Increased treatment of hypertension does not explain the decline in stroke mortality in the United States, 1970-1980. *Hypertension* 13 (Suppl. 1): 169-173.

Bonjer, F.H. (1968). Relationship between working time, physical work capacity and allowable caloric expenditure. In W. Rohmert (Ed.), *Muskelarbeit und Muskeltraining* (pp. 86-99). Stuttgart: Gentner-Verlag.

Bonneux, L., Barendredegt, J.J., Meeter, K., Bonsel, G.J., and van der Maas, P.J. (1994). Estimating clinical morbidity due to ischemic heart disease and congestive heart failure: The future rise of heart failure. *American Journal of Public Health* 84: 20-28.

Booth, F.W., Weeden, S.H., and Tseng, B.S. (1994). Effect of aging on human skeletal muscle and motor function. *Medicine and Science in Sports and Exercise* 26: 556-560.

Borchelt, M.F., and Steinhagen-Thiessen, E. (1992). Physical performance and sensory functions as determinants of independence in activities of daily living in the old and the very old. *Physiopathological Processes of Aging* 673: 350-361.

Borg, G., and Linderholm, H. (1967). Perceived exertion and pulse rate during exercise in various age groups. *Acta Medica Scandinavica* (Suppl. 472): 194-206.

Boring, C.C., Squires, T.S., Tong, T., and Montgomery, S. (1994). Cancer statistics. *Cancer* 44: 7-26.

Borkan, G.A., and Norris, A.H. (1980). Assessment of biological age using a profile of physical parameters. *Journal of Gerontology* 35: 177-184.

Borst, S.E., Millard, W.J., and Lowenthal, D.T. (1994). Growth hormone, exercise and aging: The future of therapy for the frail elderly. *Journal of the American Geriatric Society* 42: 528-535.

Bortz, W.M. (1982). Disuse and aging. *Journal of the American Medical Association* 248: 1203-1208.

Bouchard, C. (1992). Genetics, physical activity and energy balance. In V.S. Hubbard (Ed.), *NIH Workshop on Physical Activity and Obesity* (pp. 54-56). Washington, DC: National Institutes of Health.

Bouchard, C. (1994). Genetics of human obesities: Introductory notes. In C. Bouchard (Ed.), *The genetics of obesity* (pp. 1-15). Boca Raton, FL: CRC Press.

Bouchard, C., and Després, J-P. (1988). Variation in fat distribution with age and health implications. In W. Spirduso and H.M. Eckert (Eds.), *Physical activity and aging: The Academy Papers* 22 (pp. 78-106). Champaign, IL: Human Kinetics.

Bouchard, C., Després, J-P., and Tremblay, A. (1993). Exercise and obesity. *Obesity Research* 1: 133-147.

Bouchard, C., Dionne, F.T., Simoneau, J-A., and Boulay, M.R. (1992). Genetics of aerobic and anaerobic performances. *Exercise and Sport Sciences Reviews* 20: 27-58.

Bouchard, C., Shephard, R.J., and Stephens, T. (Eds.). (1994). *Physical activity, fitness and health*. Champaign, IL: Human Kinetics.

Bouchard, C., Shephard, R.J., Stephens, T., Sutton, J., and McPherson, B. (1990). *Exercise, fitness and health*. Champaign, IL: Human Kinetics.

Bourlière, F. (1982). *Gérontologie: Biologie et clinique*. Paris: Flammarion.

Boutier, V., and Payette, H. (1994). Validity of weight and height given from memory in an elderly population. *Age & Nutrition* 5: 17-21.

Bovens, I.M.P.M., van Baak, M.A., Vrencken, J.G.P.M., Wijnen, J.A.G., Saris, W.H.M., and Verstappen, F.T.J. (1993). Maximal aerobic power in cycle ergometry in middle-aged men and women, active in sports, in relation to age and physical activity. *International Journal of Sports Medicine* 14: 66-71.

Brash, D.E., and Hart, R.W. (1978). Molecular biology of aging. In J.A. Behnke, C.E. Finch, and G.B. Moment (Eds.), *The biology of aging* (pp. 247-261). New York: Plenum Press.

Braunwald, E. (1988). *Heart disease: A textbook of cardiovascular medicine*. Philadelphia: Saunders.

Bray, G. (Ed.). (1979). *Obesity in America*. Washington, DC: Department of Health, Education and Welfare.

Brendler, C.B. (1994). Disorders of the prostate. In W.R. Hazzard, E.L. Bierman, J.P. Blass, W.H. Ettinger, and J.B. Halter (Eds.), *Principles of geriatric medicine and gerontology* (pp. 657-664). New York: McGraw-Hill.

Brenner, I., Shek, P.N., and Shephard, R.J. (1994). Infection in athletes. *Sports Medicine* 17: 86-107.

Bristow, M.R., Hershberger, R.E., Port, J.D., Gilbert, E.M., Sandoval, A., Rasmussen, R., Cates, A.E., and Feldman, A.M. (1990). Beta-adrenergic pathways in nonfailing and failing human ventricular myocardium. *Circulation* 82 (Suppl. I): I12-I15.

Brody, H. (1976). An examination of cerebral cortex and brainstem aging. In R.D. Terry and S. Gershon (Eds.), *Aging 3. Neurobiology of aging* (pp. 177-181). New York: Raven Press.

Brody, S.J. (1985). Formal health support systems. In R. Andres, E.L. Bierman, and W.R. Hazzard (Eds.), *Principles of geriatric medicine* (pp. 187-198). New York: McGraw-Hill.

Brooks, S.V., and Faulkner, J.A. (1994). Skeletal muscle weakness in old age: Underlying mechanisms. *Medicine and Science in Sports and Exercise* 26: 432-439.

Brown, A.B., McCartney, N., and Sale, D.G. (1990). Positive adaptations to weight-lifting training in the elderly. *Journal of Applied Physiology* 69: 1725-1733.

Brown, C.F., and Oldridge, N.B. (1985). Exercise-induced angina in the cold. *Medicine and Science in Sports and Exercise* 17: 607-610.

Brown, D.R. (1992). Physical activity, ageing, and psychological well-being: An overview of the research. *Canadian Journal of Sport Sciences* 17: 185-193.

Brown, J.P., Delmas, P.D., Malaval, L., Edouard, C., Chapuy, M.C., and Meunier, P.J.M. (1984). Serum bone Gla protein: A specific marker for bone formation in postmenopausal osteoporosis. *Lancet* 1: 1091-1093.

Brown, J.R., and Crowden, G.P. (1963). Energy expenditure ranges and muscular work grades. *British Journal of Industrial Medicine* 20: 277-283.

Brown, M. (1985). Long-term endurance exercise effects on skeletal muscle in aging rats [Abstract]. *Medicine and Science in Sports and Exercise* 17: 245.

Brown, M., and Holloszy, J.O. (1991). Effects of a low intensity exercise program on selected physical performance characteristics of 60- to 71-year olds. *Aging* 3: 129-139.

Brown, M., and Rose, S.J. (1985). The effects of aging and exercise on skeletal muscle—clinical considerations. *Topics in Gerontology and Rehabilitation* 1: 20-30.

Brown, W.T., Zebrower, M., and Kieras, F.J. (1985). Progeria, a model disease for the study of accelerated aging. In A.V. Woodhead, A.D. Blackett, and A. Hollaender (Eds.), *Molecular biology of aging* (pp. 375-396). New York: Plenum Press.

Brown, W.W., Davis, B.B., Spry, L.A., Wonsurat, N., Malone, J.D., and Donoto, D.T. (1986). Aging and the kidney. *Archives of Internal Medicine* 146: 1790-1796.

Brownell, K.D. (1984). Behavioral and psychological aspects of motivation to exercise. *International Journal of Sports Medicine* 5 (Suppl.): 69-70.

Brownlie, L., Brown, S., Diewert, J., Good, P., Holman, G., Laue, G., and Banister, E. (1982). The evaluation of firefighter recruits [Abstract]. *Canadian Journal of Sport Sciences* 7: 231.

Bruce, R.A., and Fisher, L.D. (1987). Exercise-enhanced risk factors for coronary heart disease versus age as criteria for mandatory retirement of healthy pilots. *Journal of Cardiopulmonary Rehabilitation* 7: 383-384.

Bruera, E., Brenneis, C., Michaud, M., Chadwick, S., and MacDonald, R.N. (1987). Association between involuntary muscle function and asthenia, nutritional status, lean body mass, psychometric assessment and tumor mass in patients with advanced cancer. *Proceedings of the American Society of Clinical Oncology* 6: 261.

Bruera, E., Carraro, S., Roca, E., Cedaro, L., and Chacon, R. (1984). Association between malnutrition and calorie intake, emesis, psychological depression, glucose taste and tumor mass. *Cancer Treatment Reports* 68: 873-876.

Buchner, D.M., Beresford, S.A., Larson, E.B., LaCroix, A.Z., and Wagner, E.H. (1993). Effects of physical activity on health status in older adults II. Intervention studies. *Annual Review of Public Health* 13: 469-488.

Bugiardini, R., Borghi, A., and Pozzati, A. (1993). Treatment of ischemic heart disease in the elderly: Focus on unstable angina. *American Journal of Geriatric Cardiology* 2: 41-46.

Buist, A.S., Ghezzo, H., Anthonisen, N.R., Cherniack, R.M., Ducic, S., Macklem, P.T., Manfreda, J., Martin, R.R., McCarthy, D., and Ross, B.B. (1979). Relationship between the single breath N_2 test and age, sex and smoking habit in three North American cities. *American Review of Respiratory Diseases* 120: 305-318.

Buono, M.J., McKenzie, B.T., and Kasch, F. (1991). Effects of ageing and physical training on the peripheral sweat production of the human eccrine sweat gland. *Age and Ageing* 20: 439-441.

Burch, G.E., and Collot, C. (1972). *Elderly people in their towns*. Paris: International Center for Social Gerontology.

Burr, M.L., Phillips, K.M., and Hurst, D.N. (1985). Lung function in the elderly. *Thorax* 40: 54-59.

Burrows, B., Lebowitz, M.D., Camilli, A.E., and Knudson, R.J. (1986). Longitudinal changes in forced expiratory volume in one second in adults. *American Review of Respiratory Diseases* 133: 974-980.

Buskirk, E.R., and Hodgson, J.L. (1987). Age and aerobic power: The rate of change in men and women. *Federation Proceedings* 46: 1824-1829.

Butler, R.N. (1992). Quality of life: Can it be an end-point? *American Journal of Clinical Nutrition* 55: 1267S-1270S.

Butterworth, D.E., Nieman, D.C., Perkins, R., Warren, B.J., and Dotson, R.G. (1993). Exercise training and nutrient intake in elderly women. *Journal of the American Dietetic Association* 93: 653-657.

Buysse, D.J., Reynolds, C.F., Monk, T.H., Hoch, C.C., Yeager, A.L., and Kupfer, D.J. (1991). Quantification of subjective sleep quality in healthy elderly men and women using the Pittsburgh Sleep Quality Index (PSQI). *Sleep* 14: 331-338.

Cable, N.T., and Green, J.H. (1990). The influence of bicycle exercise with or without hand immersion in cold water, on forearm sweating in young and middle-aged women. *Experimental Physiology* 75: 505-514.

Cady, L.D., Thomas, P.C., and Karwasky, R.J. (1985). Program for increasing health and physical fitness of firefighters. *Journal of Occupational Medicine* 27: 110-114.

Calkins, E., and Challa, H.R. (1985). Disorders of the joints and connective tissues. In R. Andres, E.L. Bierman, and W.R. Hazzard (Eds.), *Principles of geriatric medicine* (pp. 813-843). New York: McGraw-Hill.

Calkins, E., Reinhard, J.D., and Vladutiu, A.O. (1994). Rheumatoid arthritis and autoimmune rheumatic diseases in the older patient. In W.R. Hazzard, E.L. Bierman, J.P. Blass, W.E. Ettinger, and J.B. Halter (Eds.), *Principles of geriatric medicine and gerontology* (pp. 961-964). New York: McGraw-Hill.

Canada Health Survey. (1982). Ottawa: Health and Welfare, Canada.

Canadian Consensus Conference on Cholesterol. (1988). Final Report. The Canadian Consensus Conference on the prevention of heart and vascular disease by altering serum cholesterol and other risk factors. *Canadian Medical Association Journal* 139 (Suppl.): 1-8.

Cannon, J.G., Meydani, S.N., Fielding, R.A., Fiatarone, M.A., Meydani, M., Farhangmehr, M., Orencole, S.F., Blumberg, J.B., and Evans, W.J. (1991). Acute phase response in exercise. II. Associations between vitamin E, cytokines, and muscle proteolysis. *American Journal of Physiology* 260: R1235-R1240.

Capuano-Pucci, D., Rheault, W., and Rudman, D. (1987). Relationship between plasma somatomedin C and muscle performance in a geriatric male population. *American Journal of Physical Medicine* 66: 364-370.

Carlos, J.P., and Wolfe, M.D. (1989). Methodological and nutritional issues in assessing the oral health of aged subjects. *American Journal of Clinical Nutrition* 50: 1210-1218.

Carmelli, D. (1982). Intrapair comparisons of total lifespan in twins and pairs of sibs. *Human Biology* 54: 525-537.

Carroll, J.F., Pollock, M.L., Graves, J.E., Leggett, S.H., Spitler, D.L., and Lowenthal, D.T. (1992). Incidence of injury during moderate and high-intensity walking training in the elderly. *Journals of Gerontology* 47: M61-M66.

Cartee, G.D. (1994). Aging skeletal muscle: Response to exercise. *Exercise and Sport Sciences Reviews* 22: 91-120.

Carter, D.R. (1984). Mechanical loading histories and cortical bone remodelling. *Calcified Tissue International* 36: S19-S61.

Carter, D.R., Fyhrie, D.P., and Whalen, R.T. (1987). Trabecular bone density and loading history: Regulation of connective tissue biology by mechanical energy. *Journal of Biomechanics* 20: 785-794.

Carter, R., and Coast, J.R. (1993). Respiratory muscle training in patients with chronic obstructive pulmonary disease. *Journal of Cardiopulmonary Rehabilitation* 13: 117-125.

Carter, R., Coast, J.R., and Idell, S. (1992). Exercise training in patients with chronic obstructive pulmonary disease. *Medicine and Science in Sports and Exercise* 24: 281-291.

Casaburi, R., Patessio, A., Ioli, F., Zanaboni, S., Donner, C.F., and Wasserman, K. (1991). Reductions in exercise lactic acidosis and ventilation as a result of exercise training in patients with obstructive lung disease. *American Review of Respiratory Diseases* 143: 9-18.

Cascells, W., Hennekens, C.H., Evans, D., Rosener, B., de Silva, R.A., Lown, B., Davies, J.E., and Jesse, M.J. (1980). Retirement and coronary mortality. *Lancet* 1: 1288-1289.

Casey, B. (1984). Recent trends in retirement policy and practice in Europe and the U.S.A.: An overview of programmes directed to the exclusion of older workers and a suggestion for an alternative strategy. In P.K. Robinson, J. Livingston, and J.E. Birren (Eds.), *Aging and technological advances* (pp. 125-138). New York: Plenum Press.

Caspersen, C.J., Bloemberg, B.P.M., Saris, W.H.M., Merritt, R.K., and Kromhout, D. (1991). The prevalence of selected physical activities and their relation with coronary heart disease risk factors in elderly men: The Zutphen Study, 1985. *American Journal of Epidemiology* 133: 1-15.

Caspersen, C.J., Christenson, G.M., and Pollard, R.A. (1986). Status of the 1990 physical fitness and exercise objectives—evidence from NHIS 1985. *Public Health Reports* 101: 587-592.

Caspersen, C.J., Powell, K.E., and Merritt, R.K. (1994). Measurement of health status and well-being. In C. Bouchard, R.J. Shephard, and T. Stephens (Eds.), *Physical activity, fitness and health* (pp. 180-202). Champaign, IL: Human Kinetics.

Castelli, W.P. (1993). Risk factors in the elderly: A view from Framingham. *American Journal of Geriatric Cardiology* 2: 8-19.

Cavanaugh, D.J., and Cann, C.E. (1988). Brisk walking does not stop bone loss in postmenopausal women. *Bone* 9: 201-204.

Cavanagh, P. (1980). *The running shoe book.* Mountain View, CA: Anderson World.

Celli, R. (1986). Respiratory muscle function. *Clinics in Chest Medicine* 7: 757-784.

Chappard, D., Plantard, B., Petitjean, M., Alexandre, C., and Riffat, G. (1991). Alcoholic cirrhosis and osteoporosis in men: A light and scanning electron microscopy study. *Journal of Studies in Alcohol* 52: 269-274.

Charette, S.L., McEvoy, L., Pyka, G., Snow-Harter, C., Guido, D., Wiswell, R.A., and Marcus, R. (1991). Muscle hypertrophy response to resistance training in older women. *Journal of Applied Physiology* 70: 1912-1916.

Charness, N. (1991). Cognition and aging. In C. Blais (Ed.), *Aging into the twenty-first century* (pp. 204-222). North York, ON: Captus University Publications.

Chassin, M.R., Kosecoff, J., Park, R.E., Winslow, C.M., Kahn, K.L., Merrick, N.J., Keesey, J., Fink, A., Soloman, D.H., and Brook, R.H. (1987). Does inappropriate use explain geographic variations in the use of health care services? *Journal of the American Medical Association* 258: 2533-2537.

Chauhan, J., Hawrysh, Z.J., Gee, M., Donald, E.A., and Basu, T.K. (1987). Age-related olfactory and taste changes and interrelationships between taste and nutrition. *Journal of the American Dietetic Association* 87: 1543-1550.

Cheng, S., Suominen, H., Rantanen, T., Parkatti, T., and Heikkinen, E. (1991). Bone mineral density and physical activity in 50-60-year old women. *Bone and Mineral* 12: 123-132.

Cheng, S., Suominen, H. Era, P., and Heikkinen, E. (1994). Bone density of the calcaneus and fractures of the calcaneus and fractures in 75- and 80-year-old men. *Osteoporosis International* 4: 48-54.

Chernoff, R., and Silver, A.J. (1993). Nutritional intervention in the frail elderly. In H.M. Perry, J.E. Morley, and R.M. Coe (Eds.), *Aging and musculoskeletal disorders* (pp. 243-254). New York: Springer.

Cheskin, L.J., and Schuster, M.H. (1994). Colonic disorders. In W.R. Hazzard, E.L. Bierman, J.P. Blass, W.H. Ettinger, and J.B. Halter (Eds.), *Principles of geriatric medicine and gerontology* (3rd ed., pp. 723-732). New York: McGraw-Hill.

Chestnut, C.H. (1994). Osteoporosis. In W.R. Hazzard, E.L. Bierman, J.P. Blass, W.H. Ettinger, and J.B. Halter (Eds.), *Principles of geriatric medicine and gerontology* (pp. 897-909). New York: McGraw-Hill.

Chi, M.M., Hintz, C.S., Coyle, E.F., Martin, W.H., Ivy, J.L., Nemeth, P.M., Holloszy, J.O., and Lowry, O.H. (1983). Effects of detraining on enzymes of energy metabolism in individual human muscle fibers. *American Journal of Physiology* 244: C276-C287.

Chiang, A.N., and Huang, P.C. (1988). Excess energy and nitrogen balance at protein intakes above the requirement level in young men. *American Journal of Clinical Nutrition* 48: 1015-1022.

Chick, T.W., Cagle, T.G., Vegas, F.A., Poliner, J.K., and Murata, G.H. (1991). The effect of aging on submaximal exercise performance and recovery. *Journals of Gerontology* 46: B34-B38.

Chilibeck, P.D., Sale, D.G., and Webber, C.E. (1995). Exercise and bone mineral density. *Sports Medicine* 19: 103-122.

Chillag, S., Bates, M., Voltin, R., and Jones, D. (1990). Sudden death: Myocardial infarction in a runner with normal coronary arteries. *Physician and Sportsmedicine* 18 (3): 89-94.

Chodzo-Zajko, W.J. (1991). Physical fitness, cognitive performance and aging. *Medicine and Science in Sports and Exercise* 23: 868-872.

Chodzo-Zajko, W.J., and Moore, K.A. (1994). Physical fitness and cognitive functioning in aging. *Exercise and Sport Sciences Reviews* 22: 195-220.

Chow, R., Harrison, J.E., Brown, C.F., and Hajek, V. (1986). Physical fitness effect on bone mass in post-menopausal women. *Archives of Physical Medicine and Rehabilitation* 67: 231-234.

Chow, R., Harrison, J.E., and Notarius, C. (1987). Effect of two randomised exercise programmes on bone mass of healthy post-menopausal women. *British Medical Journal* 295: 1441-1444.

Chow, E., Harrison, J.E., Sturtbridge, W., Josse, R., Murray, T.M., Bayley, A., Dornan, J., and Hammond, T. (1987). The effect of exercise on bone mass of osteoporotic patients in fluoride treatment. *Clinical and Investigative Medicine* 10: 59-63.

Chown, S.M. (1983). Profiles of abilities. In J.E. Birren, J.M.A. Munnichs, H. Thomae, and M. Minors (Eds.), *Aging: A challenge to science and society* (pp. 2264-2275). Oxford: Oxford University Press.

Chrétien, R., Simard, C.P., and Dorion, A. (1987). Effects of relaxation on the peripheral chronaxie of persons having multiple sclerosis. In G. Ward and M. Berridge (Eds.), *International perspectives on adapted physical activity* (pp. 65-72). Champaign, IL: Human Kinetics.

Chumlea, W.C., and Baumgartner, R.N. (1990). Bioelectric impedance methods for the estimation of body composition. *Canadian Journal of Sport Sciences* 15: 172-179.

Chumlea, W.C., Roche, A.F., and Mukherjee, D. (1984). *Nutritional assessment of the elderly through anthropometry*. Columbus, OH: Ross Laboratories.

Ciocon, J.O., Galindo-Ciocon, D., and Galindo, D.J. (1995). Raised leg exercises for leg edema in the elderly. *Angiology* 46: 19-25.

Clark, R.L. (1984). Aging and labor force participation. In P.K. Robinson, J. Livingston, and J.E. Birren (Eds.), *Aging and technological advances* (pp. 39-54). New York: Plenum Press.

Clarke, D.H., Hunt, M.Q., and Dotson, C.O. (1992). Muscular strength and endurance as a function of age and activity level. *Research Quarterly* 63: 302-310.

Clarke-Williams, M.J. (1978). The management of aged amputees. In J.C. Brocklehurst (Ed.), *Textbook of geriatric medicine and gerontology* (2nd ed., pp. 556-569). Edinburgh: Churchill Livingstone.

Clarkson-Smith, L., and Hartley, A.A. (1989). Relationships between physical exercise and cognitive abilities in older adults. *Psychology and Aging* 4: 183-189.

Clarkson-Smith, L., and Hartley, A.A. (1990). Structural equation models of relationships between exercise and cognitive abilities. *Psychology and Aging* 5: 437-446.

Clement, F.J. (1974). Longitudinal and cross-sectional assessments of age changes in physical strength as related to sex, social class and mental ability. *Journal of Gerontology* 29: 423-429.

Coats, A.J.S. (1993). Physical exercise and training in elderly patients with heart failure. *Cardiology in the Elderly* 1: 569-573.

Coats, A.J.S., Adamopoulos, S., Radaelli, A., McCance, A., Meyer, T.E., Bernardi, L., Solda, P.L., Davey, P., Ormerod, O., Forfar, C., Conway, J., and Sleight, P. (1992). Controlled trial of physical training in chronic heart failure: Exercise performance, hemodynamics, ventilation and autonomic function. *Circulation* 85: 2119-2131.

Coe, C.I., Watson, A., Joyce, H., and Pride, N.B. (1989). Effects of smoking on changes in respiratory resistance with increasing age. *Clinical Science* 76: 487-494.

Coggan, A.R., Spina, R.J., King, D.S., Rogers, M.A., Brown, M., Nemeth, P.M., and Holloszy, J.O. (1992). Skeletal muscle adaptations to endurance training in 60- to 70-yr-old men and women. *Journal of Applied Physiology* 72: 1780-1786.

Colandrea, M.A., Friedman, G.D., Nichaman, M.Z., and Lynd, C.N. (1970). Systolic hypertension in the elderly: An epidemiologic assessment. *Circulation* 41: 239-245.

Cole, K.J. (1991). Grasp force control in older adults. *Journal of Motor Behavior* 23: 251-258.

Cole, K.J., and Beck, C.L. (1994). The stability of precision grip force in older adults. *Journal of Motor Behavior* 26: 171-177.

Cole, T.R., and Meyer, D.G. (1991). Aging, metaphor and meaning: A view from cultural history. In G.M. Kenyon, J.E. Birren, and J.J.F. Schroots (Eds.), *Metaphors of aging in science and the humanities* (pp. 57-82). New York: Springer.

Coles, R.R.A. (1981). *Tinnitus*. London: CIBA Foundation.

Collins, K.J. (1987). Effects of cold on old people. *British Journal of Hospital Medicine* 38: 506-514.

Collins, K.J., Exton-Smith, A., and Doré, C. (1981). Urban hypothermia: Prefered temperature and thermal perception in old age. *British Medical Journal* 282: 157-177.

Collishaw, N.E., and Myers, G. (1984). Dollar estimates of the consequences of tobacco use in Canada, 1979. *Canadian Journal of Public Health* 75: 192-199.

Colsher, P.L., Dorfman, L.T., and Wallace, R.B. (1988). Specific health conditions and work-retirement status among the elderly. *Journal of Applied Gerontology* 7: 485-503.

Colvez, A., and Blanchet, M. (1983). Potential gains in life expectancy free of disability: A tool for health planning. *International Journal of Epidemiology* 12: 86-91.

Comfort, A. (1979). *The biology of senescence* (3rd ed.). New York: Elsevier Science.

Conn, E.H., Williams, R.S., and Wallace, R.G. (1982). Exercise responses before and after physical conditioning in patients with severely depressed left ventricular function. *American Journal of Cardiology* 49: 296-300.

Connidis, I. (1989). *Family ties and aging*. Toronto, ON: Butterworths.

Cononie, C., Graves, J.E., Pollock, M.L., Phillips, I., Summers, C., and Hagberg, J.M. (1991). Effect of exercise training on blood pressure in 70- to 79-year-old men and women. *Medicine and Science in Sports and Exercise* 23: 505-511.

Cononie, C.C., Goldberg, A.P., Rogus, A., and Hagberg, J.M. (1994). Seven consecutive days of exercise lowers plasma insulin responses to an oral glucose challenge in sedentary elderly. *Journal of the American Geriatric Society* 42: 394-398.

Coon, P.J., Bleecker, E.R., Drinkwater, D.T., Meyers, D.A., and Goldberg, A.P. (1990). Effects of body composition and exercise capacity on glucose tolerance, insulin and lipoprotein lipids in healthy older men: A cross-sectional and longitudinal intervention study. *Metabolism* 38: 1201-1209.

Cooper, C., Barker, D.J.P., and Wickham, C. (1988). Physical activity, muscle strength and calcium intake in fracture of the proximal femur in Britain. *British Medical Journal* 297: 1443-1446.

Cooper, C.B. (1995). Determining the role of exercise in patients with chronic pulmonary disease. *Medicine and Science in Sports and Exercise* 27: 147-157.

Copeland, K.C., Colletti, R.B., Devlin, J.D., and McAuliffe, T.L. (1990). The relationship between insulin-like growth factor-1, adiposity and aging. *Metabolism* 39: 584-587.

Coroni-Huntley, J., Brock, D.B., Ostfeld, A.M., Taylor, J.O., and Wallace, R.B. (1986). *Established populations for epidemiological studies of the elderly: Resource data book* (NIH Publication No. 86-2443). Washington, DC: U.S. Public Health Service, National Institute on Aging.

Costa, P.T., and McCrae, R.R. (1985). Concepts of functional or biological age: A critical view. In R. Andres, E.L. Bierman, and W.R. Hazzard (Eds.), *Principles of geriatric medicine* (pp. 30-37). New York: McGraw-Hill.

Cotes, J.E. (1993). *Lung function* (5th ed.). Oxford: Blackwell Scientific.

Cottreau, M., Chambers, L.F., Gordon, C.L., Martin, J., Hicks, A.L., McCartney, N., and Webber, C.E. (1995). Lumbar spine and total body bone mass in healthy elderly men and women. *Canadian Journal on Aging* 14: 553-563.

Courtois, Y. (1982). Vieillissement cellulaire et moleculaire [Cellular and molecular aging]. In F. Bourlière (Ed.), *Gérontologie: Biologie et clinique*, (pp. 5-25). Paris: Flammarion.

Cox, J.R., Macias-Nunez, J.F., and Dowd, A.B. (1991). Renal disease. In J.S. Pathy (Ed.), *Principles and practice of geriatric medicine* (2nd. ed., pp. 1159-1163). Chichester: Wiley.

Cox, J.R., and Shalaby, W.A. (1981). Potassium changes with age. *Gerontology* 27: 340-344.

Crapo, R.O. (1993). The aging lung. In D.A. Mahler (Ed.), *Pulmonary disease in the elderly* (pp. 1-25). New York: Marcel Dekker.

Crepaldi, G., and Manzato, E. (1993). Cardiovascular risk factors in the elderly in Italy. *American Journal of Geriatric Cardiology* 2: 20-23.

Cress, M.E., Byrnes, W.C., Dickinson, A.L., and Foster, V.L. (1984). Modification of Type II fiber atrophy and LDH isozyme component of an 8 week endurance training program in elderly women [Abstract]. *Medicine and Science in Sports and Exercise* 16: 105.

Cress, M.E., and Schultz, E. (1985). Aging muscle: Functional, morphologic, biochemical and regenerative capacity. In E.L. Smith (Ed.), *Exercise and Aging. Topics in Geriatric Rehabilitation* 1: 11-19.

Cress, M.E., Thomas, D.P., Johnson, J., Kasch, F.W., Cassens, R.G., Smith, E.L., and Agre, J.C. (1991). Effect of training on VO_2max, thigh strength, and muscle morphology in septuagenarian women. *Medicine and Science in Sports and Exercise* 23: 752-758.

Crilly, R.G., Richardson, L.D., Roth, J.H., Vandervoort, A.A., Hayes, K.C., and Mackenzie, R.A. (1987). Postural stability and Colles' fracture. *Age and Ageing* 16: 133-138.

Crilly, R.G., Willems, D.A., Trenholm, K.J., Hayes, K.C., and Delaquierre-Richardson, L.F.O. (1989). Effect of exercise on postural sway in the elderly. *Gerontology* 35: 137-143.

Crimi, E., Bartalucci, C., and Brusasco, V. (1996). Asthma, exercise and immune function. *Exercise Immunology Review* 2: 45-64.

Crist, D.M., Mackinnon, L.T., Thompson, R.F., Atterbom, H.A., and Egan, P.A. (1989). Physical exercise increases natural killer-cell mediated tumor cytotoxicity in elderly women. *Gerontology* 35: 66-71.

Cristofalo, V.J., Phillips, P.D., and Brooks, K.M. (1985). Cellular senescence: Factors modulating cellular proliferation in vitro. In A.V. Woodhead, A.D. Blackett, and A. Hollaender (Eds.), *Molecular biology of aging* (pp. 241-254). New York: Plenum Press.

Cruts, H.E.P., Van Alste, J.E., de Vries, J., and Huisman, K. (1985). Cardiac loads during prosthetic training in leg amputees. In J.H. Haeberigs and H. Vorsteveld (Eds.), *Workshop on Disabled Sports* (pp. 60-78). Amersfoort, Netherlands: Nederlandse Invaliden Sportbond.

Cullinan, P. (1988). Respiratory disease in England and Wales. *Thorax* 43: 949-954.

Culver, B.H., and Butler, J. (1985). Alterations in pulmonary function. In R. Andres, E.L. Bierman, and W.R. Hazzard (Eds.), *Principles of geriatric medicine* (pp. 280-287). New York: McGraw-Hill.

Cummings, S.R., Black, D., Arnaud, C., Browner, W.S., Cauley, J.A., Genant, H.K., Mascioli, S., Nevitt, M.C., Scott, J., Seeley, D., Sherwin, P., Steiger, P., and Vogt, T. (1989). Appendicular densiometry predicts hip fractures. *Journal of Bone and Mineral Research* 4: S327.

Cummings, S.R., Kelsey, J.L., Nevitt, M.C., and O'Dowd, K. (1985). Epidemiology of osteoporosis and osteoporotic fractures. *Epidemiological Reviews* 7: 178-208.

Cunningham, D.A., Montoye, H.J., Metzner, H.L., and Keller, J.B. (1969). Physical activity at work and at leisure as related to occupation. *Medicine and Science in Sports* 1: 165-170.

Cunningham, D.A., Paterson, D.H., Himann, J.E., and Rechnitzer, P.A. (1993). Determinants of independence in the elderly. *Canadian Journal of Applied Physiology* 18: 243-254.

Cunningham, D.A., Rechnitzer, P., Howard, J.H., and Donner, A.P. (1987). Exercise training of men at retirement: A clinical trial. *Journals of Gerontology* 42: 17B-23B.

Cunningham, D.A., Rechnitzer, P.A., and Donner, A.P. (1986). Exercise training and the speed of self-selected walking pace in men at retirement. *Canadian Journal on Aging* 5: 19-26.

Cutler, R.G. (1985). Evolutionary biology of senescence. In R. Andres, E.L. Bierman, and W.R. Hazzard (Eds.), *Principles of geriatric medicine* (pp. 22-29). New York: McGraw-Hill.

Dalsky, G.P., Stocke, K.S., Ehsani, A.A., Slatopolsky, E., Lee, W.C., and Birge, S.J. (1988). Weight-bearing exercise training and lumbar bone mineral content in post-menopausal women. *Annals of Internal Medicine* 108: 824-828.

Danielson, M.E., Cauley, J.A., and Rohay, J.M. (1993). Physical activity and its association with plasma lipids and lipoproteins in elderly women. *Annals of Epidemiology* 3: 351-357.

Dannefer, D. (1991). The race is to the swift: Images of collective aging. In G.M. Kenyon, J.E. Birren, and J.J.F. Schroots (Eds.), *Metaphors of aging in science and the humanities* (pp. 155-172). New York: Springer.

Danneskold-Samsoe, B., Kofod, V., Munter, J., Grimby, G., Schnohr, P., and Jensen, G. (1984). Muscle strength and functional capacity in 78-81-year-old men and women. *European Journal of Applied Physiology* 52: 310-314.

Dardevet, D., Sornet, C., Attaix, D., Baracos, V.E., and Grizard, J. (1994). Insulin-like growth factor 1 and insulin resistance in skeletal muscles of adults and old rats. *Endocrinology* 134: 1475-1484.

Davey, P., Meyer, T., Coats, A., Adamopoulos, S., Casedi, B., Conway, J., and Sleight, P. (1992). Ventilation in chronic heart failure: Effects of physical training. *British Heart Journal* 68: 473-477.

Davidson, M.B. (1982). Diabetes in the elderly. Diagnosis and treatment. *Hospital Practice* 17: 113-129.

Davidson, S.M., and Marmor, T.R. (1980). *The cost of living longer.* Lexington, MA: Lexington Books.

Davidson, W.A.S. (1991). Metaphors of health and aging: Geriatrics as metaphor. In G.M. Kenyon, J.E. Birren, and J.J.F. Schroots (Eds.), *Metaphors of aging in science and the humanities* (pp. 173-184). New York: Springer.

Davidson, W.R., and Fee, E.C. (1990). Influence of aging on pulmonary hemodynamics in a population free of coronary artery disease. *American Journal of Cardiology* 65: 1454-1458.

Davies, B.H. (1991). The respiratory system. In M.S.J. Pathy (Ed.), *Principles and practice of geriatric medicine* (2nd ed., pp. 663-681). Chichester: Wiley.

Davies, C.T.M., Thomas, D.O., and White, M.J. (1986). Mechanical properties of young and elderly human muscle. *Acta Medica Scandinavica* 711 (Suppl.): 219-226.

Davies, H.E.F. (1975). Respiratory changes in heart rate, sinus arrhythmia in the elderly. *Gerontologia Clinica* 17: 96-100.

Davis, A. (1987). Epidemiology of hearing disorders. In A. Kerr (Ed.), *Scott Brown's otolaryngology* (5th ed., Vol. 2, pp. 90-126). London: Butterworths.

Davis, M.A. (1988). Epidemiology of OA. *Clinics in Geriatric Medicine* 4: 241-255.

Davis, M.A., Ettinger, W.H., and Neuhaus, J.M. (1991). Obesity and osteoarthritis of the knee: Evidence from the National Health & Nutrition Examination Survey (NHANES I). *Seminars in Arthritis and Rheumatology* 20 (Suppl.): 34-41.

Davis, P.O., and Dotson, C.O. (1987). Job performance testing: An alternative to age discrimination. *Medicine and Science in Sports and Exercise* 19: 179-185.

Davis, P.O., Dotson, C.O., and Santa-Maria, D.L. (1982). Relationship between simulated firefighting tasks and physical performance measures. *Medicine and Science in Sports and Exercise* 14: 65-71.

Debry, G. (1982). Nutrition: De la carence à la surcharge [Nutrition: From famine to over-eating]. In F. Bourlière (Ed.), *Gérontologie: Biologie et clinique* (pp. 191-212). Paris: Flammarion.

Debry, G., Bleyer, R., and Martin, J.M. (1977). Nutrition of the elderly. *Journal of Human Nutrition* 31: 195-203.

Decker, D.L. (1980). *Social gerontology. An introduction to the dynamics of aging.* Boston: Little, Brown.

Delafuente, M., Ferrandez, M.D., Miguel, J., and Hernanz, A. (1992). Changes with aging and physical exercise in ascorbic acid content and proliferative response of murine lymphocytes. *Mechanisms of Ageing and Development* 65: 177-186.

del Roso, A., de Tata, V., Gori, Z., and Bergamini, E. (1990). Lipofuscin pigment accumulation across the free wall of the left ventricle of the aging rat. In H.L. Segal, M. Rothstein, and E. Bergamini (Eds.), *Protein metabolism in aging* (pp. 371-374). New York: Wiley-Liss.

De Meersman, R.E. (1993). Heart rate variability and aerobic fitness. *American Heart Journal* 125: 726-731.

Dempsey, J.A., Powers, S., and Gledhill, N. (1990). Discussion: Cardiovascular and pulmonary adaptation to physical activity. In C. Bouchard, R.J. Shephard, T. Stephens, J. Sutton, and B. McPherson (Eds.), *Exercise, fitness and health* (pp. 205-216). Champaign, IL: Human Kinetics.

Dempsey, J.A., and Seals, D.R. (1995). Aging, exercise and cardiopulmonary function. In D.R. Lamb, C.V. Gisolfi, and E. Nadel (Eds.), *Perspectives in exercise science and sports medicine: Vol. 8. Exercise in older adults* (pp. 237-297). Indianapolis: Benchmark Press.

Denahan, T., Barney, J.A., Sheldahl, L.M., and Ebert, T.J. (1993). Lack of changes in cardiac vagal activity in older males following 12 weeks of aerobic training [Abstract]. *Medicine and Science in Sports and Exercise* 25: S55.

Denis, C., and Chatard, J-C. (1992). Entrainabilité du sujet agé [Trainability of the elderly subject]. In *La revue de gériatrie, Proceedings of Euromedicine 92* (pp. 203-204). Montpellier: Le Corum.

Denton, F., and Spencer, B. (1980). Canada's population and labour force. Past, present and future. In V.W. Marshall (Ed.), *Aging in Canada. Social perspectives* (pp. 232-247). Toronto, ON: Fitzhenry & Whiteside.

Department of Health and Social Security. (1972). Nutrition survey of the elderly. *Reports on Public Health and Medical Subjects* 123. London: Her Majesty's Stationery Office.

Department of Health and Social Security. (1979). *Reports on Health and Social Subjects* 16. London: Her Majesty's Stationery Office.

Dequeker, J., Tobing, L., Rutten, V., Geusens, P., Medos Study Group. (1991). Relative risk factors for osteoporotic fracture: A pilot study of the MEDOS questionnaire. *Clinical Rheumatology* 10: 49-53.

Derks, C.M. (1980). Ventilation/perfusion distribution in young and old volunteers during mild exercise. *Bulletin Européan de Physiopathologie Respiratoire* 16: 145-154.

D'Errico, A., Scarani, P., Colosimo, E., Spina, M., Grigoni, W.F., and Mancini, A.M. (1989). Changes in the alveolar connective tissue of the ageing lung. *Virchow's Archives. A. Pathological Anatomy and Histopathology* 415: 137-144.

Després, J-P. (1994). Physical activity and adipose tissue. In C. Bouchard, R.J. Shephard, and T. Stephens (Eds.), *Physical activity, fitness and health* (pp. 358-368). Champaign, IL: Human Kinetics.

DeStephano, F., Coulehan, J., and Wiant, J.K. (1979). Blood pressure survey on the Navajo Indian reservation. *American Journal of Epidemiology* 109: 335-345.

de Vries, J.H., Noorda, R.J.P., Voetberg, C.A., and van der Veen, E.A. (1991). Growth hormone release after the sequential use of growth hormone releasing factor and exercise. *Hormone and Metabolic Research* 23: 397-398.

Dewys, W., and Kisner, D. (1982). Principles of nutritional care of the cancer patient. In K. Carter, E. Glatstein, and R.B. Livingston (Eds.), *Principles of cancer treatment* (pp. 252-259). New York: McGraw-Hill.

Diamond, M.C., Johnson, R.E., Protti, A.M., Ott, C., and Kajisa, L. (1985). Plasticity in the 904-day-old rat cerebral cortex. *Experimental Neurology* 87: 309-317.

Di Bello, V., Lattanzi, F., Picano, E., Talarico, L., Caputo, M.T., Di Muro, C., Santoro, G., Lunardi, M., Distante, A., and Giusti, C. (1993). Left ventricular performance and ultrasonic myocardial quantitative reflectivity in endurance senior athletes: An echocardiographic study. *European Heart Journal* 14: 358-363.

Diesel, W., Noakes, T.D., Swanepoel, C., and Lambert, M. (1990). Isokinetic muscle strength predicts maximum exercise tolerance in renal patients on chronic hemodialysis. *American Journal of Kidney Diseases* 16: 109-114.

Dietz, J.H. (1981). *Rehabilitation oncology*. New York: Wiley.

Dill, D.B., Hillyard, S.D., and Miller, J. (1980). Vital capacity, exercise performance and blood gases at altitude as related to age. *Journal of Applied Physiology* 48: 6-9.

Dill, D.B., Robinson, S., and Ross, J.C. (1967). A longitudinal study of 16 champion runners. *Journal of Sports Medicine* 7: 4-27.

Dillard, S. (1983). *Durée ou qualité de la vie. Conseil des affaires sociales et de la famille* [Duration or quality of life. Council of Social and Family Affairs]. Québec, PQ: Les Publications de Québec.

DiPietro, L. (1995). Physical activity, body weight, and adiposity: An epidemiologic perspective. *Exercise and Sport Sciences Reviews* 23: 275-303.

DiPietro, L., Williamson, D.F., Caspersen, C.J., and Eaker, E. (1993). The descriptive epidemiology of selected physical activities and body weight among adults trying to lose weight: The Behavioral Risk Factor Surveillance System Survey, 1989. *International Journal of Obesity* 17: 69-76.

Dobbs, R.J., Charlett, A., Bowes, S.G., O'Neill, C.J.A., Weller, C., Hughes, J., and Dobbs, S.M. (1993). Is this walk normal? *Age and Ageing* 22: 27-30.

Doherty, T.J., Vandervoort, A.A., and Brown, W.F. (1993). Effects of ageing on the motor unit: A brief review. *Canadian Journal of Applied Physiology* 18: 331-358.

Domino, E.F. (1988). Present status of tardive dyskinesia. In R. Strong, W.G. Wood, and W.J. Burke (Eds.), *Aging: Vol. 33. Central nervous system disorders of aging. Clinical intervention and research* (pp. 117-126). New York: Raven Press.

Donahue, R.P., Abbott, R.D., Reed, D.M., and Yano, K. (1988). Physical activity and coronary heart disease in middle-aged and elderly men: The Honolulu Heart Study. *American Journal of Public Health* 78: 683-685.

Donaldson, C., and Mooney, G. (1991). Needs assessment, priority setting, and contracts for health care: An economic view. *British Medical Journal* 303: 1529-1530.

Donnelly, J.E. (1992). Role of physical activity in short-term weight loss. In V.A. Hubbard (Ed.), *NIH Workshop on Physical Activity and Obesity* (pp. 75-79). Washington, DC: National Institutes of Health.

Dorgan, J.F., Brown, C., Barrett, M., Splansky, G.L., Kreger, B.E., D'Agostino, R.B., Albanes, D., and Schatzkin, A. (1994). Physical activity and risk of breast cancer in the Framingham Heart Study. *American Journal of Epidemiology* 139: 662-669.

Douglas, P.S., and O'Toole, M. (1992). Aging and physical activity determine cardiac structure and function in the older athlete. *Journal of Applied Physiology* 72: 1969-1973.

Downes, T.R., Nomeir, A., Smith, K.M., Stewart, K.P., and Little, W.C. (1989). Mechanism of altered pattern of left ventricular filling with aging in subjects without cardiac disease. *American Journal of Cardiology* 64: 523-527.

Drenick, E.J., Bale, G.S., Seltzer, F.S.A., and Johnson, D.G. (1980). Excessive mortality and causes of death in morbidly obese men. *Journal of the American Medical Association* 243: 443-445.

Drinkwater, B. (1994). Physical activity, fitness and osteoporosis. In C. Bouchard, R.J. Shephard, and T. Stephens (Eds.), *Physical activity, fitness and health* (pp. 724-736). Champaign, IL: Human Kinetics.

Dublin, L.I., Lotka, A.J., and Spiegelman, M. (1949). *Length of life: A study of the life table* (chap. 6). New York: Ronald Press.

Duffy, M.E., and MacDonald, E. (1990). Determinants of functional health of older persons. *Gerontologist* 30: 503-509.

Dugan, D., Walker, R., and Monroe, D.A. (1995). The effects of a 9-week program of aerobic and upper body exercise on the maximal voluntary ventilation of chronic obstructive pulmonary disease patients. *Journal of Cardiopulmonary Rehabilitation* 15: 130-133.

Dummer, G.M., Clarke, D.H., Vaccaro, P., Velden, L.V., Goldfarb, A.H., and Sockler, J.M. (1985). Age related differences in muscular strength among female masters swimmers. *Research Quarterly* 56: 97-110.

Duncan, J.J., Gordon, N.F., and Scott, C.B. (1991). Women walking for health and fitness. How much is enough? *Journal of the American Medical Association* 266: 3295-3299.

Duncan, P.W., Chandler, J., Studenski, S., Hughes, M., and Prescott, B. (1993). How do physiological components of balance affect mobility in elderly men? *Archives of Physical Medicine and Rehabilitation* 74: 1343-1349.

Dupler, T.L., and Cortes, C. (1993). Effects of whole-body resistive training in the elderly. *Gerontology* 39: 314-319.

Dupree, L., Broskowski, H., and Schonfeld, L. (1984). The gerontology alcohol project: A behavioral treatment program for elderly alcohol abusers. *Gerontologist* 24 (5): 510-516.

Durak, E. (1989). Exercise for specific populations: Diabetes mellitus. *Sports Training, Medicine and Rehabilitation* 1: 175-180.

Durenberg, P., van der Kooy, K., Hulshof, T., and Evers, P. (1988). Body mass index as a measure of body fatness in the elderly. *European Journal of Clinical Nutrition* 43: 231-236.

Durnin, J.V.G.A., and Passmore, R. (1967). *Energy, work, and leisure*. London: Heinemann.

Durnin, J.V.G.A., and Womersley, J.A. (1974). Body fat assessed from total body density and its estimation from skinfold thickness: Measurements on 481 men and women aged from 16-72 years. *British Journal of Nutrition* 32: 77-97.

Durstine, J.L., and Haskell, W.L. (1994). Effects of exercise training on plasma lipids and lipoproteins. *Exercise and Sport Sciences Reviews* 22: 477-521.

Dustman, R.E., Emmerson, R., and Shearer, D. (1994). Physical activity, age, and cognitive neuropsychological function. *Journal of Aging and Physical Activity* 2: 143-181.

Easterlin, R.A., Crimmins, E.M., and Ohanian, L. (1984). Changes in labor force participation of persons 55 and over since World War II: Their nature and causes. In P.K. Robinson, J. Livingston, and J.E. Birren (Eds.), *Aging and technological advances* (pp. 89-98). New York: Plenum Press.

Effros, R.B., and Walford, R.W. (1983). The immune response of aged mice to influenza: Diminished T-cell proliferation, interleukin-2 production and cytotoxicity. *Cellular Immunology* 81: 298-305.

Ehsani, A.A. (1993). Physiologic adaptations to exercise in the hypertensive elderly. *Cardiology in the Elderly* 1: 558-563.

Ehsani, A.A., Ogawa, T., Miller, T.R., Spina, R.J., and Jilka, S.M. (1991). Exercise training improves left ventricular systolic function in older men. *Circulation* 83: 96-103.

Ekblöm, B. (1982). Short and long-term physical training in patients with rheumatoid arthritis. *Annals of Clinical Research* 14 (Suppl. 34): 109-110.

Ekblöm, B. (1985). Exercise and rheumatoid arthritis. In P. Welsh and R.J. Shephard (Eds.), *Current therapy in sports medicine 1985-6* (pp. 108-110). Burlington, ON: BC Decker.

Ekdahl, C., and Broman, G. (1992). Muscle strength, endurance, and aerobic capacity in rheumatoid arthritis: A comparative study with healthy subjects. *Annals of the Rheumatic Diseases* 51: 35-40.

Elahi, D., Herschoff, R., Muller, D.C., Tobin, J.D., and Andres, R. (1982). Insulin sensitivity and age. *Diabetes* 32: 195A.

Ellestad, M.H. (1985). *Stress testing—principles and practice* (2nd ed.). Philadelphia: Lea & Febiger.

Ellis, B., and Ries, A.L. (1991). Upper extremity exercise training in pulmonary rehabilitation. *Journal of Cardiopulmonary Rehabilitation* 11: 227-231.

Ellis, K.J., Yasumura, S., Vartsky, A.N., and Cohn, S.H. (1982). Total body nitrogen in health and disease: Effects of age, weight, height and sex. *Journal of Laboratory and Clinical Medicine* 99: 917-926.

Elveback, L., and Lie, J.T. (1984). Combined high incidence of coronary artery disease in Olmstead County, Minnesota, 1950-1979. *Circulation* 70: 345-349.

Elwood, P.C. (1971). Epidemiological aspects of iron deficiency in the elderly. *Gerontological Clinics* 13: 2-11.

Emery, C.F. (1994). Effects of age on physiological and psychological functioning among COPD patients in an exercise program. *Journal of Aging and Health* 6: 3-16.

Emery, C.F., and Blumenthal, J.A. (1991). Effects of physical exercise on psychological and cognitive functioning of older adults. *Gerontologist* 30: 516-521.

Emery, C.F., and Gatz, M. (1990). Psychological and cognitive effects of an exercise program for community-residing older adults. *Gerontologist* 30: 184-188.

Emmett, J.D., and Hodgson, J.L. (1993). Cardiovascular responses to snow-shoveling in a thermoneutral, cold and cold with wind environment. *Journal of Cardiopulmonary Rehabilitation* 13: 43-50.

Era, P., and Heikkinen, E. (1985). Postural sway during standing and unexpected disturbance of balance in random samples of men of different ages. *Journals of Gerontology* 40: 287M-295M.

Era, P., Jokela, J., and Heikkinen, E. (1986). Reaction and movement time in men of different ages. A population survey. *Perceptual and Motor Skills* 63: 111-130.

Era, P., Lyra, A.L., Viitasalo, J.T., and Heikkinen, E. (1992). Determinants of isometric muscle strength in men of different ages. *European Journal of Applied Physiology* 64: 84-91.

Era, P., Rantanen, T., Avlund, K., Gause-Nilsson, I., Heikkinen, E., Schroll, M., Steen, B., and Suominen, H. (1994). Maximal isometric muscle strength and anthropometry in 75-year-old men and women in three Nordic localities. *Scandinavian Journal of Medicine, Science and Sports* 4: 26-31.

Erickson, A.V., Isberg, B.O., and Lindgren, J.U. (1989). Prediction of vertebral strength by dual photon absorptiometry and quantitative computed tomography. *Calcified Tissue International* 44: 243-250.

Ericsson, K.A. (1990). Peak performance and age: An examination of peak performance in sports. In P.B. Baltes and M.M. Baltes (Eds.), *Successful aging: Perspectives from the behavioral sciences*. Cambridge: Cambridge University Press.

Eriksson, K-F., and Lindgärde, F. (1991). Prevention of Type 2 (non-insulin-dependent) diabetes mellitus by diet and physical exercise. *Diabetologia* 34: 891-898.

Erschler, W.B. (1988). Biomarkers of aging: Immunological events. *Experimental Gerontology* 23: 387-389.

Eskelinen, L., Kohvakka, A., Merisalo, T., Hurri, H., and Wägar, G. (1991). Relationship between the self-assessment and clinical assessment of health status and work ability. *Scandinavian Journal of Work, Environment & Health* 17 (Suppl. 1): 40-47.

Etnier, J.L., and Landers, D.M. (1995). Brain function and exercise. Current perspectives. *Sports Medicine* 19: 81-85.

Ettinger, W.H., and Fried, L.P. (1991). Aerobic exercise as therapy to prevent functional decline in patients with osteoarthritis. In M. Ory and R. Weindruch (Eds.), *Preventing frailty and falls in the elderly* (pp. 210-218). Springfield, IL: Charles C Thomas.

Ettinger, W.H., Wahl, P.W., Kuller, L.H., Bush, T.L., Tracy, R.P., Manolio, T.A., Borhani, N.O., Wong, N.D., and O'Leary, D.H. (1992). Lipoprotein lipids in older people: Results from the Cardiovascular Health Study. *Circulation* 86: 858-869.

Evans, D.M.D. (1971). Haematological aspects of iron deficiency in the elderly. *Gerontologia Clinica* 13: 12-30.

Evans, J.G. (1991). Challenge of aging. *British Medical Journal* 303: 408-409.

Evans, R.W., Manninen, D.L., Garrison, L.P., Hart, L.G., Blagg, C.R., Gutman, R.A., Hull, A.R., and Lowrie, E.G. (1985). The quality of life of patients with end-stage renal disease. *New England Journal of Medicine* 312: 553-559.

Eveleth, P. (1994). *Uses and interpretation of anthropometry in the elderly for the assessment of physical status*. Geneva: World Health Organization.

Everhart, J., Knowler, W.C., and Bennett, P.H. (1985). Incidence and risk factors for non-insulin dependent diabetes. In M.I. Harris and R.F. Hamman (Eds.), *Diabetes in America* (US DHHS, National Diabetes Data Group, NIH Publication No. 85-1468, pp. 1-35). Washington, DC: U.S. Government Printing Office.

Ewart, C.K. (1989). Psychological effects of resistance weight training: Implications for cardiac patients. *Medicine and Science in Sports and Exercise* 21: 683-688.

Exton-Smith, A.N., and Collins, K.J. (1991). The autonomic nervous system. In M.S.J. Pathy (Ed.), *Principles and practice of geriatric medicine* (2nd ed., pp. 817-840). Chichester: Wiley.

Eyre, D.R., Paz, M.A., and Gall, P.M. (1984). Cross-linking in collagen and elastin. *Annual Reviews of Biochemistry* 53: 717-748.

Fagard, R., Thijs, L., and Amery, A. (1993). Age and the hemodynamic response to posture and to exercise. *American Journal of Geriatric Cardiology* 2 (2): 23-30.

Fagard, R., and Tipton, C.M. (1994). Physical activity, fitness and hypertension. In C. Bouchard, R.J. Shephard, and T. Stephens (Eds.), *Physical activity, fitness and health* (pp. 633-655). Champaign, IL: Human Kinetics.

Fallentin, N., Nielsen, J., and Sogaard, K. (1993). Physical work load and functional capacity among cleaning workers. A case of age-related mismatch and disproportion [Abstract]. In J. Ilmarinen (Ed.), *Aging and work* (p. 41). Helsinki: Institute for Occupational Medicine.

Farrar, R.P., Martin, T.P., and Ardies, C.M. (1981). The interaction of aging and endurance exercise upon the mitochondrial function of skeletal muscle. *Journal of Gerontology* 36: 642-647.

Feibusch, J.M., and Holt, P.R. (1982). Impaired absorption capacity for carbohydrate in the aging human. *Digestive Disease Science* 27: 1095-1100.

Feinleib, M. (1985). Epidemiology of obesity in relation to health hazards. *Annals of Internal Medicine* 106: 1019-1024.

Feinleib, M., Rifkind, B., Sempos, C., Johnson, C., Bachorik, P., Lippel, K., Carroll, M., Ingster-Moore, L., and Murphy, R. (1993). Methodological issues in the measurement of cardiovascular risk factors: Within person variability in selected serum lipid measures—results from the third National Health and Nutrition Examination Survey (NHANES III). *Canadian Journal of Cardiology* 9 (Suppl. D): 87D-88D.

Feldman, M.L. (1976). Aging changes in the morphology of cortical dendrites. In R.D. Terry and S. Gershon (Eds.), *Neurobiology of aging* (pp. 211-227). New York: Raven Press.

Feldman, R.D. (1986). Physiological and metabolic correlates of age-related changes in the human beta-adrenergic receptor system. *Federation Proceedings* 45: 48-50.

Ferland, M., Després, J-P., Tremblay, A., Pinault, S., Nadeau, A., Moorjani, S., Lupien, P.J., Thériault, G., and Bouchard, C. (1989). Assessment of adipose tissue distribution by computed axial tomography in obese women: Association with body density and anthropometric measurements. *British Journal of Nutrition* 61: 139-148.

Ferretti, G., Narici, M.V., Binzoni, T., Gariod, L., Le Bas, J.F., Reutenauer, H., and Cerretelli, P. (1994). Determinants of peak muscle power: Effects of age and physical conditioning. *European Journal of Applied Physiology* 68: 111-115.

Feskens, E.J., Loeber, J.G., and Kromhout, D. (1994). Diet and physical activity as determinants of hyperinsulinemia: The Zutphen elderly study. *American Journal of Epidemiology* 140: 350-360.

Fiatarone, M., O'Neill, E.F., Ryan, N.D., Clements, K.M., Solares, G.R., Nelson, M.E., Roberts, S.B., Kehayias, J.J., Lipsitz, L.A., and Evans, W.J. (1994). Exercise training and nutritional supplementation for physical frailty in very elderly people. *New England Journal of Medicine* 330: 1769-1775.

Fiatarone, M.A., Marks, E.C., Ryan, N.D., Meredith, C.N., Lipsitz, L.A., and Evans, W.J. (1990). High-intensity strength training in nonagenarians: Effects on skeletal muscle. *Journal of the American Medical Association* 263: 3029-3034.

Fiatarone, M.A., Morley, J.E., Bloom, E.T., Benton, D., Solomon, G.F., and Makinodan, T. (1989). The effect of exercise on natural killer cell activity in young and old subjects. *Journals of Gerontology* 44: M37-M45.

Fields, K.B., DeLaney, M., and Hinckle, J.S. (1990). A prospective study of type A behavior and running injuries. *Journal of Family Practice* 30: 425-429.

Fiessinger, J.N., Carmer, J.M., and Housset, E. (1982). Artériopathies athéroscleroteuses des membres inférieures [Atherosclerotic arteriopathology of the lower limbs]. In F. Bourlière (Ed.), *Gérontologie: Biologie et clinique* (pp. 157-163). Paris: Flammarion.

Finch, C.E., Johnson, S., Kohama, S., Lerner, S., Masters, J., May, P., Morgan, D., Nichols, N., Pasinetti, G., and Telford, N. (1987). Physiological approaches to the roles of gene regulation in the brain during aging. In P. Davies and C. Finch (Eds.), *Molecular neuropathology of aging* (pp. 143-158). Plainview, NY: Cold Spring Harbor Laboratory Press.

Fink, R.I., Kolterman, O.G., Griffin, J., and Olefsky, J.M. (1983). Mechanisms of insulin resistance on aging. *Journal of Clinical Investigation* 71: 1523-1535.

Fisher, E., Nelson, M., and Evans, W. (1989). Effects of diet and exercise on bone health. In R. Harris and S. Harris (Eds.), *Physical activity, aging and sports* (pp. 301-315). Albany, NY: Center for Studies of Aging.

Fisher, N.M., Gresham, G.E., Abrams, M., Hicks, J., Horrigan, D., and Pendergast, D.R. (1993). Quantitative effects of physical therapy on muscular and functional performance in subjects with osteo-arthritis of the knees. *Archives of Physical Medcine and Rehabilitation* 74: 840-847.

Fisher, N.M., Kame, V.D., Rouse, L., and Pendergast, D.R. (1994). Quantitative evaluation of a home exercise program on muscle and functional capacity of patients with osteoarthritis. *American Journal of Physical Medicine and Rehabilitation* 73: 413-420.

Fisher, N.M., and Pendergast, D.R. (1994). Effects of a muscle exercise program on exercise capacity in subjects with osteoarthrosis. *Archives of Physical Medicine and Rehabilitation* 75: 792-797.

Fisher, N.M., Pendergast, D.R., and Calkins, E.C. (1990). Maximal isometric torque of knee extension as a function of muscle length in subjects of advancing age. *Archives of Physical Medicine and Rehabilitation* 71: 729-734.

Fisher, N.M., Pendergast, D.R., and Calkins, E.C. (1991). Muscle rehabilitation in impaired elderly nursing home residents. *Archives of Physical Medicine and Rehabilitation* 72: 181-185.

Fisher, N.M., Pendergast, D.R., Gresham, G.E., and Calkins, E.C. (1991). Muscle rehabilitation: Its effect on muscular and functional performance of patients with knee osteoarthritis. *Archives of Physical Medicine and Rehabilitation* 72: 367-374.

Fitness Canada. (1983). *Fitness and lifestyle in Canada.* Ottawa, ON: Government of Canada.

Fitness Canada. (1986). *Canadian Standardized Test of Fitness (CSTF) operations manual* (3rd ed.). Ottawa, ON: Government of Canada.

Fitzpatrick, R., Fletcher, A., Gore, S., Jones, D., Spiegelhalter, D., and Cox, D. (1992). Quality of life measures in health care: 1. Applications and issues of assessment. *British Medical Journal* 305: 1074-1077.

Fleg, J.L., Schulman, S., Gerstenblith, G., Goldberg, A., Tankersley, C., Becker, L., Clulow, J., Drinkwater, D., Lakatta, L., and Lakatta, E.G. (1988). Central versus peripheral adaptations in highly trained seniors [Abstract]. *Physiologist* 31: A158.

Fleg, J.L., Schulman, S., O'Connor, F., Becker, L.C., Gerstenblith, G., Clulow, J.F., Renlund, D.G., and Lakatta, E.F. (1994). Effects of acute beta-adrenergic receptor blockade on age-associated changes in cardiovascular performance during dynamic exercise. *Circulation* 90: 2333-2341.

Fleg, J.L., Schulman, S.P., Gerstenblith, G., Becker, L.C., O'Connor, F.C., and Lakatta, E.G. (1993). Additive effects of age and silent myocardial ischemia on the left ventricular response to upright cycle exercise. *Journal of Applied Physiology* 75: 499-504.

Fleg, J.L., Tzankoff, S.P., and Lakatta, E.G. (1985). Age-related augmentation of plasma catecholamines during dynamic exercise in healthy males. *Journal of Applied Physiology* 59: 1033-1039.

Fletcher, A., Gore, S., Jones, D., Fitzpatrick, R., Spiegelhalter, D., and Cox, D. (1992). Quality of life measures in health care: II. Design, analysis and interpretation. *British Medical Journal* 305: 1145-1148.

Florini, J.R., and Roberts, S.B. (1980). Effect of rat age on blood levels of somatomedin-like growth factors. *Journal of Gerontology* 35: 23-30.

Flynn, M.A., Nolph, G.B., Baker, A.S., Martin, W.M., and Krause, G. (1989). Total body potassium in aging humans: A longitudinal study. *American Journal of Clinical Nutrition* 50: 713-717.

Fogelholm, M., Kaprio, J., and Sarna, S. (1994). Healthy lifestyles of former Finnish world class athletes. *Medicine and Science in Sports and Exercise* 25: 224-229.

Folgering, H., and Van Herwaarden, C. (1994). Exercise limitations in patients with pulmonary diseases. *International Journal of Sports Medicine* 15: 107-111.

Forbes, G.B. (1987). *Human body composition: Growth, aging, nutrition and activity*. New York: Springer-Verlag.

Forbes, G.B., Brown, M.R., Welle, S.L., and Lipinski, B.A. (1986). Deliberate overfeeding in women and men: Energy cost and composition of weight gain. *British Journal of Nutrition* 56: 1-9.

Ford, G.A., Blaschke, T.F., Wiswell, R., and Hoffman, B.B. (1993). Effect of aging on changes in plasma potassium during exercise. *Journals of Gerontology* 48: M140-M145.

Forette, B., Tortrat, D., and Wolmark, Y. (1989). Cholesterol as risk factor for mortality in elderly women. *Lancet* i: 868-870.

Forette, F., Henry, F.-J., and Hervy, M.-P. (1982). Hypertension. In F. Bourlière (Ed.), *Gérontologie: Biologie et clinique* (pp. 131-142). Paris: Flammarion.

Foreyt, J. (1992). Psychological issues in obesity and physical activity. In V.A. Hubbard (Ed.), *NIH Workshop on Physical Activity and Obesity* (pp. 83-84). Washington, DC: National Institutes of Health.

Forman, D.E., Manning, W.J., Hauser, R., Gervino, E.V., Evans, W.J., and Wei, J.Y. (1992). Enhanced left ventricular diastolic filling associated with long-term endurance training. *Journals of Gerontology* 47: M56-M58.

Forster, A., and Young, J. (1995). Incidence and consequences of falls due to stroke: A systematic enquiry. *British Medical Journal* 311: 83-86.

Forwood, M.R., and Burr, D.B. (1993). Physical activity and bone mass: Exercises in futility? *Bone and Mineral* 21: 89-112.

Foss, M.L., Lampmann, R.M., Watt, E., and Schteingart, D.E. (1975). Initial work tolerance of extremely obese patients. *Archives of Physical Medicine and Rehabilitation* 57: 63-67.

Foster, V.L., Hume, G.J.E., Byrnes, W.C., Dickinson, A.L., and Chatfield, S.J. (1989). Endurance training for elderly women: Moderate vs low intensity. *Journals of Gerontology* 44: M184-M188.

Fotherby, M.D., Harper, G.D., and Potter, J.F. (1992). General practitioners' management of hypertension in elderly patients. *British Medical Journal* 305: 750-752.

Fouillot, J-P., Benaoudia, M., Blum, R., and Rieu, M. (1992). Modification de la variabilité du rhythme cardiaque au cours du vieillissement [Modification of the variability of the heart rhythm during aging]. *La Revue de Gériatrie, Proceedings of Euromedicine* 92 (pp. 196-197). Montpellier: Le Corum.

Fox, S.M. (1986). Heavy duty truck drivers and cardiac disorders. *Proceedings of the Medical/Industry Interchange Conference.* Washington, DC: American College of Cardiology.

Fozard, J.L. (1972). Predicting age in the adult years from psychological assessment of abilities and personality. *Aging and Human Development* 3: 175-182.

Frändin, K., Grimby, G., Mellström, D., and Svänborg, A. (1991). Walking habits and health-related factors in a 70-year-old population. *Gerontology* 37: 281-288.

Franklin, B., and Kahn, J.K. (1995). Detecting the individual prone to exercise-related sudden cardiac death. *Sports Science Review* 1: 85-105.

Franklin, B.A., Bonzheim, K., Gordon, S., and Timmis, G.C. (1991). Resistance training in cardiac rehabilitation. *Journal of Cardiac Rehabilitation* 11: 99-107.

Freedson, P.S., Gilliam, T.B., Mahoney, T., Maliszewski, A.F., and Kastango, K. (1993). Industrial torque levels by age group and gender. *Isokinetics and Exercise Science* 3: 34-42.

Fries, J.F. (1980a). Aging, natural death and the compression of morbidity. *New England Journal of Medicine* 303: 130-135.

Fries, J.F. (1980b). *Aging well.* Reading, MA: Addison-Wesley.

Fries, J.F. (1992). Strategies for reduction of morbidity. *American Journal of Clinical Nutrition* 55: 1257S-1262S.

Fries, J.F., Bloch, D.A., Harrington, H., Richardson, N., and Beck, R. (1993). Two-year results of a randomized controlled trial of a health promotion program in a retiree population: The Bank of America Study. *American Journal of Medicine* 94: 455-462.

Fries, J.F., Harrington, H., Edwards, R., Kent, L.A., and Richardson, N. (1994). Randomized controlled trial of cost reductions from a health education program: The California Public Employees' Retirement System (PERS) Study. *American Journal of Health Promotion* 8: 216-223.

Frisancho, A.R., and Flegel, P.N. (1983). Elbow breadth as a measure of frame size for U.S. males and females. *American Journal of Clinical Nutrition* 37: 311-314.

Frisch, R.E., Wyshak, G., Witschi, J., Albright, N.L., Albright, T.E., and Schiff, I. (1987). Lower lifetime occurrence of breast cancer and cancers of the reproductive system among former college athletes. *British Journal of Fertility* 32: 217-225.

Frishman, W.H. (1993). Hyperlipidemia in the elderly. *American Journal of Geriatric Cardiology* 2 (4): 22-27.

Froelich, C.J., Burkett, J.S., Guiffaut, S., Kingsland, R., and Brauner, D. (1988). Phytohemagglutinin induced proliferation by aged lymphocytes: Reduced expression of high affinity interleukin-2 receptors and interleukin-2 secretion. *Life Sciences* 43: 1583-1590.

Froelicher, V.F., Jensen, D., Gentner, F., Sullivan, M., McKirnan, M.D., Witztum, K., Scharf, J., Strong, M.L., and Ashburn, W. (1984). A randomized trial of exercise training in patients with coronary heart disease. *Journal of the American Medical Association* 252: 1291-1297.

Frontera, W.R., Hughes, V.A., Dallal, G.E., and Evans, W.R. (1993). Reliability of isokinetic muscle strength testing in 45 to 78-year old men and women. *Archives of Physical Medicine and Rehabilitation* 74: 1181-1185.

Frontera, W.R., Hughes, V.A., Lutz, K.J., and Evans, W.J. (1991). A cross-sectional study of muscle strength and mass in 45- to 78-yr old men and women. *Journal of Applied Physiology* 71: 644-650.

Frontera, W.R., Meredith, C.N., O'Reilly, K.P., and Evans, W.J. (1988). Strength conditioning in older men: Skeletal muscle hypertrophy and improved function. *Journal of Applied Physiology* 64: 1038-1044.

Fuchi, T., Iwaoka, K., Higuchi, M., and Kobayashi, S. (1989). Cardiovascular changes associated with increased aerobic capacity and aging in long-distance runners. *European Journal of Applied Physiology* 58: 884-889.

Fuller, J.J., and Winters, J.M. (1993). Assessment of 3-D joint contact load predictions during postural/stretching exercises in aged females. *Annals of Biomedical Engineering* 21: 277-288.

Fullerton, H.N. (1984). Demographic trends affecting the age structure of the labor force: 1950-2000. In P.K. Robinson, J. Livingston, and J.E. Birren (Eds.), *Aging and technological advances* (pp. 55-74). New York: Plenum Press.

Furberg, C.D., and Black, D.M. (1988). The systolic hypertension in the elderly pilot program: Methodological issues. *European Heart Journal* 9: 223-227.

Furukawa, T. (1994). Assessment of the adequacy of the multiple regression model to estimate biological age. In A.K. Balin (Ed.), *Practical handbook of human biologic age determination* (pp. 471-484). Boca Raton, FL: CRC Press.

Gafni, A., and Yu, K. (1989). A comparative study of the Ca^{2+}-Mg^{2+} dependent ATPase from skeletal muscles of young, adult and old rats. *Mechanisms in Ageing and Development* 49: 105-117.

Gaido, M.L., Schwartzman, R.A., Caron, L-A. M., and Cidlowski, J.A. (1990). Glucocorticoids and cell death: Biochemical mechanisms. In C.E. Finch and T.E. Johnson (Eds.), *Molecular biology of aging* (pp. 299-310). New York: Liss.

Gardsell, P., Johnell, O., and Nilsson, B.E. (1991). The predictive value of bone loss for fragility fractures in women: A longitudinal study over 15 years. *Calcified Tissue International* 49: 90-94.

Garn, S.M. (1975). Bone loss and aging. In R. Goldman and M. Rockstein (Eds.), *The physiology and pathology of human aging* (pp. 39-58). New York: Academic Press.

Garn, S.M., Leonard, W.R., and Hawthorne, V.M. (1986). Three limitations of the body mass index. *American Journal of Clinical Nutrition* 44: 996-997.

Garn, S.M., Sullivan, T.V., and Hawthorne, V. (1988). Evidence against functional differences between central and peripheral fat. *American Journal of Clinical Nutrition* 47: 836-839.

Garrow, J.S. (1994). Should obesity be treated? Treatment is necessary. *British Medical Journal* 309: 654-656.

Garry, P.J. (1994). Nutrition and aging. In W.R. Faulkner and S. Meites (Eds.), *Geriatric clinical chemistry*. Washington, DC: American Association for Clinical Chemistry.

Gavras, I., and Gavras, H. (1980). Special considerations in treating hypertension in the elderly. *Geriatrics* 35: 34-40.

Gayle, R.C., Spitler, D.L., Karper, W.B., Jaeger, R.M., and Rice, S.N. (1988). Psychological changes in exercising COPD patients. *International Journal of Rehabilitation Research* 11: 335-342.

Gelman, R., Watson, A., Bronson, R., and Yunis, E. (1988). Murine chromosomal regions correlated with longevity. *Genetics* 118: 693-704.

Genant, H.K., Cann, C.E., and Faul, D.D. (1982). Quantitative computed tomography for assessing vertebral bone mineral. In J. Dequecker and C.C. Johnston (Eds.), *Noninvasive bone measurements: Methodological problems* (pp. 215-249). Oxford: IRL Press.

General Mills (1979). *Family health in an era of stress.* Survey conducted by Yankevitch, Skelly & White, Inc. for General Mills, Minneapolis. Minneapolis: Author.

Gensler, H.L., and Bernstein, H. (1981). DNA damage as the primary cause of aging. *Quarterly Review of Biology* 56: 279-303.

Geographic profile of the aged. *Statistical Bulletin* 74 (1): 2-9.

Gerhardsson, M., Norrell, S.E., Kiviranta, H., Pederssen, N.L., and Ahlbom, A. (1986). Sedentary jobs and colon cancer. *American Journal of Epidemiology* 123: 775-780.

Gerstenblith, G. (1980). Non-invasive assessment of cardiac function in the elderly. In M.L. Weisfeldt (Ed.), *The aging heart* (pp. 247-267). New York: Raven Press.

Gerstenblith, G., Fredericksen, J., Yin, F.C., Fortuin, N.J., Lakatta, E.G., and Weisfeldt, M.L. (1977). Echocardiographic assessment of a normal adult aging population. *Circulation* 56: 273-278.

Gerstenblith, G., Weisfeldt, M.L., and Lakatta, E.G. (1985). Disorders of the heart. In R. Andres, E.L. Bierman, and W.R. Hazzard (Eds.), *Principles of geriatric medicine* (pp. 515-526). New York: McGraw-Hill.

Ghigo, E., Goffi, S., Nicolosi, M., Arvat, E., Valente, F., Mazza, E., Ghigo, M.C., and Camanni, F. (1990). Growth hormone (GH) responsiveness to combined administration of arginine and GH-releasing hormone does not vary with age in man. *Journal of Clinical Endocrinology and Metabolism* 71: 1481-1485.

Gianuzzi, P., Tavazzi, L., Temporelli, P.L., Corra, U., Imparato, A., Gattone, M., Giordano, A., Sala, L., Schweiger, C., and Malinverni, C. (1993). Long-term physical training and left ventricular remodelling after anterior myocardial reinfarction: Results of the Exercise in Anterior Myocardial Infarction (EAMI) Trial. *Journal of the American College of Cardiology* 22: 1821-1829.

Gibson, M.C., and Schultze, E. (1983). Age-related differences in absolute numbers of skeletal muscle satellite cells. *Muscle and Nerve* 6: 574-580.

Gibson, R.F., and Fisher, C.R. (1979). Age differences in health care spending, Fiscal Year 1977. *Social Security Bulletin* 42 (1): 12.

Giglia, L. (1992). *The relationship between physical activity and the risk of developing breast cancer.* Unpublished M.Sc. dissertation, University of Toronto, Toronto, ON.

Gilders, R.M., and Dudley, G.A. (1992). Endurance exercise training and treatment of hypertension. The controversy. *Sports Medicine* 13: 71-77.

Giraud, G.D., Morton, M.J., Davis, L.E., Paul, M.S., and Thornburg, K.L. (1993). Estrogen-induced left ventricular chamber enlargement in ewes. *American Journal of Physiology* 264: E490-E496.

Gitlin, L.N., Lawton, M.P., Windsor-Landsberg, L.A., Kleban, M.H., Sands, L.P., and Posner, J. (1992). In search of psychological benefits: Exercise in healthy older adults. *Journal of Aging and Health* 4: 174-192.

Glaser, R.M. (1985). Exercise and locomotion for the spinal cord injured. *Exercise and Sport Sciences Reviews* 13: 263-304.

Goedhard, W.J.A. (1993). Psycho-social stress in relation to age in a working population. In J. Ilmarinen (Ed.), *Aging and work.* Helsinki: Institute for Occupational Medicine.

Going, S.B., Williams, D.P., Lohman, T.G., and Hewitt, M.J. (1994). Aging, body composition, and physical activity: A review. *Journal of Aging and Physical Activity* 2: 38-66.

Goldberg, A.P., Andres, R., and Bierman, E.L. (1985). Diabetes mellitus in the elderly. In R. Andres, E.L. Bierman, and W.R. Hazzard (Eds.), *Principles of geriatric medicine* (pp. 750-763). New York: McGraw-Hill.

Goldberg, A.P., and Harter, H.R. (1994). Physical activity, fitness and kidney disease. In C. Bouchard, R.J. Shephard, and T. Stephens (Eds.), *Physical activity, fitness and health* (pp. 762-773). Champaign, IL: Human Kinetics.

Goldberg, P.B., Kreider, M.S., McLean, M.R., and Roberts, J. (1986). Effects of aging at the adrenergic cardiac neuroeffector junction. *Federation Proceedings* 45: 45-47.

Goldfarb, A.H., Vaccaro, P., and Ostrove, S.M. (1989). Effects of age and body composition on the blood glucose response during exercise. In R. Harris and S. Harris (Eds.), *Physical activity, aging and sports* (pp. 251-258). Albany, NY: Center for Studies of Aging.

Goldstein, R.S., Gort, E.H., Stubbing, D., Avendano, M.A., and Guyatt, G.H. (1994). Randomized controlled trial of respiratory rehabilitation. *Lancet* 344: 1394-1397.

Goldstein, S. (1990). Replicative senescence: The human fibroblast comes of age. *Science* 249: 1129-1133.

Goldstein, S., Murano, S., Benes, H., Moerman, E.J., Jones, R.A., Thweatt, R., Shmookler-Reis, R.J., and Howard, B.H. (1990). On the molecular-genetic mechanism of the human fibroblast senescence. In H.L. Segal, M. Rothstein, and E. Bergamini (Eds.), *Protein metabolism in aging* (pp. 189-194). New York: Wiley-Liss.

Goldstein, S., Wojtyk, R.I., Harley, C.B., Pollard, J.W., Chamberlain, J.W., and Stanners, C.P. (1985). Protein synthetic fidelity in aging human fibroblasts. In D. Salk, Y. Fujiwara, and G.M. Martin (Eds.), *Werner's syndrome and human aging*. New York: Plenum Press.

Gompertz, B. (1825). On the nature of the function expressive of the law of human mortality and a new method of expressing the value of life contingencies. *Philosophical Transactions of the Royal Society of London A* 15: 513-585.

Goodman, J. (1995a). Exercise and congestive heart failure. In J. Torg and R.J. Shephard (Eds.), *Current therapy in sports medicine* (3rd ed., pp. 658-663). Philadelphia: Mosby–Yearbook.

Goodman, J. (1995b). Exercise and sudden cardiac death. Etiology in apparently healthy individuals. *Sports Science Review* 4: 14-30.

Goodrick, C.L., Ingram, D.K., Reynolds, M.A., Freeman, J.R., and Cider, N.L. (1983). Differential effects of intermittent feeding and voluntary exercise on body weight and lifespan in adult rats. *Journal of Gerontology* 38: 36-45.

Goodwin, T.S., Searles, R.P., and Tung, S.K. (1982). Immunological responses of a healthy population. *Clinical and Experimental Immunology* 48: 403-410.

Goran, M.I., and Poehlman, E.T. (1992a). Endurance training does not enhance total energy expenditure in healthy elderly persons. *American Journal of Physiology* 263: E950-E957.

Goran, M.I., and Poehlman, E.T. (1992b). Total energy expenditure and energy requirements in healthy elderly persons. *Metabolism* 41: 744-753.

Goranzon, H., and Forsum, E. (1985). Effect of reduced energy intake versus increased physical activity on the outcome of nitrogen balance experiments in man. *American Journal of Clinical Nutrition* 41: 919-928.

Gordon, D.J., and Rifkind, B. (1989). Treating high blood cholesterol in the older patient. *American Journal of Cardiology* 63: 48H-63H.

Gosselin, L.E., Bohlmann, T., and Thomas, D.P. (1988). Effects of age and endurance training on capillary density and fiber type distribution in rat diaphragm muscle [Abstract]. *Medicine and Science in Sports and Exercise* 20: S9.

Gotfredsen, A., Jensen, J., Borg, J., and Christiansen, C. (1986). Measurement of lean body mass and total body fat using dual photon absorptiometry. *Metabolism* 35: 88-93.

Gottfries, C.G. (1986). Monoamines and myelin components in aging and dementia disorders. In D.F. Swaab, E. Fliers, W. Miriam, W.A. Van Gool, and F. Van Haaren (Eds.), *Progress in brain research* 70 (pp. 133-140). New York: Elsevier.

Gould, R., and Takala, M. (1993). Pension or work—the preferences of older workers. In J. Ilmarinen (Ed.), *Aging and work* (pp. 67-73). Helsinki: Institute for Occupational Medicine.

Govindasamy, D., Paterson, D.H., Poulin, M.J., and Cunningham, D.A. (1992). Cardiorespiratory adaptation with short term training in older men. *European Journal of Applied Physiology* 65: 203-208.

Graham, P.A. (1991). The eye. In M.S.J. Pathy (Ed.), *Principles and practice of geriatric medicine* (2nd ed., pp. 985-993). Chichester: Wiley.

Grand, A., Groscaude, P., Bocquet, J., Pous, J., and Albarede, J.L. (1990). Disability, psychosocial factors and mortality among the elderly in a rural French sample. *Journal of Clinical Epidemiology* 43: 773-782.

Granger, C.V., Albrecht, G.L., and Hamilton, B.B. (1979). Outcome of comprehensive medical rehabilitation measurements by PULSES profile and Barthel Index. *Archives of Physical Medicine and Rehabilitation* 60: 145-154.

Granger, C.V., Hamilton, B.B., and Fiedler, R.C. (1992). Discharge outcome after stroke rehabilitation. *Stroke* 23: 978-982.

Granhed, H., Johnson, R., and Hansson, T. (1987). The loads on the lumbar spine during extreme weight-lifting. *Spine* 12: 146-149.

Green, M.F. (1991). The endocrine system. In M.S.J. Pathy (Ed.), *Principles and practice of geriatric medicine* (2nd ed., pp. 1061-1121). Chichester: Wiley.

Green, J.S., and Crouse, S.F. (1993). Endurance training, cardiovascular function and the aged. *Sports Medicine* 16: 331-341.

Green, J.S., and Crouse, S.F. (1995). The effects of endurance training on functional capacity in the elderly: A meta-analysis. *Medicine and Science in Sports and Exercise* 27: 920-926.

Greendale, G.A., Barrett-Connor, E., Edelstein, S., Ingles, S., and Haile, R. (1995). Lifetime leisure exercise and osteoporosis. *American Journal of Epidemiology* 141: 951-959.

Greendale, G.A., Hirsch, S.H., and Hahn, T.J. (1993). The effects of a weighted vest on perceived health status and bone density in older persons. *Quality of Life Research* 2: 141-152.

Greenwald, P., Kelloff, G., Bruch-Witman, C., and Kramer, B.S. (1995). Chemoprevention. *CA: A Cancer Journal for Clinicians* 45: 31-49.

Griffiths, A., and Pathy, M.S.J. (1991). Neurological disorders of the elderly. In M.S.J. Pathy (Ed.), *Principles and practice of geriatric medicine* (2nd ed., pp. 683-801). Chichester: Wiley.

Grigliatti, T.A. (1987). Programmed cell death and aging in Drosophila melanogaster. In A.D. Woodhead and K.H. Thompson (Eds.), *Evolution of longevity in animals. A comparative approach* (pp. 193-208). New York: Plenum Press.

Grimby, G., Danneskold-Samsoe, B., Hvid, K., and Saltin, B. (1982). Morphology and enzymatic capacity in arm and leg muscles in 78-81 year old men and women. *Acta Physiologica Scandinavica* 115: 125-134.

Grimby, G., and Saltin, B. (1966). A physiological analysis of physically well-trained middle-aged and old athletes. *Acta Medica Scandinavica* 179: 513-526.

Grove, K.A., and Londeree, B.R. (1992). Bone density in post-menopausal women: High impact vs low impact exercise. *Medicine and Science in Sports and Exercise* 24: 1190-1194.

Grover, R.F., Tucker, C.E., McGroarty, S.R., and Travis, R.R. (1990). The coronary stress of skiing at high altitude. *Archives of Internal Medicine* 150: 1205-1208.

Gruber, J.J. (1986). Physical activity and self-esteem development in children: A meta-analysis. In G.A. Stull and H.M. Eckert (Eds.), *Effects of physical activity on children* (pp. 30-48). Champaign, IL: Human Kinetics.

Gudat, U., Berger, M., and Lefèbvre, P. (1994). Physical activity, fitness and non-insulin dependent (Type II) diabetes mellitus. In C. Bouchard, R.J. Shephard, and T. Stephens (Eds.), *Physical activity, fitness and health* (pp. 669-683). Champaign, IL: Human Kinetics.

Guenard, H., and Emeriau, J-P. (1992). Le vieillissement des fonctions cardiorespiratoires [Aging of cardiorespiratory functions]. *La Revue de Gériatrie, Proceedings of Euromedicine 92* (pp. 195-196). Montpellier: Le Corum.

Guigoz, Y., Vellas, B., and Garry, P.J. (1994). Mini nutritional assessment: A practical assessment tool for grading the nutritional state of elderly patients. *Facts and Research in Gerontology* (Suppl.: Nutrition, pp. 15-59). Paris: Serdi.

Gunby, M.C., and Morley, J.E. (1995). Calcium, vitamin D, and ostopenia. In J.E. Morley, Z. Glick, and L.Z. Rubenstein (Eds.), *Geriatric nutrition: A comprehensive review* (2nd ed., pp. 107-114). New York: Raven Press.

Guralnik, J.M., LaCroix, A.Z., Abbott, R.D., Berkman, L.F., Satterfield, S., Evans, D.A., and Wallace, R.B. (1993). Maintaining mobility in late life. *American Journal of Epidemiology* 137: 845-857.

Guralnik, J.M., LaCroix, A.Z., Everett, D.F., and Kovar, M.G. (1989). Aging in the eighties: The prevalence of comorbidity and its association with disability. *Advance Data from Vital and Health Statistics Series 3*, No. 170. Hyattsville, MD: National Center for Health Statistics.

Gutin, B., and Kasper, M.J. (1992). Can vigorous exercise play a role in osteoporosis prevention? A review. *Osteoporosis International* 2: 55-69.

Guyatt, G., Keller, J., Singer, J., Halcrow, S., and Newhouse, M. (1992). Controlled trial of respiratory muscle training in chronic airflow limitation. *Thorax* 47: 598-602.

Guyatt, G.H., Dego, R.A., Charlson, M., Levine, M.N., and Mitchell, A. (1989). Responsiveness and validity in health status measurement: A clarification. *Journal of Clinical Epidemiology* 42: 403-408.

Gwathmey, J.K., Slawsky, M.T., Perreault, C.L., Briggs, G.M., Morgan, J.P., and Wei, J.Y. (1990). Effect of exercise conditioning on excitation-contraction coupling in aged rats. *Journal of Applied Physiology* 69: 1366-1371.

Hagberg, J.M. (1987). Effect of training on the decline of $\dot{V}O_2$max with aging. *FASEB Journal* 46: 1830-1833.

Hagberg, J.M. (1989). Patients with end-stage renal disease. In B.A. Franklin, S. Gordon, and G.C. Timmis (Eds.), *Exercise in modern medicine* (pp. 146-155). Baltimore: Williams & Wilkins.

Hagberg, J.M., Allen, W.K., Seals, D.R., Hurley, B.F., Ehsani, A.A., and Holloszy, J.O. (1985). A hemodynamic comparison of young and older endurance athletes during exercise. *Journal of Applied Physiology* 58: 2041-2046.

Hagberg, J.M., Graves, J.E., Limacher, M., Woods, D.R., Leggett, S.H., Cononie, C., Gruber, J.J., and Pollock, M.L. (1989). Cardiovascular response of 70 to 79-yr-old men and women to exercise training. *Journal of Applied Physiology* 66: 2589-2594.

Hagberg, J.M., Montain, S.J., Martin, W.H., and Ehsani, A.A. (1989). Effect of exercise training in 60- to 69-year-old persons with essential hypertension. *American Journal of Cardiology* 64: 348-353.

Hagberg, J.M., Seals, D.R., Yerg, J.E., Gavin, J., Gingerich, R., Premachandra, B., and Holloszy, J.O. (1988). Metabolic responses to exercise in young and older athletes and sedentary men. *Journal of Applied Physiology* 65: 900-908.

Hagberg, J.M., Yerg, J.E., and Seals, D.R. (1988). Pulmonary function in young and older athletes and untrained men. *Journal of Applied Physiology* 65: 101-105.

Haggmark, T., Jansson, E., and Svane, B. (1978). Cross-sectional area of the thigh muscle in man measured by computed tomography. *Scandinavian Journal of Clinical and Laboratory Investigation* 38: 355-360.

Hajduczok, G., Chapleau, M.W., and Abboud, F.M. (1991). Increase in sympathetic activity with age. II. Role of impairment of cardiopulmonary baroreflexes. *American Journal of Physiology* 260: H1121-H1127.

Häkkinen, K., and Häkkinen, A. (1991). Muscle cross-sectional area, force production and relaxation characteristics in women at different age. *European Journal of Applied Physiology* 62: 410-414.

Halhuber, M.J., and Humpeler, K.J. (1985). Does altitude cause exhaustion of the heart and circulatory system? *Medicine and Science in Sports and Exercise* 19: 192-202.

Hall, D.A., Middleton, R.S.W., El-Ridi, S.S., and Zajac, A. (1980). Serum elastase levels following a stroke in elderly subjects. *Gerontology* 26: 167-173.

Hall, J.A., Dixson, G.H., Barnard, R.J., and Pritikin, N. (1982). Effects of diet and exercise on peripheral vascular disease. *Physician and Sportsmedicine* 10 (5): 90-101.

Hallinan, C.J., and Schuler, P.B. (1993). Body shape perceptions of elderly women exercisers and nonexercisers. *Perceptual and Motor Skills* 77: 451-456.

Halter, J.B. (1985). Alterations of autonomic nervous system function. In R. Andres, E.L. Bierman, and W.R. Hazzard (Eds.), *Principles of geriatric medicine* (pp. 218-230). New York: McGraw-Hill.

Hamdorf, P.A., Withers, R.T., Penhall, R.K., and Plummer, J.L. (1993). A follow-up study on the effects of training on the fitness and habitual activity patterns of 60- to 70-year-old women. *Archives of Physical Medicine and Rehabilitation* 74: 473-477.

Hamilton, M., Pickering, W.G., Fraser-Roberts, J.A., and Sowry, G.S.C. (1954). The etiology of essential hypertension. 1. The arterial pressure in the general population. *Clinical Science* 13: 11-35.

Hanawalt, P.C., Gee, P., and Ho, L. (1990). DNA repair in differentiating cells in relation to aging. In C. Finch and T.E. Johnson (Eds.), *Molecular biology of aging* (pp. 45-51). New York: Wiley-Liss.

Härmä, M., and Hakola, T. (1993). Ageing decreases sleep length and alertness after consecutive night shifts. In J. Ilmarinen (Ed.), *Aging and work* (pp. 226-231). Helsinki: Institute of Occupational Health.

Harman, D. (1981). The aging process. *Proceedings of the National Academy of Science, USA* 78: 7124-7128.

Harper, A.B., Laughlin, W.S., and Mazess, R.B. (1984). Bone mineral content in St. Lawrence Island Eskimos. *Human Biology* 56: 63-78.

Harries, U.J., and Bassey, E.J. (1990). Torque-velocity relationships for the knee extensors in women in their 3rd and 7th decades. *European Journal of Applied Physiology* 60: 187-190.

Harrill, I., and Kylen, A. (1980). Protein intake and serum protein in elderly women. *Nutrition Reports International* 21: 717-720.

Harris, E.D. (1990). Rheumatoid arthritis: Pathophysiology and implications for treatment. *New England Journal of Medicine* 322: 1277-1289.

Harris, T., Cook, E.F., Garrison, R., Higgins, M., Kannel, W., and Goldman, L. (1988). Body mass index and mortality among non-smoking older persons: The Framingham Heart Study. *Journal of the American Medical Association* 259: 1520-1524.

Harris, T., Feldman, J.J., Kleinman, J., Ettinger, W.H., Makuc, D., and Schatzkin, A.G. (1992). The low cholesterol mortality association in a national cohort. *Journal of Clinical Epidemiology* 45: 595-601.

Hart, D., Bowling, A., Ellis, M., and Silman, A. (1990). Locomotor disability in very elderly people: Value of a programme for screening and provision of aids for daily living. *British Medical Journal* 301: 216-220.

Hartley, A.A., and Hartley, J.T. (1986). Age differences and changes in sprint swimming performances. *Experimental Aging Research* 12: 65-70.

Harvey, I., Frankel, S.J., Shalam, D., and Marks, R. (1989). Non-melanoma skin cancer: Questions concerning its distribution and natural history. *British Medical Journal* 299: 118-120.

Haskell, W.L. (1994). The efficacy and safety of exercise programs in cardiac rehabilitation. *Medicine and Science in Sports and Exercise* 26: 815-823.

Haslam, D.R.S., McCartney, N., McKelvie, R.S., and MacDougall, J.D. (1988). Direct measurements of arterial blood pressure during formal weight-lifting in cardiac patients. *Journal of Cardiopulmonary Rehabilitation* 8: 213-225.

Hasling, C., Sondergaard, K., Charles, P., and Mosekilde, L. (1992). Calcium metabolism in post-menopausal osteoporotic women is determined by dietary calcium and coffee intake. *Journal of Nutrition* 122: 1119-1126.

Hassi, J., Vironkannas, H., Anttonen, H., and Järvenpää, I. (1985). Health hazards in snowmobile use. In R. Fortuine (Ed.), *Circumpolar health '84*. Seattle: University of Washington Press.

Hassmen, P., Ceci, R., and Backman, L. (1992). Exercise for older women: A training method and its influences on physical and cognitive performance. *European Journal of Applied Physiology* 64: 460-466.

Hatori, M., Hasegawa, A., Adachi, H., Shinozaki, A., Hayashi, R., Okano, H., Mizunuma, H., and Murata, K. (1993). The effects of walking at the anaerobic threshold level on vertebral bone loss in postmenopausal women. *Calcified Tissue International* 52: 411-414.

Haut, R.C., Lancaster, R.L., and DeCamp, C.E. (1992). Mechanical properties of the canine patellar tendon: Some correlations with age and the content of collagen. *Journal of Biomechanics* 25: 163-173.

Havenith, G., Inoue, Y., Luttikholt, V., and Kenney, W.L. (1995). Age predicts cardiovascular, but not thermoregulatory, responses to humid heat stress. *European Journal of Applied Physiology* 70: 88-96.

Hawkins, H.L., Kramer, A.F., and Capaldi, D. (1992). Aging, exercise, and attention. *Psychology and Aging* 7: 643-653.

Hawkins, W.E., and Duncan, T. (1991). Structural equation analysis of an exercise/ sleep health practices model on quality of life of elderly persons. *Perceptual and Motor Skills* 72: 831-836.

Hayflick, L. (1985). Theories of biological aging. In R. Andres, E.L. Bierman, and W.R. Hazzard (Eds.), *Principles of geriatric medicine* (pp. 9-19). New York: McGraw-Hill.

Hazzard, W.R. (1985). The practice of geriatric medicine. In R. Andres, E.L. Bierman, and W.R. Hazzard (Eds.), *Principles of geriatric medicine* (pp. 3-5). New York: McGraw-Hill.

Hazzard, W.R., and Ettinger, W.H. (1995). Aging and atherosclerosis: Changing considerations in cardiovascular disease prevention as the barrier to immortality is approached in old age. *American Journal of Geriatric Cardiology* 4 (4): 16-36.

Health and Welfare, Canada. (1982). *The Canada Health Survey*. Ottawa, ON: Author.

Health and Welfare, Canada. (1985). *Canada's Health Promotion Survey*. Ottawa, ON: Author.

Health and Welfare, Canada. (1986). Economic burden of illness in Canada. *Chronic Diseases in Canada* 12 (3): Suppl.

Health and Welfare, Canada. (1989). *The active health report on seniors*. Ottawa: Author.

Health and Welfare, Canada. (1993). *Aging and independence: Overview of a national survey*. Ottawa, ON: Author.

Heaney, R.P. (1989). Osteoporotic fracture space: An hypothesis. *Bone and Mineral* 6: 1-13.

Heath, G.W., Hagberg, J.M., Ehsani, A.A., and Holloszy, J.O. (1981). A physiological comparison of young and older endurance athletes. *Journal of Applied Physiology* 51: 634-640.

Heath, G.W., Leonard, B.E., Wilson, R.H., Kendrick, J.S., and Powell, K.E. (1987). Community-based exercise intervention: Zuni diabetes project. *Diabetes Care* 10: 579-583.

Hefton, J.M., Darlington, G.J., Casazza, B.A., and Weksler, M.E. (1980). Immunological studies of aging 5. Impaired proliferation of PHA responsive human lymphocytes in culture. *Journal of Immunology* 125: 1007-1110.

Hegsted, D.M. (1989). Recommended dietary intakes for elderly subjects. *American Journal of Clinical Nutrition* 50 (Suppl.): 1190-1194.

Heifets, M., Davis, T.A., Tegtmeyer, E., and Klahr, S. (1987). Exercise training ameliorates progressive renal disease in rats with subtotal nephrectomy. *Kidney International* 32: 815-820.

Heikkinen, E., Suominen, H., Era, P., and Lyra, A-L. (1994). Variations in aging parameters, their sources, and possibilities of predicting physiological age. In A.K. Balin (Ed.), *Practical handbook of human biologic age determination* (pp. 71-92). Boca Raton, FL: CRC Press.

Heinonen, A., Oja, P., Sievänen, H., and Vuori, I. (1993). Effects of equivolume strength training programmes of low, medium and high resistance on maximal isometric strength in sedentary women. *Scandinavian Journal of Medicine, Science and Sports* 3: 104-109.

Heislein, D.M., Harris, B.A., and Jette, A. (1994). A strength training study for postmenopausal women: A pilot study. *Archives of Physical Medicine and Rehabilitation* 75: 198-204.

Heitmann, B.L. (1991). Body fat in the adult Danish population aged 35-65 years: An epidemiological study. *International Journal of Obesity* 15: 535-545.

Helderman, J.H., Vestal, R.E., Rowe, J.W., Tobin, J.D., Andres, R., and Robertson, G.L. (1978). The response of arginine vasopressin to intravenous ethanol and hyertonic saline in man: The impact on aging. *Journal of Gerontology* 33: 39-47.

Helfman, P.M., and Bada, J.L. (1976). Aspartic acid racemisation in dentine as a measure of ageing. *Nature* 262: 279-281.

Helmrich, S.P., Ragland, D.R., Leung, R.W., and Paffenbarger, R.S. (1991). Physical activity and reduced occurrence of non-insulin dependent diabetes mellitus. *New England Journal of Medicine* 325: 147-152.

Henkin, Y., Como, J., and Oberman, A. (1992). Secondary dyslipidemia. Inadvertent effects of drugs in clinical practice. *Journal of the American Medical Association* 267: 961-968.

Hernandez-Avila, M., Coldlitz, G.A., Stampfer, M.J., Rosner, B., Roberts, W.N., Hennekens, C.H., and Speizer, F.E. (1992). Caffeine, moderate alcohol intake, and risk of fracture of the hip and forearm in middle-aged women. *American Journal of Clinical Nutrition* 54: 157-163.

Hespel, P., Vergauwen, L., Vandenberghe, K., and Richter, E.A. (1995). Important role of insulin and flow in stimulating glucose uptake in contracting skeletal muscle. *Diabetes* 44: 210-215.

Heuser, I.J.E., Wark, H-J., Keul, J., and Holsboer, F. (1991). Hypothalamic-pituitary-adrenal axis function in elderly endurance athletes. *Journal of Clinical Endocrinology and Metabolism* 73: 485-488.

Hiatt, W.R., Regensteiner, J.G., Hargarten, M.E., Wolfel, E.E., and Brass, E.P. (1990). Benefit of exercise conditioning for patients with peripheral arterial disease. *Circulation* 81: 602-609.

Higginbotham, M.B., Morris, K.G., Williams, R.S., Coleman, R.E., and Cobb, F.R. (1986). Physiological basis for the age-related decline in aerobic work capacity. *American Journal of Cardiology* 57: 1374-1379.

Hill, R.D., Storandt, M., and Malley, M. (1993). The impact of long-term exercise training on psychological functioning in older adults. *Journals of Gerontology* 48: P12-P17.

Hlatky, M.A., Pryor, D.B., Harrell, F.E., Califf, R.M., Mark, D.B., and Rosati, R.A. (1984). Factors affecting sensitivity and specificity of exercise electrocardiography. *American Journal of Medicine* 77: 64-71.

Hodge, G. (1987). *The elderly in Canada's small towns*. Vancouver, BC: University of British Columbia, Centre for Human Settlements.

Hoffman-Goetz, L., and Husted, J. (1995). Exercise and cancer: Do the biology and the epidemiology correspond? *Exercise Immunology Review* 1: 81-96.

Hogan, J.C., Ogden, G.D., and Fleishman, E.A. (1978). Assessing physical requirements for establishing medical standards in selected benchmark jobs. Final Report (3012/R78-8). Washington, DC: Advanced Resources Organization.

Hogan, P.I., and Santomier, J.P. (1984). Effect of mastering swim skills on older adults' self-efficacy. *Research Quarterly* 55: 294-296.

Hoiseth, A., Alho, A., Husby, T., and Engh, V. (1991). Are patients with fractures of the femoral neck more osteoporotic? *European Journal of Radiology* 13: 2-5.

Hollenbach, K.A., Barrett-Connor, E., Edelstein, S.L., and Holbrook, T. (1993). Cigarette smoking and bone mineral density in older men and women. *American Journal of Public Health* 83: 1265-1270.

Hollingsworth, D.R., Hollingsworth, J.W., Bogitsch, S., and Keehn, R.J. (1969). Neuromuscular tests of ageing in Hiroshima subjects. *Journal of Gerontology* 24: 276-283.

Holloszy, J.O. (1993). Exercise increases average longevity of female rats despite increased food intake and no growth retardation. *Journals of Gerontology* 48: B97-B100.

Holloszy, J.O., and Schectman, K.B. (1991). Interaction between exercise and food restriction: Effects on longevity of male rats. *Journal of Applied Physiology* 70: 1529-1535.

Holubarsch, C., Goulette, R.P., Litten, R.Z., Martin, B.J., Mulieri, L.A., and Alpert, N.R. (1985). The economy of isometric force development, myosin isoenzyme pattern and myofibrillar ATPase activity in normal and hypothyroid rat myocardium. *Circulation Research* 56: 78-86.

Hombach, V., Höher, M., Höpp, H.W., Peper, A., Osterhues, H-H., Eggeling, T., Kochs, M., Weismüller, P., Welz, A., Hannekum, A., and Hilger, H.H. (1990). Was leistet die hochverstärkte Elektrokardiographie zur Identifikation von gefährdeten Patienten? [Value of high resolution electrocardiography in identification of patients at risk]. *Herz* 15: 28-41.

Hopkins, D.R., Murrah, B., Hoeger, W.W.K., and Rhodes, R.C. (1990). Effect of low impact aerobic dance on the functional fitness of elderly women. *Gerontologist* 30: 189-192.

Hopsu, L., and Louhevaara, V. (1993). The developmental work research and aging in cleaning work. In J. Ilmarinen (Ed.), *Aging and work* (pp. 166-169). Helsinki: Institute for Occupational Medicine.

Hornbrook, M.C., Stevens, V.J., Wingfield, D.J., Hollis, J.F., Greenlick, M.R., and Ory, M.G. (1994). Preventing falls among community-dwelling older persons: Results from a randomized trial. *Gerontologist* 34: 16-23.

Horne, J.A. (1988). *Why we sleep: The functions of sleep in humans and other mammals.* Oxford: Oxford University Press.

Horne, J.A., and Minard, A. (1985). Sleep and sleepiness following a behaviorally "active" day. *Ergonomics* 28: 567-575.

Horowitz, D.L. (1986). Nutrition, aging and diabetes. In E.A. Young (Ed.), *Nutrition, aging and health* (pp. 145-163). New York: Liss.

Horowitz, M., Maddern, G.J., Chatterton, B.E., Collins, P.J., Harding, P.E., and Shearman, D.J.C. (1984). Changes in gastric emptying rates with age. *Clinical Science* 67: 213-218.

Horowitz, M., Need, A.G., Morris, H.A., and Nordin, B.E.C. (1993). Osteoporosis in postmenopausal women. In H.M. Perry, J.E. Morley, and R.M. Coe (Eds.), *Aging and musculoskeletal disorders* (pp. 78-98). New York: Springer.

Horstmann, T., Mayer, F., Fischer, J., Maschmann, J., Röcker, K., and Dickhuth, H.H. (1994). The cardiocirculatory reaction to isokinetic exercises in dependence on the form of exercise and age. *International Journal of Sports Medicine* 15 (Suppl. 1): S50-S55.

Horton, E.S. (1991). Exercise and decreased risk of NIDDM [Editorial]. *New England Journal of Medicine* 325: 196-197.

Horvath, S.M., and Borgia, J.F. (1984). Cardiopulmonary gas transport and aging. *American Review of Respiratory Diseases* 129: 568-571.

Howe, M.L., Stones, M.J., and Brainerd, C.J. (1990). *Cognitive and behavioral performance in atypical aging.* New York: Springer.

Howze, E.H., Smith, M., and DiGilio, D.A. (1989). Factors affecting the adoption of exercise behavior among sedentary older adults. *Health Education Research* 4: 173-180.

Hoyer, W.J., and Plude, D.J. (1980). Attention and perceptual processes in the study of cognitive aging. In L.W. Poon (Ed.), *Aging in the 1980s: Psychological issues* (pp. 207-238). Washington, DC: American Psychological Association.

Hu, M-H., and Woollacott, M.H. (1994). Multisensory training of standing balance in older adults. I. Postural stability and one-leg stance balance. *Journals of Gerontology* 49: M52-M61.

Hubert, H.B., Feinleib, M., McNamara, P.M., and Castelli, W.P. (1983). Obesity as an independent risk factor for cardiovascular disease: A 26-year follow-up of participants in the Framingham Heart Study. *Circulation* 67: 968-977.

Hughes, V.A., and Meredith, C.N. (1989). Effects of aging, exercise and diet on glucose metabolism. In R. Harris and S. Harris (Eds.), *Physical activity, aging and sports* (pp. 259-270). Albany, NY: Center for Studies of Aging.

Hugonot, R., Dubos, G., and Mathes, G. (1978). Etude expérimentale des troubles de la soif chez le vieillard [Experimental study of thirst disturbances in the old person]. *Révue de Gériatrie* 4: 179-181.

Hui, S.L., Slemenda, C.W., and Johnston, C.C. (1989). Baseline measurement of bone mass predicts fracture in white women. *Annals of Internal Medicine* 111: 355-361.

Hunt, A. (1978). *The elderly at home.* London: Her Majesty's Stationery Office.

Hunt, S., McEwen, J., and McKenna, S. (1986). *Measuring health status.* London: Croom Helm.

Hutchins, E.B. (1994). Aging and the appraisal of health risks. In A.K. Balin (Ed.), *Practical handbook of human biologic age determination* (pp. 55-67). Boca Raton, FL: CRC Press.

Huuhtanen, P., and Piispa, M. (1993). Attitudes on work and retirement by occupation. In J. Ilmarinen (Ed.), *Aging and work* (pp. 152-156). Helsinki: Institute for Occupational Medicine.

Ilmarinen, J. (1988). Physiological criteria for retirement age. *Scandinavian Journal of Work, Environment & Health* 14 (Suppl. 1): 88-89.

Ilmarinen, J. (1989). Work and cardiovascular health: Viewpoint of occupational physiology. *Annals of Medicine* 21: 209-214.

Ilmarinen, J. (1991). The aging worker. *Scandinavian Journal of Work, Environment & Health* 17 (Suppl. 1): 1-141.

Ilmarinen, J. (1993). *Aging and work.* Helsinki: Institute of Occupational Health.

Institutional care and elderly people. (1993). *British Medical Journal* 306: 806-807.

International Labor Organization. (1977). *Labor force estimates and projections* (2nd ed.). Geneva: Author.

International Labor Organization. (1992). *The ILO and the elderly.* Geneva: Author.

Israel, S. (1992). Age-related changes in strength and special groups. In P. Komi (Ed.), *Strength and power in sport* (pp. 319-328). Oxford: Blackwell Scientific.

Iverson, B.D., Gossman, M.R., Shaddea, S.A., and Turner, M.E. (1990). Balance performance, force production, and activity levels in noninstitutionalized men 60 to 90 years of age. *Physical Therapy* 70: 348-355.

Ives, D., Bonino, P., Traven, N., and Kuller, L.H. (1993). Morbidity and mortality in rural community-dwelling elderly with low total serum cholesterol. *Journals of Gerontology* 48: M103-M107.

Jackson, A.S., Beard, E.F., Wier, L.T., Ross, R.M., Stuteville, J.E., and Blair, S.N. (1995). Changes in aerobic power of men ages 25-70 yr. *Medicine and Science in Sports and Exercise* 27: 113-120.

Jackson, J.A., Klecrekoper, M., Parfitt, A.M., Rao, D.S., Villanueva, A.R., and Frame, B. (1987). Bone histomorphometry in hypogonadal and eugonadal men with spinal osteoporosis. *Journal of Clinical Endocrinology and Metabolism* 65: 53-58.

Jackson, R. (1986). The Masters knee—past, present and future. In J.R. Sutton and R.M. Brock (Eds.), *Sports medicine for the mature athlete* (pp. 257-263). Indianapolis: Benchmark Press.

Jackson, R.A., and Finucane, P. (1991). Diabetes mellitus. In M.S.J. Pathy (Ed.), *Principles and practice of geriatric medicine* (pp. 1123-1143). Chichester: Wiley.

Jaglal, S.B., Kreger, N., and Darlington, G. (1993). Past and recent physical activity and risk of hip fracture. *American Journal of Epidemiology* 138: 107-118.

Jahng, J.S., Kang, K.S., Park, H.W., and Han, M.H. (1991). Assessment of bone mineral density in post-menopausal and senile osteoporosis using quantitative CT. *Orthopedics* 14: 1101-1105.

James, S.L., Bates, B.T., and Osternig, L.R. (1978). Injuries to runners. *American Journal of Sports Medicine* 6: 40-50.

Jarvik, L., Falek, A., Kallman, F.J., and Lorge, I. (1960). Survival trends in a senescent twin population. *American Journal of Human Genetics* 12: 170-179.

Jarvik, L.F., and Neshkes, R.E. (1985). Alterations in mental function with aging and disease. In R. Andres, E.L. Bierman, and W.R. Hazzard (Eds.), *Principles of geriatric medicine* (pp. 237-247). New York: McGraw-Hill.

Jee, W.S., Wronski, T.J., Morey, E.R., and Kimmel, D.B. (1983). Effects of spaceflight on trabecular bone in rats. *American Journal of Physiology* 244: R310-R314.

Jenkins, R.R. (1988). Free radical chemistry. Relationship to exercise. *Sports Medicine* 5: 156-170.

Jensen, E.W., Espersen, K., Kanstrup, I.L., and Christensen, N.J. (1992). Age-related changes of exercise-induced plasma catecholamines and neuropeptide Y responses in normal human subjects. *Acta Physiologica Scandinavica* 144: 129-133.

Jensen, E.W., Espersen, K., Kanstrup, I-L., and Christensen, N.J. (1994). Exercise-induced changes in plasma catecholamines and neuropeptide Y: Relation to age and sampling times. *Journal of Applied Physiology* 76: 1269-1273.

Jeppesen, B.B., and Harvald, B. (1985). Low incidence of urinary calculi in Greenland Eskimos explained by a low calcium/magnesium ratio. In R. Fortuine (Ed.), *Circumpolar health '84* (pp. 288-290). Seattle: University of Washington Press.

Jette, A.M., and Branch, L.G. (1981). The Framingham Disability Study: II. Physical ability among the aging. *American Journal of Public Health* 71: 1211-1216.

Jirovec, M.M. (1991). The impact of daily exercise on the mobility, balance and urine control of cognitively impaired nursing home residents. *International Journal of Nursing Studies* 28: 145-151.

Joffres, M.R., Hamet, P., Rabkin, S.W., Gelskey, D., Hogan, K., Fodor, G., and Canadian Heart Health Surveys Research Group. (1992). Prevalence, control and awareness of high blood pressure among Canadian adults. *Canadian Medical Association Journal* (Special Suppl., June 1, pp. 28-36).

Johansson, G., and Jarnio, G.B. (1991). Balance training in 70-year-old women. *Physiotherapy Theory and Practice* 7: 121-125.

Johnson, B.D., and Dempsey, J.A. (1991). Demand vs capacity in the aging pulmonary system. *Exercise and Sport Sciences Reviews* 19: 171-210.

Johnson, B.D., Reddan, W.G., Pegelow, D.F., Scow, K.C., and Dempsey, J.A. (1991). Flow limitation and regulation of functional residual volume in a physically active aging population. *American Review of Respiratory Diseases* 143: 960-967.

Johnson, B.D., Reddan, W.G., Scow, K.C., and Dempsey, J.A. (1991). Mechanical constraints on exercise hyperpnea in a fit aging population. *American Review of Respiratory Diseases* 143: 968-977.

Johnson, L.E. (1995). Vitamin malnutrition in the elderly. In J.E. Morley, Z. Glick, and L.Z. Rubenstein (Eds.), *Geriatric Nutrition* (2nd ed., pp. 79-105). New York: Raven Press.

Johnson, R.K., Goran, M.I., and Poehlman, E.T. (1994). Correlates of overreporting and underreporting of energy intake in healthy older men and women. *American Journal of Clinical Nutrition* 59: 1286-1290.

Jones, N.L. (1984). Dyspnea in exercise. *Medicine and Science in Sports and Exercise* 16: 14-19.

Jones, P.N. (1991). On collagen fibril diameter distributions. *Connective Tissue Research* 26: 11-21.

Joos, S.K., Mueller, W.H., Hanis, C.L., and Schull, W.J. (1984). Diabetes alert study: Weight history and upper body obesity in diabetic and non-diabetic Mexican-American adults. *Annals of Human Biology* 11: 167-171.

Jorgensen, L.G., Perko, G., and Secher, N.H. (1992). Regional cerebral artery mean flow velocity and blood flow during dynamic exercise in humans. *Journal of Applied Physiology* 73: 1825-1830.

Jose, A.D., and Collison, D.L. (1970). The normal range and determinants of the intrinsic heart rate in man. *Cardiovascular Research* 4: 160-167.

Judge, J.O., Lindsey, C., Underwood, M., and Winsemius, M. (1993). Balance improvements in older women: Effects of exercise and training. *Physical Therapy* 73: 254-265.

Judge, T.E. (1980). Potassium and magnesium. In A.N. Exton-Smith and F.I. Caird (Eds.), *Metabolic and nutritional disorders in the elderly* (pp. 39-44). Bristol: Wright.

Jugdutt, B.I., Mickorowski, B.L., and Kappadoga, C.T. (1988). Exercise training after anterior Q wave myocardial infarction: Importance of regional left ventricular function and topography. *Journal of the American College of Cardiology* 12: 362-372.

Kabisch, D., and Funk, S. (1991). Todesfälle im organisierten und angeleiten Sport. [Cases of death in organized and unorganized sport]. *Deutsche Zeitschrift für Sportmedizin* 42: 464-468.

Kalache, A. (1991). Ageing in developing countries. In M.S.J. Pathy (Ed.), *Principles and practice of geriatric medicine* (2nd ed., pp. 1517-1528). Chichester: Wiley.

Kallinen, M., and Alén, M. (1994). Sports-related injuries in elderly men still active in sports. *British Journal of Sports Medicine* 28: 52-55.

Kallinen, M., and Markku, A. (1995). Aging, physical activity and sports injuries: An overview of common sports injuries in the elderly. *Sports Medicine* 20: 41-52.

Kallman, D.A., Plato, C.C., and Tobin, J.D. (1990). The role of muscle loss in age-related decline of grip strength: Cross-sectional and longitudinal perspectives. *Journal of Gerontology* 45: M82-M88.

Kallman, D.A., Wigley, F.M., Scott, W.W., Hochberg, M.C., and Tobin, J.D. (1989). New radiographic grading scales for osteoarthritis of the hand: Reliability for determining prevalence and progression. *Arthritis and Rheumatism* 32: 1584-1591.

Kallman, F.G., and Sander G. (1948). Twin studies on ageing and longevity. *Journal of Heredity* 39: 349-357.

Kanis, J.A., Johnell, O., Gullberg, B., Allander, E., Dilsen, G., Gennari, C., Vaz, A.A.L., Lyritis, G.P., Mazzuoli, G., Miravet, L., Passeri, M., Cano, R.P., Rapado, A., and Ribot, C. (1992). Evidence for efficacy of drugs affecting bone metabolism in preventing hip fracture. *British Medical Journal* 305: 1124-1128.

Kannel, W.B. (1980). Host and environmental determinants of hypertension. Perspective from the Framingham Study. In H. Kesteloot and J. Joossens (Eds.), *Epidemiology of high blood pressure* (pp. 265-295). The Hague: Martinus Nijhoff.

Kannel, W.B. (1994). Rationale for treatment of hypertension in the elderly. *American Journal of Geriatric Cardiology* 3: 33-45.

Kannel, W.B., and Agostino, R.B. (1995). The importance of cardiovascular risk factors in the elderly. *American Journal of Geriatric Cardiology* 4 (2): 10-23.

Kannel, W.B., and Brand, F.N. (1985). Cardiovascular risk factors in the elderly. In R. Andres, E.L. Bierman, and W.R. Hazzard (Eds.), *Principles of geriatric medicine* (pp. 104-119). New York: McGraw-Hill.

Kannel, W.B., Gagnon, D.R., and Cupples, L.A. (1990). Epidemiology of sudden coronary death: Population at risk. *Canadian Journal of Cardiology* 6: 439-444.

Kannel, W.B., and Gordon, T. (1978). Evaluation of cardiovascular risk in the elderly: The Framingham Study. *Bulletin of the New York Academy of Medicine* 54: 573-591.

Kannel, W.B., Plehn, J.F., and Cupples, L.A. (1988). Cardiac failure and sudden death in the Framingham Study. *American Heart Journal* 115: 869-875.

Kannel, W.B., Skinner, J.J., Schwartz, M.J., and Shurtleff, D. (1970). Intermittent claudication incidence in the Framingham Study. *Circulation* 41: 875-883.

Kannus, P., and Józsa, L. (1991). Histopathological changes preceding spontaneous rupture of a tendon: A controlled study of 891 patients. *Journal of Bone and Joint Surgery* 73A: 1507-1525.

Kaplan, G.A., Seeman, T.E., Cohen, R.D., Knudsen, L.P., and Guralnik, J. (1987). Mortality among the elderly in the Alameda County study: Behavioral and demographic risk factors. *American Journal of Public Health* 77: 307-312.

Kaplan, R.M. (1985). Quantification of health outcomes for policy studies in behavioral epidemiology. In R.M. Kaplan and M. Criqui (Eds.), *Behavioral epidemiology and disease prevention* (pp. 31-54). New York: Plenum Press.

Kaplan, R.M., Feeny, D.A., and Revicki, D.A. (1993). Methods for assessing relative importance in preference based outcome measures. *Quality of Life Research* 2: 467-475.

Karlsson, M.K., Johnell, O., and Obrant, K.J. (1993). Bone mineral density in weightlifters. *Calcified Tissue International* 52: 212-215.

Kasch, F.W., Boyer, J.L., Van Camp, S.P., Verity, L.S., and Wallace, J.P. (1990). The effect of physical activity and inactivity on aerobic power in older men (a longitudinal study). *Physician and Sportsmedicine* 18 (4): 73-83.

Kasch, F.W., Boyer, J.L., Van Camp, S.P., Verity, L.S., and Wallace, J.P. (1993). Effect of exercise on cardiovascular ageing. *Age and Ageing* 22: 5-10.

Kasch, F.W., Wallace, J.P., Van Camp, S.P., and Verity, L. (1988). A longitudinal study of cardiovascular stability in active men aged 45 to 65 years. *Physican and Sportsmedicine* 16 (1): 117-125.

Kasperczyk, W.J., Rosocha, S., Bosch, U., Oestem, H.J., and Tscheme, U. (1991). Alter, Aktivität und die Belastbarkeit von Kniebanden [Age, activity and elasticity of knee tendons]. *Umfallchirurgie* 94: 372-375.

Kasperk, C.H., Wergedal, J.E., Farley, J.R., Linkhart, T.A., Turner, R.T., and Baylick, D.J. (1989). Androgens directly stimulate proliferation of bone cells in vitro. *Endocrinology* 124: 1576-1578.

Kastello, G.M., Sothman, M.S., and Murthy, V.S. (1993). Young and old subjects matched for aerobic capacity have similar noradrenergic responses to exercise. *Journal of Applied Physiology* 74: 49-54.

Katch, V.L., Becque, M.D., Rocchini, A.B., and Allen, W. (1984). The energy cost of walking for obese and non-obese adolescents [Abstract]. *Medicine and Science in Sports and Exercise* 16: 135.

Kauffman, T.L. (1985). Strength training effect in young and aged women. *Archives of Physical Medicine and Rehabilitation* 65: 223-226.

Kavanagh, T. (1983). Exercise in cold. *Journal of Cardiac Rehabilitation* 3: 70-73.

Kavanagh, T. (1989). Does exercise training improve coronary collateralization? A new look at an old belief. *Physician and Sportsmedicine* 17 (1): 96-114.

Kavanagh, T., Lindley, L.J., Shephard, R.J., and Campbell, R. (1988). Health and sociodemographic characteristics of the Masters competitor. *Annals of Sports Medicine* 4: 55-64.

Kavanagh, T., Mertens, D.J., Matosevic, V., Shephard, R.J., and Evans, B. (1989). Health and aging of Masters athletes. *Clinical Sports Medicine* 1: 72-88.

Kavanagh, T., Myers, M.G., Baigrie, R.S., Mertens, D.J., and Shephard, R.J. (1996). Quality of life and cardiorespiratory function in congestive heart failure: Effects of 12 months of aerobic training. *Heart* 76: 42-49.

Kavanagh, T., Pandit, V., and Shephard, R.J. (1973). The application of exercise testing to the elderly amputee. *Canadian Medical Association Journal* 108: 314-317.

Kavanagh, T., and Shephard, R.J. (1977). The effects of continued training on the aging process. *Annals of the New York Academy of Sciences* 301: 656-670.

Kavanagh, T., Shephard, R.J., Doney, H., and Pandit, V. (1973). Intensive exercise in coronary rehabilitation. *Medicine and Science in Sports and Exercise* 5: 34-39.

Kavanagh, T., Shephard, R.J., Lindley, L.J., and Pieper, M. (1983). Influence of exercise and lifestyle variables upon high density lipoprotein cholesterol after myocardial infarction. *Arteriosclerosis* 3: 249-259.

Kawashima, T., and Uhthoff, H.K. (1991). Pattern of bone loss of the proximal femur: A radiologic, densitometric and histomorphometric study. *Journal of Orthopedic Research* 9: 634-640.

Kaye, S.A., Folsom, A.R., Prineas, R.J., Potter, J.D., and Gapstur, S.M. (1990). The association of body fat distribution with lifestyle and reproductive factors in a population study of premenopausal women. *International Journal of Obesity* 14: 583-591.

Kaye, S.A., Folsom, A.R., Sprafka, J.M., Prineas, R.J., and Wallace, R.B. (1991). Increased incidence of diabetes mellitus in relation to abdominal adiposity in older women. *Journal of Clinical Epidemiology* 44: 329-334.

Kayman, S., Bruvold, W., and Stern, J.S. (1990). Maintenance and relapse after weight loss in women: Behavioral aspects. *American Journal of Clinical Nutrition* 52: 800-807.

Keen, J., Jarrett, R.J., and McCartney, P. (1982). The ten year follow-up of the Bedford survey (1962-72). Glucose tolerance and diabetes. *Diabetologia* 22: 73-78.

Keene, G.S., Parker, M.J., and Prtor, G.A. (1993). Mortality and morbidity after hip fractures. *British Medical Journal* 307: 1248-1250.

Keesey, R.E. (1992). Exercise as a modifier of body weight set-point. In V.A. Hubbard (Ed.), *NIH Workshop on Physical Activity and Obesity* (pp. 70-74). Washington, DC: National Institutes of Health.

Keh-Evans, L., Rice, C.L., Noble, E.G., Paterson, D.H., Cunningham, D.A., and Taylor, A.W. (1992). Comparison of histochemical, biochemical and contractile properties of triceps surae of trained aged subjects. *Canadian Journal on Aging* 11: 412-425.

Keller, H.H. (1995). Weight gain impact morbidity and mortality in institutionalized older persons. *Journal of the American Geriatric Society* 43: 165-169.

Kelly, J., and O'Malley, K. (1984). Adrenoceptor function and aging. *Clinical Science* 66: 509-515.

Kelly, J.R., Steinkamp, M.W., and Kelly, J.R. (1987). Later-life satisfaction: Does leisure contribute? *Leisure Sciences* 9: 189-200.

Kelly, P.J., Eisman, J.A., Stuart, M.C., Pocock, N.A., Sambrook, P.I., and Gwinn, T.H. (1990). Somatomedin-C, physical fitness and bone density. *Journal of Clinical Endocrinology and Metabolism* 70: 718-723.

Kempeneers, G.L.G., Noakes, T.D., van Zyl Smit, R., Myburgh, K.H., Lambert, M., and Wiggins, T. (1990). Skeletal muscle limits the exercise tolerance of renal transplant recipients: Effects of a graded exercise training programme. *American Journal of Kidney Diseases* 16: 57-65.

Kennedy, R.D., Andrews, G.R., and Caird, F.I. (1977). Ischaemic heart disease in the elderly. *British Heart Journal* 39: 1121-1127.

Kenney, R.A. (1982). *Physiology of aging. A synopsis*. Chicago: Yearbook, 1982.

Kenney, W.L. (1995). Body fluid and temperature regulation as a function of age. In D.R. Lamb, C.V. Gisolfi, and E. Nadel (Eds.), *Exercise in older adults* (pp. 305-351). Carmel, IN: Cooper.

Kenney, W.L., and Zappe, D.H. (1994). Effect of age on renal blood flow during exercise. *Aging, Clinical and Experimental Research* 6: 293-302.

Kenyon, G.M. (1991). Homo viator: Metaphors of aging, authenticity and meaning. In G.M. Kenyon, J.E. Birren, and J.J.F. Schroots (Eds.), *Metaphors of aging in science and the humanities* (pp. 17-36). New York: Springer.

Kenyon, G.M., Birren, J.E., and Schroots, J.J.F. (1991). *Metaphors of aging in science and the humanities*. New York: Springer.

Kesteloot, H. (1991). Life expectancy and nutrition: The epidemiological evidence. In M.S.J. Pathy (Ed.), *Principles and practice of geriatric medicine* (2nd ed., pp. 165-178). Chichester: Wiley.

Keys, A. (1980). *Seven countries: A multivariate analysis of death and coronary heart disease*. Cambridge, MA: Harvard University Press.

Kiebzak, G.M. (1991). Age-related bone changes. *Experimental Gerontology* 26: 171-187.

Kilbom, Å., Baltzari, L., Ilmarinen, J., Nygard, C-H., Nörregaard, C., Solem, P.E., and Westerholm, P. (1993). Aging and retirement: An international comparison. In J. Ilmarinen (Ed.), *Aging and work* (pp. 54-62). Helsinki: Institute for Occupational Health.

Killian, K.J. (1987). Limitation of exercise by dyspnea. *Canadian Journal of Sport Sciences* 12 (Suppl. 1): 53S-60S.

Killian, K.J. (1995). Exercise-induced bronchial obstruction. In J. Torg and R.J. Shephard (Eds.), *Current therapy in sports medicine* (3rd ed., pp. 676-678). Philadelphia: Mosby-Yearbook.

Killian, K.J., and Jones, N.L. (1988). Respiratory muscles and dyspnea. *Clinics in Chest Medicine* 9: 237-248.

King, A.C., Taylor, C.B., and Haskell, W.L. (1993). Effects of differing intensities and formats of 12 months of exercise training on psychological outcomes in older adults. *Health Psychology* 12: 292-300 and erratum, 405.

Kinnunen, U., Rasku, A., and Parkatti, T. (1993). Aging in the teaching profession: Work, well-being and health among aging teachers. In J. Ilmarinen (Ed.), *Aging and work* (pp. 157-161). Helsinki: Institute for Occupational Health.

Kinsella, K.G. (1992). Changes in life expectancy. *American Journal of Clinical Nutrition* 55: 1196S-1202S.

Kirkwood, T.B.L. (1992). Comparative life spans of species: Why do specimens have the life spans they do? *American Journal of Clinical Nutrition* 55: 1191S-1195S.

Kirsteins, A.E., Dietz, F., and Hwang, S-M. (1991). Evaluating the safety and potential use of a weight-bearing exercise, tai-chi chuan, for rheumatoid arthritis patients. *American Journal of Physical Medicine and Rehabilitation* 70: 136-141.

Kirwan, J.P., Kohrt, W.M., Wojta, D.M., Bourey, R.E., and Holloszy, J.O. (1993). Endurance exercise training reduces glucose-stimulated insulin levels in 60- to 70- year-old men and women. *Journals of Gerontology* 48: M84-M90.

Kissebah, A.H., Vydelingum, N., Murray, R., Evans, D.J., Hartz, A.J., Kalkhoff, R.K., and Adams, P.W. (1982). Relation of body fat distribution to metabolic complications of obesity. *Journal of Clinical Endocrinology and Metabolism* 54: 254-260.

Kitzman, D.W., Higginbotham, M.B., and Sullivan, M.J. (1993). Aging and the cardiovascular response to exercise. *Current Science* 1: 543-550.

Klag, M.J., Whelton, P.K., and Appel, L.J. (1990). Effect of age on the efficacy of blood pressure treatment strategies. *Hypertension* 26: 700-705.

Klein, C., Cunningham, D.A., Paterson, D.H., and Taylor, H.W. (1988). Fatigue and recovery contractile properties of young and elderly men. *European Journal of Applied Physiology* 57: 684-690.

Klitgaard, H., Ausoni, S., and Damiani, E. (1989). Sarcoplasmic reticulum of human skeletal muscle: Age-related changes and effects of training. *Acta Physiologica Scandinavica* 137: 23-31.

Klitgaard, H., Mantoni, M., Schiaffino, S., Ausoni, S., Gorza, L., Laurent-Winter, C., Schnohr, P., and Saltin, B. (1990). Function, morphology and protein expression of ageing skeletal muscle: A cross-sectional study of elderly men with different training backgrounds. *Acta Medica Scandinavica* 104: 41-54.

Knudson, R.J., Lebowitz, M.D., Holberg, C.J., and Burrows, B. (1983). Changes in the normal maximal expiratory flow volume curve with growth and ageing. *American Review of Respiratory Diseases* 127: 725-734.

Kohl, H.W., Laporte, R., and Blair, S.N. (1988). Physical activity and cancer: An epidemiological perspective. *Sports Medicine* 6: 222-237.

Kohl, H.W., and McKenzie, J.D. (1994). Physical activity, fitness and stroke. In C. Bouchard, R.J. Shephard, and T. Stephens (Eds.), *Physical activity, fitness and health* (pp. 609-621). Champaign, IL: Human Kinetics.

Kohl, H.W., Moorefield, D.L., and Blair, S.N. (1987). Is cardiorespiratory fitness associated with general chronic fatigue in apparently healthy men and women? [Abstract]. *Medicine and Science in Sports and Exercise* 19: S56.

Kohrs, M.B., and Czajka-Narins, D.M. (1986). Assessing the nutritional status of the elderly. In E.A. Young (Ed.), *Nutrition, aging and health* (pp. 25-59). New York: Liss.

Kohrt, W.M., Malley, M.T., Coggan, A.R., Spina, R.J., Ogawa, T., Ehsani, A.A., Bourey, R.E., Martin, W.H., and Holloszy, J.O. (1991). Effects of gender, age and fitness level on response of VO_2max to training in 60-71 yr olds. *Journal of Applied Physiology* 71: 2004-2011.

Kohrt, W.M., Malley, M.T., Dalsky, G.P., and Holloszy, J.O. (1992). Body composition of healthy sedentary and trained young and older men and women. *Medicine and Science in Sports and Exercise* 24: 832-837.

Kohrt, W.M., Obert, K.A., and Holloszy, J.O. (1992). Exercise training improves fat distribution patterns in 60- to 70-year-old men and women. *Journals of Gerontology* 47: M99-M105.

Kohrt, W.M., and Snead, D.B. (1993). Effect of exercise on bone mass in the elderly. In H.M. Perry, J.E. Morley, and R.M. Coe (Eds.), *Aging and muscle disorders* (pp. 214-227). New York: Springer.

Kohrt, W.M., Spina, R.J., Ehsani, A.A., Cryer, P.E., and Holloszy, J.O. (1993). Effects of age, adiposity, and fitness level on plasma catecholamine responses to standing and exercise. *Journal of Applied Physiology* 75: 1828-1835.

Koller, W.C., Glatt, S.L., and Fox, J.H. (1985). Senile gait (a distinct neurologic entity). *Clinics in Geriatric Medicine* 1: 661-669.

Korenchevsky, V. (1961). In G.H Bourne (Ed.), *Physiological and pathological ageing* (pp. 40-44, 311-315). New York: Hafner.

Kostis, J.B., Moreya, A.E., Amends, M.T., DiPietro, J., Cosgrove, N., and Kuo, P.T. (1986). The effect of age on heart rate in subjects free of heart disease. *Circulation* 65: 141-145.

Kovanen, V. (1989). Effects of ageing and physical training on rat skeletal muscle. *Acta Physiologica Scandinavica* 135 (Suppl. 557): 1-56.

Kovar, M.G., and LaCroix, A.Z. (1987). Aging in the eighties: Ability to perform work-related activities. Data from the supplement on aging to the National Health Interview Survey, United States, 1984. *Advance Data from Vital and Health Statistics*, No. 136 (DHHS Publication No. PHS 87-1250). Hyattsville, MD: Department of Health and Human Services.

Kovar, P.A., Allegrante, J.P., MacKenzie, C.R., Peterson, M.G.E., Gutin, B., and Charlson, M.E. (1992). Supervised fitness walking in patients with osteoarthritis of the knee: A randomized, controlled trial. *Annals of Internal Medicine* 116: 529-534.

Kral, L.P., and Besser, R.S. (1989). *Joslin diabetes manual* (12th ed.). Philadelphia: Lea & Febiger.

Krall, E.A., and Dawson-Hughes, B. (1994). Walking is related to bone density and rates of bone loss. *American Journal of Medicine* 96: 20-26.

Kriska, A.M., Blair, S.N., and Pereira, M.A. (1994). The potential role of physical activity in the prevention of non-insulin dependent diabetes mellitus: The epidemiological evidence. *Exercise and Sport Sciences Reviews* 22: 121-143.

Krølner, B., and Toft, B. (1983). Vertebral bone loss: An unheeded side effect of therapeutic bed rest. *Clinical Science* 64: 537-540.

Krølner, B., Toft, B., Nielsen, S.P., and Tondevold, E. (1983). Physical exercise as prophylaxis against involutional vertebral bone loss: A controlled trial. *Clinical Science* 64: 541-546.

Kronmal, R., Cain, K., Ye, Z., and Omenn, G.S. (1993). Total serum cholesterol levels and mortality risk as a function of age. *Archives of Internal Medicine* 153: 1065-1073.

Krumholz, H.M., Seeman, T.E., Merrill, S.S., de Leon, C.F.M., Vaccarino, V., Silverman, D.I., Isukahara, R., Ostfeld, A.M., and Berkman, L.F. (1994). Lack of association between cholesterol and coronary heart disease mortality and morbidity and all-cause mortality in persons older than 70 years. *Journal of the American Medical Association* 272: 1335-1340.

Kuczmarski, R.J., Flegel, K.M., Campbell, S.M., and Johnson, C.L. (1994). Increasing prevalence of overweight among U.S. adults. The National Health & Nutrition Examination Surveys, 1960 to 1991. *Journal of the American Medical Association* 272: 205-211.

Kujala, U.M., Kaprio, J., and Sarna, S. (1994). Osteoarthritis of weight-bearing joints of lower limbs in former elite male athletes. *British Medical Journal* 308: 231-234.

Kukkonen, K., Rauramaa, R., Voutilainen, E., and Lansimies, E. (1982). Physical training of middle-aged men with borderline hypertension. *Annals of Clinical Research* 14 (Suppl. 34): 139-145.

Kunkel, S.R., and Applebaum, R.A. (1992). Estimating the prevalence of long-term disability for an aging society. *Journals of Gerontology* 47: S253-S260.

LaCroix, A.Z., Guralnik, J.M., Berkman, L.F., Wallace, R.B., and Satterfield, S. (1993). Maintaining mobility in later life. II. Smoking, alcohol consumption, physical activity, and body mass index. *American Journal of Epidemiology* 137: 858-869.

LaForest, S., St-Pierre, D.M.M., Cyr, J., and Gayton, D. (1990). Effects of age and regular exercise on muscle strength and endurance. *European Journal of Applied Physiology* 60: 104-111.

Lakatta, E.G. (1987). Cardiac muscle changes in senescence. *Annual Reviews of Physiology* 49: 519-531.

Lakatta, E.G. (1993a). Cardiovascular regulatory mechanisms in advanced age. *Physiological Reviews* 73: 413-467.

Lakatta, E.G. (1993b). Deficient neuro-endocrine regulation of the cardiovascular system with advancing age in healthy humans. *Circulation* 87: 631-636.

Lambert, M., and Didier, J.P. (1979). Bioénergétique de la marche chez l'artéritique amputé de membre inférieur, appareillé depuis moins d'un ans [Bioenergetics of walking in atherosclerosis of the lower limb, fitted with a prosthesis for less than one month]. *Annales de Médecine Physique* 22: 235-249.

Lampman, R.M., and Schteingart, D.E. (1991). Effects of exercise training on glucose control, lipid metabolism, and insulin sensitivity in hypertriglyceridemia and non-insulin dependent diabetes mellitus. *Medicine and Science in Sports and Exercise* 23: 703-712.

Landers, D.M., and Petruzello, S.J. (1994). Physical activity, fitness and anxiety. In C. Bouchard, R.J. Shephard, and T. Stephens (Eds.), *Physical activity, fitness and health* (pp. 868-882). Champaign, IL: Human Kinetics.

Landfield, P.W. (1987). Modulation of brain aging correlates by long-term alterations of adrenal steroids and neurally-active peptides. In E.R. de Klolt, V.N. Wiegart, and D. de Wied (Eds.), *Progress in brain research* 72. Amsterdam: Elsevier.

Landfield, P.W., Pitler, T.A., and Applegate, M.D. (1986). The effects of high Mg^{2+}/Ca^{2+} ratios on frequency potentiation in hippocampal slices of young and aged rats. *Journal of Neurophysiology* 56: 797-811.

Lane, N.E., Bloch, D.A., Jones, H., Marshall, W.H., Wood, P.D., and Fries, J.J. (1986). Long-distance running, bone density and osteoarthritis. *Journal of the American Medical Association* 255: 1147-1151.

Lane, N.E., Bloch, D.A., Wood, P.D., and Fries, J.J. (1987). Aging, long-distance running and the development of musculoskeletal disability. *American Journal of Medicine* 82: 772-780.

Lane, N., Micheli, B., Bjorkengren, A., Oehlert, J., Shi, H., Bloch, D., and Fries, J. (1993). The risk of osteoarthritis with running and aging: A 5-year longitudinal study. *Journal of Rheumatology* 20: 461-468.

Langer, R.D., Klauber, M.R., Criqui, M.H., and Barrett-Connor, E. (1994). Exercise and survival in the very old. *American Journal of Geriatric Cardiology* 3 (4): 24-34.

Lanyon, L.E. (1984). Functional strain as a determinant for bone remodelling. *Calcified Tissue International* 36: S56-S61.

LaPlante, M.P. (1988). *Data on disability from the National Health Interview Survey 1983-1985.* Washington, DC: National Institute on Disability and Rehabilitation Research.

Larsson, B., Svärdsudd, K., Welin, L., Wilhelmsen, L., Bjorntorp, P., and Tibblin, G. (1984). Abdominal adipose tissue distribution, obesity, and the risk of cardiovascular disease and death: 13-year follow-up of participants in the study of men born in 1913. *British Medical Journal* 288: 1401-1404.

Lau, E.M., Woo, J., Leung, P.C., Swaminathan, R., and Leung, D. (1992). The effects of calcium supplementation and exercise on bone density in elderly Chinese women. *Osteoporosis International* 2: 168-173.

Launer, L.J., Harris, T., Rumpel, C., and Madans, J. (1994). Body mass index, weight change and risk of mobility disability in middle-aged and older women. *Journal of the American Medical Association* 271: 1093-1098.

Lavie, C.J., and Milani, R.V. (1994). Patients with high baseline exercise capacity benefit from cardiac rehabilitation and exercise training programs. *American Heart Journal* 128: 1105-1109.

Lavie, C.J., Milani, R.V., and Littman, A.B. (1993). Benefits of cardiac rehabilitation and exercise training in secondary coronary prevention in the elderly. *Journal of the American College of Cardiology* 22: 678-683.

Lavis, V.R. (1981). Psychiatric manifestations of endocrine disease in the elderly. In A.J. Levenson and R.C. Hall (Eds.), *Neuropsychiatric manifestations of physical disease in the elderly*. New York: Raven Press.

Lawrence, R.C., Hochberg, M.C., Kelsey, J.L., McDuffie, F.C., Medsger, T.A., Felts, W.R., and Shielman, L.E. (1989). Estimates of the prevalence of selected arthritic and musculoskeletal disease in the United States. *Journal of Rheumatology* 16: 427-441.

Leach, R.E., Baumgard, S., and Broom, J. (1985). Obesity: Its relationship to OA of the knee. *Clinics in Rheumatic Diseases* 11: 203-238.

Leaf, A. (1985). Long-lived populations (extreme old age). In R. Andres, E.L. Bierman, and W.R. Hazzard (Eds.), *Principles of geriatric medicine* (pp. 82-86). New York: McGraw-Hill.

Lean, M.E.J., Han, T.S., and Morrison, C.E. (1995). Waist circumference as a measure for indicating need for weight management. *British Medical Journal* 311: 158-161.

Lee, I-M. (1994). Physical activity, fitness and cancer. In C. Bouchard, R.J. Shephard, and T. Stephens (Eds.), *Physical activity, fitness and health* (pp. 814-831). Champaign, IL: Human Kinetics.

Lee, I-M., and Paffenbarger, R.S. (1992). Changes in body weight and longevity. *Journal of the American Medical Association* 268: 2045-2049.

Lee, I-M., Paffenbarger, R.S., and Hsieh, C.C. (1992a). Physical activity and risk of prostatic cancer among college alumni. *American Journal of Epidemiology* 135: 169-179.

Lee, I-M., Paffenbarger, R.S., and Hsieh, C.C. (1992b). Time trends in physical activity among college alumni. *American Journal of Epidemiology* 135: 915-925.

Lee, J.R. (1991). Is natural progesterone the missing link in osteoporosis prevention and treatment? *Medical Hypotheses* 35: 316-318.

Legros, J.J., and Brunier, J. (1982). Vieillissement des systèmes de contrôle: Les glandes endocrines [Aging of control systems: The endocrine glands]. In F. Bourlière (Ed.), *Gérontologie: Biologie et clinique* (pp. 63-80). Paris: Flammarion.

Lehman, H.C. (1951). Chronological age vs. proficiency in physical skills. *American Journal of Physiology* 44: 161-187.

Lehman, M., and Keul, J. (1986). Age-associated changes of exercise-induced plasma catecholamine responses. *European Journal of Applied Physiology* 55: 302-306.

Leino, P., and Hänninen, K. (1993). Factors associated with decreased perceived ability in healthy lumberjacks and building construction workers. In J. Ilmarinen (Ed.), *Aging and work* (pp. 108-112). Helsinki: Institute for Occupational Health.

LeMarchand, L., Kolonel, L.N., and Yoshizawa, C.N. (1991). Lifetime occupational physical activity and prostate cancer risk. *American Journal of Epidemiology* 133: 103-111.

Lennon, D., Nagle, F., Stratrame, F., Shargo, E., and Dennis, S. (1985). Diet and exercise training effect on resting metabolic rate. *International Journal of Obesity* 9: 34-47.

Lennox, S.S., Bedell, J.R., and Stone, A.A. (1990). The effects of exercise on normal mood. *Journal of Psychosomatic Medicine* 34: 629-636.

Leon, A.S. (1987). Age and other predictors of coronary heart disease. *Medicine and Science in Sports and Exercise* 19: 159-167.

Leon, A.S. (1989). The role of physical activity in the prevention and management of obesity. In A.J. Ryan and F.L. Allman (Eds.), *Sports medicine* (2nd ed., pp. 593-618). New York: Academic Press.

Leon, A.S. (1992). The role of exercise in the prevention and management of diabetes mellitus and blood lipid disorders. In R.J. Shephard and H. Miller (Eds.), *Exercise and the heart in health and disease* (pp. 299-368). New York: Marcel Dekker.

Leon, A.S., Connett, J., Jacobs, D.R., and Rauraama, R. (1987). Leisure-time physical activity and risk of coronary heart disease and death. The Multiple Risk Factor Intervention Trial. *Journal of the American Medical Association* 258: 2388-2395.

Lerner, D.J., and Kannel, W.B. (1986). Patterns of coronary heart disease morbidity and mortality in the sexes: A 26-year follow-up of the Framingham population. *American Heart Journal* 111: 383-390.

Levi, F., LaVecchia, C., Negri, E., and Franceschi, S. (1993). Selected physical activities and risk of endometrial cancer. *British Journal of Cancer* 67: 846-851.

Levy, W.C., Cerquiera, M.D., Abrass, I.B., Schwartz, R.S., and Stratton, J.R. (1993). Endurance exercise training augments diastolic filling at rest and during exercise in healthy young and older men. *Circulation* 88: 116-126.

Lewin, T., Jurgens, H., Louekari, L. (1970). Secular trend in the adult height of Skolt Lapps. *Arctic Anthropology* 7: 53-62.

Lewis, D.S., Rollwitz, W.L., Bertrand, H.A., and Masoro, E.J. (1986). Use of NMR for measurement of total body water and estimation of body fat. *Journal of Applied Physiology* 60: 836-840.

Lexell, J. (1993). Ageing and human muscle: Observations from Sweden. *Canadian Journal of Applied Physiology* 18: 2-18.

Lexell, J., Henriksson-Larsson, K., and Sjöstrom, M. (1983). Distribution of different fiber types in human skeletal muscles. 2. A cross-sectional study of whole m. vastus lateralis. *Acta Physiologica Scandinavica* 117: 115-122.

Lexell, J., Taylor, C.C., and Sjöstrom, M. (1988). What is the cause of the ageing atrophy? Total number, size and proportion of different fibre types studied in whole vastus lateralis muscle from 15 to 83 year old men. *Journal of Neurological Science* 84: 275-294.

Lie, J.T., and Hammond, P.I. (1988). Pathology of the senescent heart: Anatomic observations on 237 autopsy studies of patients 90 to 105 years old. *Proceedings of the Mayo Clinic* 63: 552-564.

Liemohn, W.P. (1975). Strength and aging: An exploratory study. *International Journal of Aging and Human Development* 6: 347-357.

Lindheim, S.R., Notelovitz, M., Feldman, E.B., Larsen, S., Khan, F.Y., and Lobo, R.A. (1994). The independent effects of exercise and estrogen on lipids and lipoproteins in postmenopausal women. *Obstetrics and Gynecology* 83: 167-172.

Lindpaintner, K. (1995). Clinical implications of basic research. Finding an obesity gene—a tale of mice and men. *New England Journal of Medicine* 332: 679-680.

Linn, B.S. (1975). Chronologic versus biologic age in geriatric patients. In R. Goldman and M. Rockstein (Eds.), *The physiology and pathology of human aging* (pp. 9-18). New York: Academic Press.

Linos, A., Worthington, J.W., Palumbo, P.J., O'Fallon, W.M., and Kurland, L.T. (1980). The epidemiology of rheumatoid arthritis in Rochester, Minnesota. A study of incidence, prevalence and mortality. *American Journal of Epidemiology* 111: 87-98.

Linsted, K.D., Tonstad, K., and Kuzma, J. (1991). Self-report of physical activity and patterns of mortality in Seventh-Day Adventist men. *Journal of Clinical Epidemiology* 44: 355-364.

Lipschitz, D.A. (1994). Anemia. In W.R. Hazzard, E.L. Bierman, J.P. Blass, W.H. Ettinger, and J.B. Halter (Eds.), *Principles of geriatric medicine and gerontology* (3rd ed., pp. 741-747). New York: McGraw-Hill.

Lipsitz, L.A. (1989). Orthostatic hypotension in the elderly. *New England Journal of Medicine* 321: 952-957.

Livesley, B. (1992). Reducing home accidents in elderly people [Editorial]. *British Medical Journal* 305: 2-3.

Logan, M., Rubal, B., Raven, P., English, W., and Walters, N. (1981). Heart structure and function of females with multiple sclerosis: A deconditioned population [Abstract]. *Medicine and Science in Sports and Exercise* 13: 133.

Lokey, E.A., and Tran, Z.V. (1989). Effects of exercise training on serum lipid and lipoprotein concentrations in women: A meta-analysis. *International Journal of Sports Medicine* 10: 424-429.

Long, B.C. (1985). Stress-management interventions: A 15-month follow-up of aerobic conditioning and stress innoculation training. *Cognitive Therapeutic Research* 9: 471-478.

Longmuir, P., and Shephard, R.J. (1994). Reliability and validity of a modified Canadian aerobic fitness test for individuals with mobility impairments. *Adapted Physical Activity Quarterly* 12: 161-175.

Loomis, R.A., and Thomas, C.D. (1991). Elderly women in nursing home and independent residence: Health, body attitudes, self-esteem and life satisfaction. *Canadian Journal on Aging* 10: 224-231.

Lord, S.R., Caplan, G.A., and Ward, J.A. (1993). Balance, reaction time and muscle strength in exercising and nonexercising older women: A pilot study. *Archives of Physical Medicine and Rehabilitation* 74: 837-839.

Lord, S.R., and Castell, S. (1994). Physical activity program for older persons: Effect on balance, strength, neuromuscular control, and reaction time. *Archives of Physical Medicine and Rehabilitation* 75: 648-652.

Lorentz, E.J. (1985). Rehabilitation in the elderly. In R. Andres, E.L. Bierman, and W.R. Hazzard (Eds.), *Principles of geriatric medicine* (pp. 939-950). New York: McGraw-Hill.

Louhevaara, V., and Lusa, S. (1993). Guidelines on the follow-up of the firefighters' work ability. In J. Ilmarinen (Ed.), *Aging and work* (pp. 134-141). Helsinki: Institute for Occupational Medicine.

Lucy, S.D., and Hayes, K.C. (1985). Postural sway profiles: Normal subjects and subjects with cerebellar ataxia. *Physiotherapy Canada* 37: 140-148.

Ludwig, F.C. (1994). The morphometric assessment of biological age. In A.K. Balin (Ed.), *Practical handbook of human biologic age determination* (pp. 313-325). Boca Raton, FL: CRC Press.

Lupinacci, N.S., Rikli, R.E., Jessie, J.C., and Ross, D. (1993). Age and physical activity effects on reaction time and digit symbol substitution performance in cognitively active adults. *Research Quarterly* 64: 144-150.

Lyon, R.T., Rivers, S.P., and Veith, F.J. (1994). Cardiovascular disease in the elderly: Peripheral vascular disease in the elderly. *American Journal of Geriatric Cardiology* 3: 15-30.

MacDonald, S., Joffres, M.R., Stachenko, S., Horlick, L., and Foder, G. (1992). Multiple cardiovascular disease risk factors in Canadian adulls. *Canadian Medical Association Journal* 146: 2021-2029.

Macera, C.A., Pate, R.R., Powell, K.E., Jackson, K.L., Kendrick, J.S., and Craven, T.E. (1989). Predicting lower extremity injuries among habitual runners. *Archives of Internal Medicine* 149: 2565-2568.

Macey, S.M., and Schneider, D.F. (1993). Deaths from excessive heat and excessive cold among the elderly. *Gerontologist* 33: 497-500.

Macias, J.F., Bondia, A., and Rodriguez-Commes, J.L. (1987). Physiology and disorders of water balance and electrolytes in the elderly. In J.F. Macias and J.S. Cameron (Eds.), *Renal function and disease in the elderly* (pp. 67-93). London: Butterworths.

Macias, J,F., Garcia-Iglesias, C., Tabernero, J.M., Rodriguez-Commes, J.L., Corbacho, L., and de Castro, S. (1983). Behavior of the aging kidney under acute acid overload. *Nefrologia* 3: 11-16.

MacIntyre, E., Stevenson, J.C., Whitehead, M.I., Wimalawansa, S.J., Banks, L.M., and Healy, M.J.R. (1988). Calcitonin for prevention of postmenopausal bone loss. *Lancet* 2: 1481-1483.

MacRae, P.G. (1989). Physical activity and central nervous system integrity. In W.W. Spirduso and H.M. Eckert (Eds.), *Physical activity and aging* (pp. 69-77). Champaign, IL: Human Kinetics.

MacRae, P.G., Feltner, M.E., and Reinsch, S. (1994). A 1-year exercise program for older women: Effects on falls, injuries, and physical performance. *Journal of Aging and Physical Activity* 2: 127-142.

MacVicar, M.G., Winningham, M.L., and Nickel, J.L. (1989). Effects of aerobic training on cancer patients' functional capacity. *Nursing Research* 38: 348-351.

Maddocks, J. (1961). Possible absence of hypertension in two complete Pacific island populations. *Lancet* 2: 396-399.

Mader, S.L. (1989). Aging and postural hypotension. *Journal of the American Geriatric Society* 37: 129-137.

Mader, W. (1991). Aging and the metaphor of narcissism. In G.M. Kenyon, J.E. Birren, and J.J.F. Schroots (Eds.), *Metaphors of aging in science and the humanities* (pp. 131-154). New York: Springer.

Maggi, A., Schmidt, M.J., Ghetti, B., and Enna, S.J. (1979). Effect of aging on neurotransmitter receptor binding in rat and human brain. *Life Sciences* 24: 367-373.

Magnani, M., Fazi, A., Chiarantini, L., Serafini, G., and Stocchi, V. (1990). Mechanisms of enzyme decay during red blood cell aging. In H.L. Segal, M. Rothstein, and E. Bergamini (Eds.), *Metabolism in aging* (pp. 217-232). New York: Wiley-Liss.

Mahler, D.A., and O'Donnell, D.E. (1991). Alternative modes of exercise training for pulmonary patients. *Journal of Cardiopulmonary Rehabilitation* 11: 58-63.

Makinodan, T., Bloom, E.T., James, S.J., and Lubinski, J. (1991). Immunity and ageing. In M.S.J. Pathy (Ed.), *Principles and practice of geriatric medicine* (2nd ed., pp. 3-12). Chichester: Wiley.

Makinodan, T., Lubinski, J., and Fong, T.C. (1987). Cellular, biochemical and molecular basis of T-cell senescence. *Archives of Pathology and Laboratory Medicine* 111: 910-914.

Makrides, L., Heigenhauser, J.F., and Jones, N.L. (1990). High intensity endurance training in 20- to 30- and 60- 70-year old healthy men. *Journal of Applied Physiology* 69: 1792-1798.

Makrides, L., Heigenhauser, J.F., McCartney, N., and Jones, N.L. (1985). Maximal short-term exercise capacity in healthy subjects aged 15-70 years. *Clinical Science* 69: 197-205.

Makris, V.I., Yee, R.D., Langefeld, C.D., Chapell, A.S., and Slemenda, C.W. (1993). Visual loss and performance in blind athletes. *Medicine and Science in Sports and Exercise* 25: 265-269.

Mancini, D.M., Lirato, C., and Pauciullo, P. (1993). High cholesterol in the elderly: The Italian experience. *American Journal of Geriatric Cardiology* 2 (4): 28-35.

Mancini, D.M., Walter, G., Reichek, N., Lenkinski, R., McCully, K.K., Mullen, J.L., and Wilson, J.R. (1992). Contribution of skeletal muscle atrophy to exercise intolerance and altered muscle metabolism in heart failure. *Circulation* 85: 1364-1373.

Manfredi, T.G., Fielding, R.A., O'Reilly, K.P., Meredith, C.N., Lee, H.Y., and Evans, W.J. (1991). Plasma creatine kinase activity and exercise-induced muscle damage in older men. *Medicine and Science in Sports and Exercise* 23: 1028-1034.

Manning, G.F. (1991). Spinning the "Globe of Memory": Metaphor, literature, and aging. In G.M. Kenyon, J.E. Birren, and J.J.F. Schroots (Eds.), *Metaphors of aging in science and the humanities* (pp. 37-56). New York: Springer.

Manolio, T., Ettinger, W., Tracy, R., Kuller, L.H., Borhani, N.O., Lynch, J.C., and Fried, L.P. (1993). Epidemiology of low cholesterol levels in older adults: The cardiovascular health study. *Circulation* 87: 728-737.

Manolio, T.A., Pearson, T., Wenger, N., Barrett-Connor, E., Payne, G.H., and Harlan, W.R. (1992). Cholesterol and heart disease in older persons and women—review of an NHLBI workshop. *Annals of Epidemiology* 2: 161-176.

Manson, J.E., Nathan, D.M., Krolewski, A.S., Stampfer, M.U., Willett, W.C., and Hennekins, C.H. (1992). A prospective study of exercise and incidence of diabetes among U.S. male physicians. *Journal of the American Medical Association* 268: 63-67.

Manson, J.E., Rimm, E.B., Stampfer, M.U., Colditz, G.A., Willett, W.C., Krolewski, A.S., Rosner, B., Hennekins, C.H., and Speizer, F.E. (1991). Physical activity and incidence of non-insulin dependent diabetes mellitus in women. *Lancet* 338: 774-778.

Manton, K.G. (1989). Epidemiological, demographic, and social correlates of disability. *Millbank Quarterly* 67 (Suppl. 2:1): 13-58.

Manton, K.G., Corder, L.S., and Stallard, E. (1993). Disability and mortality among the oldest-old: Implications for current and future health and long-term care service needs. *Journal of the Gerontological Society* 48: S153-S166.

Mariani, E., Roda, P., Mariani, A.R., Vitale, M., Degrassi, A., Papa, S., and Facchini, A. (1990). Age-associated changes in CD8+ and CD16+ cell reactivity: Clonal analysis. *Clinical and Experimental Immunology* 48: 148-154.

Marin, R. (1986). *Occupational Mortality 1971-80*. Helsinki: Central Statistical Office of Finland.

Marti, B., and Howald, H. (1990). Long-term effects of physical training on aerobic capacity: Controlled study of former elite athletes. *Journal of Applied Physiology* 69: 1451-1459.

Marti, B., Knobloch, M., Tschopp, A., Jucker, A., and Howald, H. (1989). Is excessive running predictive of degenerative hip disease? *British Medical Journal* 229: 91-93.

Marti, B., Pekkanen, J., Nissinen, A., Ketola, A., Kivelä, S., Punsar, S., and Karvonen, M.J. (1989). Association of physical activity with coronary risk factors and physical ability: Twenty-year follow-up of a cohort of Finnish men. *Age and Ageing* 18: 103-109.

Marti, B., Vader, J.P., Minder, C.E., and Abelin, T. (1988). On the epidemiology of running injuries. The 1984 Bern Grand Prix study. *American Journal of Sports Medicine* 16: 285-294.

Martin, A.D., Silverthorn, K.G., Houston, C.S., Bernhardson, S., Wyda, A., and Roos, L.L. (1991). Trends in fracture of the proximal femur in two million Canadians; 1972 to 1984. *Clinical Orthopedics and Related Research* (Philadelphia) 266: 111-118.

Martin, D., and Notelovitz, M. (1993). Effects of aerobic training on bone mineral density of postmenopausal women. *Journal of Bone and Mineral Research* 8: 931-936.

Martin, W.H., Kohrt, W.M., Malley, M.T., Korte, E., and Stoltz, S. (1990). Exercise training enhances leg vasodilatory capacity of 65-yr-old men and women. *Journal of Applied Physiology* 69: 1804-1809.

Martin, W.H., Ogawa, T., Kohrt, W.M., Malley, M.T., Korte, E., Kieffer, P.S., and Schechtman, K.B. (1991). Effects of aging, gender and physical training on peripheral vascular function. *Circulation* 84: 654-664.

Martinsen, E.W., Strand, J., Paulson, G., and Kaggestad, J. (1989). Physical fitness levels in patients with anxiety and depressive disorders. *International Journal of Sports Medicine* 10: 58-61.

Masoro, E.J. (1985). Metabolism. In C.E. Finch and E.L. Schneider (Eds.), *Handbook of the biology of aging* (pp. 540-563). New York: Van Nostrand Reinhold.

Masoro, E.J. (1992). Retardation of aging processes by food restriction: An experimental tool. *American Journal of Clinical Nutrition* 55: 1250S-1252S.

Massé-Biron, J., Mercier, J., Collomp, K., Hardy, J.M., and Préfaut, C. (1992). Age and training effects on the lactate kinetics of master athletes during maximal exercise. *European Journal of Applied Physiology* 65: 311-315.

Master, A.M., Van Liere, E.J., Lindsay, H.A., and Hartroft, W.S. (1964). Arterial blood pressure. In P.L. Altman and D.S. Dittmer (Eds.), *Biology data book*. Washington, DC: Federation of American Societies for Experimental Biology.

Matheson, G.O., MacIntyre, J.G., Taunton, J.E., Clement, D.B., and Lloyd-Smith, T.K. (1989). Musculo-skeletal injuries associated with physical activity in older adults. *Medicine and Science in Sports and Exercise* 21: 379-385.

Maurel, E., Boissou, H., Pieraggi, M.T., Julian, M., Moczar, M., and Robert, L. (1980). Age-dependent biochemical changes in dermal connective tissue. Relationship to histological and ultrastructural observations. *Connective Tissue Research* 8: 33-39.

Mayersohn, M. (1982). The "xylose test" to assess gastrointestinal absorption in the elderly: Pharmacokinetic evaluation of the literature. *Journal of Gerontology* 37: 300-305.

Mazess, R.B., and Mathiesen, R.W. (1982). Lack of unusual longevity in Vilcabamba, Ecuador. *Human Biology* 54: 517-524.

Mazzeo, R.S., Colburn, R.W., and Horvath, S.M. (1985). Catecholamine response to strenuous exercise in trained and untrained rats 6, 15 and 27 months of age. *Medicine and Science in Sports and Exercise* 17: 261-262.

Mazzeo, R.S., and Nasrullah, I. (1992). Exercise and age-related decline in immune functions. In R.R. Watson and M. Eisinger (Eds.), *Exercise and disease* (pp. 159-178). Boca Raton, FL: CRC Press.

McAuley, E., and Rudolph, D. (1995). Physical activity, aging and psychological well-being. *Journal of Aging and Physical Activity* 3: 67-96.

McCarter, R.J.M. (1990). Age-related changes in skeletal muscle function. *Aging* 2: 27-38.

McCartney, N., Moroz, D., Garner, S.H., and McComas, A.J. (1988). The effects of strength training in patients with selected neuromuscular disorders. *Medicine and Science in Sports and Exercise* 20: 362-367.

McCauley, E. (1994). Physical activity and psychosocial outcomes. In C. Bouchard, R.J. Shephard, and T. Stephens (Ed.), *Physical activity, fitness and health* (pp. 551-568). Champaign, IL: Human Kinetics.

McClaran, S.R., Babcock, M.A., Pegelow, D.F., Reddan, W.G., and Dempsey, J.A. (1995). Longitudinal effects of aging on lung function at rest and exercise in healthy active fit elderly adults. *Journal of Applied Physiology* 78: 1957-1968.

McConnell, A.K., and Davies, C.T.M. (1992). A comparison of the ventilatory responses to exercise of elderly and younger humans. *Journals of Gerontology* 47: B137-B141.

McDonald, C.C., Alexander, F.E., Whyte, B.W., Forrest, A.P., Stewart, H.J., and Scottish Cancer Trials Breast Group. (1995). Cardiac and vascular morbidity in women receiving adjuvant tamoxifen for breast cancer in a randomised trial. *British Medical Journal* 311: 977-980.

McElvaney, G.N., Blackie, S.P., Morrison, N.J., Fairbarn, M.S., Wilcox, P.G., and Pardy, R.L. (1989). Cardiac output at rest and during exercise in elderly subjects. *Medicine and Science in Sports and Exercise* 21: 293-298.

McGandy, R.B., Burrows, C.H., Spanias, A., Meredith, A., Stone, J.L., and Norris, A.H. (1966). Nutrient intakes and energy expenditures in men of different ages. *Journal of Gerontology* 21: 581-587.

McGeer, P.L., and McGeer, E.G. (1980). Chemistry of mood and emotion. *Annual Reviews of Psychology* 31: 273-307.

McLachlan, M.S.F. (1987). Anatomic, structural and vascular changes in the aging kidney. In J.F.M. Nunez and J.S. Cameron (Eds.), *Renal function and disease in the elderly* (pp. 3-26). London: Butterworths.

McMurdo, M.E., and Rennie, L. (1993). A controlled trial of exercise by residents of old people's homes. *Age and Ageing* 22: 11-15.

McMurray, R.G., Ben-Ezra, V., Forsythe, W.A., and Smith, A.T. (1985). Responses of endurance trained subjects to caloric deficits induced by diet or exercise. *Medicine and Science in Sports and Exercise* 17: 574-579.

McNamara, P.S., Otto, R.M., and Smith, T.K. (1985). The acute response of simulated bicycle and rowing exercise on the elderly population [Abstract]. *Medicine and Science in Sports and Exercise* 17: 266.

McNeil, J.K., LeBlanc, E.M., and Joyner, M. (1991). The effect of exercise on depressive symptoms in the moderately depressed elderly. *Psychology and Aging* 6: 487-488.

McPherson, B.D. (1990). *Aging as a social process*. Toronto, ON: Butterworths.

McPherson, B.D., and Yuhasz, M. (1968). An inventory for assessing men's attitudes towards exercise and physical activity. *Research Quarterly* 39: 218-220.

Meenan, R., Gertman, P., Mason, J., and Dunaif, R. (1982). The arthritis impact measurement scales: Further investigation of a health status instrument. *Arthritis and Rheumatism* 25: 1048-1053.

Meeuwsen, H.J., Sawicki, T.M., and Stelmach, G.E. (1993). Improved foot position sense as a result of repetitions in older adults. *Journals of Gerontology* 48: P137-P141.

Mehlhorn, R.J., and Cole, G. (1985). The free radicals theory of aging: A critical review. *Advances in Free Radical Biology and Medicine* 1: 165-223.

Mehrotra, C.M.N. (1985). Appraising the performance of older workers. In P.K. Robinson, J. Livingston, and J.E. Birren (Eds.), *Aging and technological advances* (pp. 353-356). New York: Plenum Press.

Meltzer, D.E. (1993). Age dependence of Olympic weightlifting ability. *Medicine and Science in Sports and Exercise* 26: 1053-1067.

Mendez, J., Lukaski, H.C., and Buskirk, E.R. (1984). Fat-free mass as a function of max. O_2 consumption and 24-hour creatinine and 3-methyl histidine excretion. *American Journal of Clinical Nutrition* 39: 710-715.

Menkes, A., Mazel, S., Redmond, R.A., Koffler, K., Libanati, C.R., Gundberg, C.M., Zizic, T.M., Hagberg, J.M., Pratley, R.E., and Hurley, B.F. (1993). Strength training increases regional bone mineral density and bone remodeling in middle-aged and older men. *Journal of Applied Physiology* 74: 2478-2484.

Meredith, C.N., Frontera, W.R., Fisher, E., Hughes, V., Herland, J., Edwards, J., and Evans, W.R. (1989). Peripheral effects of endurance training in young and old subjects. *Journal of Applied Physiology* 66: 2844-2849.

Meredith, C.N., Frontera, W.R., O'Reilly, K.P., and Evans, W.J. (1992). Body composition in elderly men: Effect of dietary modification during strength training. *Journal of the American Geriatrics Society* 40: 155-162.

Meredith, I.T., Friberg, P., Jennings, G.L., Dewar, E.M., Fazio, V.A., Lambert, G.W., and Esler, M.D. (1991). Exercise training lowers resting renal but not cardiac sympathetic activity in humans. *Hypertension* 18: 575-582.

Mernagh, J.R., Harrison, J., Krondl, A., McNeill, K.G., and Shephard, R.J. (1986). Composition of lean tissue in health volunteers for nutritional studies in health and disease. *Nutrition Research* 6: 499-507.

Merry, B.J., and Holehan, A.M. (1981). Serum profiles of LH, FSH, testosterone and 5-alpha-DHT from 21 to 1000 days of age in ad libitum fed and dietary restricted rats. *Experimental Gerontology* 16: 431-444.

Mertens, D.M., Kavanagh, T., and Shephard, R.J. (1978). Exercise rehabilitation for chronic obstructive lung disease. *Respiration* 35: 96-107.

Mertens, D.M., Kavanagh, T., and Shephard, R.J. (1995). Exercise and fat loss in the obese cardiac patient. Manuscript in preparation.

Metropolitan Life. (1983). 1983 Metropolitan height and weight tables. *Statistical Bulletin of the Metropolitan Life Insurance Co.* 64 (2, January-June).

Meyer, H.E., Tverdal, A., and Falch, J.A. (1993). Risk factors for hip fracture in middle-aged Norwegian women and men. *American Journal of Epidemiology* 137: 1203-1211.

Miall, W.E., Ashcroft, M.T., Lovell, H.G., and Moore, F. (1967). A longitudinal study of the decline of adult height with age in two Welsh communities. *Human Biology* 39: 445-454.

Miall, W.E., and Brennan, P.J. (1981). Hypertension in the elderly: The South Wales study. In G. Ouesti and K.E. Kim (Eds.), *Hypertension in the young and the old* (p. 277). New York: Grune & Stratton.

Michaels, D.D. (1994). The eye. In W.R. Hazzard, E.L. Bierman, J.P. Blass, W.H. Ettinger, and J.B. Halter (Eds.), *Principles of geriatric medicine and gerontology* (3rd ed., pp. 441-456). New York: McGraw-Hill.

Michel, B.A., Bloch, D.A., and Fries, J.F. (1989). Weight-bearing exercise, over-exercise, and lumbar bone density over age 50 years. *Archives of Internal Medicine* 149: 2325-2329.

Michel, B.A., Lane, N.E., Björkengren, A., Bloch, D.A., and Fries, J.F. (1992). Impact of running on lumbar bone density: A 5-year longitudinal study. *Journal of Rheumatology* 19: 1759-1763.

Michelsen, S., and Otterstad, J.E. (1990). Blood pressure response during maximal exercise in apparently healthy men and women. *Journal of Internal Medicine* 227: 157-163.

Mikeski, A.E., Topp, R., Wigglesworth, J.K., Harsha, D.M., and Edwards, J.E. (1994). Efficacy of home-based training program for older adults using elastic tubing. *European Journal of Applied Physiology* 69: 316-320.

Miller, R.A. (1991). Aging and immune function. *International Review of Cytology* 124: 187-215.

Miller, T.R., Grossman, S.J., Schectman, K.B., Biello, D.R., Ludbrook, P.A., and Ehsani, A.A. (1986). Ventricular diastolic filling and its association with age. *American Journal of Cardiology* 58: 531-535.

Mills, R. (1991). The auditory system. In M.S.J. Pathy (Ed.), *Principles and practice of geriatric medicine* (pp. 995-1009). Chichester: Wiley.

Minaker, K.L., and Rowe, J.W. (1982). The gastro-intestinal system. In J.W. Rowe and R.W. Besdine (Eds.), *Health and disease of old age* (pp. 297-315). Boston: Little, Brown.

Minaker, K.L., Rowe, J.W., Tonino, R., and Pallotta, J.A. (1982). Influence of age on clearance of insulin in man. *Diabetes* 31: 851-855.

Mink, P. et al. (in press). Physical activity, waist-hip ratio and other risk factors for ovarian cancer: A prospective study of older women. *Epidemiology*.

Minor, M.A., Hewett, J.E., Webel, R.R., Anderson, S.K., and Kay, D.R. (1989). Efficacy of physical conditioning exercise in patients with rheumatoid arthritis and osteoarthritis. *Arthritis and Rheumatism* 32: 1396-1405.

Minotti, J.R., Johnson, E.C., Hudson, T.H., Zuroske, G., Murata, G., Fukushima, E., Cagle, T.G., Chick, T.W., Massie, B.M., and Icenogle, M.V. (1990). Skeletal muscle response to exercise training in congestive heart failure. *Journal of Clinical Investigation* 86: 751-758.

Misner, J.E., Massey, B.H., Bemben, M., Going, S., and Patrick, J. (1992). Long-term effects of exercise on the range of motion of aging women. *Journal of Orthopaedic and Sports Physical Therapy* 16: 37-42.

Mitchell, C.O., and Lipschitz, D.A. (1982). Detection of protein-calorie malnutrition in the elderly. *American Journal of Clinical Nutrition* 35: 398-406.

Mittelman, M.A., Maclure, M., Tofler, G.H., Sherwood, J.B., Goldberg, R.J., and Muller, J.E. (1993). Triggering of acute myocardial infarction by heavy physical exertion. Protection against triggering by regular exertion. *New England Journal of Medicine* 329: 1677-1683.

Miyatake, K., Okamoto, J., Kinoshita, N., Owa, M., Nakasone, I., Sakakibara, H., and Nimura, Y. (1984). Augmentation of atrial contribution to left ventricular flow with aging as assessed by intracardiac Doppler flowmetry. *American Journal of Cardiology* 53: 587-589.

Molander, B., and Backman, L. (1993). Performance of a complex motor skill in older and younger adults. In E. Heikkinen and S. Harris (Eds.), *Physical activity and sports for healthy aging*. Albany, NY: Center for Studies of Aging.

Moller, B.M. (1981). Hearing in 70 and 75 year old people. Results from a cross-sectional and longitudinal population study. *American Journal of Otology* 2: 22-29.

Mongeau, E. (1991). Nutrition et troisième age [Nutrition and the third age]. In C. Blais (Ed.), *Aging into the twenty-first century* (pp. 337-351). North York, ON: Captus University.

Monti, D., Troiano, L., Tropea, F., Grassili, E., Cossarizza, A., Barozzi, D., Pelloni, M.C., Tamassia, M.G., Bellomo, G., and Franceschi, C. (1992). Apoptosis—programmed cell death: A role in the aging process? *American Journal of Clinical Nutrition* 55: 1208S-1214S.

Montoye, H.J. (1975). *Physical activity and health: An epidemiological study of an entire community*. Englewood Cliffs, NJ: Prentice Hall.

Moore, G.E. (1995). Exercise and renal disease. In J. Torg and R.J. Shephard (Eds.), *Current therapy in sports medicine* (3rd ed., pp. 686-689). Philadelphia: Mosby–Yearbook.

Moore, G.E., Bertocci, L.A., and Painter, P.L. (1993). ^{31}P-Magnetic resonance spectroscopy assessment of subnormal oxidative metabolism of skeletal muscle in renal failure patients. *Journal of Clinical Investigation* 91: 420-424.

Moore, G.E., Brinker, K.R., Stray-Gundersen, J., and Mitchell, J.H. (1993). Determinants of $\dot{V}O_2$peak in patients with end-stage renal disease: On and off dialysis. *Medicine and Science in Sports and Exercise* 25: 18-23.

Moore, J.G., Tweedy, C., Christian, P.E., and Datz, F.L. (1983). Effect of age on gastric emptying of liquid-solid meals in man. *Digestive Diseases and Sciences* (New York) 28: 340-344.

Moore, K.E., Demarest, K.T., and Lookingland, K.J. (1987). Stress, prolactin and hypothalamic dopaminergic neurons. *Neuropharmacology* 26: 801-808.

Moraine, J.J., Lamotte, M., Berré, J., Niset, G., Leduc, A., and Naeije, R. (1993). Relationship of middle cerebral artery blood flow velocity to intensity during dynamic exercise in normal subjects. *European Journal of Applied Physiology* 67: 35-38.

Morey, M.C., Cowper, P.A., Feussner, J.R., DiPasquale, R.C., Crowley, G.M., Kitzman, D.W., and Sullivan, R.J. (1989). Evaluation of a supervised program in a geriatric population. *Journal of the American Geriatric Society* 37: 348-354.

Morey, M.C., Cowper, P.A., Feussner, J.R., DiPasquale, R.C., Crowley, G.M., Samsa, G.P., and Sullivan, R.J. (1991). Two-year trends in physical performance following supervised exercise among community-dwelling older veterans. *Journal of the American Geriatric Society* 39: 986-992.

Morgan, B., Alexander, J., Nicoli, S., and Brammel, H. (1990). The patient with coronary heart disease at altitude. *Journal of Wilderness Medicine* 1: 147-153.

Morgan, D.B., and Burkinshaw, L. (1983). Estimation of non-fat body tissues from measurements of skinfold thickness, total body potassium and total body nitrogen. *Clinical Science* 65: 407-414.

Morgan, D.G., Marcusson, J.O., Nyberg, P., Wester, P., Winblad, B., Gordon, M.N., and Finch, C.E. (1987). Divergent changes in D-1 and D-2 dopamine binding sites in human brain during aging. *Neurobiology of Aging* 8: 195-201.

Morgan, D.G., May, P.C., and Finch, C.E. (1988). Neurotransmitter receptors in normal human aging and Alzheimer's disease. In A.K. Sen and T.Y. Lee (Eds.), *Receptors and ligands in neurological disorders* (pp. 120-147). London: Cambridge University Press.

Morgan, K. (1987). *Sleep and ageing*. London: Croom Helm.

Morgan, W.P. (1986). Athletes and nonathletes in the middle years of life. In B.D. McPherson (Ed.), *Sport and aging* (pp. 167-186). Champaign, IL: Human Kinetics.

Morgan, W.P. (1994). Physical activity, fitness and depression. In C. Bouchard, R.J. Shephard, and T. Stephens (Eds.), *Physical activity, fitness and health* (pp. 851-867). Champaign, IL: Human Kinetics.

Morgan, W.P., and Goldstone, S.E. (1987). *Exercise and mental health*. New York: Hemisphere.

Moritani, T., and de Vries, H.A. (1980). Potential for gross muscle hypertrophy in older men. *Journal of Gerontology* 35: 672-682.

Morley, J.E., Kaiser, F.E., and Perry, H.M. (1993). The effects of testosterone and growth hormone therapy in frail elderly individuals. In H.M. Perry, J.E. Morley, and R.M. Coe (Eds.), *Aging and musculoskeletal disorders* (pp. 280-291). New York: Springer.

Morley, J.E., Perry, H.M., Kaiser, F.E., Kraenzle, D., Jensen, J., Houston, K., Mattammal, M., and Perry, H.M. (1993). Effects of testosterone replacement therapy in hypogonadal males: A preliminary study. *Journal of the American Geriatric Society* 41: 149-152.

Morris, A.F., Lussier, L., Vaccaro, P., and Clarke, D.H. (1982). Life quality characteristics of national class women masters long distance runners. *Annals of Sports Medicine* 1: 23-26.

Morris, J.N., Clayton, D.G., Everitt, M.G., Semmence, A.M., and Bargess, E.H. (1990). Exercise in leisure time: Coronary attack and death rates. *British Heart Journal* 63: 325-334.

Morris, J.N., Everitt, M.G., Pollard, R., Chave, S.P.W., and Semmence, A.M. (1980). Vigorous exercise in leisure time. Protection against coronary heart disease. *Lancet* 2: 1207-1210.

Morris, J.S., Dew, M.J., Gelb, A.M., and Clements, D.G. (1991). Age and gastrointestinal disease. In M.S.J. Pathy (Ed.), *Principles and practice of geriatric medicine* (2nd ed., pp. 417-486). Chichester: Wiley.

Moser, K.A., Goldblatt, P.O., Fox, A.J., and Jones, D.R. (1987). Unemployment and mortality: Comparison of the 1971 and 1981 longitudinal study census samples. *British Medical Journal* 294: 86-90.

Moss, A.J., and Parsons, V.L. (1986). Current estimates from the National Health Interview Survey, United States, 1985. *National Center for Health Statistics, Vital and Health Statistics Series 10*, No. 160 (DHHS Publication No. 86-1588). Washington, DC: U.S. Government Printing Office.

MRC Working Party. (1985). Hypertension. *British Medical Journal* 291: 97-104.

Mulder, M., and Härmä, M. (1992). The relation between mental and physical effort at work and sleep quality for older and younger white-collar workers. In J. Ilmarinen (Ed.), *Aging and work*. Helsinki: Institute for Occupational Health.

Mulrow, C.D., Gerety, M.B., Kanten, D., Cornell, J.E., DeNino, L.A., Chiodo, L., Aguilar, C., O'Neil, M.B., Rosenberg, J., and Solis, R.M. (1994). A randomized trial of physical rehabilitation for very frail nursing home residents. *Journal of the American Medical Association* 271: 519-524.

Murasko, D.M., Nelson, B.J., Matour, D., Goonewardene, I.M., and Kaye, D. (1991). Heterogeneity of changes in lymphoproliferative ability with increasing age. *Experimental Gerontology* 26: 269-279.

Murasko, D.M., Nelson, B.J., Silver, R., Matour, D., and Kaye, D. (1986). Immunologic response in an elderly population with a mean age of 85. *American Journal of Medicine* 81: 612-618.

Murphy, S., Khaw, K-T., May, H., and Compston, J.E. (1994). Milk consumption and bone mineral density in middle-aged and elderly women. *British Medical Journal* 308: 939-941.

Murray, D., Wood, P.J., Moriarty, J., and Clayton, B.E. (1981). Adrenocortical function in old age. *Journal of Clinical and Experimental Gerontology* 3: 255-268.

Murray, J.F. (1981). In L.H. Smith and S.O. Thiers (Eds.), *Pathophysiology: The biological principles of disease*. London: Saunders.

Murray, S., and Shephard, R.J. (1988). Possible anthropometric alternatives to skinfold measurements. *Human Biology* 60: 273-282.

Muss, H.B. (1994). Breast cancer. In W.R. Hazzard, E.L. Bierman, J.P. Blass, W.H. Ettinger, and J.B. Halter (Eds), *Principles of geriatric medicine and gerontology* (3rd ed., pp. 481-491). New York: McGraw-Hill.

Myers, A.M., and Huddy, L. (1985). Evaluating physical capabilities in the elderly. The relationship between ADL self-assessments and basic abilities. *Canadian Journal on Aging* 4: 189-200.

Nakao, M., Inoue, Y., and Murakami, H. (1989). Aging process of leg muscle endurance in males and females. *European Journal of Applied Physiology* 59: 209-214.

Narayanan, N. (1981). Differential alterations in ATP-supported calcium transport activities of sarcoplasmic reticulum and sarcolemma of aging myocardium. *Biophysica Biochemica Acta* 678: 442-459.

Naresh, M.D., and Brodsky, B. (1992). X-ray diffraction studies on human tendon show changes in collagen packing. *Biochimica Biophysica Acta* 1122: 161-166.

Nasrullah, I., and Mazzeo, R.S. (1992). Age-related immuno-senescence in Fischer 344 rats: Influence of exercise training. *Journal of Applied Physiology* 73: 1932-1938.

National Health and Welfare. (1989). *The active health report on seniors*. Ottawa: National Health and Welfare.

Need, A.G., Horowitz, M., Bridges, A., Morris, H.A., and Nordin, B.E.C. (1989). Effect of nadrolone decanoate and antiresorptive therapy on vertebral density in osteoporotic post-menopausal women. *Archives of Internal Medicine* 149: 57-60.

Nelson, M.E., Fisher, E.C., Dilmanian, F.A., Dallal, G.E., and Evans, W.J. (1991). A 1-yr walking program and increased calcium in postmenopausal women: Effects on bone. *American Journal of Clinical Nutrition* 53: 1304-1311.

Nevitt, M.C., Cummings, S.R., and Hudes, E.S. (1991). Risk factors for injurious falls: A prospective study. *Journals of Gerontology* 46: M164-M170.

Nevitt, M.C., Cummings, S.R., Kidd, S., and Black, D. (1989). Risk factors for recurrent non-syncopal falls. *Journal of the American Medical Association* 261: 2663-2668.

Newman, K.P., and Phillips, J.H. (1988). Graded exercise testing for diagnosis of coronary artery disease in elderly patients. *Southern Medical Journal* 81: 430-432.

News item: Life expectancy in Russia falls. (1994). *British Medical Journal* 308: 553.

Newsholme, E.A. (1990). Some experiments on factors that can change insulin sensitivity. *Annals of Medicine* 22: 181-184.

Nguyen, T.V., Kelly, P.J., Sambrook, P.N., Gilbert, C., Pocock, N.A., and Eisman, J.A. (1994). Lifestyle factors and bone density in the elderly: Implications for osteoporosis prevention. *Journal of Bone and Mineral Research* 9: 1339-1346.

Nicholl, J.P., and Williams, B.T. (1983). Injuries sustained by runners during a popular marathon. *British Journal of Sports Medicine* 17: 10-15.

Nichols, J.F., Omizo, D.K., Peterson, K.K., and Nelson, K.P. (1993). Efficacy of heavy-resistance training for active women over sixty: Muscular strength, body composition, and program adherence. *Journal of the American Geriatrics Society* 41: 205-210.

Nielsen, J. (1993). Work environment and health among elderly municipal cleaners. The benefits of age and the problems. In J. Ilmarinen (Ed.), *Aging and work* (pp. 48-53). Helsinki: Institute for Occupational Health.

Nieman, D.C. (1995). *Fitness and sports medicine* (3rd ed.). Palo Alto, CA: Bull.

Nieman, D.C., Butler, J., Pollett, L., Dietrich, S., and Lutz, R. (1989). Nutrient intake of marathon runners. *Journal of the American Dietetic Association* 89: 1273-1278.

Nieman, D.C., Henson, D.A., Gusewitch, G., Warren, B.J., Dotson, R.C., Butterworth, D.E., and Nehlsen-Cannarella, S.L. (1993). Physical activity and immune function in elderly women. *Medicine and Science in Sports and Exercise* 25: 823-831.

Nieman, D.C., Warren, B.J., O'Donnell, K.A., Dotson, R.G., Butterworth, D.E., and Henson, D.A. (1993). Physical activity and serum lipids and lipoproteins in elderly women. *Journal of the American Geriatric Society* 41: 1339-1344.

Niinimaa, V., and Shephard, R.J. (1978a). Training and oxygen conductance in the elderly. I. The respiratory system. *Journal of Gerontology* 33: 354-361.

Niinimaa, V., and Shephard, R.J. (1978b). Training and oxygen conductance in the elderly. II. The cardiovascular system. *Journal of Gerontology* 33: 362-367.

Noppa, H., Andersson, M., Bengtsson, C., Bruce, A., and Isaksson, B. (1979). Body composition in middle-aged women with special reference to the correlation between total body mass and anthropometric data. *American Journal of Clinical Nutrition* 32: 1388-1395.

Nordin, B.E.C., and Heaney, R.P. (1990). Calcium supplementation of the diet: Justified by present evidence. *British Medical Journal* 300: 1056-1060.

Nordin, B.E.C., Need, A.G., Morris, H.A., and Horowitz, M. (1985). New approaches to the problems of osteoporosis. *Clinics in Orthopedics* 200: 181-197.

Nordstrom, J.W. (1982). Trace mineral nutrition in the elderly. *American Journal of Clinical Nutrition* 30: 788-795.

Norman, L.G. (1960). Medical aspects of road safety. *Lancet* i: 989-994, 1039-1045.

Norvell, N., Martin, D., and Salamon, A. (1991). Psychological and physiological benefits of passive and aerobic exercise in sedentary middle-aged women. *Journal of Mental and Nervous Diseases* 179: 573-574.

Norwegian Confederation of Sports. (1984). *Physical activity in Norway, 1983*. Oslo: Norwegian Confederation of Sports.

Notelovitz, M., Martin, D., Tesa, R., McKenzie, L., and Fields, C. (1991). Estrogen therapy and variable resistance weight training increase bone mineral in surgically menopausal women. *Journal of Bone and Mineral Research* 6: 583-590.

Nottrodt, J.W., and Celentano, E.J. (1984). Use of validity measures in the selection of physical screening tests. In D.A. Attwood and C. McCann (Eds.), *Proceedings of the 1984 International Conference on Occupational Ergonomics*. Toronto, ON: Human Factors Association of Canada.

Nygard, C-H., Luopajärvi, T. Cedercreutz, G., and Ilmarinen, J. (1987). Musculo-skeletal capacity of employees aged 44 to 58 years in physical, mental and mixed types of work. *European Journal of Applied Physiology* 56: 555-561.

Nygard, C-H., Luopajärvi T., and Ilmarinen, J. (1991). Musculo-skeletal capacity and its changes among aging municipal employees in different work categories. *Scandinavian Journal of Work, Environment & Health* 17 (Suppl. 1): 110-117.

Oberling, Fr., and Sengler, J. (1982). Anémies chez le vieillard [Anemias in the old person]. In F. Bourlière (Ed.), *Gérontologie: Biologie et clinique*. Paris: Flammarion.

O'Brien-Cousins, S. (1993). The determinants of late life exercise among women over age 70. Unpublished doctoral dissertation, University of British Columbia, Vancouver, BC.

O'Connor, F., Fleg, J.L., Gerstenblith, G., Becker, L.C., Goldberg, A.P., Hagberg, J.M., Lakatta, L., Lakatta, E.G., and Schulman, S.P. (1994). Effect of body fat on exercise hemodynamics in sedentary older men. *Aging, Clinical and Experimental Research* 6: 257-265.

O'Connor, G.T., Buring, J.E., Yusuf, S., Goldhaber, S.Z., Olmstead, E.M., Paffenbarger, R.S., and Hennekens, C.H. (1989). An overview of randomized trials of rehabilitation with exercise after myocardial infarction. *Circulation* 80: 234-244.

O'Connor, P.J., Aenchbacher, L.E., and Dishman, R.K. (1993). Physical activity and depression in the elderly. *Journal of Aging and Physical Activity* 1: 34-58.

O'Donnell, D.E., and Webb, K.A. (1995). Exercise reconditioning in patients with chronic airflow limitation. In J. Torg and R.J. Shephard (Eds.), *Current therapy in sports medicine* (3rd ed., pp. 678-684). Philadelphia: Mosby–Yearbook.

Office of Population Censuses and Surveys. (1976). *Monitor*. London: Author.

Ogawa, T., Spina, R.J., Martin, W.H., Kohrt, W.M., Schectman, K.B., Holloszy, J.O., and Ehsani, A.A. (1992). Effects of aging, sex and physical training on cardiovascular responses to exercise. *Circulation* 86: 494-503.

O'Hagan, C.M., Smith, D.M., and Pileggi, K.L. (1994). Exercise classes in rest homes: Effect on physical function. *New Zealand Medical Journal* 107: 39-40.

O'Hara, W.J., Allen, C., and Shephard, R.J. (1977). Treatment of obesity by exercise in the cold. *Canadian Medical Association Journal* 117: 773-779.

Ohno, H., Yahata, T., Sato, Y., Yamamura, K., and Taniguchi, N. (1988). Physical training and fasting erythrocyte activities of free radical scavenging enzyme systems in sedentary men. *European Journal of Applied Physiology* 57: 173-176.

Oldridge, N.B., Guyatt, G., Fischer, M., and Rimm, A.A. (1988). Randomized trials of cardiac rehabilitation: Combined experience of randomized clinical trials. *Journal of the American Medical Association* 260: 945-950.

Olivetti, G., Melissari, M., Capasso, J.M., and Anversa, P. (1991). Cardiomyopathy of the aging human heart: Myocyte loss and reactive cellular hypertrophy. *Circulation Research* 68: 1560-1568.

Olseni, L., Midgren, B., and Wollmer, P. (1992). Mucus clearance at rest and during exercise in patients with bronchial hypersecretion. *Scandinavian Journal of Rehabilitation Medicine* 24: 61-64.

O'Reilly, K. (1989). Thermal regulation and hydration levels in aging. In R. Harris and S. Harris (Eds.), *Physical activity, aging, and sports* (pp. 345-359). Albany, NY: Center for Studies of Aging.

Orentreich, D.S., and Orentreich, N. (1985). Alterations in the skin. In R. Andres, E.L. Bierman, and W.R. Hazzard (Eds.), *Principles of geriatric medicine* (pp. 354-371). New York: McGraw-Hill.

Orwoll, E.S., Ferar, J., Oviatt, S.K., McClung, M.R., and Huntington, K. (1989). The relationship of swimming exercise to bone mass in men and women. *Archives of Internal Medicine* 149: 2197-2200.

Osiewacz, H.D. (1995). Aging and genetic instabilities. In K. Esser and G.M. Martin (Eds.), *Molecular aspects of aging* (pp. 29-44). New York: Wiley.

Ostfeld, A.M. (1980). A review of stroke epidemiology. *Epidemiological Reviews* 2: 136-152.

Ostrow, A.C. (1989). *Aging and motor behavior*. Indianapolis: Benchmark Press.

Ouslander, J.G. (1994). Nursing home care. In W.R. Hazzard, E.L. Bierman, J.P. Blass, W.H. Ettinger, and J.B. Halter (Eds.), *Principles of geriatric medicine and gerontology* (3rd ed., pp. 357-374). New York: McGraw-Hill.

Overend, T.J., Cunningham, D., Paterson, D.H., and Lefcoe, M.S. (1993). Anthropometric and computed tomographic assessment of the thigh in young and old men. *Canadian Journal of Applied Physiology* 18: 263-273.

Overstall, P.W. (1991). Falls. In M.S.J. Pathy (Ed.), *Principles and practice of geriatric medicine* (2nd ed., pp. 1231-1240). Chichester: Wiley.

Overstall, P.W., Exton-Smith, A.N., Imms, F.J., and Johnson, A.L. (1977). Falls in the elderly related to postural imbalance. *British Medical Journal* 1: 261-264.

Owens, J.F., Matthews, K.A., Wing, R.R., and Kuller, L.H. (1992). Can physical activity mitigate the effects of aging in middle-aged women? *Circulation* 85: 1265-1270.

Paffenbarger, R.S. (1988). Contributions of epidemiology to exercise science and cardiovascular health. *Medicine and Science in Sports and Exercise* 20: 426-438.

Paffenbarger, R.S., Hyde, R.T., Wing, A.L., Lee, I-M., Jung, D.L., and Kampert, J.B. (1993). The association of changes in physical activity level and other lifestyle characteristics with mortality among men. *New England Journal of Medicine* 328: 538-545.

Paffenbarger, R.S., Hyde, R.T., and Wing, A.L. (1987). Physical activity and incidence of cancer in diverse populations: A preliminary report. *American Journal of Clinical Nutrition*. 45: 312-317.

Paffenbarger, R.S., Hyde, R.T., Wing, A.L., Lee, I-M., and Kampert, J.B. (1994). Some interrelations of physical activity, physiological fitness, health and longevity. In C. Bouchard, R.J. Shephard, and T. Stephens (Eds.), *Physical activity, fitness and health* (pp. 119-133). Champaign, IL: Human Kinetics.

Page, L.B., Damon, A., and Moelleriag, R.C. (1974). Antecedents of cardiovascular disease in six Solomon Island societies. *Circulation* 49: 1132-1146.

Pahlavani, M.A., Cheung, T.H., Chesky, J.A., and Richardson, A. (1988). Influence of exercise on the immune function of rats of various ages. *Journal of Applied Physiology* 64: 1997-2001.

Painter, P.L. (1988). Exercise in end-stage renal disease. *Exercise and Sport Sciences Reviews* 16: 305-339.

Palmore, E.B., Fillenbaum, G.G., and George, L.K. (1984). Consequences of retirement. *Journals of Gerontology* 39: 109P-116P.

Pansu, D., and Bellaton, C. (1976). L'homéostase calcique chez le sujet agé [Calcium homeostasis in the elderly subject]. In H.P. Klotz (Ed.), *Les endocrines et l'homéostase calcique* (pp. 317-330). Paris: Expansion Scientifique Francaise.

Pantano, P., Baron, J.C., Lebrun-Grandie, P., Duquesnay, N., Bousser, M.G., and Comar, D. (1983). Effects of aging on regional CBF and CMRO2 in humans. *European Neurology* 22 (Suppl. 2): 24-31.

Panton, L.B., Graves, J.E., Pollock, M.L., Hagberg, J.M., and Chen, W. (1990). Effect of aerobic and resistance training on fractionated reaction time and speed of movement. *Journals of Gerontology* 45: M26-M31.

Panush, R.S. (1994). Physical activity, fitness and osteoarthritis. In C. Bouchard, R.J. Shephard, and T. Stephens (Eds.), *Physical activity, fitness and health* (pp. 712-723). Champaign, IL: Human Kinetics.

Panush, R.S., and Brown, D.G. (1987). Exercise and arthritis. *Sports Medicine* 4: 54-64.

Panush, R.S., and Inzinna, J.D. (1994). Recreational activities and degenerative joint disease. *Sports Medicine* 17: 1-5.

Pate, R.R., and Macera, C.A. (1994). Risks of exercising: Musculo-skeletal injuries. In C. Bouchard, R.J. Shephard, and T. Stephens (Eds.), *Physical activity, fitness and health* (pp. 1008-1018). Champaign, IL: Human Kinetics.

Pate, R.R., Pratt, M., Blair, S.N., Hookel, W.L., Macera, C.A., Bouchard, C., Buchner, D., Ettinger, W., Heath, G.W., King, A.C., Kriska, A., Leon, A.S., Marcus, B.H., Morris, J., Paffenbarger, R.S., Patrick, K., Pollock, M.L., Rippe, J.M., Sallis, J., and Wilmore, J.H. (1995). Physical activity and public health. A recommendation from the Centers for Disease Control and Prevention and the American College of Sports Medicine. *Journal of the American Medical Association* 273: 402-407.

Pate, R.R., Sargent, R., Baldwin, C., and Burgess, M. (1990). Dietary intake of women runners. *International Journal of Sports Medicine* 11: 461-466.

Paterson, D.H. (1992). Effects of ageing on the cardiovascular system. *Canadian Journal of Sport Sciences* 17: 171-177.

Paterson, D.H., Cunningham, D.A., and Babcock, M.A. (1989). On-kinetics in the elderly. In G.D. Swanson, F.S. Grodins, and R.C. Hughson (Eds.), *Respiratory Control* (pp. 171-178). New York: Plenum Press.

Patrick, D., and Deyo, R. (1989). Generic and disease-specific measures in assessing health status and quality of life. *Medical Care* 27: S217-S232.

Patrick, D.L., and Erickson, P. (1993). *Health status and health policy: Quality of life in health care evaluation and resource allocation.* New York: Oxford University Press.

Pavlou, K.N., Steffe, W.P., Lerman, R.H., and Burrows, B.A. (1985). Effects of dieting and exercise on lean body mass, oxygen uptake and strength. *Medicine and Science in Sports and Exercise* 17: 466-471.

Pawlson, L.G. (1994). Health care implications of an aging population. In W.R. Hazzard, E.L. Bierman, J.P. Blass, W.H. Ettinger, and J.B. Halter (Eds.), *Principles of geriatric medicine and gerontology* (3rd ed., pp. 167-176). New York: McGraw-Hill.

Payette, N., and Gray-Donald, K. (1994). Risk of malnutrition in an elderly population receiving home care services. *Facts and Research in Gerontology* (Suppl.: Nutrition, pp. 71-85). Paris: Serdi.

Pearlstein, E., Gold, L.I., and Garcia-Pardo, A. (1980). Fibronectine: A review of its structure and biological activity. *Molecular and Cellular Biochemistry* 29: 103-128.

Pekkanen, J., Marti, B., Nissinen, A., Tuomilehto, J., Punsar, S., and Karvonen, M.J. (1987). Reduction of premature mortality by high physical activity: A 20-year follow-up of middle-aged Finnish men. *Lancet* i: 1473-1477.

Penschow, J., and Mackay, I.R. (1980). NK and K cell activity of human blood: Differences according to sex, age and disease. *Annals of the Rheumatic Diseases* 39: 82-86.

Perk, J., and Hedback, B. (1988). Cost effectiveness of cardiac rehabilitation. *Proceedings of IV World Congress of Cardiac Rehabilitation*, Brisbane (p. 110). Canberra, Australia: National Heart Foundation of Australia.

Perkins, L.C., and Kaiser, H.L. (1961). Results of short-term isotonic and isometric exercise programs in persons over sixty. *Physical Therapy Review* 41: 633-635.

Perloff, J.J., McDermott, M.T., Perloff, K.G., Blue, P.W., Enzenhauer, R., Sieck, E., Chantelois, A.E., Dolbow, A., and Kidd, G.S. (1991). Reduced bone mineral content is a risk factor for hip fractures. *Orthopedic Review* 20: 690-698.

Perri, I.S., and Templar, D.I. (1984/1985). The effects of an aerobic exercise program on psychological variables in older adults. *International Journal of Aging and Human Development* 20: 167-172.

Perrier. (1979). *The Perrier Study: Fitness in America.* New York: Author.

Perry, B.C. (1982). Falls among the elderly: A review of the methods and conclusions of epidemiological studies. *Journal of the American Geriatric Society* 30: 367-371.

Perry, M.C. (1994). Lung cancer. In W.R. Hazzard, E.L. Bierman, J.P. Blass, W.H. Ettinger, and J.B. Halter (Eds.), *Principles and practice of geriatric medicine and gerontology* (3rd ed., pp. 607-613). Chichester: Wiley.

Peters, R.K., Garabrandt, D.H., Yu, M.C., and Mack, T.M. (1989). A case-control study of occupational and dietary factors in colorectal cancer in young men by subsite. *Cancer Research* 49: 5459-5468.

Philbin, E.F., Ries, M.D., and French, T.S. (1995). Feasibility of maximal cardiopulmonary exercise testing in patients with end-stage arthritis of the hip and knee prior to total joint arthroplasty. *Chest* 108: 174-181.

Phillips, P., Rolls, B., Ledingham, J.G., Forsling, M.L., Morton, J.H., Crowe, M.J., and Wollner, L. (1984). Reduced thirst after water deprivation in healthy elderly men. *New England Journal of Medicine* 311: 753-759.

Phillips, S., Fox, N., Jacobs, J., and Wright, W.E. (1988). The direct medical costs of osteoporosis for American women aged 45 and older, 1986. *Bone* 9: 271-279.

Pickering, T.G. (1993). Should age influence our choice of antihypertensive medications? *American Journal of Geriatric Cardiology* 2 (2): 10-17.

Piispa, M., and Huuhtanen, P. (1993). Attitudes of retired people on work. In J. Ilmarinen (Ed.), *Aging and work* (pp. 152-156). Helsinki: Institute for Occupational Health.

Pines, A., Fisman, E.Z., Levo, Y., Averbuch, M., Lidor, A., Drory, Y., Finkelstein, M., Hetman-Peri, M., Moshlowitz, M., Ben-Ari, E., and Ayalon, D. (1991). The effects of hormone replacement therapy in normal post-menopausal women: Measurements of Doppler-derived parameters of aortic flow. *American Journal of Obstetrics and Gynecology* 164: 806-812.

Pirke, K.M., Sinterman, R., and Vogt, H.J. (1980). Testosterone and testosterone precursors in the spermatic vein and in the testicular tissue of old men. *Gerontology* 26: 221-230.

Pocock, N.A., Eisman, J.A., Gwinn, T.H., Sambrook, P.N., Yeates, M.G., and Freund, J. (1988). Regional muscle strength, physical fitness and weight but not age predict femor bone mass [Abstract]. *Journal of Bone and Mineral Research* 3 (Suppl. 1): 584.

Pocock, N.A., Eisman, J.A., Sambrook, P.N., Yeates, M.G., Freund, J., and Guinn, T. (1987). Muscle strength and physical fitness in the determination of bone mass. *Journal of Bone and Mineral Research* 2(Suppl. 1). Abstract.

Pocock, N.A., Eisman, J.A., Yeates, M.G., Sambrook, P.N., and Eberl, S. (1986). Physical fitness is a major determinant of femoral neck and lumbar spine bone mineral density. *Journal of Clinical Investigation* 78: 618-621.

Poehlman, E.T. (1989). A review. Exercise and its influence on resting energy metabolism in man. *Medicine and Science in Sports and Exercise* 21: 515-525.

Poehlman, E.T., and Danforth, E. (1991). Endurance training increases metabolic rate and norepinephrine appearance rate in older individuals. *American Journal of Physiology* 24: E233-E239.

Poehlman, E.T., Gardner, A.W., Arciero, P.J., Goran, M.I., and Calles-Escandon, J. (1994). Effects of endurance training on total fat oxidation in elderly persons. *Journal of Applied Physiology* 76: 2281-2287.

Poehlman, E.T., Gardner, A.W., and Goran, M.I. (1992). Influence of endurance training on energy intake, norepinephrine kinetics, and metabolic rate in older individuals. *Metabolism* 41: 941-948.

Poehlman, E.T., McAuliffe, T.I., Van Houten, D.R., and Danforth, E. (1990). Influence of age and endurance training on metabolic rate and hormones in healthy men. *American Journal of Physiology* 259: E66-E72.

Poehlman, E.T., Melby, C.L., and Badylak, S.F. (1991). Relation of age and physical exercise status on metabolic rate in younger and older healthy men. *Journals of Gerontology* 46: B54-B58.

Poehlman, E.T., Rosen, C.J., and Copeland, K.C. (1994). The influence of endurance training on insulin-like growth factor-1 in older individuals. *Metabolism* 43: 1401-1405.

Poirier, J., and Finch, C. (1994). Neurochemistry of the aging human brain. In W.R. Hazzard, E.L. Bierman, J.P. Blass, W.H. Ettinger, and J.B. Halter (Eds.), *Principles of geriatric medicine and gerontology* (3rd ed., pp. 1005-1012). New York: McGraw-Hill.

Poitrenaud, J., Bourlière, F., and Vallery-Masson, J. (1982) Conséquences de la retraite sur la santé [Health consequences of retirement] (pp. 343-354). In F. Bourlière (Ed.), *Gérontologie: Biologie et clinique*. Paris: Flammarion.

Poitrenaud, J., Vallery-Masson, J., Darcet, P., Barrere, H., Derriennic, F., and Guez, D. (1994). Sources of individual differences in cognitive aging: A longitudinal study of an elderly French managerial population. *Facts and research in gerontology* (pp. 35-50). Paris: Serdi.

Pokorny, M.L.L., Blom, D.H.J., and Van Leeuwen, P. (1987). Shifts, duration of work and accident risk of bus drivers. *Ergonomics* 30: 61-88.

Polednak, A.P. (1976). College athletics, body size and cancer mortality. *Cancer* 38: 382-387.

Polinsky, R.J., Kopin, I.J., Ebert, M.H., and Weise, V. (1981). Pharmacologic distinction of different orthostatic hypotension syndromes. *Neurology* 31: 1-7.

Pollock, C.L. (1992). Breaking the risk of falls: An exercise benefit for older patients. *Physician and Sportsmedicine* 20 (11): 147-156.

Pollock, M.L. (1974). Physiological characteristics of older champion track athletes. *Research Quarterly* 45: 363-373.

Pollock, M.L. (1988). Exercise prescription for the elderly. In W.W. Spirduso and H.M. Eckert (Eds.), *Physical activity and aging* (pp. 163-174). Champaign, IL: Human Kinetics.

Pollock, M.L., Carroll, J.F., Graves, J.E., Leggett, S.H., Braith, R.W., Limacker, M., and Hagberg, J.M. (1991). Injuries and adherence to walk/jog and resistance training programs in the elderly. *Medicine and Science in Sports and Exercise* 23: 1194-1200.

Pollock, M.L., Foster, C., Knapp, D., Rod, J.I., and Schmidt, D.H. (1987). Effect of age and training on aerobic capacity and body composition of master athletes. *Journal of Applied Physiology* 62: 725-731.

Pollock, M.L., Gettman, L.R., Milesis, C.A., Bah, M.D., Durstine, L., and Johnson, R.B. (1977). Effects of frequency and duration of training on attrition and incidence of injury. *Medicine and Science in Sports and Exercise* 9: 31-36.

Pollock, M.L., Miller, H.S., Linnerud, A.C., Royster, C.L., Smith, W.E., and Sonner, W.E. (1974). Physiological characteristics of champion American track athletes 40-75 years of age. *Journal of Gerontology* 29: 645-649.

Pomrehn, P., Wallace, R., and Burmeister, L. (1982). Ischemic heart disease mortality in Iowa farmers. The influence of lifestyle. *Journal of the American Medical Association* 248: 1073-1076.

Ponichtera-Mulcare, J.A. (1993). Exercise and multiple sclerosis. *Medicine and Science in Sports and Exercise* 25: 451-465.

Poon, L.W. (1985). Differences in human memory with aging: Nature, causes, and clinical implications. In J.E. Birren and K.W. Schaie (Eds.), *Handbook of the psychology of aging* (pp. 427-462). New York: Van Nostrand Reinhold.

Poor, G., Jacobsen, S.J., and Melton, L.J. (1994). Mortality following hip fracture. *Facts and research in gerontology* (pp. 91-109). Paris: Serdi.

Pope, A.M., and Tarlov, A.R. (1991). *Disability in America: Towards a national agenda for prevention.* Washington, DC: Institute of Medicine, National Academy Press.

Port, S., Cobb, F.R., Coleman, R.E., and Jones, R.H. (1980). Effect of age on the response of the left ventricular ejection fraction to exercise. *New England Journal of Medicine* 303: 1133-1137.

Port, S., McEwan, P., Cobb, F.R., and Jones, R.H. (1981). Influence of resting left ventricular function on the left ventricular response to exercise in patients with coronary artery disease. *Circulation* 63: 856-863.

Posner, J.D., Gorman, K.M., Gitlin, L.N., Sands, L.P., Kleban, M., Windsor, L., and Shaw, C. (1990). Effects of exercise training in the elderly on the occurrence and time to onset of cardiovascular diagnoses. *Journal of the American Geriatric Society* 38: 205-210.

Posner, J.D., Gorman, K.M., Windsor-Landsberg, L., Larsen, J., Bleiman, M., Shaw, C., Rosenberg, B., and Knebl, J. (1992). Low to moderate intensity endurance training in healthy older adults: Physiological responses after four months. *Journal of the American Geriatric Society* 40: 1-7.

Poulin, M.J., Cunningham, D.A., Paterson, D.H., Rechnitzer, P.A., Ecclestone, N.A., and Koval, J.J. (1994). *American Journal of Respiratory and Critical Care Medicine* 149: 408-415.

Poulin, M.J., Vandervoort, A.A., Paterson, D.H., Kramer, J.F., and Cunningham, D. (1992). Eccentric and concentric torques of knee and elbow extension in young and older men. *Canadian Journal of Sport Sciences* 17: 3-7.

Powell, K.E., Stephens, T., Marti, B., Heinemann, L., and Kreuter, M. (1991). Progress and problems in the promotion of physical activity. In O. Pekka and R. Telama (Eds.), *Sport for all* (pp. 55-73). Amsterdam: Elsevier.

Powell, K.E., Thompson, P.D., Caspersen, C.J., and Kendrick, J.S. (1987). Physical activity and the incidence of coronary heart disease. *Annual Reviews of Public Health* 8: 253-287.

Pratley, R., Niclas, B., Rubin, M., Miller, J., Smith, A., Smith, M., Hurley, B., and Goldberg, A. (1994). Strength training increases resting metabolic rate and norepinephrine levels in healthy 50- to 65-yr-old men. *Journal of Applied Physiology* 76: 133-137.

Pratley, R.E., Hagberg, J.M., Rogus, E.M., and Goldberg, A.P. (1995). Enhanced insulin sensitivity and lower waist-to-hip ratio in master athletes. *American Journal of Physiology* 268: E484-E490.

Préfaut, C., Anselme, F., Caillaud, C., and Massé-Biron, J. (1994). Exercise-induced hypoxemia in older athletes. *Journal of Applied Physiology* 76: 120-126.

Prince, R.L., Smith, M., Dick, I.M., Price, R.I., Webb, P.G., Henderson, N.K., and Harris, M.M. (1991). Prevention of post-menopausal osteoporosis: A comparative study of exercise, calcium supplementation, and hormone replacement therapy. *New England Journal of Medicine* 325: 1189-1195.

Probart, C.K., Notelovitz, M., Martin, D., Khan, F.Y., and Fields, C. (1991). The effect of moderate aerobic exercise on physical fitness among women 70 years and older. *Maturitas* 14: 49-56.

Province, M.A., Hadley, E.C., Hornbrook, M.C., Lipsitz, L.A., Miller, P.J., Mulrow, C.D., Ory, M.G., Sattin, R.W., Tinetti, M.E., and Wolf, S.L. (1995). The effects of exercise on falls in elderly patients. A preplanned meta-analysis of the FICSIT Trials. *Journal of the American Medical Association* 273: 1341-1347.

Puggaard, L., Pedersen, H.P., Sandager, E., and Klitgaard, H. (1994). Physical conditioning in elderly people. *Scandinavian Journal of Medicine, Science and Sports* 4: 47-56.

Pullar, T., and Wright, V. (1991). Diseases of the joints. In M.S.J. Pathy (Ed.), *Principles and practice of geriatric medicine* (2nd ed., pp. 1237-1274). Chichester: Wiley.

Puranen, J., Ala-Ketola, L., Peltokalleo, P., and Saarela, J. (1975). Running and primary osteoarthritis of the hip. *British Medical Journal* 1: 424-425.

Purslow, P.P. (1989). Strain-induced reorientation of an intramuscular connective tissue network: Implications for passive muscle elasticity. *Journal of Biomechanics* 22: 21-31.

Pyka, G., Lindenberger, E., Charette, S., and Marcus, R. (1994). Muscle strength and fiber adaptations to a year-long resistance training program in elderly men and women. *Journals of Gerontology* 49: M22-M27.

Pyykkö, I., Aalto, H., Hytönen, M., Starck, J., Jäntti, P., and Ramsay, H. (1988). Effect of age on postural control. In B. Amblard, A. Berthoz, and F. Clarac (Eds.), *Posture and gait. Development, adaptation and modulation* (pp. 95-104). Amsterdam: Elsevier.

Quaglietti, S., and Froelicher, V. (1994). Physical activity and cardiac rehabilitation for patients with coronary heart disease. In C. Bouchard, R.J. Shephard, and T. Stephens (Eds.), *Physical activity, fitness and health* (pp. 591-608). Champaign, IL: Human Kinetics.

Quetelet, A. (1835). *Sur l'homme et le développement de ses facultés* [On man, and the development of his faculties]. Paris: Bachelier Imprimeur-Libraire.

Radin, E.L., and Rose, R.M. (1986). Role of subchondral bone in the initiation and progression of cartilage damage. *Clinics in Orthopedics* 213: 34-40.

Ragheb, M.G., and Griffith, C.A. (1982). The contribution of leisure participation and leisure satisfaction to life satisfaction of older persons. *Journal of Leisure Research* 14: 295-306.

Räihä, I.J., Piha, S.J., Seppänen, A., Puukka, P., and Sourander, L.B. (1994). Predictive value of continuous ambulatory electrocardiographic monitoring in elderly people. *British Medical Journal* 309: 1263-1267.

Rakowski, W., and Mor, V. (1992). The association of physical activity with mortality among older adults in the longitudinal study of aging (1984-1988). *Journals of Gerontology* 47: M122-M129.

Ramaiya, K.L., Swai, A.B., McLarty, D.G., and Alberti, K.G. (1991). Impaired glucose tolerance and diabetes mellitus in Hindu Indian immigrants in Dar es Salaam. *Diabetic Medicine* 8: 738-774.

Ramlow, J.M., and Kuller, J.H. (1990). Effects of the summer heat wave of 1988 on daily mortality in Allegheny County, PA. *Public Health Reports* 105: 283-289.

Ramsdale, S.J., Bassey, E.J., and Pye, D.W. (1994). Dietary calcium intake relates to bone mineral density in premenopausal women. *British Journal of Nutrition* 71: 77-84.

Rautanen, T., Sipilä, S., and Suominen, H. (1993). Muscle strength and history of heavy manual work among elderly trained women and randomly chosen sample population. *European Journal of Applied Physiology* 66: 514-517.

Ravussin, E., Valencia, M.E., Schult, L.O., Esparza, J., and Bennett, P.H. (1992). Effect of a traditional lifestyle on the physical and metabolic characteristics of Pima Indians living in Northern Mexico. *Diabetes* 41: Abstract No. 2.

Ray, W.A., Federspiel, C.F., Baugh, D.K., and Dodds, S. (1987). Impact of growing numbers of the very old on Medicaid expenditures for nursing homes. A multi-state, population-based analysis. *American Journal of Public Health* 77: 699-703.

Ray, W.A., Griffin, M.R., and Downey, W. (1989). Benzodiazepines of long and short elimination half-life and the risk of hip fracture. *Journal of the American Medical Association* 362: 3303-3307.

Reading, J.L., Goodman, J.M., Plyley, M.J., Floras, J.S., Liu, P.P., and Shephard, R.J. (1993). Vascular conductance and aerobic power in sedentary and active subjects and heart failure patients. *Journal of Applied Physiology* 74: 567-573.

Reardon, J., Patel, K., and ZuWallack, R.L. (1993). Improvement in quality of life is unrelated to improvement in exercise endurance after outpatient pulmonary rehabilitation. *Journal of Cardiopulmonary Rehabilitation* 13: 51-54.

Reaven, P.D. (1995). Insulin resistance and aging: Modulation by obesity and physical activity. In D.R. Lamb, C.V. Gisolfi, and E. Nadel (Eds.), *Perspectives in exercise science and sports medicine: Vol. 8. Exercise in older adults* (pp. 395-434). Carmel, IN: Cooper.

Reaven, P.D., Barrett-Connor, E., and Edelstein, S. (1991). Relation between leisure-time physical activity and blood pressure in older women. *Circulation* 83: 559-565.

Reaven, P.D., McPhillips, J.B., Barrett-Connor, E., and Criqui, M.H. (1990). Leisure time exercise and lipid and lipoprotein levels in an older population. *Journal of the American Geriatric Society* 38: 847-854.

Reddan, W.G. (1985). Body fluid and thermal regulation with age. *Topics in Geriatric Rehabilitation* 1: 40-48.

Reed, R.L., Hartog, R., Yochum, K., Pearlmutter, L., Ruttinger, C., and Mooradian, A.D. (1993). A comparison of hand-held isometric strength measurement with isokinetic muscle strength measurement in the elderly. *Journal of the American Geriatric Society* 41: 53-56.

Reed, R.L., Pearlmutter, L., Yochum, K., Meredith, K.E., and Mooradian, A.D. (1991). The relationship between muscle mass and muscle strength in the elderly. *Journal of the American Geriatric Society* 39: 555-561.

Reeder, B.A. (1991). *Cardiovascular disease in Canada 1991* (pp. 1-34). Ottawa, ON: Heart and Stroke Foundation of Canada.

Regensteiner, J.G. (1991). Relationship between habitual physical activity and insulin levels among non-diabetic men and women. San Luis Valley diabetes study. *Diabetes Care* 14: 1066-1074.

Reinsch, S., MacRae, P., Lachenbruch, P.A., and Tobis, J.S. (1992). Attempts to prevent falls and injury: A prospective community study. *Gerontologist* 32: 450-456.

Reiser, K.M., Hennesy, S.M., and Last, J.A. (1987). Analysis of age-associated changes in collagen cross-linking in the skin and lung in monkeys and rats. *Biochemica et Biophysica Acta* 926: 339-348.

Rejeski, W.J., Brawley, L.R., and Shumaker, S.A. (1996). Relationships between physical activity and health-related quality of life. *Exercise and Sport Sciences Reviews* 24: 71-108.

Reker, G.T., and Wong, P.T.P. (1984). Psychological and physical well-being in the elderly: The perceived well-being scale (PWB). *Canadian Journal on Aging* 3: 23-32.

Renold, A.E. (1981). Epidemiological considerations of overweight and obesity. In G. Enzi, G. Crepaldi, G. Pozza, and A.E. Renold (Eds.), *Obesity: Pathogenesis and treatment* (pp. 1-6). London: Academic Press.

Reuben, D.B., Laliberte, L., Hiris, J., and Mor, V. (1990). A hierarchical exercise scale to measure function at the Advanced Activities of Daily Living (AADL) level. *Journal of the American Geriatric Society* 38: 855-861.

Rice, C.L., Cunningham, D.A., Paterson, D.H., and Lefcoe, M.S. (1989). Arm and leg composition determined by computed tomography in young and elderly men. *Clinical Physiology* 9: 207-220.

Rice, D.P., Hodgson, T.A., and Kopstein, A.N. (1985). The economic costs of illness: A replication and update. *Health Care Financing Review* 7: 61-80.

Richardson, M.L., Genant, H.K., Cann, C.E., Ettinger, B., Gordan, G.S., Kolb, F.O., and Reiser, U.J. (1985). Assessment of metabolic bone disease by quantitative computed tomography. *Clinics in Orthopedics* 195: 224-238.

Riddick, C.C., and Daniel, S.N. (1984). The relative contribution of leisure activities and other factors to the mental health of older women. *Journal of Leisure Research* 16: 136-148.

Rider, R.A., and Daly, J. (1991). Effects of flexibility training on enhancing spinal mobility in older women. *Journal of Sports Medicine and Physical Fitness* 31: 213-217.

Ries, W. (1994). The determination of biological age. In A.K. Balin (Ed.), *Practical handbook of biologic age determination* (pp. 173-180). Boca Raton, FL: CRC Press.

Riggs, B.L., and Melton, L.J. (1992). The prevention and treatment of osteoporosis. *New England Journal of Medicine* 327: 620-627.

Riggs, B.L., Wahner, H.W., Seeman, E., Offord, K.P., Dunn, W.L., Mazess, R.B., Johnson, K.A., and Melton, L.J. (1982). Changes in bone mineral density of the proximal femur with aging: Differences between the postmenopausal and senile osteoporosis syndromes. *Journal of Clinical Investigation* 70: 716-723.

Rikli, R.E., and Edwards, D.J. (1991). Effects of a three year exercise program on motor function and cognitive processing speed in older women. *Research Quarterly* 62: 61-67.

Rikli, R.E., and McManis, B.G. (1990). Effects of exercise on bone mineral content in post-menopausal women. *Research Quarterly* 61: 243-249.

Rinne, J. (1987). Muscarinic and dopaminergic receptors in aging human brain. *Brain Research* 404: 161-168.

Rissanen, A., Heliovaraa, M., Kneckt, P., Reunanen, A., and Aromaa, A. (1991). Determinant of weight gain and overweight in adult Finns. *European Journal of Clinical Nutrition* 45: 419-430.

Rivera, A.M., Pels, E.A., Sady, S.P., Cullinane, E.M., and Thompson, P.D. (1989). Physiological factors associated with the lower maximal oxygen consumption of masters runners. *Journal of Applied Physiology* 66: 949-954.

Rivlin, R.S. (1981). Nutrition and aging: Some unanswered questions. *American Journal of Medicine* 71: 337-340.

Road, J.D., Newman, S., Derenne, J.P., and Grassino, A. (1986). The in vivo length-force relationship of the canine diaphragm. *Journal of Applied Physiology* 60: 63-70.

Robert, L. (1982). Vieillissement de la matrice intercellulaire [Aging of the intercellular matrix]. In F. Bourlière (Ed.), *Gérontologie: Biologie et clinique* (pp. 26-36). Paris: Flammarion.

Roberts, B.L. (1989). Effects of walking on balance among elders. *Nursing Research* 38: 180-182.

Roberts, B.L. (1990). Effects of walking on reaction and movement times among elders. *Perceptual and Motor Skills* 71: 131-140.

Robertson, H.T., Haley, N.R., Guthrie, M., Cardenas, D., Eschbach, J.W., and Adamson, J.W. (1990). Recombinant erythropoietin improves exercise capacity in anemic hemodialysis patients. *American Journal of Kidney Diseases* (Duluth) 16: 325-332.

Robertson-Tschabo, E., and Arenberg, D. (1985). Mental function and aging. In R. Andres, E.L. Bierman, and W.R. Hazzard (Eds.), *Principles of geriatric medicine* (pp. 129-140). New York: McGraw-Hill.

Robine, J.M., and Ritchie, K. (1991). Healthy life expectancy: Evaluation of global indicator of change in population health. *British Medical Journal* 302: 457-460.

Robinson, K., and Mulcahy, R. (1986). Return to employment of professional drivers following myocardial infarction. *Irish Medical Journal* 79: 31-34.

Robinson, P.K., Livingston, J., and Birren, J. (1985). *Aging and Technological Advances*. New York: Plenum Press.

Roche, A.F. (1994). Sarcopenia: A critical review of its measurements and health-related significance in the middle-aged and elderly. *American Journal of Human Biology* 6: 33-42.

Rode, A., and Shephard, R.J. (1994a). The aging of lung function: Cross-sectional and longitudinal studies of an Inuit population. *European Respiratory Journal* 7: 1653-1659.

Rode, A., and Shephard, R.J. (1994b). Secular and age trends in the height of adults among a Canadian Inuit community. *Arctic Medical Research* 53: 18-24.

Rode, A., and Shephard, R.J. (1995a). Body fat distribution and other cardiac risk factors among circumpolar Inuit and nGanasan. *Arctic Medical Research* 54: 125-133.

Rode, A., and Shephard, R.J. (1995b). Basal metabolic rate of the Inuit. *American Journal of Human Biology* 7: 723-729.

Rode, A., and Shephard, R.J. (1996). Lung volumes of Igloolik Inuit and Volochanka nGanasan. *Arctic Medical Research* 55: 4-13.

Rode, A., Shephard, R.J., Vloshinsky, P.E., and Kuksis, A. (1995). Plasma fatty acid profiles of Canadian Inuit and Siberian nGanasan. *Arctic Medical Research* 54: 10-20.

Rodeheffer, R.J., Gerstenblith, G., Becker, L.C., Fleg, J.L., Weisfeldt, M.L., and Lakatta, E.G. (1984). Exercise cardiac output is maintained with advancing age in healthy human subjects. Cardiac dilatation and increased stroke volume compensate for a diminished heart rate. *Circulation* 69: 203-213.

Rogers, H.B., Schroeder, T., Secher, N.H., and Mitchell, J.H. (1990). Cerebral blood flow during static exercise in humans. *Journal of Applied Physiology* 68: 2358-2361.

Rogers, M.A. (1989). Acute effects of exercise on glucose tolerance in non-insulin dependent diabetics. *Medicine and Science in Sports and Exercise* 21: 362-368.

Rogers, M.A., and Evans, W.J. (1993). Changes in skeletal muscle with aging: Effects of exercise training. *Exercise and Sport Sciences Reviews* 21: 65-102.

Rogers, M.A., Hagberg, J.M., Martin, W.H., Ehsani, A.A., and Holloszy, J.O. (1990). Decline in $\dot{V}O_2$max with aging in masters athletes and sedentary men. *Journal of Applied Physiology* 68: 2195-2199.

Roghmann, K.J. (1987). Immune response of elderly patients to pneumococcus. *Journals of Gerontology* 42: 265B-270B.

Rogol, A.D., Weltman, J.Y., Evans, W.S., Veldhuis, J.D., and Weltman, A.L. (1992). Long-term endurance training alters the hypothalamic-pituitary axes for gonadotrophins and growth hormone. *Endocrinology and Metabolism Clinics of North America* (Philadelphia) 21: 817-832.

Rokaw, S.M., Detels, R., Coulson, A.H., Sayre, J.W., Tashkin, D.P., Allwright, S.S., and Massey, F.J. (1980). The UCLA population studies of chronic obstructive respiratory disease. *Chest* 78: 252-262.

Roland, M., and Morris, R. (1983). A study of the natural history of back pain. 1. Development of a reliable and sensitive measure of disability in low back pain. *Spine* 8: 141-144.

Rosano, G.M.C., Sarrel, P.M., Poole-Wilson, P.A., and Collins, P. (1993). Beneficial effects of estrogen on exercise-induced myocardial ischemia in women with coronary artery disease. *Lancet* 342: 133-136.

Rose, M.R., and Graves, J.L. (1989). What evolutionary biology can do for gerontology. *Journals of Gerontology* 44: B27-B29.

Rosenberg, E. (1986). Sport voluntary association involvement and happiness among middle-aged and elderly Americans. In B. McPherson (Ed.), *Sport and aging* (pp. 45-52). Champaign, IL: Human Kinetics.

Ross, D.L., Grabeau, G.M., Smith, S., Seymour, M., Knierim, N., and Pitetti, K.H. (1989). Efficacy of exercise for end-stage renal disease patients immediately following high-efficiency hemodialysis: A pilot study. *American Journal of Nephrology* 9: 376-383.

Rossman, I. (1977). Anatomic and body composition changes with aging. In C.E. Finch and L. Hayflick (Eds.), *Handbook of the biology of aging* (pp. 189-221). New York: Van Nostrand Reinhold.

Rothstein, M. (1987). Evidence for and against the error catastrophe hypothesis. In H.R. Warner, R.N. Butler, R.L. Sprott, and E.L. Schneider (Eds.), *Modern biological theories of aging* (pp. 139-154). New York: Raven Press.

Rothstein, M. (1990). Altered proteins, errors and aging. In H.L. Segal, M. Rothstein, and E. Bergamini (Eds.), *Protein metabolism in aging* (pp. 3-14). New York: Wiley-Liss.

Rowe, J.W. (1985). Alterations in renal function. In R. Andres, E.L. Bierman, and W.R. Hazzard (Eds.), *Principles of geriatric medicine* (pp. 319-324). New York: McGraw-Hill.

Rowe, J.W., Andres, R., Tobin, J.D., Norris, A.H., and Shock, N.W. (1976). The effect of age on creatinine clearance in men: A cross-sectional and longitudinal study. *Journal of Gerontology* 31: 155-163.

Rowe, J.W., and Troen, B.R. (1980). Sympathetic nervous system and aging in man. *Endocrinology Reviews* 1: 167-179.

Rozanski, A., Diamond, G.A., Forrester, J.S., Berman, D.S., Morris, D., and Swan, H.J. (1984). Alternative referent standards for cardiac normality. *Annals of Internal Medicine* 101: 164-171.

Rubenstein, L.Z., and Josephson, K.R. (1993). Epidemiology and prevention of falls in the nursing home. In H.M. Perry, J.E. Morley, and R.M. Coe (Eds.), *Aging and musculoskeletal disorders* (pp. 123-146). New York: Springer.

Rubenstein, L.Z., Robbins, A.S., Schulman, B.L., Rosado, J., Osterweil, D., and Joseph-son, K.R. (1988). Falls and instability in the elderly. *Journal of the American Geriatric Society* 36: 226-278.

Rubenstein, L.Z., Schairer, C., Wieland, G.D., and Kane, R. (1984). Systematic biases in functional status assessment of elderly adults. Effects of different data sources. *Journals of Gerontology* 39: 686M-691M.

Rubin, C.T., Bain, S.D., and McLeod, K.J. (1992). Suppression of the osteogenic re-sponse in the aging skeleton. *Calcified Tissue International* 50: 306-313.

Rubin, S.M., Sidney, S., Black, D.M., Browner, W.S., Hulley, S.B., and Cummings, S.R. (1990). High blood cholesterol in elderly men and the excess risk for coronary heart disease. *Annals of Internal Medicine* 113: 916-920.

Rudman, D. (1985). Growth hormone, body composition and aging. *Journal of the American Geriatric Society* 33: 800-807.

Rudman, D., Feller, A.G., Cohn, L., Shetty, K.R., Caindec, N., and Rudman, I.W. (1993). Growth hormone in elderly men. In H.M. Perry, J.E. Morley, and R.M. Coe (Eds.), *Aging and musculoskeletal disorders* (pp. 267-279). New York: Springer.

Rudman, D., Feller, A.G., Ngraj, H.S., Gergans, G.A., Lalitha, P.Y., Goldberg, A.F., Schlenker, R.A., Cohn, L., Rudman, I.W., and Mattson, D.E. (1990). Effects of hu-man growth hormone in men over 60 years old. *New England Journal of Medicine* 323: 1-6.

Ruegsegger, P., Dambacher, M.A., Ruegsegger, E., Fischer, J.A., and Anliker, M. (1984). Bone loss in premenopausal and postmenopausal women. *Journal of Bone and Joint Surgery* 66A: 1015-1023.

Rundgren, A., Aniansson, A., Ljungberg, P., and Wetterqvist, H. (1984). Effects of a training programme for elderly people on mineral content of the heel bone. *Ar-chives of Gerontology and Geriatrics* 3: 243-248.

Russell, E.S. (1978). Genes and aging. In J.A. Behnke, C.E. Finch, and G.B. Moment (Eds.), *The biology of aging* (pp. 235-245). New York: Plenum Press.

Rutenfranz, J., Ilmarinen, J., Klimmer, F., and Kylian, H. (1990). Work load and de-manded physical work capacity under different industrial working conditions. In Kaneko, M. (Ed.), *Fitness for the aged, disabled, and industrial worker* (pp. 217-238). Champaign, IL: Human Kinetics.

Rutenfranz, J., Klimmer, F., and Ilmarinen, J. (1982). Arbeitsphysiologische Uberlegungen zur Beschaftigung von wiblicher Jugendlichen und Frauen im Bauhauptgewerbe [Work physiology considerations in the employment of young-sters and women in heavy industry]. *Arbeitsmedizin, Sozialmedizin und Präventivemedizin* 70: 1-48.

Ryan, M. (1988). Life expectancy and mortality data from the Soviet Union. *British Medical Journal* 296: 1513-1515.

Sacher, G.A. (1982). Evolutionary theory in gerontology. *Perspectives in Biology and Medicine* 25: 339-353.

Sachs, C., Hamberger, B., and Kaijser, L. (1985). Cardiovascular responses and plasma catecholamines in old age. *Clinical Physiology* 5: 553-565.

Safran, M.R., Seaber, A.V., and Garrett, W.E. (1989). Warm-up and muscular injury prevention: An update. *Sports Medicine* 8: 239-249.

Salk, D., Fujiwara, Y., and Martin, G.M. (1985). *Werner's syndrome and human aging*. New York: Plenum Press.

Sallis, J.F., Haskell, W.L., Wood, P.D., Fortmann, S.P., Rogers, T., Blair, S.N., and Paffenbarger, R.S. (1985). Physical activity assessment methodology in the five city project. *American Journal of Epidemiology* 121: 91-106.

Salminen, S. (1993). Aging and occupational safety. In J. Ilmarinen (Ed.), *Aging and work* (pp. 209-214). Helsinki: Institute for Occupational Health.

Salthouse, T.A. (1982). *Adult Cognition: An experimental psychology of human aging.* New York: Springer-Verlag.

Saltin, B. (1986). Physiological characteristics of the masters athlete. In J.R. Sutton and R.M. Brock (Eds.), *Sports medicine for the mature athlete* (pp. 59-80). Indianapolis: Benchmark Press.

Saltin, B., and Grimby, G. (1968). Physiological analysis of middle-aged and old former athletes. Comparison of still active athletes of the same ages. *Circulation* 38: 1104-1115.

Sandler, R.B. (1989). Muscle strength assessments and the prevention of osteoporosis: A hypothesis. *Journal of the American Geriatric Society* 37: 1192-1197.

Sandler, R.B., Burdett, R., Zaleskiewicz, M., Sprowls-Repcheck, C., and Harwell, M. (1991). Muscle strength as an indicator of the habitual level of physical activity. *Medicine and Science in Sports and Exercise* 23: 1375-1381.

Sans, S. (1993). Risk factor prevalence from the WHO-MONICA project. *Canadian Journal of Cardiology* 9 (Suppl. D): 85D-86D.

Sara, V.R., and Hall, K. (1990). Insulin-like growth factors and their binding proteins. *Physiological Reviews* 70: 591-613.

Sarafino, E.P. (1994). *Health psychology: Biopsychosocial interactions.* New York: Wiley.

Sarna, S., and Kaprio, J. (1994). Life expectancy of former athletes. *Sports Medicine* 17: 149-151.

Sato, T., Fuse, A., and Kuwata, T. (1979). Enhancement by interferon of natural cytotoxic activities of lymphocytes from human cord blood and peripheral blood of aged persons. *Cellular Immunology* 45: 458-463.

Scarpace, P.J. (1986). Decreased beta-adrenergic responsiveness during senescence. *Federation Proceedings* 45: 51-54.

Scarpace, P.J., Lowenthal, D.T., and Tümer, N. (1992). Influence of exercise and age on myocardial beta-adrenergic receptor properties. *Experimental Gerontology* 27: 169-177.

Scarpace, P.J., Mader, S.L., and Tümer, N. (1993). Adrenergic receptors: Implications for falls. In H.M. Perry, J.E. Morley, and R.M. Coe (Eds.), *Aging and musculoskeletal disorders* (pp. 147-166). New York: Springer.

Schaie, K.W. (1989). Perceptual speed in adulthood: Cross-sectional and longitudinal studies. *Psychology and Aging* 4: 443-453.

Schauffler, H.H., Agostino, R.B., and Kannel, W.B. (1993). Risk for cardiovascular disease in the elderly and associated Medicare costs: The Framingham Study. *American Journal of Preventive Medicine* 9: 146-154.

Schiffman, S.S., and Gatlin, C.A. (1993). Clinical physiology of taste and smell. *Annual Reviews of Nutrition* 13: 405-436.

Schmidt, R.A. (1987). *Motor control and learning* (2nd ed.). Champaign, IL: Human Kinetics.

Schneider, S.H., Amorosa, L.F., Clemow, L., Khachadurian, A.V., and Ruderman, N.B. (1992). Ten-year experience with an exercise-based outpatient lifestyle modification program in the treatment of diabetes mellitus. *Diabetes Care* 15: 1800-1809.

Schols, A.M.W., Mostert, R., Soeters, P.B., and Wouters, E.F.M. (1991). Body composition and exercise performance in patients with chronic obstructive pulmonary disease. *Thorax* 46: 695-699.

Schroots, J.J.F. (1991). Metaphors of aging and complexity. In G.M. Kenyon, J.E. Birren, and J.J.F. Schroots (Eds.), *Metaphors of aging in science and the humanities* (pp. 219-244). New York: Springer.

Schroots, J.J.F., Birren, J.E., and Kenyon, G.M. (1991). Metaphors of aging: An overview. In G.M. Kenyon, J.E. Birren, and J.J.F. Schroots (Eds.), *Metaphors of aging in science and the humanities* (pp. 1-16). New York: Springer.

Schulman, S.P., Lakatta, E.G., Fleg, J.L., Lakatta, L. Becker, L.C., and Gerstenblith, G. (1992). Age-related decline in left ventricular filling at rest and exercise. *American Journal of Physiology* 263: H1932-H1938.

Schultz, E., and Lipton, B.H. (1982). Skeletal muscle satellite cells: Changes in proliferative potential as a function of age. *Mechanisms in Ageing and Development* 20: 377-383.

Schulz, R., and Curnow, C. (1988). Peak performance and age among superathletes: Track and field, swimming, baseball, tennis and golf. *Journals of Gerontology* 43: P113-P120.

Schuster, E.H., and Bulkley, B.H. (1980). Ischemic cardiomyopathy: A clinico-pathological study of fourteen patients. *American Heart Journal* 100: 506-512.

Schwartz, R.S., Cain, K.C., Shuman, W.P., Larson, V., Stratton, J.S., Beard, J.C., Kahn, S.E., Cerquiera, M.D., and Abrass, I.B. (1992). Effect of intensive endurance training on lipoprotein profiles in young and older men. *Metabolism* 41: 649-654.

Schwartz, R.S., Shuman, W.P., Larson, V., Cain, K.C., Fellingham, G.W., Beard, J.C., Kahn, S.E., Stratton, J.R., Cerquiera, M.D., and Abrass, I.B. (1991). The effect of intensive endurance training on body fat distribution in young and older men. *Metabolism* 40: 545-551.

Scottish Health Service (1981). *Scottish health statistics, 1979.* Edinburgh: Her Majesty's Stationery Office.

Seals, D.R., Hagberg, J.M., Allen, W.K., Hurley, B.F., Dalsky, G.P., Ehsani, A.A., and Holloszy, J.O. (1984). Glucose tolerance in young and older athletes and sedentary men. *Journal of Applied Physiology* 56: 1521-1525.

Seals, D.R., Hagberg, J.M., Hurley, B.F., Ehsani, A.A., and Holloszy, J.O. (1984a). Effects of endurance training on glucose tolerance and plasma lipid levels in older men and women. *Journal of the American Medical Association* 252: 645-649.

Seals, D.R., Hagberg, J.M., Hurley, B.F., Ehsani, A.A., and Holloszy, J.O. (1984b). Endurance training in older men and women. I. Cardiovascular responses to exercise. *Journal of Applied Physiology* 57: 1024-1029.

Seals, D.R., Hagberg, J.M., Spina, R.J., Rogers, K.B., Schectman, K.B., and Ehsani, A.A. (1994). Enhanced left ventricular performance in endurance trained older men. *Circulation* 89: 198-205.

Seals, D.R., Taylor, J.A., Ng, A.V., and Esler, M.D. (1994). Exercise and aging: Autonomic control of the circulation. *Medicine and Science in Sports and Exercise* 26: 568-576.

Sedgwick, A.W., Taplin, R.E., Davidson, A.H., and Thomas, D.W. (1988). Effects of physical activity on risk factors for coronary heart disease in previously sedentary women: A five-year longitudinal study. *Australia and New Zealand Journal of Medicine* 18: 600-605.

Seely, S. (1990). The gender gap: Why do women live longer than men? *International Journal of Cardiology* 29: 113-119.

Segal, K.R., Gutin, B., Albu, J., and Pi-Suner, X. (1987). Thermic effect of food and exercise in lean and obese men of similar lean body mass. *American Journal of Physiology* 252: E110-E117.

Seidell, J.C., Cigolini, M., Deslypere, J-P., Charzewska, J., Ellsinger, B-M., and Cruz, A. (1991). Body fat distribution in relation to physical activity and smoking habits in 38-year-old European men. *American Journal of Epidemiology* 133: 257-265.

Sem, S.W., Nes, M., Engedal, K., Pedersen, J.I., and Trygg, K. (1988). An attempt to identify and describe a group of non-institutionalized elderly with the lowest nutrient score. *Comprehensive Gerontology* 2: 60-66.

Semble, E.L., Loeser, R.F., and Wise, C.M. (1990). Therapeutic exercise for rheumatoid arthritis and osteoarthritis. *Seminars in Arthritis and Rheumatism* 20: 32-39.

Sempos, C.T., Cleeman, J.I., Carroll, M.D., Johnson, C.L., Bachorik, P.S., Gordon, D.J., Burt, V.L., Briefel, R.R., Brown, C.D., Lippel, K., and Rifkind, B.M. (1993). Prevalence of high blood cholesterol among U.S. adults. *Journal of the American Medical Association* 269: 3009-3014.

Setaro, J.F., Soufer, R., Remetz, M.S., Perlmutter, R.A., and Zaret, B.L. (1992). Long-term outcome in patients with congestive failure and intact systolic left ventricular performance. *American Journal of Cardiology* 69: 1212-1216.

Seto, J.L., and Brewster, C.E. (1991). Musculoskeletal conditioning of the older athlete. *Clinical Sports Medicine* 10: 401-429.

Severson, R.K., Nomura, A.M.Y., Grove, J.S., and Stemmerman, G.N. (1989). A prospective analysis of physical activity and cancer. *American Journal of Epidemiology* 130: 522-529.

Shalom, R., Blumenthal, J.A., Williams, R.S., McMurray, R.G., and Dennis, V.W. (1984). Feasibility and benefits of exercise training in patients on maintenance dialysis. *Kidney International* 25: 958-963.

Shanas, E. (1980). Older people and their families: The new pioneers. *Journal of Marriage and Family* 42: 9-15.

Shanas, E., Townsend, P., Wedderburn, D., Friis, H., Stehouwer, J., and Milhøj, P. (1968). *Old people in three industrial societies*. London: Routledge, Kegan.

Shank, R.E. (1985). Nutrition principles. In R. Andres, E.L. Bierman, and W.R. Hazzard (Eds.), *Principles of geriatric medicine* (pp. 444-460). New York: McGraw-Hill.

Shannon, D.C., Carley, D.W., and Benson, H. (1987). Aging of modulation of heart rate. *American Journal of Physiology* 253: H874-H877.

Shaver, J.L.F., Giblin, E., and Paulsen, V. (1991). Sleep quality sub-types in midlife women. *Sleep* 14: 18-23.

Shaw, L.J., and Miller, D. (1994). Noninvasive coronary risk stratification of elderly patients. *American Journal of Geriatric Cardiology* 3: 12-21.

Shay, K.A., and Roth, D.L. (1992). Association between aerobic fitness and visuo-spatial performance in healthy older adults. *Psychology and Aging* 7: 15-24.

SHEP Cooperative Research Group (1991). Prevention of stroke by antihypertensive drug treatment in older persons with isolated systolic hypertension. Final results of the systolic hypertension in the elderly program. *Journal of the American Medical Association* 265: 3255 3264.

Shephard, R.J. (1977). *Endurance fitness* (2nd ed.). Toronto, ON: University of Toronto Press.

Shephard, R.J. (1978a). *Human physiological work capacity.* London: Cambridge University Press.

Shephard, R.J. (1978b). *Physical activity and aging* (1st ed.). London: Croom Helm.

Shephard, R.J. (1980). Work physiology and activity patterns. In F.A. Milan (Ed.), *The human biology of circumpolar populations* (pp. 305-338). London: Cambridge University Press.

Shephard, R.J. (1981). *Ischemic heart disease and exercise.* London: Croom Helm.

Shephard, R.J. (1982a). Are we asking the right questions? *Journal of Cardiac Rehabilitation* 2: 21-26.

Shephard, R.J. (1982b). The daily workload of the postal carrier. *Journal of Human Ergology* 11: 157-164.

Shephard, R.J. (1982c). *Physiology and biochemistry of exercise.* New York: Praeger.

Shephard, R.J. (1983a). *Biochemistry of Exercise.* Springfield, IL: Charles C Thomas.

Shephard, R.J. (1983b). Equal opportunity for a geriatric labor force: Some observations on marine surveying. *Journal of Occupational Medicine* 25: 211-214.

Shephard, R.J. (1983c). The value of exercise in ischemic heart disease: A cumulative analysis. *Journal of Cardiac Rehabilitation* 3: 294-298.

Shephard, R.J. (1984a). Can we identify those for whom exercise is hazardous? *Sports Medicine* 1: 75-86.

Shephard, R.J. (1984b). Management of exercise in the elderly. *Canadian Journal of Applied Sport Sciences* 9: 109-120.

Shephard, R.J. (1985a). Physical activity for the senior: A role for pool exercises? *Canadian Association for Health, Physical Education and Recreation Journal* 50 (6): 2-5, 20.

Shephard, R.J. (1985b). Technological change and the aging of working capacity. In P.K. Robinson, J. Livingston, and J.E. Birren (Eds.), *Aging and technological advances* (pp. 195-208). New York: Plenum Press.

Shephard, R.J. (1986a). Cardiovascular risk and truck driving. *Journal of Cardiopulmonary Rehabilitation* 6: 260-262.

Shephard, R.J. (1986b). *Economic benefits of enhanced fitness.* Champaign, IL: Human Kinetics.

Shephard, R.J. (1986c). *Fitness of a nation.* Basel: Karger.

Shephard, R.J. (1986d). Nutrition and physiology of aging. In E.A. Young (Ed.), *Nutrition, aging and health* (pp. 1-24). New York: Liss.

Shephard, R.J. (1987a). *Physical activity and aging* (2nd ed.). London: Croom Helm.

Shephard, R.J. (1987b). Respiratory factors limiting prolonged effort. *Canadian Journal of Sport Sciences* 12 (Suppl.): 45S-52S.

Shephard, R.J. (1988). Effects of exercise on biological features of aging. In R.S. Williams and A.G. Wallace (Eds.), *Biological effects of physical activity* (pp. 55-70). Champaign, IL: Human Kinetics.

Shephard, R.J. (1989a). Exercise and lifestyle change. *British Journal of Sports Medicine* 23: 11-22.

Shephard, R.J. (1989b). Habitual physical activity levels and perception of exertion in the elderly. *Journal of Cardiopulmonary Rehabilitation* 9: 17-23.

Shephard, R.J. (1990). Assessment of occupational fitness in the context of human rights legislation. *Canadian Journal of Sports Sciences* 15: 89-95.

Shephard, R.J. (1991a). *Body composition in biological anthropology.* London: Cambridge University Press.

Shephard, R.J. (1991b). An exercise physiologist's perspective on metaphors of health and aging. In G.M. Kenyon, J.E. Birren, and J.J.F. Schroots (Eds.), *Metaphors of aging in science and the humanities* (pp. 185-198). New York: Springer.

Shephard, R.J. (1991c). Fitness and aging. In C. Blais (Ed.), *Aging into the twenty-first century* (pp. 22-35). Downsview, ON: Captus University.

Shephard, R.J. (1991d). Occupational demand and human rights. Public safety officers and cardiorespiratory fitness. *Sports Medicine* 12: 94-109.

Shephard, R.J. (1992a). Does exercise reduce all-cancer death rates? *British Journal of Sports Medicine* 26: 125-128.

Shephard, R.J. (1992b). Exercise in old age (65-85). In R.J. Shephard and H.J. Miller (Eds.), *Exercise and the heart in health and disease* (pp. 187-231). New York: Marcel Dekker.

Shephard, R.J. (1992c). How cold weather affects the heart. *Perspectives in Cardiology* 8: 35-51.

Shephard, R.J. (1992d). Public safety officers and cardiac disease. *Journal of Cardiopulmonary Rehabilitation* 12: 51-55.

Shephard, R.J. (1993a). *Aerobic Fitness and Health.* Champaign, IL: Human Kinetics.

Shephard, R.J. (1993b). Aging, respiratory function and exercise. *Journal of Aging and Physical Activity* 1: 59-83.

Shephard, R.J. (1993c). Economic benefits of secondary and tertiary cardiac rehabilitation: A critical study. *Annals of the Academy of Medicine, Singapore,* 21: 57-62.

Shephard, R.J. (1993d). Exercise compliance: The challenge of an aging population. *Canadian Medical Association Journal* 9: 72D-74D.

Shephard, R.J. (1993e). Exercise in the prevention and treatment of cancer: An update. *Sports Medicine* 15: 258-280.

Shephard, R.J. (1994). Determinants of exercise in people aged 65 years and older. In R. Dishman (Ed.), *Advances in exercise adherence* (pp. 343-360). Champaign, IL: Human Kinetics.

Shephard, R.J. (1995a). Exercise and cancer: Linkages with obesity? *International Journal of Obesity* 19: S63-S68.

Shephard, R.J. (1995b). Review essay: A personal perspective on aging and productivity with particular reference to physically demanding work. *Ergonomics* 38: 617-636.

Shephard, R.J. (1995c). Worksite health promotion and productivity. In R.L. Kaman (Ed.), *Worksite health promotion economics* (pp. 147-173). Champaign, IL: Human Kinetics.

Shephard, R.J. (1996). Exercise and Cancer: Linkages with obesity. *Critical Reviews in Food Science and Nutrition* 36: 321-339.

Shephard, R.J. (in press-a). Exercise and the quality of life. *Quest.*

Shephard, R.J. (in press-b). Secondary rehabilitation. In D. Ashton and A. Rickards (Eds.), *Coronary artery disease (CAD) in women.* London: Churchill Livingstone.

Shephard, R.J., Berridge, M., and Montelpare, W. (1990). On the generality of the "sit and reach" test: An analysis of flexibility data for an aging population. *Research Quarterly* 61: 326-330.

Shephard, R.J., Bouhlel, E., Vandewalle, H., and Monod, H. (1988). Muscle mass as a factor limiting physical work. *Journal of Applied Physiology* 64: 1472-1479.

Shephard, R.J., Goodman, J., Rode, A., and Schaefer, O. (1984). Snowmobile use and decrease of stature among the Inuit. *Arctic Medical Research* 38: 32-36.

Shephard, R.J., Kavanagh, T., Campbell, R., and Lorenz, B. (1994). Net energy cost of stair climbing and ambulation in subjects with hemiplegia. *Sports Medicine, Training and Rehabilitation* 5: 199-210.

Shephard, R.J., Kavanagh, T., Campbell, R., and Lorenz, B. (1995). Net oxygen costs of ambulation in normal subjects and subjects with lower limb amputations. *Canadian Journal of Rehabilitation*: 8: 97-108.

Shephard, R.J., Kavanagh, T., and Mertens, D.J. (1995). Personal health benefits of Masters athletic competition. *British Journal of Sports Medicine*: 29: 35-40.

Shephard, R.J., Kavanagh, T., Tuck, J., and Kennedy, J. (1983). Marathon jogging in postmyocardial infarction patients. *Journal of Cardiopulmonary Rehabilitation* 3: 321-329.

Shephard, R.J., Kofsky, P.R., Harrison, J.E., McNeill, K.G., and Krondl, A. (1985). Body composition of older female subjects: New approaches and their limitations. *Human Biology* 57: 671-686.

Shephard, R.J., and LaBarre, R. (1978). Attitudes of the public towards cigarette smoke in public places. *Canadian Journal of Public Health* 69: 302-310.

Shephard, R.J., and Lavalleé, H. (in press). Effects of enhanced physical education, gender and environment on lung volumes of primary school children. *Journal of Sports Medicine and Physical Fitness*.

Shephard, R.J., and Leith, L. (1990). Physical activity and cognitive changes with aging. In M.L. Howe, M.J. Stones, and C.J. Brainerd (Eds.), *Cognitive and behavioral performance factors in atypical aging* (pp. 153-180). New York: Springer-Verlag.

Shephard, R.J., Montelpare, W., Berridge, M., and Flowers, J. (1986). Influence of exercise and of lifestyle education upon attitudes to exercise of older people. *Journal of Sports Medicine and Physical Fitness* 26: 175-179.

Shephard, R.J., and Montelpare, W.M. (1988). Geriatric benefits of exercise as an adult. *Journals of Gerontology* 43: M86-M90.

Shephard, R.J., Montelpare, W.M., Plyley, M.J., McCracken, D., and Goode, R.C. (1991). Handgrip dynamometry, Cybex measurements and lean mass as markers of the ageing of muscle function. *British Journal of Sports Medicine* 25: 204-208.

Shephard, R.J., Prien, E., and Hughes, G. (1988). Age restrictions on bus driver selection. *Journal of Human Ergology* 17: 119-138.

Shephard, R.J., and Rode, A. (1996). *The effects of modernization upon an Inuit community*. London: Cambridge University Press.

Shephard, R.J., and Shek, P.N. (1995a). Cancer, immune function and physical activity. *Canadian Journal of Applied Physiology* 20: 1-25.

Shephard, R.J., and Shek, P.N. (1995b). Exercise and the aging of immune function. *International Journal of Sports Medicine* 16: 1-6.

Shephard, R.J., Vandewalle, H., Gil, V., Bouhlel, E., and Monod, H. (1992). Respiratory, muscular and overall perceptions of effort: The influence of hypoxia and muscle mass. *Medicine and Science in Sports and Exercise* 24: 556-567.

Sheppard, H.L. (1985). Health, work and retirement. In R. Andres, E.L. Bierman, and W.R. Hazzard (Eds.), *Principles of geriatric medicine* (pp. 150-153). New York: McGraw-Hill.

Shimura, S., Boatman, E.S., and Martin, C.J. (1986). Effects of aging on the alveolar pores of Kohn and on the cytoplasmic components of alveolar type II cells in monkey lungs. *Journal of Pathology* 148: 1-11.

Shinkai, S., Kohno, H., Komura, T., Asai, H., Inai, R., Oka, K., Kurokawa, Y., and Shephard, R.J. (1995). Physical activity and immunosenescence in elderly men. *Medicine and Science in Sports and Exercise* 27: 1516-1526.

Shinton, R., and Sagar, G. (1993). Lifelong exercise and stroke. *British Medical Journal* 307: 231-234.

Shipley, M.J. (1991). Does plasma cholesterol concentration predict mortality from coronary heart disease in elderly people? 18 year follow up in Whitehall study. *British Medical Journal* 303: 89-92.

Shock, N.W., Greulich, R.C., Andres, R., Arenberg, D., Costa, P.T., Lakatta, E.G., and Tobin, J.D. (1984). *Normal human aging. The Baltimore Longitudinal Study of Aging* (NIH Publication No. 84-2450). Washington, DC: U.S. Government Printing Office.

Shock, N.W., and Norris, A.H. (1970). Neuromuscular coordination as a factor in age changes in muscular exercise. In D. Brunner and E. Jokl (Eds.), *Physical Activity and Aging*. Baltimore: University Park Press.

Shumaker, S.A., Anderson, R.T., and Czajkowski, S.M. (1990). Psychological tests and scales. In B. Spilker (Ed.), *Quality of life assessments in clinical trials* (pp. 95-113). New York: Raven Press.

Sidell, M. (1995). *Health in old age: Myth, mystery and management*. Buckingham, U.K.: Open University.

Sidney, K.H., Niinimaa, V., and Shephard, R.J. (1983). Attitudes towards exercise and sports: Sex and age differences and changes with endurance training. *Journal of Sports Sciences* 1: 194-210.

Sidney, K.H., and Shephard, R.J. (1977a). Attitudes towards health and physical activity in the elderly: Effects of a physical training programme. *Medicine and Science in Sports and Exercise* 8: 246-252.

Sidney, K.H., and Shephard, R.J. (1977b). Training and e.c.g. abnormalities in the elderly. *British Heart Journal* 39: 1114-1120.

Sidney, K.H., and Shephard, R.J. (1978a). Frequency and intensity of exercise training for elderly subjects. *Medicine and Science in Sports and Exercise* 10: 125-131.

Sidney, K.H., and Shephard, R.J. (1978b). Growth hormone and cortisol: Age differences, effects of exercise and training. *Canadian Journal of Applied Sport Sciences* 2: 189-193.

Sidney, K.H., Shephard, R.J., and Harrison, J. (1977). Endurance training and body composition of the elderly. *American Journal of Clinical Nutrition* 30: 326-333.

Siegel, J. (1981). Demographic background for international gerontological studies. *Journal of Gerontology* 36: 93-102.

Silderberg, R. (1979). Obesity and osteoarthrosis. In M. Mancini, B. Lewis, and F. Contaldo (Eds.), *Medical Complications of Obesity* (pp. 310-315). London: Academic Press.

Silver, A.J., Guillen, C.P., Kahl, M.J., and Morley, J.E. (1993). Effect of aging on body fat. *Journal of American Geriatric Society* 41: 211-213.

Simkin, A., Ayalon, J., and Leichter, I. (1987). Increased trabecular bone density due to bone-loading exercises in post-menopausal osteoporotic women. *Calcified Tissue International* 40: 59-63.

Singh, R.B., Singh, N.K., Rastogi, S.S., Mani, U.V., and Niaz, M.A. (1993). Effects of diet and lifestyle changes on atherosclerotic risk factors after 24 weeks on the Indian Diet Heart study. *American Journal of Cardiology* 71: 1283-1288.

Singh, S.J., Morgan, M.D.L., Scott, S., Walters, D., and Hardman, A.E. (1992). Development of a shuttle-walking test of disability in patients with chronic airways obstruction. *Thorax* 47: 1019-1024.

Sipilä, S., Viitsalo, J., Era, P., and Suominen, H. (1991). Muscle strength in male athletes aged 70-81 years and a population sample. *European Journal of Applied Physiology* 63: 399-403.

Siscovick, D.S., Ekelund, L.G., Johnson, J.L., Truong, Y., and Adler, A. (1991). Sensitivity of exercise electrocardiography for acute cardiac events during moderate and strenuous physical activity. The Lipid Research Clinics Coronary Primary Prevention Trial. *Archives of Internal Medicine* 151: 325-330.

Siscovick, D.S., Weiss, N.S., Fletcher, R.H., and Lasky, T. (1984). The incidence of primary cardiac arrest during vigorous exercise. *New England Journal of Medicine* 311: 874-877.

Skarfors, E.T., Lithell, H., Silenius, I., and Wegener, T.A. (1987). Physical training as treatment for type II (non-insulin dependent) diabetes in elderly men. *Diabetologia* 30: 930-933.

Skinner, H.B., Barrack, R.L., and Cook, S.D. (1984). Age-related decline in proprioception. *Clinics in Orthopedics and Related Research* 184: 208-211.

Skinner, J.S. (1988). Biological, functional and chronological age. In W.W. Spirduso and H.M. Eckert (Eds.), *Physical activity and aging: The academy papers* 22 (pp. 65-68). Champaign, IL: Human Kinetics.

Slattery, M.L., McDonald, A., Bild, D.E., Caan, B.J., Hilner, J.E., Jacobs, D.R., and Liu, K. (1992). Associations of body fat distribution with dietary intake, physical activity, alcohol and smoking in blacks and whites. *American Journal of Clinical Nutrition* 55: 943-950.

Slemenda, C.W., Hui, S.L., Longcope, C., and Johnston, C.C. (1987). Sex steroids and bone mass: A study of changes about the time of the menopause. *Journal of Clinical Investigation* 80: 1261-1269.

Slemenda, C.W., and Johnson, C.C. (1994). Epidemiology of osteoporosis. In R.A. Lobo (Ed.), *Treatment of the post-menopausal woman: Basic and clinical aspects* (pp. 161-168). New York: Raven Press.

Slemenda, C.W., Miller, J.Z., Hui, S.L., Reister, T.K., and Johnston, C.C. (1991). The role of physical activity in the development of skeletal mass in children. *Journal of Bone Mineral Research* 6: 1227-1233.

Slemenda, C.W., Miller, J.Z., Reister, T.K., Hui, S.L., and Johnston, C.C. (1991). Calcium supplementation enhances bone mineral accretion in growing children. *Journal of Bone Mineral Research* 6: S136.

Smidt, G.L., Lin, S.-Y., O'Dwyer, K., and Blanpied, P.R. (1992). The effect of high intensity trunk exercise on bone mineral density of postmenopausal women. *Spine* 17: 280-285.

Smith, C.H. (1995). Drug-food/food-drug interactions. In J.E. Morley, Z. Glick, and L.Z. Rubenstein (Eds.), *Geriatric nutrition* (2nd ed., pp. 311-328). New York: Raven Press.

Smith, E.L., and Gilligan, C. (1989). Osteoporosis, bone mineral and exercise. In W.W. Spirduso and H.M. Eckert (Eds.), *Physical activity and aging* (pp. 107-119). Champaign, IL: Human Kinetics.

Smith, E.L., Gilligan, C., McAdam, M., Ensign, C.P., and Smith, P.E. (1989). Deterring bone loss by exercise intervention in premenopausal and postmenopausal women. *Calcified Tissue International* 44: 312-321.

Smith, E.L., Raab, D.M., Zook, S.K., and Gilligan, C. (1989). Bone changes with aging and exercise. In R. Harris and S. Harris (Eds.), *Physical activity, aging and sports* (pp. 287-294). Albany, NY: Center for Studies of Aging.

Smith, E.L., Reddan, W., and Smith, P.E. (1981). Physical activity and calcium modalities for bone mineral increase in aged women. *Medicine and Science in Sports and Exercise* 13: 60-64.

Smith, E.L., Sempos, C.T., and Purvis, R.W. (1981). Bone mass and strength decline with age. In E.L. Smith and R.C. Serfass (Eds.), *Exercise and aging: The scientific basis* (pp. 59-88). Hillside, NJ: Enslow.

Smith, G.D., Bartley, M., and Blane, D. (1990). The Black report on socioeconomic inequalities in health 10 years on. *British Medical Journal* 301: 373-376.

Smith, J.R., Ning, Y., and Pereira-Smith, O.M. (1992). Why are the transformed cells immortal? Is the process reversible? *American Journal of Clinical Nutrition* 55: 1215S-1221S.

Smith, K., Cook, D., Guyatt, G.H., Madhavan, J., and Oxman, A.D. (1992). Respiratory muscle training in chronic airflow limitation. A meta-analysis. *American Review of Respiratory Diseases* 145: 533-539.

Smith, L.K. (1992). Exercise in patients with heart failure. In R.J. Shephard and H.J. Miller (Eds.), *Exercise and the heart in health and disease* (pp. 397-412). New York: Marcel Dekker.

Smith, S.C., Gilpin, E., Ahnve, S., Dittrich, H., Nicod, P., Henning, H., and Ross, J. (1990). Outlook after acute myocardial infarction in the very elderly compared with that in patients aged 65 to 75 years. *Journal of the American College of Cardiology* 16: 784-792.

Sohal, R., and Allen, R.G. (1985). Relationship between metabolic rate, free radicals, differentiation and aging: A unified theory. In A.D. Woodhead, A.D. Blackett, and A. Hollaender (Eds.), *Molecular Biology of Aging* (pp. 75-104). New York: Plenum Press.

Sohal, R., and Wolfe, L. (1986). Lipofuscin characteristics and significance. In D.F. Swaab, E. Fliers, M. Mirmiran, W.A. van Gool, and F. van Haaren (Eds.), *Progress in brain research* 70 (pp. 171-183). Amsterdam: Elsevier.

Sohn, R.S., and Micheli, L.J. (1985). The effect of running on the pathogenesis of osteoarthritis of the hips and knees. *Clinical Orthopedics* 198: 106-109.

Solomon, G.F. (1991). Psychosocial factors, exercise and immunity. Athletes, elderly persons and AIDS patients. *International Journal of Sports Medicine* 12: S50-S52.

Sonstroem, R.J. (1984). Exercise and self-esteem. In R.L. Terjung (Ed.), *Exercise and Sport Sciences Reviews* 12: 123-155.

Sorlie, D., and Myhre, K. (1978). Effects of physical training in intermittent claudication. *Scandinavian Journal of Clinical and Laboratory Investigation* 38: 217-222.

Speake, D.L., Cowart, M.E., and Stephens, R. (1991). Healthy lifestyle practices of rural and urban elderly. *Health Values* 15: 45-51.

Sperling, L. (1980). Evaluation of upper extremity function in 70 year old males and females. *Scandinavian Journal of Rehabilitation Medicine* 12: 139-144.

Spiegel, R., Azcona, A., and Morgan, K. (1991). Sleep and its disorders. In M.S.J. Pathy (Ed.), *Principles and practice of geriatric medicine* (2nd ed., pp. 253-264). Chichester: Wiley.

Spiegelhalter, D.J., Gore, S.M., Fitzpatrick, R., Fletcher, A.E., Jones, D.R., and Cox, D.R. (1992). Quality of life measures in health care. III. Resource allocation. *British Medical Journal* 305: 1205-1209.

Spina, M., Volpin, D., and Giro, M.G. (1980). Age-related changes in the content of cross-links and their precursors in elastin of human thoracic aortae. In A.M. Robert and L.

Robert (Eds.), *Biochimie des tissus conjunctifs normaux et pathologiques* [Biochemistry of normal and pathological connective tissues] (pp. 125-129). Paris: CNRS.

Spina, R.J., Bourey, R.E., Ogawa, T., and Ehsani, A.A. (1994). Effects of exercise training on alpha-adrenergic mediated pressor responses and baroreflex function in older subjects. *Journals of Gerontology* 49: B277-B281.

Spina, R.J., Ogawa, T., Kohrt, W.M., Martin, W.H., Holloszy, J.O., and Ehsani, A.A. (1993). Differences in cardiovascular adaptations to endurance exercise training between older men and women. *Journal of Applied Physiology* 75: 849-855.

Spirduso, W. (1988). Physical activity and aging: Introduction. In W.W. Spirduso and H. Eckert (Eds.), *Physical activity and aging: The academy papers* 22 (pp. 1-5). Champaign, IL: Human Kinetics.

Spirduso, W. (1995). *Physical dimensions of aging*. Champaign, IL: Human Kinetics.

Spitzer, W.O., Dobson, A.J., Hall, J., Chesterman, E., Levi, J., Shepherd, R., Battista, R.N., and Catchlove, B.R. (1981). Measuring the quality of life of cancer patients; a concise QL index for use by physicians. *Journal of Chronic Diseases* 34: 585-597.

Sports Council and the Health Education Authority. (1992). *The Allied Dunbar National Fitness Survey: The main findings*. Summary report. London: Author.

Squires, R.W., Lavie, C.J., Brandt, T.R., Gau, G.T., and Bailey, K.R. (1987). Cardiac rehabilitation in patients with severe ischemic left ventricular function. *Mayo Clinic Proceedings* 62: 997-1002.

Stampfer, M.J., Coldlitz, G.A., Willett, W.C., Manson, J.E., Rosner, B., Speizer, F.E., and Hennekens, C.H. (1991). Postmenopausal oestrogen therapy and cardiovascular disease. *New England Journal of Medicine* 325: 756-762.

Stanley, S.N., and Taylor, N.A.S. (1993). Isokinematic muscle mechanics in four groups of women of increasing age. *European Journal of Applied Physiology* 66: 178-184.

Star, V.L., and Hockberg, M.C. (1993). Osteoporosis: Treat current injury, retard future loss. *Internal Medicine* 14: 32-41.

Statistics Canada. (1984). *Population labour force activity* (Catalogue 92-915). Ottawa, ON: Minister of Supply and Services.

Statistics Canada. (1985). *General social survey*. Ottawa, ON: Minister of Supply and Services.

Statistics Canada. (1986). *Health and activity limitations survey*. Ottawa, ON: Author.

Statistics Canada. (1990). *A portrait of seniors in Canada* (Catalogue 89-519). Ottawa, ON: Minister of Supply and Services.

Statistics Canada. (1991). *Workforce 2000*. Ottawa, ON: Minister of Supply and Services.

Stebbins, C.L., Schultz, E., Smith, R.T., and Smith, E.L. (1985). Effects of chronic exercise during aging on muscle end-plate morphology in rats. *Journal of Applied Physiology* 58: 45-51.

Stefanick, M.L., and Wood, P.D. (1994). Physical activity, lipid and lipoprotein metabolism, and lipid transport. In C. Bouchard, R.J. Shephard, and T. Stephens (Eds.), *Physical activity, fitness and health* (pp. 417-431). Champaign, IL: Human Kinetics.

Steinberg, F.U., Sunwoo, I., and Roettger, R.F. (1985). Prosthetic rehabilitation of geriatric amputee patients: A follow-up study. *Archives of Physical Medicine and Rehabilitation* 66: 742-745.

Steinhaus, L.A., Dustman, R.E., Ruhling, R.O., Emmerson, R.Y., Johnson, S.C., Shearer, D.E., Latin, R.W., Shigeoka, J.W., and Bonekat, W.H. (1990). Aerobic capacity of older adults: A training study. *Journal of Sports Medicine and Physical Fitness* 30: 163-172.

Stelmach, G.E. (1994). Physical activity and aging: Sensory and perceptual processing. In C. Bouchard, R.J. Shephard, and T. Stephens (Eds.), *Physical activity, fitness and health* (pp. 509-510). Champaign, IL: Human Kinetics.

Stelmach, G.E., and Worringham, C.J. (1985). Sensorimotor deficits related to postural stability. *Clinics in Geriatric Medicine* 1: 679-694.

Stephens, T. (1988). Physical activity and mental health in the United States and Canada: Evidence from four population surveys. *Preventive Medicine* 17: 35-47.

Stephens, T., and Craig, C. (1986). Fitness and activity measurement in the 1981 Canada Fitness Survey. In T. Drury (Ed.), *Proceedings of NHCS workshop on assessing physical fitness and activity patterns in general population surveys*. Washington, DC: U.S. National Center for Health Statistics.

Stephens, T., and Craig, C. (1990). *The well-being of Canadians: The 1988 Campbell's survey*. Ottawa, ON: Canadian Fitness and Lifestyle Research Institute.

Sternfeld, B. (1992). Cancer and the protective effect of physical activity: The epidemiological evidence. *Medicine and Science in Sports and Exercise* 24: 1195-1209.

Sternfeld, B., Quesenberry, C.P., Williams, C.S., Sataiano, W.A., and Sidney, S. (1995). A case-control study of lifetime physical activity and risk of breast cancer. Paper under review, cited by I-M. Lee (1995), personal communication.

Sterns, H.L., and Patchett, M.B. (1984). Technology and the aging adult: Career development and training. In P.K. Robinson, J. Livingston, and J.E. Birren (Eds.), *Aging and technological advances* (pp. 261-278). New York: Plenum Press.

Stevenson, E.T., Davy, K.P., Reiling, M.J., and Seals, D.R. (1995). Maximal aerobic capacity and total blood volume in highly trained middle-aged and older female endurance athletes. *Journal of Applied Physiology* 77: 1691-1696.

Stevenson, J.S., and Topp, R. (1990). Effects of moderate and low intensity long-term exercise by older adults. *Research in Nursing and Health* 13: 209-218.

Stewart, A.L., King, A.C., and Haskell, W.L. (1993). Endurance exercise and health-related quality of life in 50- to 60-year-old adults. *Gerontologist* 33: 782-789.

Stillman, R.J., Lohman, T.G., Slaughter, M.H., and Massey, B.H. (1986). Physical activity and bone mineral content in women aged 30 to 85 years. *Medicine and Science in Sports and Exercise* 18: 576-580.

Stini, W.A., Chen, Z., and Stein, P. (1994). Aging, bone loss, and the body mass in Arizona retirees. *American Journal of Human Biology* 6: 43-50.

Stones, M.J., and Dawe, D. (1993). Acute exercise facilitates semantically cued memory in nursing home residents. *Journal of the American Geriatric Society* 41: 531-534.

Stones, M.J., and Kozma, A. (1982). Sex differences in changes with age in record running performances. *Canadian Journal on Aging* 1: 12-16.

Stones, M.J., and Kozma, A. (1986). Age trends in maximal physical performance: Comparison and evaluation of models. *Experimental Aging Research* 12: 207-215.

Stones, M.J., and Kozma, A. (1988). Physical activity, age, and cognitive/motor performance. In M.J. Howe and C.J. Brainerd (Eds.), *Cognitive development in adulthood: Progress in cognitive development and research* (pp. 273-321). New York: Springer-Verlag.

Stratton, J.R., Cerqueira, M.D., Schwartz, R.S., Levy, W.C., Veith, R.C., Kahn, S.E., and Abrass, I.B. (1992). Differences in cardiovascular responses to isoproterenol in relation to age and exercise training in healthy men. *Circulation* 86: 504-512.

Stratton, J.R., Dunn, J.F., Adamopoulos, S., Kemp, G.J., Coats, A.J.S., and Rajagopolan, B. (1994). Training partially reverses skeletal muscle abnormalities during exercise in heart failure. *Journal of Applied Physiology* 76: 1575-1582.

Stratton, J.R., Levy, W.C., Schwartz, R.S., Abrass, I.B., and Cerqueira, M.D. (1994). Beta-adrenergic effects on left ventricular filling: Influence of aging and exercise training. *Journal of Applied Physiology* 77: 2522-2529.

Strawbridge, W.J., Kaplan, G.A., Camacho, T., and Cohen, R.D. (1992). The dynamics of viability and functional change in an elderly cohort: Results from the Alameda County Study. *Journal of the American Gerontological Society* 40: 799-806.

Strong, M.J., and Garruto, R.M. (1994). Neuronal aging and age-related disorders of the human nervous system. In D.E. Crews and R.M. Garruto (Eds.), *Biological anthropology and aging: Perspectives on human variation over the lifespan* (pp. 214-231). New York: Oxford University Press.

Strong, R., Wood, W.G., and Samorajski, T. (1991). Neurochemistry of Ageing. In M.S.J. Pathy (Ed.), *Principles and practice of geriatric medicine* (2nd ed., pp. 69-97). Chichester: Wiley.

Stunkard, A.J. (1983). Physical activity and obesity. *Finnish Journal of Sports and Experimental Medicine* 2: 99-111.

Sudarsky, L., and Rosenthal, M. (1983). Gait disorders among elderly patients (a survey study of 50 patients). *Archives of Neurology* 40: 740-743.

Suderam, S.G., and Manikar, G.D. (1983). Hyponatremia in the elderly. *Age and Ageing* 12: 77-80.

Sullivan, D.H., Moroarty, M.S., Chernoff, R., and Lipschitz, D.A. (1988) Patterns of care: An analysis of the quality of nutritional care routinely provided to elderly hospitalized veterans. *Journal of Parenteral and Enteral Nutrition* 13: 249-254.

Sullivan, M.J., Higginbotham, M.B., and Cobb, F.R. (1989). Exercise training in patients with chronic heart failure delays ventilatory anaerobic threshold and improves submaximal exercise performance. *Circulation* 79: 324-329.

Sulman, J., and Wilkinson, S. (1989). An activity group for long-stay elderly patients in an acute care hospital: Program evaluation. *Canadian Journal on Aging* 8: 34-50.

Sun, A.Y., and Seaman, R.N. (1977). The effect of aging on synaptosomal Ca^2 transport in the brain. *Experimental Aging Research* 3: 107-116.

Sun, J.C.L., Eiken, O., and Mekjavic, I.B. (1993). Autonomic nervous control of heart rate during blood flow restricted exercise in man. *European Journal of Applied Physiology* 66: 202-206.

Sundstrom, E. (1986). *Work places: The psychology of the physical environment in offices and factories.* London: Cambridge University Press.

Suominen, H. (1994). Bone mineral density and long-term exercise: An overview of cross-sectional athlete studies. *Sports Medicine* 16: 316-330.

Suominen, H., and Rahkila, P. (1991). Bone mineral density of the calcaneus in 70- to 81-yr-old male athletes and a population sample. *Medicine and Science in Sports and Exercise* 23: 1227-1233.

Superko, H.R. (1991). Exercise training, serum lipids, and lipoprotein particles: Is there a change threshold? *Medicine and Science in Sports and Exercise* 23: 677-685.

Suurnakki, T., Nygard, C-H., and Ilmarinen, J. (1991). Stress and strain of elderly employees in municipal occupations. *Scandinavian Journal of Work, Environment & Health* 17 (Suppl. 1): 30-39.

Suvanto, S., Huuhtanen, P., Nygard, C-H., and Ilmarinen, J. (1991). Performance efficiency and its changes among aging municipal employees. *Scandinavian Journal of Work, Environment & Health* 17 (Suppl. 1): 118-121.

Suwalski, M. (1982). Importance of physical training of rheumatic patients. *Annals of Clinical Research* 14 (Suppl. 34): 107-109.

Suzuki, S., Sato, M., and Okubo, T. (1995). Expiratory muscle training and sensation of respiratory effort during exercise in normal subjects. *Thorax* 50: 366-370.

Suzuki, Y., Kuwajima, I., Hoshino, S., Kanemaru, A., Shimozawa, T., Matsushita, S., and Kuramoto, K. (1991). Cardiac performance in elderly hypertensive patients with left ventricular hypertrophy: Responses to isometric exercise and beta-agonists. *Journal of Cardiovascular Pharmacology* 17 (Suppl. 2): S129-S132.

Svänborg, A. (1985). Ecology, aging and health in a medical perspective. In P.K. Robinson, J. Livingston, and J.E. Birren (Eds.), *Aging and technological advances* (pp. 159-168). New York: Plenum Press.

Svänborg, A., Eden, S., and Mellstrom, D. (1991). Metabolic changes in aging as predictors of disease: The Swedish experience. In D.K. Ingram, G.T. Baker, and N.W. Shock (Eds.), *The potential for nutritional modulation of aging* (pp. 81-90). Trumbull, CT: Food & Nutrition Press.

Svanstrom, L. (1990). Simply osteoporosis—or a multifactorial genesis for the increasing incidence of fall injuries in the elderly? *Scandinavian Journal of Social Medicine* 18: 165-169.

Swartz, H.M., and Mäder, K. (1995). Free radicals in aging: Theories, facts and artifacts. In K. Esser and G.M. Martin (Eds.), *Molecular aspects of aging* (pp. 77-97). New York: Wiley.

Swerts, P.M.J., Kretzers, L.M.J., Trepstra-Lindeman, E., Verstappen, F.T.J., and Wouters, E.F.M. (1990). Exercise reconditioning in the rehabilitation of patients with chronic obstructive pulmonary disease: A short and long-term analysis. *Archives of Physical Medicine and Rehabilitation* 71: 570-573.

Swinne, C.J., Shapiro, E.P., Lima, S.D., and Fleg, J.L. (1992). Age-associated changes in left ventricular diastolic performance during isometric exercise in normal subjects. *American Journal of Cardiology* 69: 823-826.

Szathmary, E.J.E., and Holt, N. (1983). Hyperglycemia in Dogrib Indians of the North West Territories, Canada: Association with age and a centripetal distribution of body fat. *Human Biology* 55: 493-515.

Taaffe, D.R., Pruitt, L., Reim, J., Hintz, R.L., Butterfield, G., Hoffman, A.R., and Marcus, R. (1994). Effect of recombinant human growth hormone on the muscle strength response to resistance exercise in elderly men. *Journal of Clinical Endocrinology and Metabolism* 79: 1361-1366.

Taeuber, C. (1985). Older workers: Force of the future? In P.K. Robinson, J. Livingston, and J.E. Birren (Eds.), *Aging and technological advances* (pp. 75-88). New York: Plenum Press.

Tager, I.B., Segal, M.R., Speizer, F.E., and Weiss, S.T. (1988). The natural history of forced expiratory volumes; effects of cigarette smoking and respiratory symptoms. *American Review of Respiratory Diseases* 138: 837-849.

Takeda, S., and Matsuzawa, J. (1985). Age related brain atrophy: A study with computed tomography. *Journals of Gerontology* 40: 159M-163M.

Takemoto, K.A., Bernstein, L., Lopez, J.F., Marshak, D., Rahimtoola, S.H., and Chandraratna, N. (1992). Abnormalities of diastolic filling of the left ventricle associated with aging are less pronounced in exercise-trained individuals. *American Heart Journal* 124: 143-148.

Tandan, R., and Bradley, W.G. (1985). Amyotrophic lateral sclerosis. 1. Clinical features, pathology, and ethical issues in management. *Annals of Neurology* 18: 271-280.

Tankersley, C.G., Smolander, J., Kenney, W.L., and Fortney, S.M. (1991). Sweating and skin blood flow during exercise: Effects of age and maximal oxygen uptake. *Journal of Applied Physiology* 71: 236-242.

Tate, C.A., Hyek, M.F., and Taffet, G.E. (1994). Mechanisms for the responses of cardiac muscle to physical activity in old age. *Medicine and Science in Sports and Exercise* 26: 561-567.

Taylor, D.J., Crowe, M., Bore, P.J., Styles, P., Arnold, D.L., and Radda, G.K. (1984). Examination of the energetics of aging skeletal muscle using nuclear magnetic resonance. *Gerontology* 30: 2-7.

Taylor, J.A., Hand, G.A., Johnson, D.G., and Seals, D.R. (1991). Sympathoadrenal-circulatory regulation during sustained isometric exercise in young and older men. *American Journal of Physiology* 26: R1061-R1069.

Taylor, J.A., Hand, G.A., Johnson, D.G., and Seals, D.R. (1992). Augmented forearm vasoconstriction during dynamic exercise in healthy older men. *Circulation* 86: 1789-1799.

Tenette, M., and Cuny, G. (1982). Rééducation fonctionelle [Functional reeducation]. In F. Bourlière (Ed.), *Gérontologie: Biologie et clinique* (pp. 328-342). Paris: Flammarion.

Teramoto, S., Fukuchi, Y., Nagase, T., Matsuse, T., and Orimo, H. (1995). A comparison of ventilatory components in young and elderly men during exercise. *Journal of Gerontology* 50A: B34-B39.

Terry, P., and Tockman, M.S. (1985). Chronic airways obstruction. In R. Andres, E.L. Bierman, and W.R. Hazzard (Eds.), *Principles of geriatric medicine* (pp. 571-578). New York: McGraw-Hill.

Thiele, B.L., and Strandness, D.E. (1994). Peripheral vascular disease. In W.R. Hazzard, E.L. Bierman, J.P. Blass, W.E. Ettinger, and J.B. Halter (Eds.), *Principles of geriatric medicine and gerontology* (3rd ed., pp. 533-540). New York: McGraw-Hill.

Thomas, D.P., McCormick, R.J., Zimmerman, S.D., Vadlamudi, R.K., and Gosselin, L.E. (1992). Aging and training-induced alterations in collagen characteristics of rat left ventricle and papillary muscle. *American Journal of Physiology* 263: H778-H783.

Thomas, D.R. (1994). Outcome from protein-energy malnutrition in nursing home residents. *Facts and Research in Gerontology* (Suppl.: Nutrition, pp. 87-95). Paris: Serdi.

Thomas, J.R., Landers, D.M., Salazar, W., and Etnier, J. (1994). Exercise and cognitive function. In C. Bouchard, R.J. Shephard, and T. Stephens (Eds.), *Physical activity, fitness and health* (pp. 521-529). Champaign, IL: Human Kinetics.

Thompson, C.H., Davies, R.J.O., Kemp, G.J., Taylor, D.J., Radda, G.K., and Rajagoplan, B. (1993). Skeletal muscle metabolism during exercise and recovery in patients with respiratory failure. *Thorax* 48: 486-490.

Thompson, H.J., Ronan. A.M., Ritacco, K.A., Tagliaferro, A.R., and Meeker, L.D. (1988). Effects of exercise on the induction of mammary carcinogenesis. *Cancer Research* 48: 2720-2723.

Thompson, P.D., and Dorsey, D.L. (1986). The heart of the Masters athlete. In J.R. Sutton and R.M. Brock (Eds.), *Sports medicine for the mature athlete* (pp. 309-318). Indianapolis: Benchmark Press.

Thompson, P.D., and Fahrenbach, M.C. (1994). Risks of exercising: Cardiovascular, including sudden death. In C. Bouchard, R.J. Shephard, and T. Stephens, (Eds.),

Physical activity, fitness and health (pp. 1019-1028). Champaign, IL: Human Kinetics.

Thompson, P.D., Funk, E.J., Carleton, R.A., and Sturner, W.Q. (1982). Incidence of death during jogging in Rhode Island from 1975 through 1980. *Journal of the American Medical Association* 242: 1265-1267.

Thompson, P.D., Stern, M.P., Williams, P., Duncan, K., Haskell, W.L., and Wood, P.D. (1979). Death during jogging or running. *Journal of the American Medical Association* 242: 1265-1267.

Thomsen, K.K., Larsen, S., Schroll, M. (1995). Cardiovascular risk factors and age: A cross-sectional survey of Danish men and women from the Glostrup population studies, 1991. *American Journal of Geriatric Cardiology* 3 (1): 31-41.

Thune, I., and Lund, E. (1994). Physical activity and the risk of prostate and testicular cancer: A cohort study of 53,000 Norwegian men. *Cancer Causes and Control* 5: 549-556.

Thurlbeck, W.M. (1991). Morphology of the aging lung. In R.G. Crystal and J.B. West (Eds.), *The lung* (pp. 1743-1748). New York: Raven Press.

Tiidus, P., Shephard, R.J., and Montelpare, W. (1989). Overall intake of energy and key nutrients: Data for middle-aged and older middle-class adults. *Canadian Journal of Sport Sciences* 14: 173-177.

Timiras, P.S. (1988). *Physiological basis of geriatrics*. New York: Macmillan.

Timiras, P.S. (1991). Physiology of ageing: Aspects of neuroendocrine regulation. In M.S.J. Pathy (Ed.), *Principles and practice of geriatric medicine* (pp. 31-54). Chichester: Wiley.

Timmons, B.A., Araujo, J., and Thomas, T.R. (1985). Fat utilization enhanced by exercise in a cold environment. *Medicine and Science in Sports and Exercise* 17: 673-678.

Timpl, R., Rohde, H., Robey, P.G., Rennard, S.I., Foidart, J.M., and Martin, G.R. (1979). Laminin. A glycoprotein from basement membranes. *Journal of Biological Chemistry* 254: 9933-9937.

Tinetti, M.E., Speechley, M., and Ginter, S.F. (1988). Risk factors for falls among elderly persons living in the community. *New England Journal of Medicine* 319: 1701-1707.

Ting, A.J. (1991). Running and the older athlete. *Clinics in Geriatric Medicine* 10: 319-325.

Tipton, C.M. (1991). Exercise, training and hypertension: An update. *Exercise and Sport Sciences Reviews* 19:447-505.

Tockman, M.S. (1994). Aging of the respiratory system. In W.R. Hazzard, E.L. Bierman, J.P. Blass, W.H. Ettinger, and J.B. Halter (Eds.), *Principles of geriatric medicine and gerontology* (3rd ed., pp. 555-564). New York: McGraw-Hill.

Todd, C.J., Freeman, C.J., Camilleri-Ferrante, C., Palmer, C.R., Hyder, A., Laxton, C.E., Parker, M.J., Payne, B.V., and Rushton, N. (1995). Differences in mortality after fracture of the hip: the East Anglian audit. *British Medical Journal* 310: 904-908.

Tomporowski, P.D., and Ellis, N.R. (1986). Effects of exercise on cognitive processes: A review. *Psychological Bulletin* 99: 338-346.

Tonkin, A.L., Wing, L.M.H., Morris, M.J., and Kapoor, V. (1991). Afferent baroreflex dysfunction and age-related orthostatic hypotension. *Clinical Science* 81: 531-538.

Toole, T., and Abourezk, T. (1989). Aerobic function, information processing and aging. In A.C. Ostrow (Ed.), *Aging and motor behavior* (pp. 37-65). Indianapolis: Benchmark Press.

Topp, R., Mikesky, A., Wigglesworth, J., Holt, W., and Edwards, J.E. (1993). The effect of a 12-week dynamic resistance strength training program on gait velocity and balance of older adults. *Gerontologist* 33: 501-506.

Torg, J. (1995). Sudden cardiac death in the athlete. In J. Torg and R.J. Shephard (Eds.), *Current therapy in sports medicine* (3rd ed., pp. 8-10). Philadelphia: Mosby–Yearbook.

Torgen, M., Nygard, C-H., and Wahlstedt, K. (1993). Health and work satisfaction among postal workers in relation to age. In J. Ilmarinen (Ed.), *Aging and work* (pp. 33-38). Helsinki: Institute for Occupational Health.

Torrance, G.W. (1987). Utility approach to measuring health-related quality of life. *Journal of Chronic Diseases* 40: 593-600.

Toshima, M.T., Kaplan, R.M., and Ries, A.L. (1990). Experimental evaluation of rehabilitation in chronic obstructive pulmonary disease: Short-term effects on exercise endurance and health status. *Health Psychology* 9: 237-252.

Toth, M.J., Gardner, A.W., Ades, P.A., and Poehlman, E.T. (1994). Contribution of body composition to age-related decline in peak VO_2 in men and women. *Journal of Applied Physiology* 77: 647-652.

Tran, Z.V., and Weltman, A. (1985). Differential effects of exercise on serum lipids and lipoprotein levels seen with changes in body weight. A meta-analysis. *Journal of the American Medical Association* 254: 919-924.

Tremblay, A., Després, J-P., and Bouchard, C. (1985). The effects of exercise training on energy balance and adipose tissue morphology and metabolism. *Sports Medicine* 2: 223-233.

Tremblay, A., Després, J-P., LeBlanc, C., Craig, C.L., Ferris, B., Stephens, T., and Bouchard, C. (1990). Effect of intensity of physical activity on body fatness and fat distribution. *American Journal of Clinical Nutrition* 51: 153-157.

Tremblay, A., Nadeau, A., Fournier, G., and Bouchard, C. (1987). Effect of a three-day interruption of exercise training on resting metabolic rate and glucose-induced thermogenesis in trained individuals. *International Journal of Obesity* 12: 163-168.

Treton, J., and Courtois, Y. (1991). Evolution of the distribution, proliferation, UV repair capacity of rat lens epithelium cells as a function of maturation and aging. *Mechanisms in Ageing and Development* 15: 251-267.

Triosi, R.J., Heinold, J.W., Vokonas, P.S., and Weiss, T.S. (1993). Cigarette smoking, dietary intake, and physical activity: Effects on body fat distribution—the normative aging study. *American Journal of Clinical Nutrition* 53: 1104-1111.

Truswell, A.F. (1985). Obesity: Diagnosis and risks. *British Medical Journal* 291: 655-657.

Tsuchida, M., Miura, T., and Aibara, K. (1987). Lipofuscin and lipofuscin-like substances. *Chemistry and Physics of Lipids* 44: 297-325.

Tucker, R.M. (1980). Is hypertension different in the elderly? *Geriatrics* 35: 28-32.

Tuomi, K., Eskelinen, L., Toikannen, J., Järvinen, E., Ilmarinen, J., and Klockars, M. (1991). Work load and individual factors affecting work ability among municipal employees. *Scandinavian Journal of Work, Environment & Health* 17 (Suppl. 1): 128-134.

Tuomi, K., Ilmarinen, J., Eskelinen, L., Järvinen, E., Toikkanen, J., and Klockars, M. (1991). Prevalence and incidence rates of diseases and work ability in different work categories of municipal occupations. *Scandinavian Journal of Work, Environment & Health* 17 (Suppl. 1): 67-74.

Tuomi, K., Järvinen, E., Eskelinen, L., Ilmarinen, J., and Klockars, M. (1991). Effect of retirement on health and work ability among municipal employees. *Scandinavian Journal of Work, Environment & Health* 17: (Suppl. 1): 75-81.

Tuomi, K., Toikkanen, J., Eskelinen, L., Backman, A-L., Ilmarinen, J., Järvinen, E., and Klockars, M. (1991). Mortality, disability and changes in occupation among aging municipal employees. *Scandinavian Journal of Work, Environment & Health* 17 (Suppl. 1): 58-66.

Turchetta, A., Calzolari, A., Donfrancesco, A., Drago, F., Miano, C. et al. (1990). Physical activity and sport in youngs with leukemia "off therapy." *Proceedings of the World Congress on Sport for All*, Tampere, Finland (O-FR-220). Poster presentation. Tampere: Institute for Health Promotion Research.

Turner, T.R., and Weiss, M.L. (1994). The genetics of longevity in humans. In D.E. Crews and R.M. Garruto (Eds.), *Biological anthropology and aging: Perspectives on human variation over the lifespan* (pp. 76-100). New York: Oxford University Press.

Uebelhart, D., Schlemmer, A., Johansen, J.S., Gineyts, E., Christiansen, C., and Delmas, P.D. (1991). Effect of menopause and hormone replacement therapy on the urinary excretion of pyridinium cross-links. *Journal of Clinical Endocrinology and Metabolism* 72: 367-373.

Uhlenbruck, G. (1993). Sport, Alter und Immunsystem [Sport, age and the immune system]. *Sport Medwelt* 44: 303-308.

United Kingdom Testicular Cancer Study Group. (1994). Aetiology of testicular cancer: Association with congenital abnormalities, age at puberty, infertility and exercise. *British Medical Journal* 308: 1393-1399.

United Nations. (1981). *Bulletin on Aging* 6 (January): 7-16.

United Nations, Department of International Economic and Social Affairs. (1988). Sex differentials in survivorship in the developing world: Levels, regional patterns and demographic determinants. *Population Bulletin of the United Nations* 25: 51-64.

U.S. Bureau of Labor Statistics. (1982). *Employment and training report of the President* (p. 155). Washington, DC: U.S. Government Printing Office.

U.S. Centers for Disease Control. (1986). 1990 Physical Fitness and Exercise Objectives. Summary of current status and recommendations for 2000. In T. Drury, G.V. Swengross, and K.E. Powell (Eds.), *Assessing physical fitness and activity patterns in general population surveys*. Hyattsville, MD: National Center for Health Statistics.

U.S. Department of Commerce. (1994). *Statistical abstract of the United States, 1994.* Washington, DC: Author.

U.S. Department of Health and Human Services. (1981). *Disability Survey 72.* Washington, DC: Author.

U.S. Department of Health and Human Services. (1991a). *Healthy people 2000: National health promotion and disease prevention objectives—full report with commentary* (DHHS Publication No. PHS 91-50212). Washington, DC: Author.

U.S. Department of Health and Human Services. (1991b). *Osteoporosis research, education and health promotion* (NIH Publication No. 91-3216). Bethesda, MD: National Institute of Arthritis and Musculoskeletal and Skin Diseases.

U.S. Department of Health and Human Services. (1992). *Vital and Health Statistics Series 10* (No. 184, December 1992). Washington, DC: Author.

U.S. Food and Nutrition Board. (1989). *Recommended dietary allowances* (10th ed.). Washington, DC: Author.

U.S. National Center for Health Statistics. (1975). Exercise and participation in sports among persons 20 years of age and over: United States, 1975. *Advanced Data*, 19. Washington, DC: Author.

U.S. National Center for Health Statistics. (1981). Basic data from wave I of the National Survey of Personal Health Practices and Consequences: United States, 1979.

Vital and Health Statistics Series 15, Nos. 1 and 2. Hyattsville, MD: U.S. Department of Health and Human Services.

U.S. National Center for Health Statistics. (1987). Aging in the eighties: Ability to perform work-related activities. Data from the supplement on aging of the National Health Interview Survey: United States, 1984. *Advance Data from Vital and Health Statistics*, No. 136 (DHHS Publication No. PHS 87-1250). Hyattsville, MD: U.S. Public Health Service.

U.S. National Center for Health Statistics. (1991). *Health, United States, 1990* (DHHS Publication No. PHS 91-1232). Hyattsville, MD: Author.

U.S. National Center for Health Statistics. (1992). *Vital Statistics of the United States, 1989* (Vol. II, Section 6. Life Tables). Hyattsville, MD: Author.

U.S. National Center for Health Statistics. (1993). Prevalence of selected chronic conditions, United States, 1986-88. *Vital Statistics* 10, No. 182. Hyattsville, MD: Author.

U.S. National Center for Health Statistics. (1994). *United States, 1992*. Hyattsville, MD: Author.

U.S. National Cholesterol Education Program (NCEP). (1993). Expert panel on detection, evaluation and treatment of high blood cholesterol in adults. *Journal of the American Medical Association* 269: 3015-3023.

U.S. National Council on Aging. (1978). *Fact book on aging: A profile of America's older population*. Washington, DC: Author.

U.S. National Council on Aging. (1981). *Aging in the eighties*. Washington, DC: Author.

U.S. National Diabetes Data Group. (1979). Classification and diagnosis of diabetes and other categories of glucose intolerance. *Diabetes* 28: 1039-1057.

U.S. National Institute for Occupational Safety and Health. (1981). *Work practice guides for manual lifting* (DHHS [NIOSH] Publication No. 81-122). Washington, DC.

U.S. National Institutes of Health. (1984). Consensus Conference. Osteoporosis. *Journal of the American Medical Association* 252: 797-802.

U.S. National Research Council, National Academy of Sciences, Food and Nutrition Board. (1980). *Committee on dietary allowances* (9th ed.). Washington, DC: National Academy of Sciences.

U.S. President's Council on Physical Fitness and Sports. (1973). *National Adult Physical Fitness Survey* (*Newsletter*, Special Edition, May, pp. 1-27). Washington, DC: The Council.

U.S. Senate Special Committee on Aging. (1972). *Developments in aging. Every tenth American*. (Report 92-784, p. 21). Washington, DC: Author.

U.S. Senate Special Committee on Aging. (1987). *Developments in aging: Vol. 1* (Report 100-291). Washington, DC: Author.

U.S. Surgeon General. (1996). *Report on physical activity and health*. Washington, DC: U.S. Public Health Service.

Uson, P.P., and Larrosa, V.R. (1982). Physical activities in retirement age. In J. Partington, T. Orlick, and J. Samela (Eds.), *Sport in perspective* (pp. 149-151). Ottawa, ON: Coaching Association of Canada.

Vailas, A.C., Pedrini, V.A., Pedrini-Mille, A., and Holloszy, J.O. (1985). Patellar-tendon matrix changes associated with aging and voluntary exercise. *Journal of Applied Physiology* 58: 1572-1576.

Vaillant, G.E. (1991). The association of ancestral longevity with successful aging. *Journals of Gerontology* 46: P292-P298.

Vaitkevicius, P.V., Fleg, J.L., Engel, J.H., O'Connor, F.C., Wright, J.G., Lakatta, L.E., Yin, F.C.P., and Lakatta, E.G. (1993). Effects of age and aerobic capacity on arterial stiffness in healthy adults. *Circulation* 88: 1456-1462.

Välimäki, M.J., Kärkkäinen, M., Lamberg-Allardt, C., Laitinen, K., Alhavra, E., Heikkinen, J., Impivaara, O., Mäkelä, P., Palmgren, J., Seppänen, R., Vuori, I., and the Cardiovascular Risk in Young Finns Study Group. (1994). Exercise, smoking, and calcium intake during adolescence and early adulthood as determinants of peak bone mass. *British Medical Journal* 309: 230-235.

Vallery-Masson, J., Poitrenaud, J., Burnat, G., and Lion, M.R. (1981). Retirement and morbidity: A three-year longitudinal study of a French managerial population. *Age and Ageing* 10: 271-276.

Valliant, P.M., and Asu, M.E. (1985). Exercise and its effects on cognition and physiology in older adults. *Perceptual and Motor Skills* 61: 1031-1038.

Van Camp, S.P., and Peterson, R.A. (1986). Cardiovascular complications of outpatient cardiac rehabilitation programs. *Journal of the American Medical Association* 256: 1160-1163.

Vandervoort, A.A. (1992). Effects of ageing on human neuromuscular function: Implications for exercise. *Canadian Journal of Sport Sciences* 17: 178-184.

Vandervoort, A.A., and McComas, A.J. (1986). Contractile changes in opposing muscles of the ankle joint with aging. *Journal of Applied Physiology* 61: 361-367.

van Gool, W.A., and Mirmiran, M. (1986). Aging and circadian rhythms. In D.F. Swaab, E. Fliers, M. Mirmiran, W.A. van Gool, and F. van Haaren (Eds.), *Progress in brain research* 70 (pp. 255-277). Amsterdam: Elsevier.

van Herwaarden, C.L.A. (1984). Exercise and training in chronic non-specific lung disease (CNSLD). *International Journal of Sports Medicine* 5 (Suppl.): 54-58.

van Saase, J.C.L.M., Noteboom, W.M.P., and Vandenbroucke, J.P. (1990). Longevity of men capable of prolonged vigorous physical exercise: A 32 year follow-up of 2259 participants in the Dutch eleven cities ice skating tour. *British Medical Journal* 301: 1409-1411.

Vartiainen, E., Puska, P., Pekkanen, J., Tuomilehto, J., and Jousilahti, P. (1994). Changes in risk factors explain changes in mortality from ischaemic heart disease in Finland. *British Medical Journal* 309: 23-27.

Verde, T., Shephard, R.J., Corey, P., and Moore, R. (1983). Exercise and heat-induced sweat. In H.G. Knuttgen, J.A. Vogel, and J.R. Poortmans (Eds.), *Biochemistry of exercise* (pp. 618-622). Champaign, IL: Human Kinetics.

Vico, L., Pouget, J.F., Calmels, P., Chatard, J.C., Rehailia, M., Minairie, P., Geyssant, A., and Alexandre, C. (1995). The relationship between physical ability and bone mass in women aged over 65 years. *Journal of Bone and Mineral Research* 10: 374-383.

Videman, T., Sarna, S., Battié, M.C., Koskinen, S., Gill, K., Paananen, H., and Gibbons, L. (1995). The long-term effects of physical loading and exercise lifestyles on back-related symptoms, disability and spinal pathology among men. *Spine* 20: 699-709.

Viidik, A. (1986). Adaptability of connective tissue. In B. Saltin (Ed.), *Biochemistry of exercise VI* (pp. 545-562). Champaign, IL: Human Kinetics.

Viitsala, J.J., Era, P., Leskinen, A.L., and Heikkinen, E. (1985). Muscle strength profiles and anthropometry in random samples of men aged 31-35, 51-55 and 71-75 years. *Ergonomics* 28: 1563-1574.

Vingârd, E., Alfredsson, L., Goldie, I., and Hogstedt, C. (1993). Sports and osteoarthrosis of the hip: An epidemiologic study. *American Journal of Sports Medicine* 21: 195-200.

Vinni, K., and Hakama M. (1980). Healthy worker effect in the total Finnish population. *British Journal of Industrial Medicine* 37: 180-184.

Vitarelli, A., Fedele, F., Montesano, T., Dagianti, A., and Dagianti, A. (1995). Echocardiographic and therapeutic approach to heart failure in the elderly. *American Journal of Geriatric Cardiology* 3: 5-16.

Vitti, K.A., Bayles, C.M., Carender, W.J., Prendergast, J.M., and D'Amico, F.J. (1993). A low-level strength training program for frail elderly adults living in an extended attention facility. *Aging Clinical and Experimental Research* 5: 363-369.

Vlassara, H. (1990). Advanced non-enzymatic tissue glycolysation: Mechanism implicated in the complications associated with aging. In C.E. Finch and T. E. Johnson (Eds.), *Molecular biology of aging* (pp. 171-185). New York: Wiley-Liss.

Vokonas, P.S., Kannel, W.B., and Cupples, L.A. (1988). Epidemiology and risk of hypertension in the elderly: The Framingham Study. *Journal of Hypertension* 6 (Suppl. 1): S3-S9.

Volden, C., Langemo, D., Adamson, M., and Oeschle, L. (1990). The relationship of age, gender, and exercise practices to measures of health, lifestyle, and self-esteem. *Applied Nursing Research* 3: 20-26.

Vollmer, W.M., Johnson, R.L., McCamant, L.E., and Buist, A.S. (1988). Longitudinal versus cross-sectional estimation of lung function decline—further insights. *Statistics in Medicine* 7: 685-696.

Voorips, L.E., Lemmink, K.A., van Heuvelen, M.J.G., Bult, P., and van Staveren, W.A. (1993). The physical condition of elderly women differing in habitual activity. *Medicine and Science in Sports and Exercise* 25: 1152-1157.

Voorips, L.E., van Staeveren, W.A., and Hautvast, J.G.A.J. (1991). Are physically active elderly women in a better nutritional condition than their sedentary peers? *European Journal of Clinical Nutrition* 45: 545-552.

Vuori, I. (1995). Exercise and sudden cardiac death: Effects of age and type of activity. *Sports Science Review* 4: 46-84.

Wagner, J.A., and Horvath, S.M. (1985). Influence of age and gender on human thermoregulatory responses to cold exposures. *Journal of Applied Physiology* 58: 180-186.

Wahrenberg, H., Bolinder, J., and Arner, P. (1991). Adrenergic regulation of lipolysis in human fat cells during exercise. *European Journal of Clinical Investigation* 21: 534-541.

Walford, R.L. (1980). Immunology and aging. *American Journal of Clinical Pathology* 74: 247-253.

Walford, R.L. (1982). Henderson Award Lecture: Studies in immunogerontology. *Journal of the American Geriatric Society* 30: 617-625.

Wallberg-Henriksson, H. (1989). Acute exercise, fuel homeostasis and glucose transport in insulin-dependent diabetes mellitus. *Medicine and Science in Sports and Exercise* 21: 356-361.

Wallberg-Henriksson, H. (1992). Exercise and diabetes mellitus. *Exercise and Sport Sciences Reviews* 20: 339-368.

Walsh, B.W., Schiff, I., Rosner, B., Greenberg, L., Ravnikar, V., and Sacks, F.M. (1991). Effects of post-menopausal estrogen replacement on the concentrations and metabolism of plasma lipoproteins. *New England Journal of Medicine* 325: 1196-1204.

Walter, S.D., Hart, L.E., McIntosh, J.M., and Sutton, J.R. (1989). The Ontario cohort study of running-related injuries. *Archives of Internal Medicine* 149: 2561-2564.

Wang, K., McCarter, R., Wright, J., Beverly, J., and Ramirez-Mitchell, R. (1991). Regulation of skeletal muscle stiffness and elasticity by titin isoforms—a test of the segmental extension model of resting tension. *Proceedings of the National Academy of Science, USA* 88: 7101-7105.

Wankel, L., and Kreisel, P.S. (1985). Factors underlying enjoyment of youth sports: Sport and age group comparisons. *Journal of Sport Psychology* 7: 51-64.

Wannamethee, G., and Shaper, A.G. (1992). Physical activity and stroke in British middle aged men. *British Medical Journal* 304: 597-601.

Wannamethee, G., Shaper, A.G., and MacFarlane, P.W. (1993). Heart rate, physical activity, and mortality from cancer and other noncardiovascular diseases. *American Journal of Epidemiology* 137: 735-748.

Ware, J.H., Dockery, D.W., Louis, T.A., Xu, X., Ferris, B.G., and Speizer, F.E. (1990). Longitudinal and cross-sectional estimates of pulmonary function decline in never smoking adults. *American Journal of Epidemiology* 132: 685-700.

Warner, K.E. (1987). Selling health promotion to corporate America: Uses and abuses of the economic argument. *Health Education Quarterly* 14: 39-55.

Warner, K.E., Wickizer, T.M., Wolfe, R.A., Schidroth, J.E., and Samuelson, M.H. (1988). Economic implications of worksite health promotion programmes: Review of the literature. *Journal of Occupational Medicine* 30: 106-112.

Warren, B.J., Nieman, D.C., Dotson, R.G., Adkins, C.H., O'Donnell, K.A., Haddock, B.L., and Butterworth, D.E. (1993). Cardiorespiratory responses to exercise training in septuagenarian women. *International Journal of Sports Medicine* 14: 60-65.

Waterbor, J., Cole, P., Delzell, E., and Andjelkovich, D. (1988). The mortality experience of major-league baseball players. *New England Journal of Medicine* 318: 1278-1280.

Weaver, T.E., and Narsavage, G.L. (1992). Physiological and psychological variables related to functional status in chronic obstructive pulmonary disease. *Nursing Research* 41: 286-291.

Webb, G.D., Poehlman, E.T., and Tonino, R.P. (1993). Dissociation of changes in metabolic rate and blood pressure with erythrocyte Na-K pump activity in older men after endurance training. *Journals of Gerontology* 48: M47-M52.

Webb, W.B. (1981). Sleep stage response of older and younger subjects after sleep deprivation. *Electroencephalography and Clinical Neurophysiology* 52: 368-371.

Weber, F., Barnard, R.J., and Roy, D. (1983). Effects of a high-complex-carbohydrate, low-fat diet and daily exercise on individuals 70 years of age and older. *Journal of Gerontology* 38: 155-161.

Wei, J.Y. (1994). Disorders of the heart. In W.R. Hazzard, E.L. Bierman, J.P. Blass, W.H. Ettinger, and J.B. Halter (Eds.), *Principles of geriatric medicine and gerontology* (3rd ed., pp. 517-532). New York: McGraw-Hill.

Weigle, D.S. (1988). Contribution of decreased body mass to diminished thermic effect of exercise in reduced-obese men. *International Journal of Obesity* 12: 567-578.

Weindruch, R., and Walford, R.L. (1988). *The retardation of aging and disease by dietary restriction.* Springfield, IL: Charles C Thomas.

Weiner, P., Azgad, Y., and Ganam, R. (1992). Inspiratory muscle training combined with general exercise reconditioning in patients with COPD. *Chest* 102: 1351-1356.

Weintraub, N., Dolan, G., and Stratmann, H. (1993). Hemodynamic and respiratory responses to maximal treadmill and arm ergometry exercise in men with chronic obstructive pulmonary disease. *Journal of Cardiopulmonary Rehabilitation* 13: 25-30.

Weisfeldt, M.L., Gerstenblith, G., and Lakatta, E.G. (1985). Alterations in circulatory function. In R. Andres, E.L. Bierman, and W.R. Hazzard (Eds.), *Principles of geriatric medicine* (pp. 248-279). New York: McGraw-Hill.

Welford, A.T. (1983). Perception, memory, and motor performance in relation to age. In J.E. Birren, J.M.A. Munnichs, H. Thomae, and M. Minors (Eds.), *Aging: A challenge to science and society* (pp. 297-311). Oxford: Oxford University Press.

Welford, A.T. (1984). Between bodily changes and performance. Some possible reasons for slowing with age. *Experimental Aging Research* 10: 73-88.

Welle, S., Thornton, C., Jozefowicz, R., and Statt, M. (1993). Myofibrillar protein synthesis in young and old men. *American Journal of Physiology* 264: E693-E698.

Wells, C.L., Boorman, M.A., and Riggs, D.M. (1992). Effect of age and menopausal status on cardiorespiratory fitness in masters women runners. *Medicine and Science in Sports and Exercise* 24: 1147-1154.

Weltman, A., Weltman, J.Y., Schurrer, R., Evans, W.S., Veldhuis, J.D., and Rogol, A.D. (1992). Endurance training amplifies the pulsatile release of growth hormone: Effects of training intensity. *Journal of Applied Physiology* 72: 2188-2196.

Wenger, N. (1992). The elderly patients with cardiovascular disease: Determining optimal components of care and access to care. *American Journal of Geriatric Cardiology* 1: 8-14.

Wesmiller, S.W., and Hoffmann, L.A. (1994). Evaluation of an assistive device for ambulation in oxygen dependent patients with COPD. *Journal of Cardiopulmonary Rehabilitation* 14: 122-126.

Whelton, P.K. (1985). Hypertension in the elderly. In R. Andres, E.L. Bierman, and W.R. Hazzard (Eds.), *Principles of geriatric medicine* (pp. 536-551). New York: McGraw-Hill.

White, C.C., Powell, K.E., Hogelin, G.C., Gentry, E.M., and Forman, M.R. (1987). The behavioral risk factor surveys: IV. The descriptive epidemiology of exercise. *American Journal of Preventive Medicine* 3: 304-310.

White, L.R., Losonczy, K.G., and Wolf, P.A. (1990). Cerebrovascular Disease. In J.C. Coroni-Huntley, R.R. Huntley, and J.J. Feldman (Eds.), *Health status and well-being of the elderly* (pp. 115-135). New York: Oxford University Press.

White, M. (1995). *Water exercise.* Champaign, IL: Human Kinetics.

White, M.J., and Carrington, C.A. (1993). The pressor response to involuntary isometric exercise of young and elderly human muscle with reference to muscle contractile characteristics. *European Journal of Applied Physiology* 66: 338-342.

Whitehurst, M. (1991). Reaction time unchanged in older women following aerobic training. *Perceptual and Motor Skills* 72: 251-256.

Whittaker, J.L., Baracos, V.E., Haennel, R.G., Brown, B.E., Humen, D.P., and Urtasun, R.C. (1991). Exercise training in the post-treatment remission period of patients with limited small cell lung cancer (SCLC). *Proceedings of the Annual Meeting, Canadian Association of Sport Sciences*, Kingston, ON.

Whittington, R.M., and Banerjee, A. (1994). Sport-related sudden natural death in the city of Birmingham. *Journal of the Royal Society of Medicine* 87: 18-21.

Wickham, C.A.C., Walsh, K., Cooper, C., Parker, D.J.P., Margetts, B.M., Morris, J., and Bruce, S.A. (1989). Dietary calcium, physical activity and risk of hip fracture. A prospective study. *British Medical Journal* 299: 889-892.

Wijkstra, P.J., Van Altena, R., Kraan, J., Otten, V., Postma, D.S., and Koeter, G.H. (1994). Quality of life in patients with chronic obstructive lung disease improves after rehabilitation at home. *European Respiration Journal* 7: 269-273.

Wilking, S.V., Belanger, A.L., Kannel, W.B., D'Agostino, R.B., and Steel, K. (1988). Determinants of isolated systolic hypertension. *Journal of the American Medical Association* 260: 3451-3455.

Wilkins, M.F. (1991). Cancer in the elderly patient. In M.S.J. Pathy (Ed.), *Principles and practice of geriatric medicine* (pp. 1385-1396). Chichester: Wiley.

Wilkins, R., and Adams, O. (1983). *Healthfulness of life*. Montréal, PQ: Institute of Research in Public Policy.

Will, B.E., Schmitt, P., and Dalrymple-Alford, J.D. (1985). *Brain plasticity, learning and memory*. New York: Plenum Press.

Williams, M.A., Maresh, C.M., Esterbrooks, D.J., Harkbrecht, J.T., and Sketch, M.H. (1985). Early exercise training in patients older than age 65 compared with that in younger patients after myocardial infarction or coronary artery bypass grafting. *American Journal of Cardiology* 55: 263-266.

Williams, P.T., Wood, P.D., Haskell, W.L., and Vranizan, K. (1982). The effects of running mileage and duration on plasma lipoprotein levels. *Journal of the American Medical Association* 247: 2672-2679.

Williamson, D.F., Madams, J., Anda, R.F., Kleinman, J.C., Kahn, H.S., and Byers, T. (1993). Recreational physical activity and 10-year weight-change in a U.S. national cohort. *International Journal of Obesity* 17: 279-286.

Willis, P., and Parkhouse, W. (1994). The effect of acute and chronic exercise on rates of protein synthesis and skeletal muscle sensitivity to insulin-like growth factor-1 in aged mice. Paper presented at the 9th International Symposium on the Biochemistry of Exercise, July, Aberdeen.

Wilson, D., and Bracci, R. (1982). The police agility test. *Law and Order* 30: 36-42.

Wilson, P.W., Anderson, K.M., and Kannel, W. (1986). Epidemiology of diabetes mellitus in the elderly. The Framingham Study. *American Journal of Medicine* 80 (5A): 3-9.

Wing, R.R., Epstein, L.H., Bayles, M.P., Kriska, A.M., Nowalk, M.P., and Gooding, W. (1988). Exercise in a behavioural weight control programme for obese patients with type 2 (non-insulin-dependent) diabetes. *Diabetologia* 31: 902-909.

Wing, R.R., Matthews, K.A., Kuller, L.H., Meilahn, E.N., and Plantinga, P. (1991). Waist to hip ratio in middle-aged women. Associations with behavioral and psychosocial factors and with changes in cardiovascular risk factors. *Arteriosclerosis and Thrombosis* 11: 1250-1257.

Wingo, P.A., Layde, P.M., Lee, N.C., Queener, S.F., Edmondson, J., and Johnston, C.C. (1979). Increases in immunoreactive parathyroid hormone with age. *New England Journal of Medicine* 300: 1419-1421.

Winningham, M.L., MacVicar, M.G., and Burke, C.A. (1986). Exercise for cancer patients: Guidelines and precautions. *Physician and Sportsmedicine* 14 (10): 125-134.

Wissler, R.W. (1985). The evolution of the atherosclerotic plaque and its complications. In W.E. Connor and J.D. Bristow (Eds.), *Coronary heart disease: Prevention, complications and treatment* (pp. 193-210). Philadelphia: Lippincott.

Wolf, P.A., D'Agostino, R.B., Belanger, A.J., and Kannel, W.B. (1991). Probability of a stroke: A risk profile from the Framingham Study. *Stroke* 22: 312-318.

Wolf, S.L., Coogler, C.E., Green, R.C., and Xu, T. (1993). Novel interventions to prevent falls in the elderly. In H.M. Perry, J.E. Morley, and R.M. Coe (Eds.), *Aging and musculoskeletal disorders* (pp. 178-195). New York: Springer.

Wolfson, L., Whipple, R., Amerman, P., and Tobin, J.N. (1990). Gait assessment in the elderly: A gait abnormality rating scale and its relation to falls. *Journals of Gerontology* 45: M12-M19.

Woo, R., Garrow, J.S., and Pi-Sunyer, F.X. (1982). Effect of exercise on spontaneous calorie intake in obesity. *American Journal of Clinical Nutrition* 36: 470-477.

Wood, P.D., Stefanick, M.L., Dreon, D.M., Frey-Hewitt, B., Garay, S.C., Williams, P.T., Superko, H.R., Fortmann, S.P., Albers, J.J., Vranizan, K.M., Ellsworth, N.M., Terry, R.B., and Haskell, W.L. (1988). Changes in plasma lipids and lipoproteins in overweight men during weight loss through dieting as compared with exercise. *New England Journal of Medicine* 319: 1173-1179.

Woodcock, A.A., Johnson, M., and Geddes, D. (1983). Cycling in patients with chronic airflow limitation. *British Medical Journal* 286: 1184.

Wood-Dauphinee, S., and Küchler, T. (1992). Quality of life as a rehabilitation outcome: Are we missing the boat? *Canadian Journal of Rehabilitation* 6: 3-12.

Woollacott, M.H. (1993). Age-related changes in posture and movement. *Journal of Gerontology* 48: 56-60.

World Health Organization. (1948). *Official Records, No. 2.* Geneva: Author.

World Health Organization. (1980). Second report on diabetes mellitus. *Technical Report Series* 646. Geneva: Author.

World Health Organization. (1984). The uses of epidemiology in the study of the elderly. *Technical Report Series* 6. Geneva: Author.

Wright, K. (1988). Nature, nurture and death. *Scientific American* 258: 34-38.

Wright, G.R., and Shephard, R.J. (1978). Brake reaction time—effects of age, sex and carbon monoxide. *Archives of Environmental Health* 33: 141-150.

Wyshak, G., Frisch, R.E., Albright, T.E., Albright, N.L., and Schiff, I. (1987). Bone fractures among former college athletes compared with non-athletes in the menopausal and postmenopausal years. *Obstetrics and Gynecology* 69: 121-126.

Xusheng, S., Yugi, X., and Ronggang, Z. (1990). Detection of AC rosette-forming lymphocytes in the healthy aged with Taichiquan (88 style) exercise. *Journal of Sports Medicine and Physical Fitness* 30: 401-405.

Yarasheski, K.E. (1993). Effect of exercise on muscle mass in the elderly. In H.M. Perry, J.E. Morley, and R.M. Coe (Eds.), *Aging and musculoskeletal disorders* (pp. 199-213). New York: Springer.

Yarasheski, K.E., Zachwieja, J.J., and Bier, D.M. (1993). Acute effect of resistance exercise on muscle protein synthesis rate in young and elderly men and women. *American Journal of Physiology* 265: E210-E214.

Yaron, M., Hultgren, H.N., and Alexander, J.K. (1995). Low risk of myocardial ischemia in the elderly visiting moderate altitude. *Wilderness and Environmental Medicine* 6: 20-28.

Yates, F.E. (1991). Aging as prolonged morphogenesis: A topological sorcerer's apprentice. In G.M. Kenyon, J.E. Birren, and J.J.F. Schroots (Eds.), *Metaphors of aging in science and the humanities* (pp. 199-218). New York: Springer.

Yerg, J.E., Seals, D.R., Hagberg, J.M., and Holloszy, J.O. (1985). Effect of endurance exercise training on ventilatory function in older individuals. *Journal of Applied Physiology* 58: 791-794.

Yoshikawa, M., Okano, K., Nakai, R., Tomori, T., and Takenaka, M. (1978). Aging and nutrition. *Asian Medical Journal* 21: 359-378.

Young, A. (1988). Exercise, fitness and recovery from surgery, disease or infection. In C. Bouchard, R.J. Shephard, T. Stephens, J. Sutton, and B. McPherson (Eds.), *Exercise, fitness and health* (pp. 589-600). Champaign, IL: Human Kinetics.

Young, A., Hughes, I., Russell, P., Parker, M.J., and Nicholls, P.J.R. (1980). Measurements of quadriceps muscle wasting by ultrasonography. *Rheumatology and Rehabilitation* 19: 141-148.

Young, A., and Skelton, D.A. (1994). Applied physiology of strength and power in old age. *International Journal of Sports Medicine* 15: 149-151.

Young, A., Stokes, M., and Crowe, M. (1985). The size and strength of quadriceps muscles of old and young men. *Clinical Physiology* 5: 145-154.

Young, D.R., and Steinhardt, M.A. (1993). The importance of physical fitness versus physical activity for coronary artery disease risk factors: A cross-sectional analysis. *Research Quarterly* 64: 377-384.

Young, E.A., and Urban, E. (1986). Aging, the aged and the gastrointestinal tract. In E.A. Young (Ed.), *Nutrition, aging and health* (pp. 91-131). New York: Liss.

Young, J.B., Rowe, J.W., Pallotta, J.A., Sparrow, D., and Landsberg, L. (1980). Enhanced plasma norepinephrine response to upright posture and oral glucose administration in elderly subjects. *Metabolism* 29: 532-539.

Young, J.C., Chen, M., and Holloszy, J.O. (1983). Maintenance of the adaptation of skeletal muscle mitochondria to exercise in rat. *Medicine and Science in Sports and Exercise* 15: 243-246.

Young, T.K., Nikitin, Y.P., Shubnikov, E.V., Astakhova, T.I., Moffatt, M.E.K., and O'Neil, J.D. (1995). Plasma lipids in two indigenous arctic populations with low risk for cardiovascular diseases. *American Journal of Human Biology* 7: 223-236.

Yousef, M., Dill, D.B., Vitez, S.D., Hillyard, S.D., and Goldman, A.S. (1984). Thermoregulatory responses to desert heat: Age, race and sex. *Journal of Gerontology* 39: 406-414.

Yu, B.P., Masoro, E.J., and McMahan, C.A. (1985). Nutritional influences on aging of Fischer 344 rats: I. Physical, metabolic and longevity characteristics. *Journal of Gerontology* 40: 657-670.

Zackin, M.J., and Meredith, C.N. (1989). Protein metabolism in aging: Effects of exercise and training. In R. Harris and S. Harris (Eds.), *Physical activity, aging and sports* (pp. 271-283). Albany, NY: Center for Studies of Aging.

Zadai, C.C. (1985). Pulmonary physiology of aging. The role of rehabilitation. *Topics in Geriatric Rehabilitation* 1: 49-57.

Zepelin, H., McDonald, C.S., and Zammit, G.K. (1984). Effects of age on auditory awakening thresholds. *Journal of Gerontology* 39: 294-300.

Zerzawy, R. (1987). Hämodynamische Reaktionen unter verschiedenen Belastungsformen [Hemodynamic reactions to different types of work]. In R. Rost and F. Webering (Eds.), *Kardiology im Sport* [Cardiology in Sport]. Cologne: German Sports Medicine Federation.

Zharhary, D., and Gershon, H. (1981). Allogenic T cytotoxic reactivity of senescent mice: Affinity for target cells and determination of cell number. *Cellular Immunology* 60: 470-479.

Zheng, W., Shu, X.O., McLaughlin, J.K., Chow, W.H., Gao, Y.T., and Blot, W.J. (1993). Occupational physical activity and the incidence of cancer of the breast, corpus uteri and ovary in Shanghai. *Cancer* 71: 3620-3624.

Zylstra, S., Hopkins, A., Erk, M., Hreshchyshyn, M.M., and Anbar, M. (1989). Effect of physical activity on lumbar spine and femoral neck bone densities. *International Journal of Sports Medicine* 10: 181-186.

Author Index

Subject Index

About the Author

Roy J. Shephard, MD, PhD, DPE, is professor emeritus of Applied Physiology at the University of Toronto and resident scholar in Health Studies at Brock University in St. Catharines, Ontario. He has spent more than three decades as a researcher, consultant, teacher, and administrator exploring the relationships among regular physical activity, aging, and health.

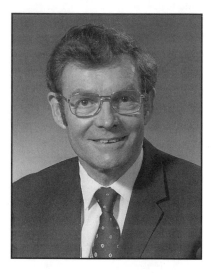

Dr. Shephard has held many distinguished positions and has received many honors. He has served as the president of the American College of Sports Medicine (ACSM), president of the Canadian Association of Sports Sciences (CASS—now known as the Canadian Society of Exercise Physiology), and vice president of the International Committee for Physical Fitness Research. In 1985 he was given the CASS Honor Award, and in 1991 he received a Citation from ACSM. He is also a two-time recipient of the Philip Noel Baker Research Prize, and he has received honorary doctorates from the University of Ghent (Belgium) and the University of Montreal.

Dr. Shephard is the author of more than 1,200 publications, including nearly 70 books, and he has served as editor-in-chief of the *Canadian Journal of Applied Physiology*. In his leisure time, Dr. Shephard enjoys walking, swimming, cycling, choral singing, and stamp collecting.